Sideline Management in Sports

Sérgio Rocha Piedade
Mark R. Hutchinson
David Parker
João Espregueira-Mendes
Philippe Neyret
Editors

Sideline Management in Sports

ISAKOS
International Society of Arthroscopy, Knee Surgery and Orthopaedic Sports Medicine

Springer

Editors
Sérgio Rocha Piedade
Exercise and Sports Medicine
Department of Orthopedics
Rheumatology, and Traumatology
University of Campinas
Campinas, Brazil

David Parker
Sydney Orthopaedic Research Institute
Sydney, NSW, Australia

Philippe Neyret
La Tour De Salvagny, France

Mark R. Hutchinson
Department of Orthopaedics
University of Illinois at Chicago
Elmhurst, IL, USA

João Espregueira-Mendes
FIFA Medical Centre of Excellence
Espregueira-Mendes Sports Centre
Porto, Portugal

ISBN 978-3-031-33866-3 ISBN 978-3-031-33867-0 (eBook)
https://doi.org/10.1007/978-3-031-33867-0

This Springer imprint is published by the registered company Springer Nature Switzerland AG
The registered company address is: Gewerbestrasse 11, 6330 Cham, Switzerland

Paper in this product is recyclable.

Preface

As in the Godfather movie, ISAKOS Sports Medicine Committee has a Trilogy. It started in 2019 with *The Sports Medicine Physician*, a book exploring the different aspects of the sports medicine physician's work. It continued in 2021 with *Specific Sports-Related Injuries*, approaching and discussing particular features of sports modalities and related injuries. Now we proudly close the ISAKOS Sports Medicine Book Trilogy with *Sideline Management in Sports*.

Even though athletes believe in the mantra "what does not kill you makes you stronger", they must keep in mind that they are also human beings. The *Sideline Management in Sports* book, organized into four sections and a total of 34 chapters, is a reference guide in managing common and specific clinical conditions that affect athletes in training and sports competition—sideline management.

Like the previous books, this project involved outstanding world references in Sports Medicine and Orthopaedics, Mark R. Hutchinson, David Parker, Joao Espregueira-Mendes, and Phillippe Neyret; thank you all for the fantastic work and contribution to this book. A special thanks to the ISAKOS President Guilhermo Arce, Former ISAKOS President Willem M. van der Merwe, and ISAKOS Board for supporting this book, and also thanks to Daniel Miranda Ferreira, Marc Safran, Andreas Imhoff, David Figueroa, Jacques Menetrey, Committee members, and all health professionals participating in this book, sharing their academic and clinical knowledge as well as experience in Orthopaedic Sports Medicine.

Thanks to my Team, Ge, Mariana, Cezar, and Magda S. Kimoto, for supporting me on this *ISAKOS Book Trilogy project.*

I would also like to thank my wife, Ana Karina Piedade, for keeping pushing me to fight for my dreams and work to make them come true. As Tina said, "You are simply the best."

In sports, we will never walk alone because passion, disappointment, defeats, victories, and friendship go together. Challenges drive us to teamwork, fighting for achievements, losing and winning battles, and making us stronger to go forward and build the future! And more than that, we learn that resilience and hard work build up a champion.

Campinas, Brazil — Sérgio Rocha Piedade

Contents

Part I

Overview: Sports Physical Demands and Injury-Related and Illness-Related Risks

1 Pediatric Athlete (Overview)

Samantha Tayne

1.1 Introduction

Youth and adolescent sports participation has increased over the past several decades, with approximately 30–45 million children participating in organized sports in the United States, which includes at least half of the children aged 5–18 years old [1–6]. There are at least two million children participating in Little League activities [7], and more than three million children participating in youth tackle football [8]. The number of participants in youth US soccer increased by almost 90% from 2000 to 2014, and the number of high school soccer participants more than doubled from 1990 to 2003, with expected continual growth of 11–21% annually [9, 10]. Pediatric athletes are training and competing with increased intensity than previously seen. Young athletes are often competing year-round, either participating in multiple sports or are specializing early in one sport. They are training 20 or more hours per week to specialize in a particular sport, and sometimes even attending sports centered boarding schools for elite training [5, 11–14]. With the increased participation and intensity of training, the injuries in pediatric athletes have also increased. Two to three million emergency department visits per year in the US for pediatric and adolescent sports related injuries have been reported [2, 15]. While there are a number of injuries unique to the pediatric athlete, the number of adult injuries such as anterior cruciate ligament (ACL) injuries in children is also rising [16]. Delay in the treatment of injury in the pediatric athlete can lead to further injury and prevent the athlete from returning to sport.

Children can be more susceptible to injury as compared to adults due to a number of factors, including a larger surface area to mass ratio, proportionally larger heads, lack of appropriate protective equipment for size, growing cartilage and long bones, and the development of complex motor skills needed to succeed in certain sports [1, 3, 17, 18]. Therefore, children and adolescents can experience unique injuries while participating in athletics, which must be considered when evaluating and managing pediatric athletes on the sidelines.

1.2 Epidemiology

Epidemiological studies have evaluated the risk of injury in pediatric and adolescent athletes and have noted that the risk of injury differs with age, gender, sport, and type of injury [10–12, 19–21]. Overall, studies have reported injury incidence ranging anywhere from 2.38 to 142.86 injuries per 1000 participation hours in adolescent ath-

S. Tayne (✉)
Department of Orthopaedic Surgery, University of North Carolina, Chapel Hill, NC, USA
e-mail: samantha_tayne@med.unc.edu

S. Rocha Piedade et al. (eds.), *Sideline Management in Sports*,
https://doi.org/10.1007/978-3-031-33867-0_1

letes, with increasing risk associated with increasing age [19]. Injury rates often follow a pattern based on school sport participation, as increased injury rates are often seen with fall sports as compared to the winter or spring [22].

While younger age athletes tend to experience less injury overall, pediatric athletes less than 12 years old appear to sustain more traumatic injuries, and more commonly to the upper extremity. This group more frequently sustained physeal fractures, apophysitis or apophyseal avulsions, and osteochondritis dissecans lesions [19, 20, 22]. Over one-third of athletes less than 12 years old who experience spine injuries, have been found to have spondylolysis, or a stress fracture of the pars interarticularis of the lumbar vertebrae [20]. The acute injuries in older adolescent athletes, aged 13–17 years, are more frequently soft tissue rather than bony in origin, such as ACL tears, meniscal tears, or shoulder instability. A greater proportion of adolescent athletes also experienced overuse injuries than the younger age group. Further, this older age group is more likely to experience injuries to the chest, pelvic region, and spine [19, 20, 22].

Injuries also vary by sex. Male athletes experience injury at a rate of 2–3 times the rate of female athletes [22]. Both female and male athletes most commonly experience injury to the lower extremity—68.5% and 53.7% of injuries, respectively, however, the type of lower extremity injury may be different [21]. Females experience patellofemoral knee pain at a rate of three times that of their male counterparts. Males are diagnosed with osteochondritis dissecans and fractures twice as often as females. And though there is a higher rate among male athletes of acute knee injuries, female athletes who sustain an acute knee injury are twice as likely to have an injury that requires surgery [23]. Female athletes appear to experience higher rates of injury to the pelvis and spine, while male athletes experience higher rates of upper extremity injury [21].

Different studies have found variations in the rate of injury by sport, but generally, males experience the highest rates of injury with ice hockey, football, rugby, basketball, and soccer, while female athletes experience the highest rates of injury with gymnastics, basketball, and soccer [11, 12, 19]. One study looking at injuries in children presenting to the emergency department over a 13-year period with soccer-related injuries found that the wrist and hand, ankle, and knee were the most commonly injured body parts, with the most common diagnoses of sprain/strain (35.9%), contusion/abrasion (24.1%), and fracture (23.2%) [9]. Sports with injuries that require surgery tend to be contact, such as football, rugby, or ice hockey, as well as sports where there may be a fall from a height, such as equestrianism, gymnastics, and ice skating [22]. For contact sports, the difference in maturity, and therefore size and strength, of adolescent boys may contribute to the risk of injury [12].

1.3 Unique Injury Risks of Pediatric Athletes

Pediatric athletes experience different patterns of injury than adult athletes due to many factors affecting both physical and psychological development. There is a difference in the relative strength of bone in children versus adults, with children having a weak point of bone at the physis, which can result in growth plate injury [2, 6, 18, 24]. The cortex is also more malleable in children than adults, which can result in plastic deformity or buckle-type fractures with mild injury. The bone is relatively weak as compared to the attached ligaments or tendons, leading to potential avulsion fractures in children, whereas an adult with a similar injury is more likely to have tearing of the soft tissue. Thick periosteum in children can also result in periosteal sleeve avulsion fractures or difficult reduction of fractures due to periosteal entrapment [18].

As pediatric athletes transition through puberty, there are many fast-occurring changes to body composition and neuromuscular development that affect coordination, strength, endurance, flexibility, joint mobility, and overall exercise capacity. During the pubescent or adolescent growth spurt, athletes can develop muscle imbalance and become less flexible as the soft tissues passively stretch over the actively grow-

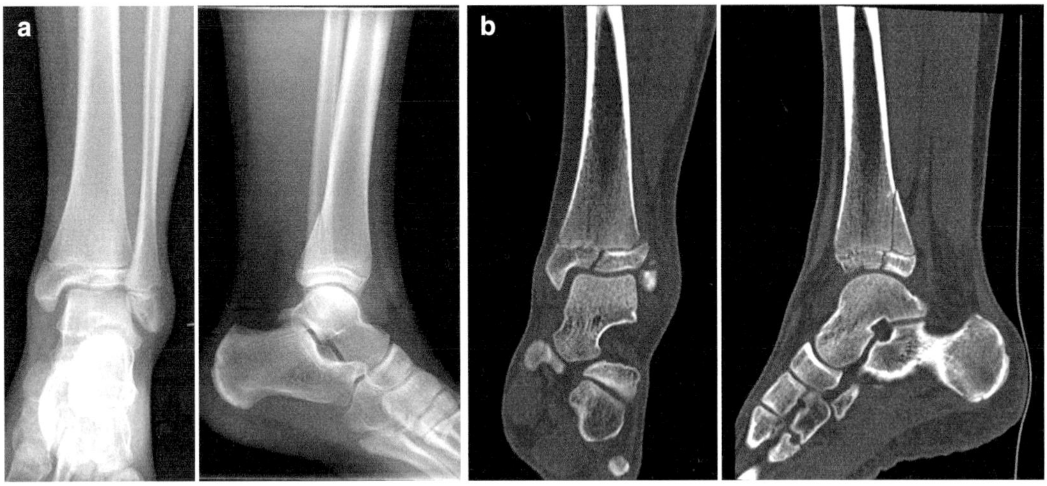

Fig. 1.1 Thirteen-year-old female gymnast after a fall. (**a**) AP and lateral radiographs and (**b**) coronal and sagittal CT slices show a triplane ankle fracture, Salter-Harris IV equivalent

ing long bones [8, 14]. Bone mineralization may lag behind bone growth, leaving the bone more porous and more vulnerable to injury [12]. Studies have also shown that changes in cognitive development during puberty affects the risk of injury, as athletes in this age group will perceive a low level of risk and overestimate their physical ability. Consequently, there is an almost two times increased risk of significant injury between 11 and 14 years old [8, 19].

1.3.1 Physeal Fractures

Pediatric athletes experience traumatic injuries that result in fractures at increased rates as compared to older or adult athletes, and many of these fractures are specific to the pediatric population. Common areas of acute physeal injury are in the wrist, ankle, and knee, though physeal fractures can be seen at any growth plate and carry the risk of growth arrest or deformity. Physeal injuries are typically described using the Salter-Harris classification system: Salter-Harris I fracture is across the physis, Salter-Harris II extends into the metaphysis, Salter-Harris III extends into the epiphysis, and Salter-Harris IV crosses the growth plate through both the metaphysis and the epiphysis. There is also a Salter-Harris V fracture, which is considered a crush injury to the growth plate [25]. Suspicion for a fracture warrants urgent imaging, especially if there is concern that a reduction may be needed.

The wrist and ankle are very common sites of fracture in the pediatric athlete, and both the distal radius or distal tibia/fibula fractures may be physeal or extraphyseal. Distal radius fractures are commonly associated with sports such as soccer, gymnastics, and snowboarding [14, 26]. Several studies have shown that there are a few key findings with a high positive predictive value for diagnosing wrist fractures in pediatric athletes including deformity, focal tenderness, edema, pain with passive motion, pain or weakness with grip, and pain with supination, indicating radiographs are needed [27–29]. Ankle fractures account for 9–18% of physeal injuries [19]. The distal fibular physeal fracture is typically a Salter-Harris type 1, and therefore may not be visible on radiographs. It is considered the equivalent of a lateral ankle sprain in an adult and requires a period of immobilization to allow for bone healing. Young adolescents experience unique patterns of distal tibial fractures, for example, triplane or tillaux fractures (Fig. 1.1), due to the order of closure of the distal tibial physis. These patterns typically affect the articular surface and therefore require appropriate evaluation and imaging for possible surgical fixation.

1.3.2 Avulsion/Apophyseal Injury

Apophyses are small, rounded ossification centers at the ends of long bones or the pelvis, which typically fuse after the long bone epiphysis. The elbow, for example, has multiple ossification centers or apophyses (Fig. 1.2). Avulsion or apophyseal injury in the pediatric and adolescent athlete is commonly seen in the knee, elbow, and hip/pelvis with forceful contraction or eccentric loading. A review of the common locations of an apophyseal avulsion and apophysitis is shown in Table 1.1.

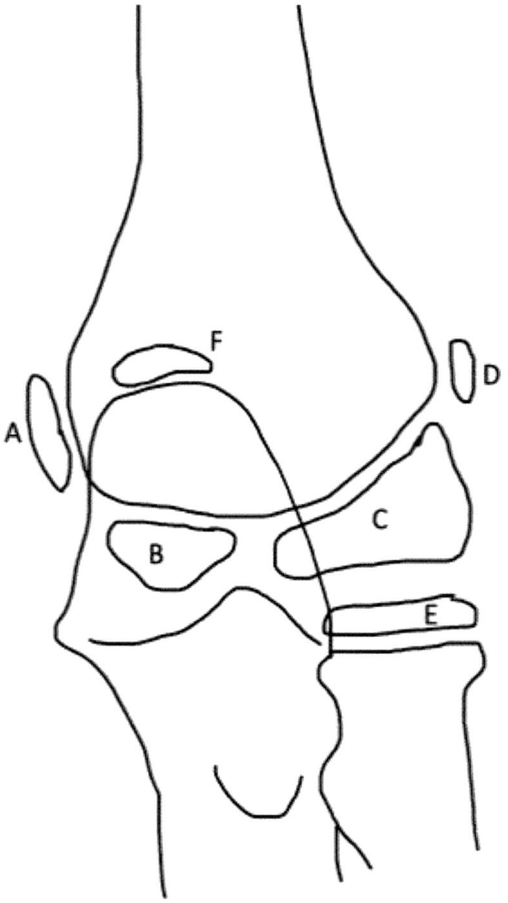

Fig. 1.2 Pediatric elbow apophyses. (**a**) Medial epicondyle: ossifies by 5 years, fuses at 16–18 years. (**b**) Trochlea: ossifies by 7 years, fuses at 12–14 years. (**c**) Capitellum: ossifies by 1 year, fuses at 12–14 years. (**d**) Lateral epicondyle: ossifies by 11 years, fuses at 12–14 years. (**e**) Olecranon: ossifies by 9 years, fuses at 15–17 years

In the elbow, the medial epicondyle or olecranon are the most common areas of acute apophyseal injury, with the forceful pull of the ulnar collateral ligament or triceps, respectively [30]. Throwing athletes may also experience more chronic inflammation or apophysitis in the elbow, which can precede an acute avulsion. Apophyseal avulsion in the knee is seen in jumping sports such as basketball with acute contraction of the extensor mechanism leading to a tibial tubercle fracture, extending to the proximal tibial physis. Though not really an apophysis, the knee can also see tibial spine avulsion fractures, as the tibial spine is often weaker than the ACL in children [23].

Apophyseal avulsions around the pelvis may involve any of several areas, including the anterosuperior iliac spine (origin of the sartorius), anteroinferior iliac spine (origin of the rectus femoris), ischial tuberosity (origin of the hamstring), iliac crest (attachment site of the tensor fascia latae and abdominal muscles), and the lesser trochanter (insertion of the iliopsoas). Avulsions occur more commonly in male athletes between the ages of 14–17 years old. These injuries are caused by indirect trauma with a sudden, violent, or unbalanced muscle contraction in sports that involve running, jumping, kicking, pivoting, and twisting with rapid acceleration and deceleration, such as soccer, football, rugby, ice hockey, sprinting gymnastics, and hockey [3, 14, 31, 32].

Importantly, apophyseal avulsions may even be seen in the spine with spinous process avulsion fractures. This occurs in adolescent athletes due to traction on the spinous process apophysis and is typically seen in the lower thoracic vertebrae or thoracolumbar junction [33].

1.3.3 Chronic or Overuse Injury

While athletes may experience acute avulsion of an apophysis or an acute physeal fracture, chronic inflammation of the apophysis or physis is also seen in the pediatric athlete due to repetitive microtrauma. There are multiple common locations for apophysitis, including the tibial tubercle

Table 1.1 Review of apophyseal avulsion and apophysitis

Location	Acute versus chronic	Description	Treatment	Common sports
Iliac crest	Acute or chronic	Attachment site of tensor fascia latae and abdominal muscles. Forceful sudden contraction causes avulsion. Repetitive twisting or bending may cause inflammation	<2 cm displacement treated conservatively with protected weight bearing. >2 cm displacement may require surgical fixation	Running, soccer, dance
Anterior superior iliac spine (ASIS)	Acute	Origin of sartorius. Forceful sudden contraction with hip extended and knee flexed causes avulsion	<2 cm displacement treated conservatively with protected weight bearing. >2 cm displacement may require surgical fixation	Soccer, rugby, ice hockey, gymnastics
Anterior inferior iliac spine (AIIS)	Acute	Origin of rectus femoris. Forceful sudden contraction with hip extended and knee flexed causes avulsion	<2 cm displacement treated conservatively with protected weight bearing. >2 cm displacement may require surgical fixation	Soccer, rugby, ice hockey, gymnastics
Ischial tuberosity	Acute	Origin of hamstring. Forceful sudden contraction with hip flexion and extended knee causes avulsion	<2 cm displacement treated conservatively with protected weight bearing. >2 cm displacement may require surgical fixation	Soccer, rugby, ice hockey, gymnastics
Lesser trochanter	Acute	Insertion of iliopsoas. Forceful sudden contraction causes avulsion	<2 cm displacement treated conservatively with protected weight bearing. >2 cm displacement may require surgical fixation	Soccer, sprinting
Tibial tubercle	Acute or chronic (Osgood Schlatter's disease)	Acute injury caused by concentric or eccentric quadriceps contraction during jumping or landing. Chronic injury from repetitive microtrauma caused by the traction of the extensor mechanism	Acute injury often requires surgical fixation if physis is involved or there is any displacement. Osgood Schlatter's is typically treated conservatively with symptom management	Basketball, sprinting, high jump, football
Distal patellar pole (Sinding–Larsen–Johansson syndrome)	Chronic	Overuse injury due to repetitive traction of the extensor mechanism	Conservative treatment with symptom management	Basketball, sprinting, high jump, football
Calcaneus (sever's disease)	Chronic	Repetitive microtrauma due to running and jumping sports	Conservative treatment with symptom management	Basketball, sprinting
Medial epicondyle of elbow	Acute or chronic (Little Leaguer's elbow)	Acute avulsion occurs due to a large valgus stress with contraction of the flexor-pronator mass. Chronic apophysitis is due to repetitive valgus stress	Surgical treatment for an acute avulsion with fragment caught in the joint. Otherwise surgical treatment is somewhat controversial with debate over displacement and ulnar nerve dysfunction. Chronic apophysitis treated with symptom management and cessation from throwing	Baseball

(continued)

Table 1.1 (continued)

Location	Acute versus chronic	Description	Treatment	Common sports
Olecranon	Acute or chronic	Repetitive contraction of the triceps. Acute forceful contraction may cause an acute avulsion, but rare and should raise suspicion of osteogenesis imperfecta	Chronic apophysitis treated with symptom management and cessation from sport. Acute displaced fracture requires surgical fixation	Baseball, gymnastics
Spinous process	Acute or chronic	Forceful, repetitive flexion of the spine	Typically treated with conservative management and cessation of sport	Gymnastics, dance

(Osgood Schlatter's Disease), distal patellar pole (Sinding–Larsen–Johansson Syndrome), calcaneus (Sever's Disease), and the medial epicondyle of the elbow (Little Leaguer's elbow). Epiphysitis or chronic physeal injury is seen in the proximal humerus (Little Leaguer's shoulder) or the distal radius (Gymnast's wrist). These injuries can result in growth arrest or deformity at any of these joints and therefore should be evaluated and treated appropriately [2, 3, 14, 18, 24].

1.3.4 Osteochondritis Dissecans (OCD)

While osteochondritis dissecans (OCD) is an injury that is more chronic in nature, it can present acutely during training or competition. A sudden or awkward movement can cause the lesion to become painful or even lead a piece of cartilage to dislodge, turning a stable lesion into an unstable one. Symptoms of locking or catching are concerning for a loose body. The etiology of OCD is not completely understood but is considered to be due to repetitive microtrauma causing a change in the vascularity of the bone.

In the knee, there is a frequent association of OCD with discoid meniscus [23, 34, 35, 36]. OCD of the knee is more common in males than females, with an incidence of 15.4 and 3.3 per 100,000 patients aged 6–19 years, respectively. They are most commonly found in adolescents aged 12–19 years old, and more commonly in black athletes over other ethnic groups [36]. OCD of the talar dome is also seen in the lower extremity. Lesions typically involve either the anterolateral or posteromedial dome, while central lesions are rare [6]. Athletes will often describe the pain after an acute inversion ankle injury or persistent symptoms after a remote injury. They describe lateral or medial ankle pain with swelling, as well as mechanical symptoms, including instability, locking, or clicking.

OCDs seen in the elbow of pediatric athletes tend to be in throwers or gymnasts over 10 years old, due to microtrauma to the radiocapitellar joint. They are most commonly found in the capitellum, but rarely can also be seen in the radial head. Athletes will describe lateral elbow pain with throwing or weight bearing and have a clear difference in range of motion as compared to the contralateral elbow, particularly with extension and pronosupination. An acute inability to extend the elbow is a strong predictor of an OCD [3, 7, 30]. Panner disease is a similar phenomenon seen in athletes typically under 10 years old in which there is damage to the posterior arterial supply to the capitellum also from abnormal radiocapitellar compression during a vulnerable period of growth, compromising endochondral ossification. These athletes will also describe lateral elbow pain and may develop a flexion contracture, but not typically as acute as seen in OCD [7].

1.4 Sideline Considerations for Pediatric Athletes

There are multiple unique considerations for the sideline management of pediatric and adolescent athletes. First of all, it is important that athletes have correct fitting equipment, and constant reassessment of equipment given the growth and changes to the pediatric athlete's body. Heat and weather also need to be considered for the pediatric athlete. The risk of heat illness is highest at the beginning of the season before the athlete is appropriately conditioned. It is important to allow athletes a week or two to acclimate to the weather and season, and it is recommended that all youth sports teams have a policy for heat conditions, allowing for adjustments to training and the competitive schedule if necessary. Hydration for youth athletes is key [8, 10].

If there is an injury during play, and there is a concern for a physeal fracture, reduction should not be attempted on the field. Too many reduction attempts at the physis can cause further damage leading to growth arrest or deformity. Therefore, reduction should be attempted after appropriate imaging has been obtained and ideally with adequate sedation to allow for the greatest chance of success. Similarly, if there is a question of dislocation versus physeal fracture, such as in the shoulder or hip, reduction should not be attempted until imaging is obtained to avoid further injury. For example, attempted reduction of a hip in a skeletally immature patient could knock off the proximal femur epiphysis, thereby causing a Delbet type 1 proximal femur fracture, or essentially an acute slipped capital femoral epiphysis (SCFE).

1.4.1 Acute Lower Extremity Injuries

Acute ankle injuries are very common in pediatric and adolescent athletes. The majority of injuries require removal from play for further evaluation if there is swelling or difficulty weight bearing. Ankle sprains are the most common reason for missed athletic participation in adolescent athletes and may result in long-term dysfunction with chronic instability if not treated appropriately [6, 14]. Recurrent ankle sprains may indicate incompetence of the ankle ligamentous stabilizers, a syndesmotic injury, or more rarely a tarsal coalition. In the pediatric or skeletally immature athlete, a distal fibular physeal fracture must be ruled out, and any swelling or tenderness of the lateral malleolus in a pediatric athlete should be treated as a Salter-Harris type I fracture even if radiographs are negative [2, 6]. Distal tibial injuries should be assessed with radiographs due to potential injury of the physis and may require CT to evaluate displacement given the intra-articular nature of triplane (Fig. 1.1) and tillaux fractures [18].

The Ottawa Foot and Ankle Rules were established to evaluate the need for radiographs in acute foot and ankle injuries. The guidelines indicate that foot radiographs should be obtained when the athlete is unable to bear weight immediately after the injury, on the sidelines, and for four steps, and when bone tenderness of the navicular bone or base of the fifth metatarsal is present; ankle radiographs should be obtained if the patient is unable to bear weight immediately after the injury or after a period of rest on the sideline, or if there is bone tenderness at the posterior edge or tip of either malleolus. These rules have been validated in both adults and pediatrics and are still the most sensitive guidelines available [29, 37]. A boot or splint and crutches can be utilized on the sideline while waiting for transfer or imaging.

Acute knee injuries (Fig. 1.3) should first be evaluated for deformity and effusion. Deformity of either the distal thigh or proximal tibia should prompt urgent evaluation for fracture or dislocation. Depending on displacement, both distal femur physeal and tibial tubercle fractures may require reduction with surgical fixation. Acute effusion of the knee can indicate a multitude of pathologies, including fracture, ACL tear or meniscal tear, patellar dislocations, and cartilage injuries. Radiographs are indicated to rule out fracture, especially given the risk of tibial spine fracture and patellar sleeve avulsion fracture in the pediatric athlete [13, 14]. Patellar dislocations are one of the most common acute knee disorders of pediatric and adolescent athletes and require imaging even in the setting of acute reduction to evaluate for loose body or cartilage injury [2, 14, 23]. In addition, a locked knee needs further evaluation for a bucket handle meniscus, discoid meniscus, or loose body [34, 35].

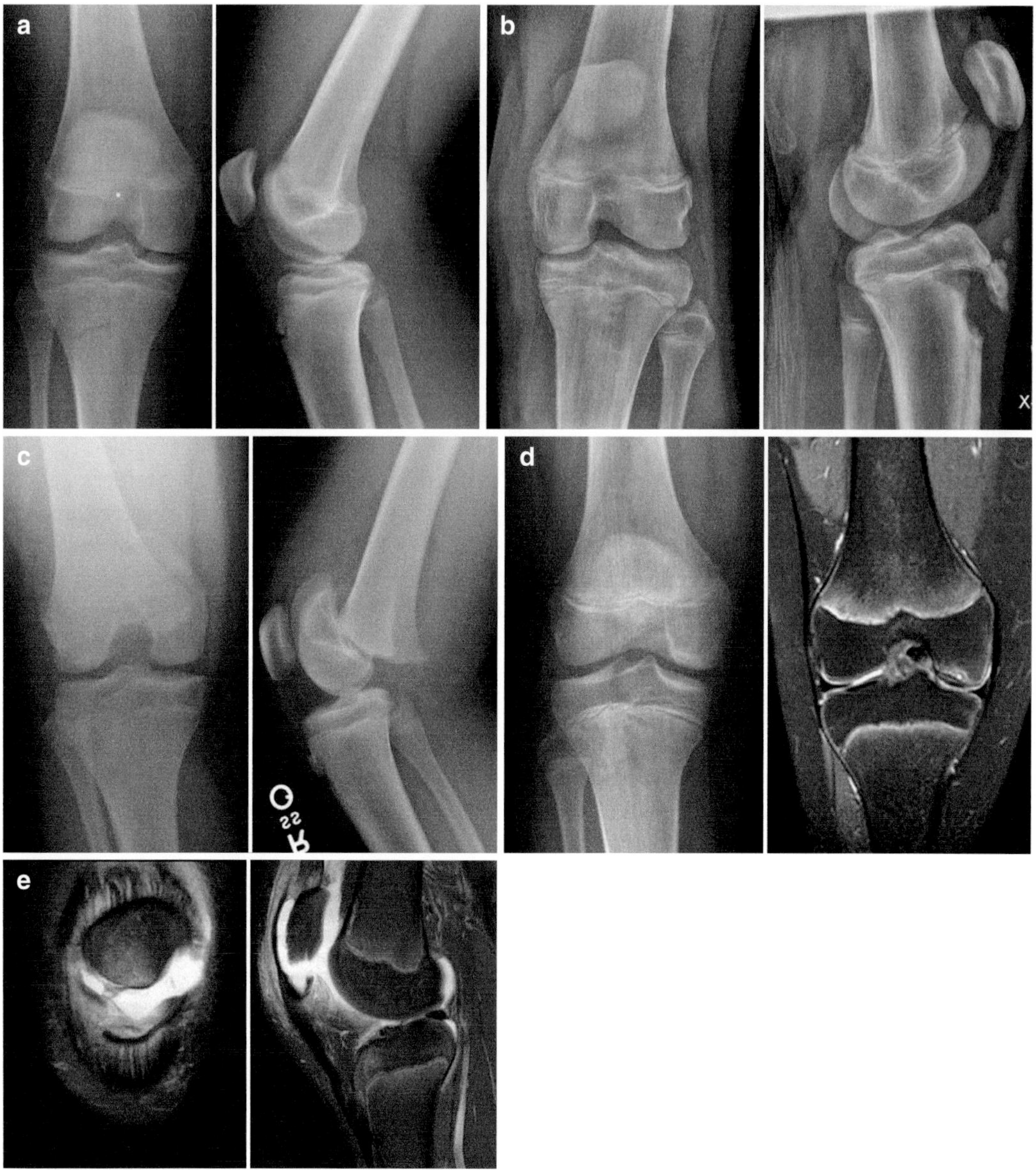

Fig. 1.3 Examples of pediatric knee injuries in sports. (**a**) AP and lateral radiographs of a 16-year-old male football player with a fracture of the tibial spine. (**b**) AP and lateral radiographs of a 14-year-old male basketball player with a tibial tubercle fracture after a dunk. (**c**) AP and lateral radiographs of a 11-year-old female with a distal femoral physeal fracture after a fall while sprinting. (**d**) AP radiograph and coronal MRI slice of a 13-year-old male football player with an OCD of the medial femoral condyle. (**e**) Coronal and sagittal MRI slices of a 12-year-old male basketball player with a patellar sleeve fracture

Similar to the foot and ankle, the Ottawa knee rules were created to indicate the need for radiographs of the knee. The Ottawa knee rules suggest that radiographs are indicated in an athlete age 55 years or older, tenderness at the head of the fibula, isolated tenderness of the patella, inability to flex to 90°, and inability to bear weight for four steps both immediately and after a period of observation on the sideline. Though not specifically designed for pediatric athlete, the Ottawa knee rules had a sensitivity of 100% and a specificity of 48.2% for children aged

2–16 years [29, 38, 39]. Pittsburgh knee rules are a separate set of indications for imaging of the knee and recommend radiographs when the mechanism of injury is blunt trauma or fall and one or more of the following factors are present: (1) age < 12 years or > 50 years and (2) inability to walk four weight-bearing steps in the emergency department or after a period of observation on the sideline [29, 40, 41]. Importantly, children will typically require radiographs regardless of physical examination. Often further imaging such as MRI will also be necessary, especially as injuries such as ACL tears in the pediatric population increase and to evaluate for cartilage injury.

While acute hip injuries are less common than ankle or knee, the sideline coverage of pediatric athletes requires awareness of specific hip conditions. The most common hip disorder in adolescents in an SCFE occurs in 10–11 per 100,000 children. It is most common among black and Hispanic males, at about 11 years of age. While many SCFE are chronic, they can also present acutely or as an acute on chronic injury due to a shearing force at the epiphysis with extension and external rotation of the femoral neck and shaft. An athlete with acute hip pain, or knee pain with a negative knee workup, should be evaluated with hip/pelvis radiographs, including a frogleg lateral. SCFE requires urgent surgical fixation and diagnosis should not be delayed due to the risk of avascular necrosis to the femoral head [3, 14, 18, 31]. Adolescents may also suffer acute apophyseal avulsion fractures with forceful contraction, and while these typically do not require surgical fixation, the athlete does need to be removed from play and protect weight bearing with crutches [3, 14, 31, 32].

1.4.2 Acute Upper Extremity Injuries

As reviewed for lower extremities most acute injuries will require removal from play and further evaluation, especially if there is any deformity or swelling. Almost half of the upper extremity injuries in pediatric athletes have been found to be fractures, therefore radiographs are typically indicated [21].

Any acute inability to extend the elbow compared to contralateral side indicates the need for removal from play and radiographs [29, 42, 43]. Knowledge of the ossification centers helps differentiate normal anatomy from fractures and avulsions. If there is uncertainty, the injured elbow can be compared to radiographs of the contralateral elbow. There is an increased risk of elbow injury in throwing athletes with inappropriate throwing volume such as pitching more than 8 months a year or 80 pitches per game. Pitching fatigue can increase the risk of injury from four to seven fold [7, 14].

The most common injury of the shoulder girdle is a clavicle fracture in the pediatric and adolescent athletes and will generally be fairly obvious on an exam. The athlete is removed from play and placed in a sling for immobilization until radiographic evaluation can be attained. If there is any tenting of the skin, transfer to the emergency department should be done urgently.

While rare in skeletally immature athletes, concern for dislocation of the shoulder may require imaging prior to attempted reduction to rule out proximal humerus fracture. In addition, adequate sedation is needed for reduction to reduce risk to the physis [2, 44, 45]. However, in adolescent athletes shoulder dislocation is more common, and the rate of recurrence has been estimated to be between 60% and 100% with a large percent of athletes suffering from glenoid bone loss [13, 30, 44, 45]. In older adolescent or high school athletes, an obvious shoulder dislocation can be reduced on the sidelines without radiographs. Shoulder harness bracing is often used for young football players, or other contact athletes such as hockey and lacrosse players, who seek to return to play during the same season, or occasionally the same game. The option to return to play with an unstable shoulder requires a full understanding by both the player and their parents of the risk of recurrence, an ability to wear the brace, and when painless range of motion and comparable strength to the contralateral side is achieved [44].

1.4.3 Facial Injuries

Sports related facial injuries have the highest frequency in pediatric and adolescent male athletes 11–20 years old. Fractures of the nasal bone are the most common facial fractures across all sports, while mandibular and zygoma fractures are more common in martial arts and soccer, and orbital fractures are more common in basketball, ice sports, and baseball [46]. The incidence of eye injuries is fairly low, with one 10-year study of soccer players showing an incidence of about 1 per 100,000 athletic exposures, however the injuries can be catastrophic. High-risk sports include basketball, baseball/softball, lacrosse, hockey, squash, racquetball, fencing, boxing, wrestling, and full-contact martial arts [10, 47, 48]. The best way to prevent eye injury is to utilize eye protection or facemasks, which can prevent about 90% of serious injuries [10]. Dental injuries are also possible with a facial injury. They account for just 0.2% of high school athletic injuries due to prevention with the use of mouth guards [10].

In the event of facial injury, first hemostasis should be achieved, especially given the rich blood supply to the face. Facial symmetry should be compared, and eyelids should be opened to check for an ocular injury. Nerve territories are assessed with motor and sensation, and bony prominences are palpated. Pupillary reflex and a brief visual acuity test are performed in case of an orbital fracture. When there is an eye injury ophthalmic ointment, and an eye protector should be placed, and the athlete taken to the emergency department for urgent care. For a nasal fracture, immediate reduction is only necessary if the airway is compromised. If there is malocclusion, or the athlete's bite does not properly align, a mandible fracture should be suspected and can be immobilized with a facial band [46].

1.4.4 Concussion

According to an estimate from 2006, about 3.8 million concussions occur during athletics annually in the United States, and 1.1–1.9 million of those are in children under 18 years old [49, 50]. Concussions have received a lot of media attention over the past two decades, and therefore a lot of research has gone into protecting athletes from concussion, however data indicate that concussion rates may still be increasing in youth and adolescent soccer players [10]. Pediatric athletes must be considered and treated differently than adults in terms of concussions. Children have different abilities to protect their heads and to take on impact due to their physiological development. Young children have poorly developed cervical musculature, an increased head-to-neck ratio, a thinner skull, as well as developing myelination, leading to increased vulnerability and greater injury to a pediatric athlete's brain than an adult's for the same force. Younger athletes also have a longer recovery. High school athletes have been found to have twice as long a recovery than college or professional athletes, 10–14 days as compared to 3–7 days, respectively [17]. This creates a longer window for a second impact, further prolonging symptoms. Concussions affect the pediatric and adolescent athlete's ability to participate in school and have the potential for long-term sequelae [17, 49, 50].

Historically there have been many tests available for the sideline assessment of concussion, but few have been specifically developed for the sideline assessment of concussion in children. There is now the SCAT-5 and SCAT-5 child available, and the Post-Concussion Symptom Scale and Post-Concussion Symptom Inventory for clinical use [50]. Perhaps even more important is the evaluation of symptoms of headache, dizziness, photophobia, and balance issues. If there is any question of concussion on the sideline for a pediatric athlete, they should be removed from play and monitored. There is now concussion training for all youth football coaches in the United States and the majority of states require routine concussion education. There should also be a preseason exam for each athlete and an emergency action plan in the case of life-threatening associated injuries, such as cervical trauma [8, 49].

1.4.5 Catastrophic Injuries

Catastrophic sports injuries are devasting in any athlete, especially in pediatric athletes. While rare overall, one study found that about 40% of life-threatening injuries in pediatrics are actually sport-related [51]. They can range from severe without permanent disability to fatal. These injuries can occur directly from sports participation or as sequelae from exertion during sport. Catastrophic injuries involving the brain and/or spinal cord occur due to compression, tensile, or shearing forces. Previous studies have indicated that about 7% of the 2500 new cases of paraplegia and 7% of the 1050 new cases of quadriplegia annually in the United States are related to sports injury [47, 51]. Catastrophic injury to the head can also involve any type of intracranial hemorrhage—epidural, subdural, intracerebral, and subarachnoid—and needs to be recognized quickly.

Cardiac and medical issues can also be the reason for a catastrophic event during sport. Sudden death can occur due to hypertrophic cardiomyopathy, coronary artery anomalies, myocarditis, aortic stenosis, aortic rupture, or right ventricular cardiomyopathy. Dysrhythmias can occur due to various underlying syndromes such as Ebstein's anomaly with pre-excitation, long QT syndromes, and Brugada syndrome. And rarely, commotio cordis is possible in an athlete who is hit directly in the chest. Exertional rhabdomyolysis can occur in athletes when overexerting in hot conditions and/or when underconditioned [47]. Emergent issues may arise in young athletes with chronic conditions, such as asthma or diabetes, if they are not appropriately managed or prepared for athletic exertion.

The best management of catastrophic injuries is prevention. Prevention is achieved through appropriate protective equipment, training of the athletes on proper technique, knowledge of the athlete's personal and family history through preparticipation physicals, and sometimes even further preparticipation workup with labs or imaging. These injuries and issues can happen quickly. Therefore, it is essential when on the sideline to be aware of the surroundings, to know where emergency medical services and automatic defibrillators can be found, and to have an emergency action plan in place for catastrophic events.

1.5 Summary

Pediatric and adolescent sports participation continues to rise, and while participation in athletics offers many benefits, there is also an increased risk of injury. In addition to the common injuries seen in adult athletes such as ACL or meniscal injury and shoulder instability, injury to the pediatric athlete often involves different injuries than in adults including physeal fracture, acute or chronic apophysitis, and OCD. An understanding of pediatric injury is essential in order to properly assess and treat pediatric athletes on the sidelines. Radiographs are typically needed to assess for fracture or physeal injury or to help prevent further injury with reduction. Concussions in children have increased the severity and duration of symptoms. Therefore, pediatric athletes need to be removed from play and assessed promptly. The best management for most injuries, especially catastrophic injury and medical emergency, is through prevention and preparation with appropriate equipment, preparticipation screening, and an emergency action plan.

References

1. Adirim TA, Cheng TL. Overview of injuries in the young athlete. Sports Med. 2003;33:75–81.
2. Soprano JV. Musculoskeletal injuries in the pediatric and adolescent athlete. Curr Sports Med Rep. 2005;4(6):329–43.
3. Coleman N. Sports injuries. Pediatr Rev. 2019;40(6):278–90.
4. Sheu Y, Chen LH, Hedegaard H. Sports- and recreation-related injury episodes in the United States, 2011–2014. Natl Health Stat Report. 2016;(99):1–12.
5. Popkin CA, Bayomy AF, Ahmad CS. Early sport specialization. J Am Acad Orthop Surg. 2019;27:e995–e1000.
6. Erickson JB, Samora WP, Klingele KE. Ankle injuries in the pediatric athlete. Sports Med Arthrosc Rev. 2016;24:170–7.

7. Greiwe RM, Saifi C, Ahmad CS. Pediatric sports elbow injuries. Clin Sports Med. 2010;29:677–703.
8. Rizzone K, Diamond A, Gregory A. Sideline coverage of youth football. Curr Sports Med Rep. 2013;12(3):143–9.
9. Leininger RE, Knox CL, Comstock RD. Epidemiology of 1.6 million pediatric soccer-related injuries presenting to US emergency departments from 1990 to 2003. Am J Sports Med. 2007;35(2):288–93.
10. Watson A, Mjaanes JM. Soccer injuries in children and adolescents. Pediatrics. 2019;144(5):e20192759.
11. Caine D, Caine C, Maffulli N. Incidence and distribution of pediatric sport-related injuries. Clin J Sports Med. 2006;16(6):500–13.
12. Caine D, Maffulli N, Caine C. Epidemiology of injury in child and adolescent sports: injury rates, risk factors, and prevention. Clin Sports Med. 2008;27(1):19–50.
13. Striano BM, Aoyama JT, Ellis HB, Kocher MS, Shea KG, Ganley TJ. Complications and controversies in the management of 5 common pediatric sports injuries. JBJS Rev. 2020;8(12):e20.00013.
14. Trentacosta N. Pediatric sports injuries. Pediatr Clin N Am. 2020;67:205–21.
15. Burt CW, Overpeck MD. Emergency visits for sports-related injuries. Ann Emerg Med. 2001;37:301–8.
16. Ardern CL, Ekas G, Grindem H, Moksnes H, Anderson A, Chotel F, Cohen M, Forssblad M, Ganley TJ, Feller JA, Karlsson J, Kocher MS, LaPrade RF, McNamee M, Mandelbaum B, Micheli L, Mohtadi M, Reider B, Roe J, Seil R, Siebold R, Silvers-Granelli HJ, Soligard T, Witvrouw E, Engebretsen L. 2018 International Olympic Committee consensus statement on prevention, diagnosis, and management of paediatric anterior cruciate ligament (ACL) injuries. Knee Surg Sports Traumatol Arthrosc. 2018;26:989–1010.
17. Davis GA, Purcell LK. The evaluation and management of acute concussion differs in young children. Br J Sports Med. 2014;48:98–101.
18. Samet JD. Pediatric sports injuries. Clin Sports Med. 2021;40:781–99.
19. Emery CA. Risk factors for injury in child and adolescent sport: a systematic review of the literature. Clin J Sport Med. 2003;13:256Y68.
20. Stracciolini A, Casciano R, Friedman HL, Meehan WP, Micheli LJ. Pediatric sports injuries: an age comparison of children versus adolescents. Am J Sports Med. 2013;41(8):1922–9.
21. Stracciolini A, Casciano R, Friedman HL, Stein CJ, Meehan WP, Micheli LJ. Pediatric sports injuries: a comparison of males versus females. Am J Sports Med. 2014;42(4):965–72.
22. Mitchell PD, Pecheva M, Modi N. Acute musculoskeletal sports injuries in school age children in Britain. Injury. 2021;52:2251–6.
23. Beck NA, Patel NM, Ganley TJ. The pediatric knee: current concepts in sports medicine. J Pediatric Orthop. 2014;23:59–66.
24. Longo UG, Ciuffreda M, Locher J, et al. Apophyseal injuries in children's and youth sports. Br Med Bull. 2016;120(1):139–59.
25. Cepela DJ, Tartaglione JP, Dooley TP, Patel PN. Classifications in brief: Salter-Harris classification of pediatric physeal fractures. Clin Orthop Relat Res. 2016;474:2531–7.
26. Russell K, Selci E. Pediatric and adolescent injury in snowboarding. Res Sports Med. 2018;26(51):166–85.
27. Pershad J, Monroe K, King W, Bartle S, Hardin E, Zinkan L. Can clinical parameters predict fractures in acute pediatric wrist injuries? Acad Emerg Med. 2000;7:1152–5.
28. Webster AP, Goodacre S, Walker D, Burke D. How do clinical features help identify paediatric patients with fractures following blunt wrist trauma? Emerg Med J. 2006;23:354–7.
29. Gould SJ, Cardone DA, Munyak J, Underwood PJ, Gould SA. Sideline coverage: when to get radiographs? A review of clinical decision tools. Sports Health. 2014;6(3):274–8.
30. Beck JJ, Richmond CG, Tompkins MA, Heyer A, Shea KG, Cruz AI. What's new in pediatric upper extremity sports injuries? J Pediatr Orthop. 2018;38:e73–7.
31. Kocher MS, Tucker R. Pediatric athlete hip disorders. Clin Sports Med. 2006;25:41–253.
32. Schroeder PB, Nicholes MA, Schmitz MR. Hip injuries in the adolescent athlete. Clin Sports Med. 2021;40:385–98.
33. Waicus KM, Smith BW. Back injuries in the pediatric athlete. Curr Sports Med Rep. 2002;1:52–8.
34. Francavilla ML, Restrepo R, Zamora KW, et al. Meniscal pathology in children: differences and similarities with the adult meniscus. Pediatr Radiol. 2014;44(8):910–25.
35. Kushare I, Klingele K, Samora W. Discoid meniscus: diagnosis and management. Orthop Clin North Am. 2015;46(4):533–40.
36. Kessler JI, Nikizad H, Shea KG, et al. The demographics and epidemiology of osteochondritis dissecans of the knee in children and adolescents. Am J Sports Med. 2014;42(2):320–6.
37. Stiell IG, Greenberg GH, McKnight RD, et al. Decision rules for the use of radiography in acute ankle injuries. Refinement and prospective validation. JAMA. 1993;269:1127–32.
38. Stiell IG, Greenberg GH, Wells GA, et al. Prospective validation of a decision rule for the use of radiography in acute knee injuries. JAMA. 1996;275:611–5.
39. Bulloch B, Neto G, Plint A, et al. Pediatric emergency researchers of Canada. Validation of the Ottawa knee rule in children: a multi-center study. Ann Emerg Med. 2003;42:48–55.
40. Bauer SJ, Hollander JE, Fuchs SH, Thode HC Jr. A clinical decision rule in the evaluation of acute knee injuries. J Emerg Med. 1995;13:611–5.
41. Seaberg DC, Yealy DM, Lukens T, Auble T, Mathias S. Multicenter comparison of two clinical decision rules for the use of radiography in acute, high-risk knee injuries. Ann Emerg Med. 1998;32:8–13.
42. Appelboam A, Reuben AD, Benger JR, et al. Elbow extension test to rule out elbow fracture: multicenter, prospective validation and observational study of

diagnostic accuracy in adults and children. BMJ. 2008;337:a2428.
43. Lamprakis A, Vlasis K, Siampou E, Grammatikopoulos I, Lionis C. Can elbow extension test be used as an alternative to radiographs in primary care? Eur J Gen Pract. 2007;13:221–4.
44. Milewski MD, Nissen CW. Pediatric and adolescent shoulder instability. Clin Sports Med. 2013;32:761–79.
45. Reid S, Liu M, Ortega H. Anterior shoulder dislocations in pediatric patients: are routine prereduction radiographs necessary? Pediatr Emerg Care. 2013;29:39–42.
46. Hwang K. Field management of facial injuries in sports. J Craniofac Surg. 2020;31(2):e179–82.
47. Luckstead EF, Patel DR. Catastrophic pediatric sports injuries. Pediatr Clin N Am. 2002;49:581–91.
48. Boden BP, Pierpoint LA, Boden RG, Comstock RD, Kerr ZY. Eye injuries in high school and collegiate athletes. Sports Health. 2017;9(5):444–9.
49. Resch JE, Kutcher JS. The acute management of sport concussion in pediatric athletes. J Child Neurol. 2015;20(12):1686–94.
50. Podolak OE, Arbogast KB, Master CL, Sleet D, Grady MF. Pediatric sports-related concussion: an approach to care. Am J Lifestyle Med. 2021;16(4):469–84.
51. Meehan WP 3rd., Mannix R. A substantial proportion of life-threatening injuries are sport-related. Pediatr Emerg Care. 2013;29(5):624–7.

Elderly/Masters Athlete (Overview) 2

Sérgio Rocha Piedade, Rogerio Carvalho Teixeira, Leonardo Augusto de Souza Beck, and Daniel Miranda Ferreira

2.1 Introduction

In a lifetime, the human body experiences a biological process of development, growth, and strengthening, followed by progressive tissue and organ deterioration over time—the human biological law [1, 2].

Even though young adulthood is, for most people, the moment of their muscle strength and physical apex, this equation does not work for everyone; therefore, it will not necessarily affect all of us similarly [3, 4]. A real example of successful aging is veterans or master athletes.

Decade after decade, an increasing life expectancy has impacted our lives positively, but, at the same time, it has become a challenge to live longer, physically and mentally healthy [5, 6].

This biological event has triggered elderly athletes to make their athletic careers longer. In addition, it has also played an essential role in stimulating the elderly to practice sports. A clear sign is that the number of master competitions has grown exponentially in the last decades, as well as the increasing interest of sponsors and participants independently of the modality of practiced sport.

In this context, the sports medicine physician should be familiar with the aging biological process and elderly athletes' needs by analyzing three scenarios: the athlete becoming aged, the elderly who decided to become regular sports practitioners or even an athlete, and the master athlete. This chapter approaches the biological process of aging,

2.2 Three Different Clinical Scenarios

1. **Elderly and sedentary adults who have become regular sports practitioners or even real athletes**

   Increasing life expectancy and a better understanding of the effects of aging are making people more conscious of the importance of sports practice and regular physical exercises for health and quality of life. In this context, more and more people who have not practised any sport or physical activity in their

S. R. Piedade (✉)
Exercise and Sports Medicine, Department of Orthopedics, Rheumatology, and Traumatology, University of Campinas—UNICAMP, Campinas, SP, Brazil
e-mail: piedade@unicamp.br

R. C. Teixeira
Knee Surgery Group from Servidor Público Estadual and Albert Einstein Hospitals, São Paulo, SP, Brazil

L. A. de Souza Beck
Department of Radiology, University of Campinas—UNICAMP, Campinas, SP, Brazil

D. M. Ferreira
Department of Radiology, University of Campinas—UNICAMP, Campinas, SP, Brazil

São Leopoldo Mandic, Faculty of Medicine, Campinas, SP, Brazil

S. Rocha Piedade et al. (eds.), *Sideline Management in Sports*,
https://doi.org/10.1007/978-3-031-33867-0_2

youth or adulthood are now beginning their journey against a sedentary lifestyle at an advanced age [7–9].

Although sports and physical activity promote health benefits in the elderly population, the physician should pay close attention to the aging physiological aspects and individual's clinical conditions [10–12]. With aging, we lose muscle and bone mass, increase adipose tissue and consequently decrease muscle strength, power, endurance, and flexibility [13].

Therefore, before prescribing sports or physical exercise training, attention to the intensity, charge, and frequency of activity should be carefully analyzed to potentialize the achievements in the musculoskeletal system and avoid injuries.

2. **Athletes that are getting older**

   With aging, athletes' bodies will experience a gradual loss of muscle mass and disturbed sensorimotor control changes take place with advancing age and can compromise the function of skeletal muscles. The most commonly observed changes are muscle and myofibril atrophy, a decrease in contractile muscle content, and a reduction in vascular capillarization that diminishes the delivery of nutrients. This process is more pronounced in the lower limbs [14], and its leading causes are due to metabolical and endocrinological changes with circadian disruption.

3. **Master athletes**

   The term master's athletes refer to men and women older than 35 years who participate in competitive athletics. There has been a continued increase in the number of master athletes in sporting such as running, swimming, cycling, rowing, and weightlifting. Some of these athletes come from a background with years of training and competition experience, while others have only begun to compete as they approach middle-aged and older [15].

   Masters' athletes demonstrate markedly greater physiological function and lower risk factors for cardiovascular disease, osteoporosis, frailty, and cognitive dysfunction than their sedentary counterparts [16].

   These athletes decline more slowly than those with younger ages and are examples of "successful ageing." Their physical fitness over a long period of time is ideal for studying the effects of ageing independently of factors that might affect their peers, such as obesity and other health conditions, or lifestyle choices like smoking and drinking alcohol.

   Prof. Stones reports that performance declines more quickly in older athletes, and that the decline is greater in women than in men, indicating that continued, consistent participation is an effective way to maintain performance [17–19].

   It is important to understand this population's special needs to adequately care for them, so they can participate at a high level and be injury-free. A suggested training program considering the biology of aging and injury prevention may be always suggested [20].

   Some authors propose that a given threshold of physical activity is needed to age optimally and to maximize the health quality. Exercising below the threshold will result in aging being affected by the unpredictable and pathological effects of inactivity. Exercise above this threshold stimulates adaptations toward maximizing athletic performance but is unlikely to have further beneficial effects on health [21].

2.3 Metabolic and Physiological Changes of Aging

With aging, the athlete's body will progressively experience metabolic and physiological changes, triggering a reduction in the levels of anabolic and sex hormones, and consequently reducing mass muscle. This process defines the pathophysiology of sarcopenia, a clinical condition that, if inadequately addressed, will predispose athletes to injuries.

2.3.1 Anabolic and Sex Hormones in Aging

Aging triggers a loss of anabolic and sex hormones, both androgens and estrogens, which influence energy storage and play a role in muscle deterioration. The lipid metabolism changes with aging and contributes to an increase in muscle fat mass and low energy production (ATP). The progressive loss of motoneurons is related to reduced muscle fibers (mainly fast twitch type II) and size, decrease in myosin heavy chains IIa and IIx mRNA levels, reduction of elastic properties, and balance capacities of connective tissues leading to impaired functional performance [22].

The microscopic mechanisms are associated with increased levels of nuclear apoptosis, mitochondrial dysfunction (biogenesis, degradation, and protein expression), muscle fiber denervation, and reduced regenerative potential. Neuromuscular junctions exhibit synaptic detachment, axonal swellings, the fragmentation of the acetylcholine receptors, and sprouting. At the molecular level, muscle protein breakdown increases and muscle protein synthesis decreases [23].

The oxidative stress occurs due to free radical accumulation (superoxide anion, nitric oxide, nitric dioxide radicals) and can generate cell toxicity and dysfunction in signaling pathways. The subsequent harmful effects are mitochondrial membrane damage and immune system with cell inflammation leading to an increased production rate of reactive oxygen species (ROS). ROS can oxidize proteins with deleterious transformations inside the healthy myofascial tissues. This mechanism is responsible for the breakdown of oxidative metabolism homeostasis, generating a chronic inflammatory response that predisposes cells to modification due to the induction of recurrent DNA disturbance with a higher mutation frequency. The growth of oxidative stress can stimulate hormonal secretion with proinflammatory activity like eicosanoids, cortisol, and insulin. This process is associated with the genesis or advancement of diseases, including type 2 diabetes, atherosclerosis, and chronic pain syndrome [24, 25].

The decline in immunological regulation, called immunosenescence, results from the accumulation of senescent T cells, thymic atrophy, and dysfunction of immune cells such as neutrophils and macrophages, NK-cells, and defective conservation of lymphocytes. This condition affects multiple pathways, including insufficient myokine signaling (IL-6, IL-7, IL-15) and shifting of membrane-bound regulatory factors toward a chronic low-grade inflammatory pattern. The consequences are lower immunological protection, impaired muscle regeneration, and enhanced skeletal muscle wasting with loss of muscle strength and function [26].

The adaptative changes in catabolic mediators such as TNF-α, TGF-β, IGF-I, glucorticoid, and C-reactive protein showed a consistent association with muscle loss and reduced levels of myogenic regulatory factors (MRFs) with the inhibition of myostatin expression.

2.4 Mass Muscle Reduction

The reduced muscle mass size can generate consequences of the aging biological process, including reduced maximal muscle strength, slower contractile velocity, and increased fatigue because of a decline in muscle protein turnover and mitochondrial disorder. From a neural perspective, there is a decreased rate of axoplasmic transport, axonal degeneration, myelin sheet irregularities with low speed of nerve regeneration, and axonal conduction velocity. The low force-generating capacity with shortening velocity can be associated with the low recruitment of motoneurons units with reduced peak and power output [23].

The altered physiological muscle mechanisms involved in phosphocreatine kinetics and pulmonary oxygen uptake have been attributed to exercise and subsequent muscle recovery. Some validated techniques to measure muscle performance are: (I) the gait speed test can be performed with short distances (2.4 m, 4 m, 6 m, 10 m distance) or long distances (at least 400-m walk test and 6-min walk test); (II) the 30-second chair stand test (CST); (III) short physical performance battery (SPPB); and (IV) timed-get-up and go-test (TUG) can be used to classify and quantify lower body power, balance, and endurance. The muscle strength can be evaluated with the hand grip strength test during isotonic contraction and can be considered reliable.

Due to limited metabolic resources, cognitive impairment can be observed during aging and high-intensity exercise. A diminished processing speed motion, hypotrophy of temporal and temporal lobes, changes in white matter, and a reduction in neuronal connectivity are observed [27].

Dopaminergic and noradrenergic systems are required for an appropriate prefrontal cortex function and can be affected during physical activity. Low leptin levels and altered glucose metabolism can lead to insulin resistance and metabolic syndrome [28].

The increase in body mass index (BMI) is considered a risk factor for atrial fibrillation. Visceral adiposity is associated with incident cardiovascular disease. Obesity is recognized as a chronic, low-grade systemic inflammatory state with a sympathovagal imbalance of the interatrial conduction delay, increased P-wave duration, terminal duration, and PR interval [29].

The aerobic muscle capacity, measured by the peak treadmill oxygen consumption (peak VO2) decline, reflects cardiovascular adaptation to transport less oxygen within the muscle to meet the energy demands of physical activity [30].

2.5 Pathophysiology of Sarcopenia

Sarcopenia is defined as a progressive and global loss of skeletal muscle mass that involves endocrine, metabolic and nutritional factors, and cytological aspects of the senescence of muscle cells.

From the endocrinological viewpoint, the progressive reduction of the secretion and sensitivity to anabolic hormones (growth hormone, testosterone, and insulin-like growth factor) affects the maintenance of muscle mass. Due to a lower degradation of pro-inflammatory cytokines (mainly, interleukin 6), the catabolic action is enhanced, consequently increasing muscle loss [31–33].

Imbalance progressively grows owing to lower muscle function and a decrease in anabolic hormone production. This apart, a remarkable progressive loss of the absorption capacity and protein synthesis in muscle cells occurs in the elderly [34].

The protein metabolism falls because of the low response to hyperaminoacidemia, causing an enhancement of adipose deposition and, consequently, a lower muscle mass per body mass takes place. This process potentializes the deleterious effects of obesity in the population named "sarcopenic obesity" [35–38].

At the age of 60 s, the lower muscle stimulation and direct denervation cause a progressive loss of motor neurons in the spinal cord, loss of peripheral neurons, and degeneration of the neuromuscular units. Consequently, sarcopenia takes place at the cellular level [39].

Some studies have shown up to 25% of motor functioning unit loss in senility, which is a valuable marker in the differentiation between other causes of muscle function loss [3, 40].

2.6 The Senescence of the Metabolic Axis and Sarcopenia

A remarkable decline of anabolic hormone production is expected in advanced ages, and a stressed decrease of total testosterone level, particularly their metabolic active portion (free portion), in elderly men [41, 42].

Although this mechanism has not been fully understood, it seems to have a cross-reaction with exercise practice and this hormone level, as observed by its increased response to sports and physical activity, suggests that the sarcopenia cycle, activity, and muscle function loss can be directly related to sports and physical activity practice.

The decline of the hypothalamic-pituitary-gonadal axis as well as the insulin-like growth factor 1 (IGF-1), both linked to loss of muscle mass in the elderly, is more pronounced in women, given its relevance to an anabolic hormone in this group [43–45].

Moreover, the skeletal muscle shows an increase in insulin resistance and a closer relationship to the loss of muscle function and the development of diabetes type II, especially among the obese sarcopenic [46].

It results in muscle contraction and increased glucose uptake into the muscle cell, a process that involves adenosine 5′-monophosphate-activated protein kinase (AMPK), related to increased insulin secretion, activation of adipose metabolism, cholesterol, and triglycerides [47].

Although multiple attempts at supplementing these hormones were tested to treat sarcopenia, the isolated approach did not have a satisfactory response [48], possibly due to other mechanisms involved in the perpetuation of the sarcopenic cycle.

2.7 Potential Red Flags in Elderly Athletes

The clinical problems affecting elderly athletes are related to the cardiovascular and musculoskeletal systems and hydroelectric disorders (dehydration) [49].

Even though sports and physical activity play an essential role in reducing global cardiovascular risk through a protective effect on coronary artery disease, acting against the formation, growth, and rupture of cholesterol plaques, strenuous activity is a concern regarding the potential risk for sudden cardiac arrest and harmful cardiovascular events [50], significantly higher in the elderly with coronary disease [51, 52].

However, it is essential to state that standardized ischemia provocative tests may not reproduce the symptoms during the session due to their low sensitivity [53].

An increasing number of studies have shown that elderly individuals who practice sports or strenuous physical exercise, especially muscular resistance training, have a higher risk of developing atrial fibrillation than those who perform physical activity at baseline levels. This finding may be related to exercise-induced cardiac remodelings, such as atrial dilation and fibrosis, increased vagal tone, and changes in left atrial pressure, which arise with physical activity [54–57].

However, further studies are needed to clarify why this population is at greater risk of developing atrial fibrillation. Elderly athletes are also more susceptible to dehydration and hyperthermia. The sensation of thirst and heat exchange through perspiration undergo significant physiological changes with age, and consequently, they tend to feel less thirsty and sweat than young athletes.

2.8 Predisposing Injury Risk in Elderly Athletes

With aging, athletes will go through the harmful effects of progressive changes in the musculoskeletal system, such as muscle and bone loss, reduction in collagen turnover, and lower concentration and reaction time, creating a scenario for injury.

Between ages 30 and 60, an estimated muscle mass loss of 15% occurs, reaching a loss of 30% of the previous muscle mass after 60, because of a reduction in the size and number of muscle fibers, so-called sarcopenia [58].

This process has a complex origin related to several factors, such as increased insulin resistance, and decreased energy and strength with age. There is a tendency for more pronounced loss of fast twitch muscle fibers (type 2) than slow twitch muscle fibers (type 1), mainly impairing speed. Although physical activity can reduce and delay the sarcopenia process, it cannot stop it completely. The elderly athlete's performance may be reduced due to sarcopenia [59].

On the other hand, the elderly athlete's concentration and reaction time decrease, becoming less efficient in decision-making in the field of play. In this context, physical demands involving high motor coordination and quick reaction time are most related to injuries [58–60].

Changes in the composition of tendons, such as a reduction in collagen turnover and an increase in elastin, can make them more rigid. Type I collagen is reduced while type III collagen is increased, conferring less resistance. In addition, there is an increase in collagen reticulation, making the tendon less flexible and the healing capacity more difficult—the risk of the rupture of the tendon structure increases [61].

Chronic Achilles tendon disorders are much more common in elderly athletes. Both degenerative alterations, known as tendinosis, affect the biomechanics of movement, predisposing to injuries. Cartilages also suffer modifications, such as reducing the number of chondrocytes and regenerative capacity [62, 63].

2.9 Main Clinical Complaints of Elderly Athletes

2.9.1 Lower Limbs

2.9.1.1 Calf Pain

A common symptom in elderly athletes is calf pain, usually reported in a more distal topography in the calf. Running, basketball, volleyball, and tennis are the sports modality commonly related to this pathology. The Achilles tendon is the largest and strongest tendon in the body, standing loads around or ten-fold greater than the body weight during jumping. This tendon function is to protect the muscles by absorbing shock during running or jumping [64].

However, the blood supply to the tendon decreases with age, and changes in tendon composition can make it less resistant, flexible, and with less regenerative capacity. Calf pain may result from an injury involving the medial portion of the gastrocnemius and may occur with ankle dorsiflexion with the knee extended in running. Consequently, the injury to the Achilles tendon is higher in elderly patients, typically in the mid to late 40s [65, 66] (Fig. 2.1).

Another common complaint of elderly athletes in the doctor's office is foot pain, usually related to pathologies of the metatarsophalangeal, metatarsal, and tarsometatarsal joints. Some frequent clinical conditions are capsular rupture, turf toe (injury to the first metatarsophalangeal joint), plantar fasciitis, impingement syndrome, stress fractures, bursitis, Morton's neuroma, fractures, sesamoiditis, plantar fibromatosis, and arthritis. At the same time, knee pain is commonly reported as a complaint in elderly athletes resulting from overuse injuries and degenerative changes of joint arthritis [67] (Fig. 2.2).

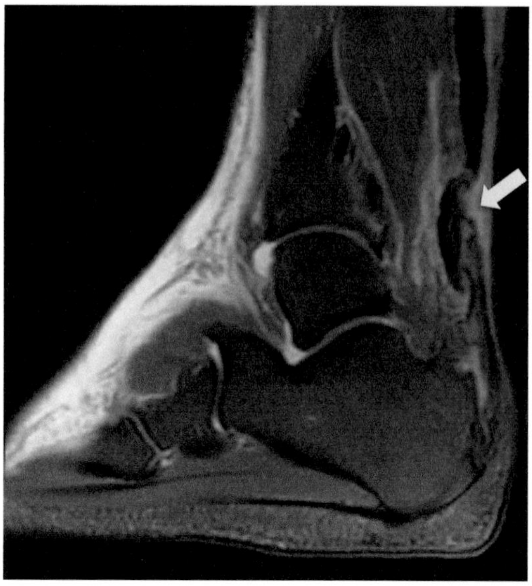

Fig. 2.1 Achilles tendon rupture in an elderly runner during a 15-km race

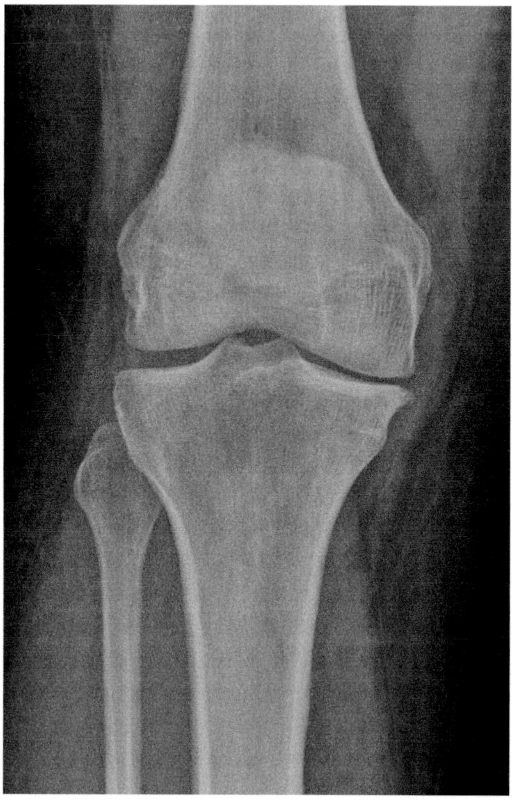

Fig. 2.2 Medial gonarthrosis with reduction of medial joint line in an elderly soccer player

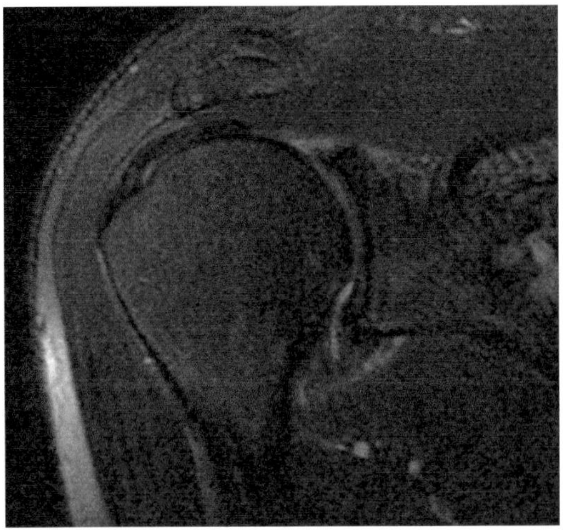

Fig. 2.3 MRI image of frozen shoulder syndrome (adhesive capsulitis) shows edema in the axillary recess

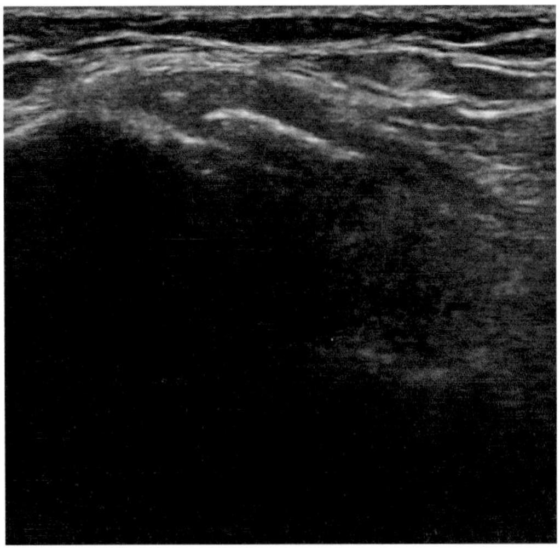

Fig. 2.4 An ultrasound image of elbow medial epicondylitis shows thickening and calcified foci of the common flexor tendon

Even though epidemiological data suggest that elderly athletes may present more pronounced degenerative changes in their spine and joints, in clinical practice, they often sustain good muscle function due to the heritage of their high physical activity developed over time [68].

2.9.2 Upper Limbs

As for the upper limbs, the most frequent complaints are pain and loss of strength. Several pathologies can be considered. Arthritis, for example, is more prevalent with age but may be related to trauma, repetitive use, and overload. It should also be remembered senile arthropathy, which is the deposition of calcium pyrophosphate, in the context of endocrine-metabolic diseases. Adhesive capsulitis or "frozen shoulder syndrome" is characterized by pain and reduced range of motion, and it is also a significant cause of shoulder pain in elderly athletes. The cause of this pathology is unknown [69] (Fig. 2.3).

Collagen alterations, already mentioned, also affect tendons in the upper limbs. The tendons that make up the rotator cuff are surrounded by lubricin, a type of heavy glycoprotein that acts as a lubricant. There is a reduction of this substance with age and a consequent increase in friction. In addition to changes in collagen, which make tendons less resistant and reduce healing capacity, complaints of pain in the shoulders involving the rotator cuff become more common in elderly athletes.

As shown in anatomopathological studies, the elderly may be predisposed to epicondylitis and pain in the elbow joint. The entheses of the tendons of both epicondyles tend to merge with the respective collateral ligament. In addition, cumulative changes have been found, through use, in the microscopic architecture of the entheses [70, 71] (Fig. 2.4).

Complaints of pain in the topography of the wrist joints should lead to suspicion of injuries to the triangular fibrocartilage complex, impingement syndrome (especially ulnar impaction), instability of the distal radio-ulnar joint, avascular necrosis, and fractures.

Injuries to the triangular fibrocartilage complex may occur due to trauma (a fall with an outstretched hand in ulnar deviation) or a degenerative process. The pain usually appears in the ulnar portion of the wrist and may be associated with complaints of weakness and loss of grip strength.

2.10 Managing the Harmful Effects of Aging

Aging is a biological process affecting all of us, sedentary and athletes, professional, or recreational—life rules. During a lifetime, athletes' sports performance suffers a slow and progressive drop reflecting the physiologic consequence of aging. And how the athletes could manage it, minimizing these harmful effects. The management strategy may vary according to the sports modality because they may differ in different aspects, such as the field of play, clothing (kimono, uniforms), rules, racquet use, ball, specific physical demands, etc. Moreover, medical decision-making cannot be standard for team and individual sports athletes.

In team sports, the athlete sometimes may change their function and role in the field of play, adopting a more favorable condition of physical stress, adaptable to their actual clinical and health situation. A clear example is the soccer player attacker who starts playing further back in the midfield or even in the defense. In contrast, their adaptation to aging seems less adaptable in individual sports, and keeping their sports performance level is a challenge.

Athletes at an advanced age should pay even more attention to the warning signs of excessive physical activity or risk injury. Overtraining syndrome is characterized by performing activity above the body's ability to recover. The rest time between sessions must be respected according to the needs of each individual.

Some *red flags* can help identify if the activity has been in excess. In the psychological field, the athlete may have difficulty sleeping and changes in mood, such as irritability, anxiety, and depressive symptoms. Headache, persistent muscle pain, and fatigue are also common. Another meaningful sign is an increase in heart rate at rest. Insufficient recovery increases the risk of overuse and repetitive strain injuries. Ultimately, the athlete's performance and income drop, generating frustration and worsening psychological symptoms.

Specifically, in athletes, close attention to nutrition, adequate training (periodization, individualization training, adequate rest), and inherent physical demands of sports modality play an essential role in extending the athlete's career at a high level and minimizing the effects of an athlete's sports performance decline. Moreover, chronic diseases, sports injuries, and mental and psychological balance may present adverse clinical conditions to potentialize the harmful effect of aging, mainly because athletes constantly work on challenging their body limits. However, genetics plays a vital role in athletes' sports performance and career and, therefore, it may sometimes surprise us, creating sports legends.

In clinical practice, the effects of aging may differ from one athlete to another. Therefore, the sports physician cannot standardize the management of all the abovementioned aspects. A close and periodical medical team surveillance of athletes' health conditions remains the best strategy to be adopted to define and guide physical performance and sports careers in elderly athletes.

Take-Home Message

- Sports training should be balanced with the elderly athlete's health condition.
- Aging triggers a loss of anabolic and sex hormones influencing energy storage and muscle deterioration.
- Although physical activity can reduce and delay the sarcopenia process, it cannot stop it completely.
- The low response to hyperaminoacidemia causes an enhancement of adipose deposition resulting in a lower muscle mass per body, potentializing the harmful effects of "sarcopenic obesity."
- Cardiovascular and musculoskeletal systems and hydroelectric disorders (dehydration) are the main clinical problems affecting elderly athletes.
- Calf pain and Achilles tendon disorders are prevalent in the mid to late 40s in elderly athletes.

References

1. DiLoreto R, Murphy CT. The cell biology of aging. Mol Biol Cell. 2015;26:4524–31.
2. Piedade SR, Inada MM, Laurito GM, Navarro e Paiva D, Fraga GP, Pagnano RG, de Andrade AL, Cardoso TP. Physical activity at adulthood and old age BT. In: Rocha Piedade S, Imhoff AB, Clatworthy M, Cohen M, Espregueira-Mendes J, editors. The sports medicine physician. Cham: Springer International Publishing; 2019. p. 59–69.
3. Faulkner JA, Larkin LM, Claflin DR, Brooks SV. Age-related changes in the structure and function of skeletal muscles. Clin Exp Pharmacol Physiol. 2007;34:1091–6.
4. Campbell MJ, McComas AJ, Petito F. Physiological changes in ageing muscles. J Neurol Neurosurg Psychiatry. 1973;36:174–82.
5. Aburto JM, Villavicencio F, Basellini U, Kjærgaard S, Vaupel JW. Dynamics of life expectancy and life span equality. Proc Natl Acad Sci U S A. 2020;117:5250–9.
6. Goodpaster BH, Park SW, Harris TB, Kritchevsky SB, Nevitt M, Schwartz AV, Simonsick EM, Tylavsky FA, Visser M, Newman AB. The loss of skeletal muscle strength, mass, and quality in older adults: the health, aging and body composition study. J Gerontol A Biol Sci Med Sci. 2006;61:1059–64.
7. Stenner BJ, Buckley JD, Mosewich AD. Reasons why older adults play sport: a systematic review. J Sport Heal Sci. 2020;9:530–41.
8. Cunningham C, O'Sullivan R, Caserotti P, Tully MA. Consequences of physical inactivity in older adults: a systematic review of reviews and meta-analyses. Scand J Med Sci Sports. 2020;30:816–27.
9. Jenkin CR, Eime RM, Westerbeek H, O'Sullivan G, van Uffelen JGZ. Sport and ageing: a systematic review of the determinants and trends of participation in sport for older adults. BMC Public Health. 2017;17:976.
10. Kehler DS, Theou O. The impact of physical activity and sedentary behaviors on frailty levels. Mech Ageing Dev. 2019;180:29–41.
11. McPhee JS, French DP, Jackson D, Nazroo J, Pendleton N, Degens H. Physical activity in older age: perspectives for healthy ageing and frailty. Biogerontology. 2016;17:567–80.
12. Warburton DER, Nicol CW, Bredin SSD. Health benefits of physical activity: the evidence. CMAJ. 2006;174:801–9.
13. Englund DA, Zhang X, Aversa Z, LeBrasseur NK. Skeletal muscle aging, cellular senescence, and senotherapeutics: current knowledge and future directions. Mech Ageing Dev. 2021;200:111595.
14. Janssen I, Heymsfield SB, Wang ZM, Ross R. Skeletal muscle mass and distribution in 468 men and women aged 18–88 yr. J Appl Physiol. 2000;89:81–8.
15. Trappe S. Master athletes. Int J Sport Nutr Exerc Metab. 2001;11(Suppl. 1):S196–207.
16. Tanaka H, Tarumi T, Rittweger J. Aging and physiological lessons from master athletes. Compr Physiol. 2019;10:261–96.
17. Stones MJ, Kozma A. Adult age trends in athletic performances. Exp Aging Res. 1981;7:269–80.
18. Stones MJ. Age differences, age changes, and generalizability in marathon running by master athletes. Front Psychol. 2019;10:2161.
19. Baker J, Horton S, Weir P. The masters athlete: understanding the role of sport and exercise in optimizing aging. New York: Routledge; 2009. p. 1–204.
20. Loudon JK. The master female triathlete. Phys Ther Sport Off J Assoc Chart Physiother Sport Med. 2016;22:123–8.
21. Lazarus NR, Harridge SDR. Declining performance of master athletes: silhouettes of the trajectory of healthy human ageing? J Physiol. 2017;595:2941–8.
22. Delbono O. Neural control of aging skeletal muscle. Aging Cell. 2003;2:21–9.
23. Keller K, Engelhardt M. Strength and muscle mass loss with aging process. Age and strength loss. Muscles Ligaments Tendons J. 2013;3:346–50.
24. Siddiqui A, Desai NG, Sharma SB, Aslam M, Sinha UK, Madhu SV. Association of oxidative stress and inflammatory markers with chronic stress in patients with newly diagnosed type 2 diabetes. Diabetes Metab Res Rev. 2019;35:e3147.
25. Khansari N, Shakiba Y, Mahmoudi M. Chronic inflammation and oxidative stress as a major cause of age-related diseases and cancer. Recent Patents Inflamm Allergy Drug Discov. 2009;3:73–80.
26. Fulop T, Larbi A, Dupuis G, Le Page A, Frost EH, Cohen AA, Witkowski JM, Franceschi C. Immunosenescence and inflamm-aging as two sides of the same coin: friends or foes? Front Immunol. 2017;8:1960.
27. Sogaard I, Ni R. Mediating age-related cognitive decline through lifestyle activities: a brief review of the effects of physical exercise and sports-playing on older adult cognition. Acta Psychopathol. 2018; https://doi.org/10.4172/2469-6676.100178.
28. Craft S, Watson GS. Insulin and neurodegenerative disease: shared and specific mechanisms. Lancet Neurol. 2004;3:169–78.
29. Magnani JW, Wang N, Benjamin EJ, et al. Atrial fibrillation and declining physical performance in older adults: the health, aging, and body composition study. Circ Arrhythm Electrophysiol. 2016;9:e003525.
30. Hollenberg M, Yang J, Haight TJ, Tager IB. Longitudinal changes in aerobic capacity: implications for concepts of aging. J Gerontol A Biol Sci Med Sci. 2006;61:851–8.
31. Vermeulen A. Ageing, hormones, body composition, metabolic effects. World J Urol. 2002;20:23–7.
32. Ferrucci L, Penninx BWJH, Volpato S, Harris TB, Bandeen-Roche K, Balfour J, Leveille SG, Fried LP, Md JMG. Change in muscle strength explains accelerated decline of physical function in older women with

high interleukin-6 serum levels. J Am Geriatr Soc. 2002;50:1947–54.
33. Zoico E, Roubenoff R. The role of cytokines in regulating protein metabolism and muscle function. Nutr Rev. 2002;60:39–51.
34. Skelton DA, Kennedy J, Rutherford OM. Explosive power and asymmetry in leg muscle function in frequent fallers and non-fallers aged over 65. Age Ageing. 2002;31:119–25.
35. Polyzos SA, Margioris AN. Sarcopenic obesity. Hormones. 2018;17:321–31.
36. Barazzoni R, Bischoff S, Boirie Y, Busetto L, Cederholm T, Dicker D, Toplak H, Van Gossum A, Yumuk V, Vettor R. Sarcopenic obesity: time to meet the challenge. Obes Facts. 2018;11:294–305.
37. Batsis JA, Villareal DT. Sarcopenic obesity in older adults: aetiology, epidemiology and treatment strategies. Nat Rev Endocrinol. 2018;14:513–37.
38. Choi KM. Sarcopenia and sarcopenic obesity. Korean J Intern Med. 2016;31:1054–60.
39. Rowan SL, Rygiel K, Purves-Smith FM, Solbak NM, Turnbull DM, Hepple RT. Denervation causes fiber atrophy and myosin heavy chain co-expression in senescent skeletal muscle. PLoS One. 2012;7:e29082.
40. Edström E, Altun M, Bergman E, Johnson H, Kullberg S, Ramírez-León V, Ulfhake B. Factors contributing to neuromuscular impairment and sarcopenia during aging. Physiol Behav. 2007;92:129–35.
41. Stanworth RD, Jones TH. Testosterone for the aging male; current evidence and recommended practice. Clin Interv Aging. 2008;3:25–44.
42. Craig BW, Brown R, Everhart J. Effects of progressive resistance training on growth hormone and testosterone levels in young and elderly subjects. Mech Ageing Dev. 1989;49:159–69.
43. Veldhuis JD. Aging and hormones of the hypothalamo-pituitary axis: gonadotropic axis in men and somatotropic axes in men and women. Ageing Res Rev. 2008;7:189–208.
44. Kraemer WJ, Gordon SE, Fleck SJ, Marchitelli LJ, Mello R, Dziados JE, Friedl K, Harman E, Maresh C, Fry AC. Endogenous anabolic hormonal and growth factor responses to heavy resistance exercise in males and females. Int J Sports Med. 1991;12:228–35.
45. Rudman D. Growth hormone, body composition, and aging. J Am Geriatr Soc. 1985;33:800–7.
46. Cleasby ME, Jamieson PM, Atherton PJ. Insulin resistance and sarcopenia: mechanistic links between common co-morbidities. J Endocrinol. 2016;229: R67–81.
47. Ryan AS. Insulin resistance with aging: effects of diet and exercise. Sports Med. 2000;30:327–46.
48. Corpas E, Harman SM, Blackman MR. Human growth hormone and human aging. Endocr Rev. 1993;14:20–39.
49. Moorman AJ, Dean LS, Yang E, Drezner JA. Cardiovascular risk assessment in the older athlete. Sports Health. 2021;13:622–9.
50. Palmefors H, DuttaRoy S, Rundqvist B, Börjesson M. The effect of physical activity or exercise on key biomarkers in atherosclerosis—a systematic review. Atherosclerosis. 2014;235:150–61.
51. Bergström G, Persson M, Adiels M, et al. Prevalence of subclinical coronary artery atherosclerosis in the general population. Circulation. 2021;144:916–29.
52. Deligiannis A, Kouidi E. Sudden cardiac death in sports: could we save Pheidippides? Acta Cardiol. 2021;76:945–59.
53. Stern S. State of the art in stress testing and ischaemia monitoring. Card Electrophysiol Rev. 2002;6: 204–8.
54. Newman W, Parry-Williams G, Wiles J, Edwards J, Hulbert S, Kipourou K, Papadakis M, Sharma R, O'Driscoll J. Risk of atrial fibrillation in athletes: a systematic review and meta-analysis. Br J Sports Med. 2021;55:1233–8.
55. Wilhelm M. Atrial fibrillation in endurance athletes. Eur J Prev Cardiol. 2014;21:1040–8.
56. Drca N, Wolk A, Jensen-Urstad M, Larsson SC. Atrial fibrillation is associated with different levels of physical activity levels at different ages in men. Heart. 2014;100:1037–42.
57. Flannery MD, Kalman JM, Sanders P, La Gerche A. State of the art review: atrial fibrillation in athletes. Heart Lung Circ. 2017;26:983–9.
58. Gomes, TL, Viana LO, Ferreira DM, Inada MM, Laurito GM, Piedade SR. The Aging Athlete: Influence of Age on Injury Risk and Rehabilitation. In: Canata GL, D'Hooghe P, Hunt KJ, Kerkhoffs G, Longo UG (eds) Management of track and field injuries. Springer, Cham. https://doi.org/10.1007/978-3-030-60216-1_31.
59. Piedade SR, Viana LO, Arruda BPL. Age and running: children and adolescents, elder people. In: The running athlete: a comprehensive overview of running in different sports. Berlin, Heidelberg: Springer; 2022. p. 29–34.
60. Piedade SR, Inada MM, Laurito GM, Navarro e Paiva D, Fraga GP, Pagnano RG, de Andrade AL, Cardoso TP. (2019). Physical Activity at Adulthood and Old Age. In: Rocha Piedade S, Imhoff A, Clatworthy M, Cohen M, Espregueira-Mendes J (eds) The Sports Medicine Physician. Springer, Cham. https://doi.org/10.1007/978-3-030-10433-7_6.
61. Svensson RB, Heinemeier KM, Couppé C, Kjaer M, Magnusson SP. Effect of aging and exercise on the tendon. J Appl Physiol. 2016;121:1237–46.
62. Maffulli N, Via AG, Oliva F. Chronic achilles tendon disorders: tendinopathy and chronic rupture. Clin Sports Med. 2015;34:607–24.
63. Touzell A. The Achilles tendon: Management of acute and chronic conditions. Aust J Gen Pract. 2020;49:715–9.
64. Fields KB, Rigby MD. Muscular calf injuries in runners. Curr Sports Med Rep. 2016;15:320–4.
65. Carmont MR, Silbernagel KG, Edge A, Mei-Dan O, Karlsson J, Maffulli N. Functional outcome of percutaneous achilles repair: improvements in achilles tendon total rupture score during the first year. Orthop J Sport Med. 2013;1:2325967113494584.
66. Maffulli N, Waterston SW, Squair J, Reaper J, Douglas AS. Changing incidence of Achilles tendon rupture in Scotland: a 15-year study. Clin J Sport Med Off J Can Acad Sport Med. 1999;9:157–60.

67. Kannus P, Niittymäki S, Järvinen M, Lehto M. Sports injuries in elderly athletes: a three-year prospective, controlled study. Age Ageing. 1989;18:263–70.
68. Kujala U, Orava S, Parkkari J, Kaprio J, Sarna S. Sports career-related musculoskeletal injuries: long-term health effects on former athletes. Sports Med. 2003;33:869–75.
69. Randelli P, Ragone V, Menon A, et al. Upper limb injuries in athletes. ESSKA Instr Course Lect B Amsterdam. 2014;2014:211–31.
70. Fejer R, Ruhe A. What is the prevalence of musculoskeletal problems in the elderly population in developed countries? A systematic critical literature review. Chiropr Man Therap. 2012;20:31.
71. Yamada E, Thomas DC. Common musculoskeletal diagnoses of upper and lower extremities in older patients. Mt Sinai J Med. 2011;78:546–57.

Paralympic Athletes

3

Lucas Paladino, Stephanie Tow, Cheri Blauwet, and Mark R. Hutchinson

3.1 Introduction

The beginning of widespread competitive and organized sporting events for individuals with disabilities traces back to the Stoke Mandeville Hospital in Great Britain. In 1944, Dr. Ludwig Guttmann was directed by the British Government to establish a dedicated spinal injury center for the rehabilitation of World War II veterans. Although their prognosis was grim, Dr. Guttman was motivated to pioneer a new approach to caring for spinal cord injury patients. He emphasized early physical and social rehabilitation coupled with aggressive avoidance and treatment of decubitus ulcers and urinary tract infections [1].

L. Paladino · M. R. Hutchinson (✉)
Department of Orthopaedic Surgery, University of Illinois Chicago, Chicago, IL, USA
e-mail: lpp@uic.edu; mhutch@uic.edu

S. Tow
Department of Physical Medicine & Rehabilitation, University of Texas Southwestern Medical Center, Dallas, TX, USA

C. Blauwet
Department of Physical Medicine & Rehabilitation, University of Texas Southwestern Medical Center, Dallas, TX, USA

Spaulding Rehabilitation Hospital and Brigham and Women's Hospital, Harvard Medical School, Boston, MA, USA
e-mail: CBLAUWET@bwh.harvard.edu

As a part of rehabilitation at Stoke Mandeville, Gutmann introduced sports, such as darts, wheelchair polo, badminton, and basketball, to his patients. This ultimately led to the integration of competitive sports, such as wheelchair archery, fencing, athletics, and swimming. Dr. Guttmann noted that his patients manifested both physical and psychological benefits. He introduced the world to the abilities of his patients in sport in 1948, intentionally at the Opening Ceremony Day of the London Summer Olympic Games, with a wheelchair archery competition among 16 patients with spinal cord injuries [2].

By 1952, this small exhibition grew into a yearly Stoke Mandeville Games drawing competitors from around the world [2]. In 1960, this sporting event was held in Rome alongside the Summer Olympics, and the Paralympic Games were born. Four hundred athletes from 23 countries competed in 57 events [3]. The event garnered strong praise, with the Pope likening Guttmann to the founder of the International Olympic Committee [2]. Since then, the Paralympic Movement and Para sport have grown exponentially. During the 2020 Tokyo Summer Paralympic Games, 4393 athletes from 162 countries competed in 539 events over 22 sports [4].

The Paralympic Games have inspired and motivated individuals with disabilities around

S. Rocha Piedade et al. (eds.), *Sideline Management in Sports*,
https://doi.org/10.1007/978-3-031-33867-0_3

the world to incorporate sporting activities into their lives. Recognizing the benefits of Para sports, there has been an increase in organizations providing sporting opportunities to athletes with disabilities, leading to an increase in sports participation across all ages and competition levels, from novice to elite. This increase in the Para sport footprint may present challenges to a sideline healthcare provider who is not familiar with working with athletes with disabilities. The medical conditions of Para athletes encompass a wide array of pathologies with varying degrees of severity and complexity. Assessing and addressing Para athletes' injuries and illnesses during competition requires an understanding of altered physiologies, sport-related injury, illness incidence and risk, prevention strategies, and sport-specific equipment. Additionally, a care giver must consider the unique impact of an athlete's impairment on their biomechanics within each sport when providing a Para athlete an individualized evaluation and treatment plan specific to their needs.

Table 3.1 Opitimizing communication and avoiding negative labels in paralympic athletes

Terms to avoid	
Avoid these phrases	Reason/alternative
Abnormal	Not appropriate in reference to a person
Afflicted with	Defines a person as their disability
Able-bodied	Implies people with disabilities lack the ability to use their body well
Confined to a wheelchair	May define a person as being restricted by a liberating piece of equipment
Deaf and dumb, deaf-mute	Often used incorrectly and may be offensive
Defect, defective, birth defect	Implies a person is somehow
Epileptic fit	Seizure
Mentally retarded	Specify the type of disability, else intellectual/developmental disability
Midget	Short stature
Paraplegic	Person with paraplegia
Quadraplegic	Person with quadriplegia
Spastic/spaz	Acceptable if used in reference to spastic palsy, but is derogatory in other contexts
Stricken with, suffers from, victim of	Assumes that a person with a disability has a reduced quality of life

3.2 Key Terminology (to Appear Alongside Introduction)

The principles of inclusion and equity are paramount to the culture of sports for persons with disabilities. Social dynamics and language surrounding disability are subject to rapid change. It can be a difficult or frustrating experience for even the most well-intentioned provider or coach to use appropriate language and terminology. The National Center on Disability and Journalism offers some basic guidelines to help anyone be mindful of appropriate language. Table 3.1 outlines several of these terms [5].

In alignment with the UN Convention on the Rights of Persons with Disabilities, the International Paralympic Committee (IPC) has also outlined several correct and incorrect or outdated terms in the setting of sport for persons with physical, visual, and/or intellectual impairment [6].

- Para sport: Any sport in which an athlete with a disability can participate. It follows the IPC Athlete classification code
  - Correct terms: Sport for athletes with a disability
  - Incorrect terms: disabled sport, disability sport, and able-bodied sport (when referring to sports for athletes without disabilities)
- Paralympic sport: A Para sport that has taken place at the Paralympic Games
- Para athlete: an athlete with a disability who participates in sport but may not have competed in the Paralympic Games
  - Correct terms: Athlete/person with disability, athlete/person with vision impairment, athlete/person with physical impairment, and athlete/person with intellectual impairment
  - Incorrect terms: disabled athlete, disabled person, blind athlete, blind person, and able-bodied athlete/person
- Paralympian/Paralympic Athlete: an athlete who has competed in the Paralympic Games.

3.3 Impairment Classification

Classifying athletes in Para sports based on the athlete's underlying medical condition(s), type of impairment, and severity of the impairment's impact on their sport(s) is necessary to create a fair and equitable landscape of competition. Furthermore, proper classification promotes participation at all levels since excellence in sport, rather than limitations, dictates the outcomes [7]. Providers should familiarize themselves with the classification system of every Para sport where they will participate in sideline medical care. This section will provide a brief overview of the general concept of classification. Details regarding classification are sport-specific, and full information regarding each sport's classification system can be found through their International Federation.

In the 1950s, classification was simply divided into athletes with upper and athletes with lower spinal cord injuries [8]. Now, each Para sport's governing body is responsible for outlining classification divisions, which accounts for the degree to which impairment affects the fundamental activity of their sport. These individual International Sports Federations are also responsible for appointing a panel of personnel with appropriate medical and technical qualifications to determine eligibility and classification [9]. The IPC outlines three steps to athlete classification [10]:

1. Athlete determined to have one of 10 Eligible Impairments, which must be secondary to an eligible medical condition that leads to permanent or progressive impairment
2. Athlete meets an objective set of Minimum Impairment Criteria for their sport
3. Assign the athlete to a Class that matches the athlete's activity function and limitation most accurately

3.3.1 Eligible Impairments

The International Standard for Eligible Impairments, developed and written by the IPC, establishes 10 categories of impairments that form the basis of classification in Para sport. Table 3.2 outlines each category. The categories are based

Table 3.2 Impairments that may qualify athletes for paralympic participation

Eligible impairment	Description
Impaired muscle power	Athletes with Impaired Muscle Power have a Health Condition that either reduces or eliminates their ability to voluntarily contract their muscles in order to move or to generate force. Examples: spinal cord injury, brachial plexopathy
Impaired passive range of movement	Athletes with Impaired Passive Range of Movement have a restriction or a lack of passive movement in one or more joints. Examples: arthrogryposis, club foot, contracture
Limb deficiency	Athletes with Limb Deficiency have total or partial absence of bones or joints as a consequence of trauma (for example traumatic amputation), illness (for example amputation due to bone cancer) or congenital limb deficiency (for example dysmelia). Examples: traumatic above knee amputation, proximal femoral focal deficiency
Leg length difference	Athletes with Leg Length Difference have a difference in the length of their legs as a result of a disturbance of limb growth, or as a result of trauma.
Short stature	Athletes with Short Stature have a reduced length in the bones of the upper limbs, lower limbs and/or trunk. Examples: achondroplasia, growth hormone dysfunction, and osteogenesis imperfecta.
Hypertonia	Athletes with hypertonia have an increase in muscle tension and a reduced ability of a muscle to stretch caused by damage to the central nervous system. Examples: cerebral palsy, traumatic brain injury and stroke.
Ataxia	Athletes with Ataxia have uncoordinated movements caused by damage to the central nervous system. Examples: cerebral palsy, traumatic brain injury, stroke and multiple sclerosis.
Athetosis	Athletes with Athetosis have continual slow involuntary movements. Examples: cerebral palsy, traumatic brain injury and stroke.

(continued)

Table 3.2 (continued)

Eligible impairment	Description
Vision Impairment	Athletes with Vision Impairment have reduced or no vision caused by damage to the eye structure, optical nerves or optical pathways, or visual cortex of the brain. Examples: retinitis pigmentosa and diabetic retinopathy.
Intellectual impairment	Athletes with an Intellectual Impairment have a restriction in intellectual functioning and adaptive behavior which affects conceptual, social and practical adaptive skills required for everyday life. This Impairment must be present before the age of 18.

on the nature of an athlete's impairment rather than specific underlying medical condition(s). Each grouping has an objective description that helps guide baseline eligibility determination. Eligibility by impairment category is also sport-specific: some Para sports include all 10 impairment categories, while other Para sports may use fewer categories for eligibility [9].

3.3.2 Sport Specific Classification

Following the determination that an athlete has an Eligible Impairment and has met the Minimum Impairment Criteria, they must be placed into an appropriate sport-specific classification. Each Para sport's international governing body is responsible for defining its classifications and aligning athletes within them [7]. The number of classifications can vary greatly by sport but allows for all events to be competitive. Each sport will define a broad impairment classification using letters and further divide based on the severity of impairment with a number.

Decreasing the number of values indicates more severe impairment. For example, Para Archery divides athletes between standing (ST), wheelchair (W), and visually impaired (V). The visual impairment category is further divided into V1 for those with near or total visual impairment and V2/3 with increasing levels of vision [11]. Some sports may also designate class categories based on events in the sport. Perhaps, the most comprehensive classification system has been formed for Para Athletics (Track and Field). It outlines 24 classifications for Track events and 26 for Field events [12].

Given the number of combinations of Para sports, Eligible Impairments, and severity—the extent of possible classifications can be dizzying. Following the 2000 Summer Paralympics in Sydney, Paralympic gold medalist Giles Long sought to simplify the explanation of impairment categories for each sport. He eventually developed LEXI—a visual system for communicating the complex classification system. Athletes, providers, and spectators can utilize LEXI to better understand Para sport classification [13].

During the classification process, the medical classifier determines which clinical assessments to perform based on the athlete's medical condition(s) and what Eligible Impairments are caused by that medical condition. Traditional examples of such assessments include passive range of movement, subjective strength testing, limb and trunk/height measurements, coordination testing, and other speciality testing [12]. Research in classification methods has started to focus on applying quantitative, testable, and easily reproducible measures to guide classification, such as for coordination testing, but further work is needed [14]. The IPC supports efforts to enhance the classification process, as it allows for, "...realization of the vision of the Paralympic Movement..." [7]. As research helps guide evidence-based processes for classification specific to each sport, each Para sport's classification processes have undergone updates and improvements.

3.4 Injury Incidence and Risk Factors

Understanding injury rates and patterns can help sideline practitioners feel more prepared when managing care at Para sporting events and guide injury prevention strategies. Elite-level athletes are more likely to experience an injury than elite athletes without impairment. During the 2016 Rio Summer Games, the prevalence of sport-related injury among Paralympians was 12.1% compared to 8% among Olympians [15]. This section offers a brief insight into injury incidence and trends during Para sport events.

During the 2012 Paralympic Summer Games in London, Willick et al. prospectively characterized the incidence and nature of the injury that occurred to competitors during the Games. At the time, this was the most comprehensive epidemiologic study of its kind reporting an injury incidence rate of 12.7 per 1000 athlete-days over 49,910 athlete-days [16]. Derman et al. performed a similar study during the 2016 Rio Games over 51,198 athlete days. They found that the overall incidence of injury across all sports was 10 per 1000 athlete-days, a reduction from 2012. Uniquely, they found significantly higher rates of pre-competition injury, which was attributed to many athletes quickly taking the place of the suspended Russian delegation [15].

During the Rio Games, 51.8% of injuries were acute, 34.5% were chronic overuse type injuries, and 13.7% were acute on chronic. The sports with the highest risk of injury were similar during the 2012 and 2016 Summer Games. Football 5-a-side, Judo, and Football 7-a-side were all independently associated with a higher incidence of injury. These sports all involve contact and higher intensity. Wheelchair fencing, rugby, and basketball also had high rates of injury. The shoulder (17.7–20.5%) was the most commonly affected body part overall at each Game, while the hand and wrist (11.4–12.0%), and foot, ankle, and toes (10.0–12.2%) were also frequently involved. The study of the 2016 Games reported that 88.5% of injuries involved athletes with four types of impairment or medical condition categories: limb deficiency, visual impairment, spinal cord injury, and central neurological injury (cerebral palsy, traumatic brain injury, and stroke) [15].

Winter Para sports, although not as well participated as summer sports, seem to demonstrate a significantly higher risk for injury in the Para athlete. Derman et al. found that over 6804 athlete-days during the 2018 Pyeongchang Winter Games, the incidence rate of injury was 20.9 per 1000 athlete-days—nearly double that observed during the Summer Games. Snowboard and alpine skiing were the largest contributors. Like the Summer Games, injuries were most frequently observed in the shoulder (27.4%); however, lower limb injuries were frequently observed during Para snowboarding. Acute injuries (77%) were found to occur at significantly higher rates than chronic injuries, a finding that differs from the Summer Games [17].

Pinheiro et al. performed a 2016 meta-analysis of Para athlete injury incidence that accounts for non-Paralympic Games events and delineated types of injury based on ambulant athletes and those who use a wheelchair. They report that non-ambulant athletes experienced shoulder injuries most frequently, and ambulant athletes sustained lower extremity injuries the most [18]. This detailed study revealed nuances in the types of injuries observed among different general impairments and highlights the need for high-quality epidemiological studies of Para athletes across all impairments and competition levels, not just elite sport. This type of work may have a profound impact on injury prevention programs.

Based on the work of Willick, Derman, and Pinheiro, sideline practitioners should expect to address acute injuries involving a variety of body parts. Important attention should be paid to the type of sport, equipment used, and the athlete's underlying medical condition. High-intensity ambulant sports may result in a higher rate of acute lower extremity injuries while low-intensity wheelchair sports may produce more chronic upper extremity complaints. However, it should be noted that a study of 244 athletes during a Summer Paralympic Games found that two-thirds of shoulder complaints were associated with spinal pathologies, mainly cervical [19]. Thus, as with all clinical encounters, it is important to form a wide-ranging differential diagnosis.

It must be noted that the incidence of concussion and traumatic brain injury has been previously underreported in Para athletes [15], but insights into this important area are beginning to emerge. In 2022, the Concussion in Para Sport

Group published its first position statement [20]. Discussion of this topic will occur later in the chapter.

3.4.1 Training, Illness, and Behavioral Perceptions Among Para Athletes

Para athletes are at high risk of illness, injury during training periods, and impaired mental health. Fagher et al. studied the prevalence of injury in Paralympic Athletes over a year long period and found that severe injuries occurred in 31% of athletes and, stunningly, 91% occurred during training. Regarding medical illness, 14% reported having a severe illness, mostly respiratory in nature. Nearly, half reported that illness occurred due to their impairment [21].

During the 1988 Seoul Games, 82% of the Canadian team sought some type of medical care [22]. Healthcare providers will likely be approached with a plethora of complaints ranging from acute injury to non-musculoskeletal complaints during Para sport events. However, providers should be aware that Para athletes may also be less likely to seek medical care compared to athletes without disabilities. This may be due to multiple factors. Some Para athletes experience different thresholds for symptom severity to seek medical evaluation. Others are unsure that a new medical provider will be both familiar with how to evaluate their sport-related injury and demonstrate an understanding of how their underlying medical condition(s) and impairment(s) impact them in sports [23, 24].

Fagher et al. also found that Para athletes commonly reported feeling upset or anxious when unable to train and continued to train even while injured [21]. This observation couples previous findings that Para athletes may have higher levels of resilience, and more commitment to mastery than athletes without disabilities, and consider their participation in sports as strongly linked to their self-identity [25–27].

The healthcare team caring for the Para athlete must pay mindful attention to an athlete's complete well-being. This includes continued preventative injury measures during non-competitive periods, surveillance of acute and chronic injuries during training, identification of illness, and assessment of behavioral and psychological wellness. Providers should also educate Para athletes about the signs of injury and illness and ensure they are aware of available healthcare resources.

3.5 Condition Specific Considerations

Any athlete in any sport may have a condition that predisposes them to illness or injury. Para athletes are no exception. Each IPC defined Eligible Impairment encompasses a variety of conditions that a physician must account for in providing care to an athlete. Every condition comes with a unique set of considerations that impact an athlete's physiology, biomechanics, or equipment used for their sport.

3.5.1 Impaired Muscle Power

3.5.1.1 Spinal Cord Injury

Spinal Cord Injury (SCI) is a traumatic injury that can lead to deficits in motor strength, coordination, and sensation. Within the United States, nearly 300,000 people have an SCI [28]. Maintaining exercise and physical activity have been associated with improved quality of life [29]. The benefits of Para sports for athletes with SCI are numerous; however, the condition often requires the use of a wheelchair during competition and, depending on the location of the injury, can affect an athlete's autonomic functioning. Physicians must integrate multiple domains of knowledge into their care of an athlete with SCI.

Autonomic Dysreflexia

Autonomic dysreflexia (AD) is an important condition that may affect athletes with SCI during competition. AD is found in individuals with a complete SCI at or above the level of T6 and is marked by uncontrolled sympathetic output following a noxious stimulus occurring below the level of the injury. The most common causes of

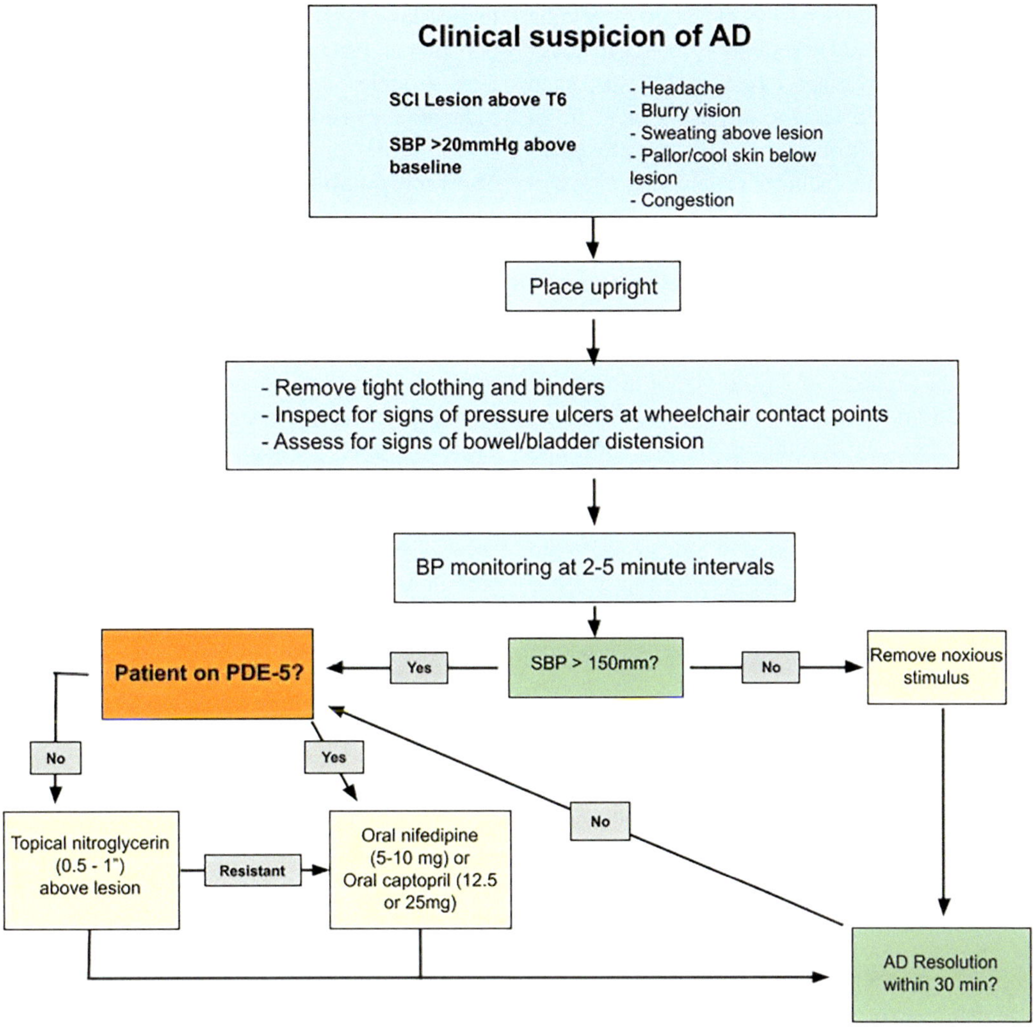

Fig. 3.1 Algorithm for treatment of autonomic dysreflexia

AD include urinary retention, constipation, and infection, but there are many other precipitating causes of AD. Figure 3.1 presents an algorithm for the treatment of autonomic dysreflexia.

The pathophysiology is rooted in both sympathetic and parasympathetic responses. AD begins with widespread splanchnic vasoconstriction that is uninhibited by descending cortical inhibition. Resultant hypertension causes vagal and aortic baroreceptors to trigger a reduction in heart rate and peripheral vasodilation. AD symptoms include hypertension >20 mmHg above baseline, headache, blurred vision, nasal congestion, flushing and sweating above the level of their SCI, and pallor and cool skin below the lesion. Since SCI often results in lower baseline systolic pressures from 90–110 mmHg, one must be suspicious of AD even when blood pressure may appear near normal [30].

AD can be a life-threatening situation, and mortality rates have been reported at 22% [30], so quick identification of the situation is crucial. Unmitigated hypertension can lead to stroke, hemorrhage, and death. An algorithm for treatment is outlined in Fig. 3.1 and described here.

The first step in management is to place the athlete in an upright position to take advantage of an orthostatic drop in blood pressure. Blood pressure measurements should be taken at short intervals, 2–5 min, and persistent elevation of systolic pressure > 150 mmHg should be noted. Next, ask the patient if they suspect a cause. If no suspected cause, perform a head-to-toe assessment in an attempt to identify and remove the causative noxious stimuli. This includes prophylactic loosening of clothing, straps, or anything causing restriction, inspecting the athlete and their wheelchair for any possible points of excess pressure or pressure sores, assessment of bowel and bladder distension, and a thorough physical exam inspecting for the presence of any source of discomfort such as in-grown toe nails [31].

If no noxious stimuli can be identified and blood pressures remain elevated >150 mmHg, pharmacologic intervention with nitroglycerin paste is warranted. Around 0.5–1 in. of paste should be applied above the level of injury. Prior to the use of any nitrate medication, a practitioner should determine if the athlete is actively taking PDE-5 inhibitors, such as sildenafil, due to the risk of precipitating severe hypotension. Some athletes may be taking these medications for erectile dysfunction secondary to their neurological impairment. In the absence of topical nitroglycerin, other fast-acting antihypertensives like nifedipine (5–10 mg) or captopril (12.5 mg, 25 mg) may be used [31]. Referral to a higher level of care needs to occur if resolution of blood pressure does not occur or the source of dysreflexia requires a higher level of care to be controlled (i.e., fractures and obstetric complications) [30].

Unfortunately, some athletes self-induce a state of AD to harness the sympathetic surge for increased performance. This is a non-substance form of doping known as "boosting." However, given the potential for harm, this is a serious issue. A survey of athletes with SCI found that 16.7% reported using boosting to enhance performance, yet less than half indicated that the act was dangerous [32]. Athletes who utilize boosting may do so by capping urinary catheters, intentionally breaking insensate toes, overtightening leg straps, twisting or sitting on the scrotum, or the usage of abdominal binders [32, 33]. Physicians and other healthcare personnel at Para sport events need to be aware of this practice and monitor athletes for any signs of boosting and resultant AD. Education on the dangers of boosting and AD should also be provided to athletes, as athlete education has proven effective in reducing the incidence of boosting [34].

Thermoregulation

The disruption of autonomic function and temperature sensation secondary to SCI can impact an athlete's ability to regulate their core body temperature. Lesions in the spinal cord can create a disconnection between afferent sensory information from the periphery and core and efferent thermoregulatory signals from the hypothalamus. Typical physiologic responses like sweating and vasodilation in response to heat or shivering and vasoconstriction in the cold are blunted in an athlete with SCI. For the Para athlete who may compete in either hot or cold environments, a shift from the normal homeostatic response needs to be considered in preventing injury and responding to illness during competition and training [35].

The degree of thermic dysregulation in those with SCI correlates with the level of spinal injury. Generally, a higher lesion is correlated with poorer temperature regulation. Higher lesions are associated with dysfunction of a greater surface area for heat dissipation and reduced muscle mass that can offer insulation and a source of metabolic warmth. It is suggested that injuries above T6 result in the greatest degree of impaired thermoregulation, secondary to the lack of sympathetic outflow on the effector side to control vasoconstriction or dilation, as well as the large surface area below the level of injury that has lost sensation and shivering ability [35, 36].

While exercising and participating in sports, it is useful to consider both the environment and level of SCI in anticipating an athlete's response. In cold conditions, it has been found that those with tetraplegia have a continual rise in core temperature whereas those without injury had a plateau in this rise. The higher level of lesion reduces the effect of heat dissipation during exercise and leads to retention [35]. Although this may be offset by convective cooling during wheelchair sports, one must be mindful that these athletes may experience a paradoxical rise in core temperature during training and competition.

Grossman et al. found through systematic review that exercise in temperate conditions, for instance, 15–25 °C (59–77 °F), resulted in increased core temperatures for participants with tetraplegia compared to those without injury but not in participants with paraplegia. In hotter conditions (>25 °C or 77 °F), the lowest levels of SCI did not differ from participants without injury, but higher-level paraplegia and tetraplegia were associated with comparatively higher core temperatures [37].

During training and competition, a provider should be aware that an athlete with SCI may retain excessive heat. Additionally, one must also assess the usage of anticholinergic medications for neurogenic bladder, which may increase susceptibility to heat-associated illness. Preventative measures, such as adequate hydration, providing access to shade, pre-competition acclimation, pre-competition cooling vests, water spray, active temperature monitoring, and other cooling measures, can help mitigate the risks of abnormal thermoregulation [38]. Due to the risk of heat exhaustion and the more severe heat stroke, physicians should monitor these athletes, especially those with higher level SCI, closely.

Heat stroke (HS) is marked by altered mental status, which is not present in heat exhaustion. Treatment of these conditions in Para athletes is similar to treatment in athletes without impairment. For athletes with SCI, care should be taken to avoid inducing autonomic dysreflexia when taking rectal temperatures by using a lidocaine lubricant. Diagnostic criteria of HS include altered mental status and core temperature $\geq$ 40 °C (104 °F). However, if HS is suspected and only a change in mental status is noted, providers may proceed with HS treatment algorithms while further workup occurs [39, 40].

The goal of any HS treatment is to lower core body temperature to 37.5–38 °C (99.5–100.4 °F) as fast as possible to reduce the risk of morbidity and mortality. Assessment of airway, breathing, and circulation is the initial step upon identification of HS. Aggressive cooling with ice–water immersion and such baths should be made available at Para sport events. Any athlete and impairment-specific equipment should be removed to ensure the maximal surface area for cooling and preservation of equipment. This includes prostheses for athletes with limb deficiencies. In the absence of an ice–water bath, or in situations where it cannot be used, ice–water dousing or layered ice–water towels can be implemented. Rectal temperatures should be consistently monitored for reduction to target and improvement of mental status achieved, with the goal of resolution of temperature within 30 min. Following resolution, athletes should be monitored for signs of hypothermia, hyponatremia, and hypoglycemia [39, 40].

Orthostatic Hypotension

Alterations to the autonomic function of athletes with SCI contribute to a higher rate of orthostatic hypotension in this community. The prevalence of this condition has been reported at 74%. However, it has been found that only 60% of those with SCI and orthostatic hypotension report symptoms. This may be due to concomitant adaptation in cerebral blood flow, which maintains cerebral oxygenation at low systemic pressures [41].

Regardless of their adaptations, athletes with SCI are more likely to experience the symptoms of orthostatic hypotension. Physicians should consider orthostatic hypotension as the etiology in an athlete reporting fatigue, light-headedness, dizziness, or syncope. Prevention is a key first step and can be accomplished through adequate hydration, salt intake, and the use of compressive stockings to encourage venous return. Should an athlete begin feeling presyncopal, assuming a recumbent or semi-recumbent position, if possible, may improve cerebral perfusion [41].

Other Conditions

Medical providers should also be aware that athletes with SCI may be at increased risk of fracture due to decreased bone mineral density. Fractures may occur in areas where the athlete is insensate, so athletes may not note a mechanism of injury or report pain at the site of injury. If swelling in an extremity becomes apparent, the provider should evaluate for fracture but also consider a broad differential diagnosis including heterotopic ossification and deep venous thrombosis. Athletes with SCI also may have spasticity on their baseline exam. Any changes in spasticity, not otherwise attributable to medication, may be due to an insidious etiology. This includes fracture, infection, or any other noxious stimuli. Appropriate treatment can be aimed at the identified cause [42].

3.5.1.2 Spina Bifida

Athletes with spina bifida, a congenital condition affecting the development of the neural tube, often participate in similar sports as athletes with SCI. Spina bifida may share similar clinical presentations to SCI, such as impaired muscle power, bowel/bladder dysfunction, and risk for pressure ulcers, and spina bifida also has unique considerations. Athletes with spina bifida are at an increased risk of latex allergy. It is important to be cautious of signs and symptoms of allergic reactions, and anaphylaxis must always be considered. While gloves are generally thought of as the most common latex-containing medical item, latex may also be present in other items in the Para sport environment like catheters, adhesive bandages, and rubber used in balls and older track construction. Unlike athletes with SCI who otherwise do not have any other medical conditions, athletes with spina bifida also may have Chiari malformations, hydrocephalus with or without a shunt, and/or neurocognitive impairment. These should all be taken into consideration when evaluating athletes with spina bifida [43].

3.5.2 Impaired Passive Range of Movement

Impaired Passive Range of Movement is an Eligible Impairment applicable to athletes who have permanent or chronic limited joint mobility. Common conditions include arthrogryposis (congenital joint contracture affecting multiple joints), severe scoliosis and kyphosis, and contracture from chronic immobilization or trauma. Chronic immobilization may be due to neurologic conditions, such as cerebral palsy, SCI, spina bifida, and others. Many conditions, such as arthritis, arthroplasty, joint hypermobility, and joint instability, limit the range of motion but are not Paralympic Eligible Impairments [9].

Impairments within this grouping can alter the biomechanics of a Para athlete compared to other athletes in their sport. For instance, Eriksson et al. found that children with arthrogryposis affecting the lower extremities relied heavily on hip musculature for gait propulsion [44]. In scoliosis, increased lateral pelvic tilt can cause an asymmetric distribution of force during competition [45]. It is important for a supervising physician to consider the athlete's entire kinetic chain, which includes affected joints and structures to anticipate where extra stress may occur during sport.

3.5.3 Limb Deficiency

Athletes competing under this Eligible Impairment will have a partial or total absence of bone or joint—whether due to trauma, congenital deficiency, or illness [9]. They utilize a variety of different prostheses, which have specific purposes for their sports. However, not all athletes with limb deficiency may use a prosthesis. Some sports do not require their usage, like alpine skiing where one may use only one ski. Other sports preclude their use, and Para swimming also does not allow the use of orthoses or prostheses in competition. Amputee soccer is competed specifically without a lower limb prosthetic device, and instead, athletes use bilateral forearm crutches [46].

The stump–socket interface and type of suspension supporting the socket are important to consider for the athlete with limb deficiency. Socket pressures vary through different knee motions in a transtibial prosthetic and differ between individuals [46, 47]. This highlights the need for proper socket fitting among these athletes. Gel liners are often used to line the socket and reduce shearing forces between the limb and the prosthesis [48]. The recommended type of socket, suspension, terminal prosthetic device, and prosthetic features will vary depending on the athlete's needs and differences in biomechanics among different sports.

Perspiration and fluctuations in limb volume can compromise an aptly fit socket and lead to changes in shearing forces. This can create altered force distribution, aggravation of existing neuromas, subsequent pain, and impaired weight bearing. Additionally, increased shearing force predisposes athletes with limb deficiency to higher rates of skin and soft tissue damage, including ulcers, dermatitis, verrucous hyperplasia, and infection [42]. Regular evaluation of socket fit and removal of prosthesis to inspect for soft tissue damage is recommended to prevent and treat injury early. If present, treatment for hyperhidrosis can be considered. This can begin conservatively with the application of topical anti-perspirants.

The absence of all or a portion of the upper limb may place asymmetric stress on the contralateral side, including the truncal muscles [49]. This may increase the risk of overuse injuries in the unaffected limb due to muscle strength imbalance. For swimmers with upper limb deficiency, an adapted paddle can be implemented during training to provide resistance on the affected side and promote hypertrophy of musculature [50]. In the event of an overuse or chronic injury, treatment plans for Para athletes should be customized to each athlete's unique needs, taking into consideration the athlete's underlying medical condition(s) and impairments. Each may have contributed to overuse or chronic injury, may increase the risk of re-injury, and may impact a treatment plan.

3.5.4 Leg Length Difference

The Minimum Impairment Criteria (MIC) for an athlete to classify under the Impairment of Leg Length Difference (LLD) varies by each Para sport. World Para Athletics defines the MIC for LLD as 7 cm [12], whereas World Para Swimming establishes that the athlete must have at least 20 cm of LLD to meet MIC [51]. Further epidemiologic studies need to be performed to delineate patterns of injury in this population during training and competition. However, it has been established that severe LLD can alter gait mechanics. In LLDs greater than 1 cm, the shorter limb has been found to experience higher peak loads during walking [52]. Although the effect of LLD on injury in athletics is not well understood, it has been suggested that chronic knee pain is more prevalent in those with LLD [53].

3.5.5 Short Stature

Osteogenesis imperfecta and achondroplasia are two common conditions seen in this category in Para sports. Due to defects in type I collagen, athletes with osteogenesis imperfecta are susceptible to fracture [54]. The sideline healthcare team should have a low threshold to suspect fracture in the case of trauma or acute onset pain during competition. Athletes with osteogenesis imperfecta may have a higher pain threshold and an atypical clinical presentation for fracture. Plain radiographs, if available at the event, can be obtained as a part of the initial work, and further CT is appropriate if suspicion remains high after a negative x ray.

Athletes with achondroplasia may be at increased risk of spinal cord injury (SCI). Due to an increased rate of multilevel cervical spine stenosis, hyperflexion and hyperextension mechanisms can lead to compression or direct injury of the spine [55]. While these athletes may have an increased hypothetical risk, any athlete during competition who has an injury worrisome for spinal cord injury needs to have an urgent, full, and thorough workup.

3.5.6 Hypertonia, Ataxia, and Athetosis

Hypertonia, ataxia, and athetosis are three Eligible Impairment categories that encompass overlapping medical conditions. This includes neurologic conditions, such as cerebral palsy, traumatic brain injury, or stroke. Often those with neurologic impairment will display some combination of these impairments. For instance, athetosis is infrequently noted in isolation but is seen in conjunction with hypertonia in cerebral palsy.

Multiple sclerosis is known to frequently present with both hypertonia and ataxia.

Hypertonia is a condition marked by spasticity, dystonia, and/or rigidity, which is the result of upper motor neuron damage. It leads to muscle tightness and can limit joint mobility [56]. Ataxia, secondary to central nervous system pathology such as cerebellar injury, leads to impaired balance and coordination [57]. Athetosis, a movement disorder characterized by slow involuntary writhing movements, may be secondary to stroke, traumatic brain injury, or cerebral palsy [58].

3.5.6.1 Cerebral Palsy

Assessing risks in athletes with cerebral palsy (CP) is dependent upon their mobility status, which will be determined by the number and severity of limb involvement. Half of athletes with CP use a wheelchair during sports [59]. These individuals are subject to the same risk of upper extremity injury and skin ulceration as athletes with SCI as we have discussed previously in this chapter. Prevention and monitoring strategies should be used to prevent the formation or progression of any pressure sores.

The knee is the most commonly injured body part for the ambulant athlete with CP [60]. Abnormal muscle tone across and around the joint alters the distribution of force throughout motion and can impair gait mechanics [61, 62]. This may also impair patellar motion and contribute to the high rates of patellofemoral pain syndrome in athletes with CP. Fatigue may exacerbate underlying gait or movement abnormalities in these athletes, so their healthcare team should have a clear understanding of their baseline function. This will help assess an athlete's risk of acute strains and sprains as well as chronic overuse [63].

Athletes with CP or other conditions that cause abnormal increases in muscle tone may have an existing treatment plan that combines a mixture of pharmacologic and non-pharmacologic treatments, with the latter possibly including interventional procedures. Other non-pharmacologic treatment modalities include stretching, serial casting, or bracing. Pharmacologic treatments for increased muscle tone include, but are not limited to, oral muscle relaxants like tizanidine or baclofen, and benzodiazepines. Interventional procedures for increased muscle tone include chemodenervation (e.g., botulinum toxin injections, phenol or alcohol neurolysis), intrathecal baclofen pump implantation and infusion, or surgical interventions such as tendon lengthening or transfer procedures [64].

Providers should be aware of what athletes' current treatment plans include and any recent procedures. It is important to be familiar with an athlete's baseline physical exam and muscle tone, which may be positionally dependent. If significant changes in tone are observed when evaluating an athlete, the provider should first consider recent changes in medications, procedures, injury, infection, illness, acute pain, noxious stimuli, environmental changes in weather, or other stressors. Addressing any underlying aggravating factor can often return an athlete to baseline muscle tone. In cases where changes in muscle tone are severe or limiting, a provider may adjust medication doses as necessary. This can help mitigate the risk of complications like rhabdomyolysis, which may occur if muscle tone remains increased for long periods of time. Changes in medications for abnormal muscle tone also may need to be titrated gradually depending on the medication. For instance, immediate discontinuation or sudden decreases in baclofen dosing may trigger withdrawal symptoms. Sideline providers should also be aware of this risk as some athletes self-limit the use of muscle relaxants to avoid competition limiting side effects, like fatigue. Identification of baclofen withdrawal may be difficult because it does not have any specific findings. Symptoms may include irritability, pruritis, nausea, vomiting, hyperthermia, hallucinations, headache, autonomic dysfunction, hypertonia that is increased from baseline, and rhabdomyolysis [65]. If withdrawal of baclofen or other medications is suspected, the athlete should be transported urgently to the nearest emergency department for further evaluation and management.

Epilepsy has been reported as a comorbidity in upwards of 49% of children with CP [66]. The use of antiepileptic medication (AED) is common among athletes with CP. While this reduces the risk of a seizure during training and competition, it does not eliminate it and physicians should be aware of the association. AEDs can detrimentally impact bone mineral density (BMD) [67]. People with CP are already at increased risk of osteopenia, and physicians should assess athletes' bone density prior to participation [42, 68].

Some athletes with CP may also have impaired cognition or communication, with up to 90% of children with CP experiencing dysarthria and subsequent motor speech impairment [69]. Communication impairments range from mild dysarthria to being non-verbal, with some using assistive technology to improve communication. The prevalence of intellectual impairment in athletes with CP is also associated with poorer communication [70]. This can limit an athlete's ability to communicate symptoms during competition or recognize signs of injury or illness, which are especially important when considering their risk of heat strain. Although they do not have the same autonomic impairment as athletes with SCI, athletes with CP produce greater amounts of metabolic heat during exercise and may be more susceptible to heat stroke and exhaustion [38].

3.5.7 Vision Impairment

Several Para sports are exclusive to athletes with Visual Impairment (VI) like football 5-a-side and goalball. The rate of injury is high for these athletes, perhaps due to the high energy nature of these sports and the deleterious effect of visual impairment on proprioception. Notable differences in injury distribution are noted for those with VI. There is a higher incidence of lower extremity injury, rather than upper, among these athletes [15, 71]. While care of these athletes is like athletes without impairment, it should be noted that ensuring the athlete is familiar with the event space may help reduce the risk of injury. Providers can offer thorough verbal descriptions and physically guide them through activity areas, such as through the long jump runway [72].

3.5.8 Intellectual Impairment

Persons with intellectual impairment have many outlets to meaningfully engage in sports—including the Special Olympics, the Paralympics, and Para sports as a whole. Athletes who opt to participate in the Olympics define excellence in their sports by personal achievement [73]. Regardless of the event these athletes compete in, their care should reflect the athlete and not the level of competition. Considerations for the care of these athletes include accounting for the number of significant comorbidities that exist in this population.

Like athletes with cerebral palsy, athletes with intellectual impairment are more likely to have seizure disorders compared to the general population. Approximately 26% are affected. The usage of antiepileptic medications may predispose to osteopenia. Athletes with underlying seizure disorders should be closely monitored for evidence or history of uncontrolled seizures, leading into periods of training and competition. The usage of antipsychotic medications is also prevalent in those with intellectual impairment and may lead to QT prolongation and disturbances in thermoregulation. Appropriate cardiac assessment should be considered for these athletes and mindful attention paid to the elevated risk of heat-associated illnesses [43].

Athletes who have Down syndrome may be more likely than other athletes to have atlantoaxial instability (range 10–40%) and may be predisposed to cervical spine subluxation. Current evidence and expert guidelines do not recommend the use of cervical spine radiography to screen atlantoaxial instability in individuals with Down syndrome who are asymptomatic. Physical exam should include a thorough evaluation for signs of potential atlantoaxial instability, such as neck pain, radiculopathy, muscle weakness, abnormally increased muscle tone, hyperreflexia, gait changes, or alterations in bowel and bladder function. If any of these signs are present, plain cervical spine radiography in the neutral position is recommended, as well as subsequent referral to a pediatric neurosurgeon or orthopedic surgeon if radiographs demonstrate abnormalities. If neutral radiographs are normal, flexion and extension radiographs may be obtained in collaboration with a subspecialist prior to referral [74]. Sports that involve high levels of neck flexion and extension or otherwise create a risk for neck injury should be avoided in those with known atlantoaxial instability [75]. Among other conditions, athletes with Down syndrome may be at increased risk of congenital heart disease, patellar instability, hip dislocation, and visual or hearing impairments—each of which should be accounted for in preparticipation physicals, competition, or assessment of medication use [59].

3.6 Concussion and Para Sport

In studying the epidemiology of injury at the 2016 Rio Summer Games, Derman et al. attempted to quantify the incidence of concussion for the first time at a Paralympic Games, but no cases were reported. In the discussion, the authors acknowledge that there were several instances of possible concussions that likely would have been reported as concussions given proper clinician education and training. The first death during a Games occurred during the study's time frame and was due to a head injury [15]. This catastrophic event emphasizes the need for continued study of the incidence of injury and education of clinicians and athletes on proper prevention and identification of concussions.

A 2021 study by Lexell et al. prospectively assessed the incidence of concussion in elite Para athletes over a 1-year period. They reported a rate of 0.5 concussions per 1000 athlete hours, 62% occurred in athletes with visual impairment, and 85% of concussions occurred due to a collision with an object or person. The overall incidence of concussion was comparable to athletes without impairment [76].

In 2022, the Concussion in Para Sport (CIPS) Group published its first position statement on concussion in Para sports. They cite a lack of research and direction provided by the Concussion in Sport (CIS) group pertaining to concussions in the Para athlete. CIPS recommends that the first consideration for a clinician is to establish a clear baseline of cognitive function and physical ability. During assessment, a clinician should use this baseline as a point of comparison in conjunction with history taken from the athlete's family and team. CIPS recommends using the Sports Concussion Assessment Tool 5 (SCAT5) as a part of athlete assessment, modified to account for the athlete's impairment, despite its known variability.

After an initial assessment, CIPS recommends following the "remove, rest, reconsider, and refer" framework for immediate management. CIPS does not believe that the Concussion In Sport Group's 2017 guidelines for return to sport (RTS) adequately address Para athletes and that their RTS timeline should be determined on an athlete-by-athlete basis [20].

3.7 Wheelchairs in Para Sport

Wheelchairs are in important piece of equipment for a large portion of Para athletes and are used in most Para sports. Athletes with SCI comprise a large proportion of wheelchair users in Para sports, but athletes also include those with cerebral palsy, limb deficiencies, and muscular dystrophy. Even athletes who primarily ambulate outside of competition may still participate in wheelchair sports depending on their functional level. Some sports are exclusively competed in by wheelchair athletes, such as wheelchair basketball or rugby. Sideline providers should become well educated about the basics of wheelchairs, their use in sports, the biomechanics of use, and the increased risk of certain injuries from their use.

Wheelchairs used in Para sports are not the same wheelchairs athletes use in their daily lives. As sporting equipment, they are designed to meet the requirements of their specific sport. For instance, in wheelchair rugby and basketball, the chair has been developed to be stable, fast, and able to withstand contact. The equipment must also meet the needs of the athlete to provide enough support while optimizing athletic and mobility. The chair should be well-fit and become an extension of the athlete's body, with the user and chair acting as a single unit. A properly fit chair will also reduce the risk of pressure sores and shearing injuries [77]. Clinicians should be aware of this and monitor athletes for injury to the skin, especially of the sacrum and ischium, and advise frequent weight shifting. Treatment of sores is relative to the severity and can range from bioocclusive dressings for less severe presentations to debridement for full-thickness sores [78].

Athlete propulsion of the wheelchair during their sport is a dynamic biomechanical action. It can be considered as having two phases: a push phase followed by a recovery phase. During the push phase, an athlete is creating force to propel their equipment. When moving forward, the push phase is largely made up of shoulder flexion with external rotation and arm extension. Shoulder flexion is achieved by the anterior deltoid and pectoralis major; constant external rotation is done by the supraspinatus and infraspinatus; extension of the arm is achieved by the biceps brachii; and scapulothoracic stability is maintained by the serratus anterior. The recovery phase finds an athlete returning the arm for the next cycle. Athletes engage the triceps to flex the arm and initiate shoulder elevation and extension while the supraspinatus and middle/posterior deltoid elevate the shoulder. The trapezius helps retract the scapula for proper return [79].

Much of the shoulder girdle is engaged during the proper wheelchair propulsion technique. This helps explain the shoulder-predominant injury patterns observed in the aforementioned epidemiological studies of Para sport. Prepared providers should become well versed in the upper extremity physical exam to best isolate sites of soft tissue injury due to acute trauma or chronic overuse. Table 3.3 provides an overview of special exam maneuvers and evaluated muscle(s) or structure(s) [80].

Many athletes also use a wheelchair outside of competition and experience increased daily demand for the upper extremity, especially the shoulder. These athletes are at the highest risk of sustaining overuse and acute upper extremity injuries [81]. Muscular strength imbalance may be a factor contributing to rotator cuff impingement syndromes in wheelchair athletes [82]. Repetitive motions of wheelchair use may contribute to an increased rate of nerve compression injuries in wheelchair athletes. Median and ulnar nerve entrapment are notable among athletes in wheelchair basketball [83].

Soft tissue injuries, including strains and sprains, are the most commonly reported in wheelchair athletes [84]. Prevention strategies aimed at strengthening and stretching the shoulder have been found to improve the range of motion and pain in wheelchair athletes [85]. Since these athletes must use the upper extremities for activities of daily living, rest can be difficult. Thus, acute management should be aimed at reducing inflammation and pain with nonsteroidal anti-inflammatories and ice. Later management may include physical therapy or corticosteroid injections when applicable [78]. Long-term management to preserve the health of the shoulder also includes evaluating the athlete's home to minimize unnecessary overhead shoulder movements that can lead to impingement. Consideration of power wheelchair use outside of sport may decrease the long-term load on the shoulder and improve the longevity of shoulder health.

Table 3.3 Comprehensive shoulder exam to assess shoulder pathologies in paralympic athletes

Test	Muscle(S) or structures tested	Maneuver	Positive if
Empty can	Supraspinatus	Arm at 90° of abduction in full internal rotation (thumb down). Patient resists downward motion	Weakness or pain
External rotation	Infraspinatus, Teres minor	Elbow in 90° of flexion, patient externall rotates against resistance	Weakness or pain
Lift off	Subscapularis	With back of hand placed of back, provider lifts hand away from back	Patient not able to maintain hand in lifted position
Belly press	Subscapularis	Patient hand on stomach with elbow forward. Resists external rotation	Weakness or pain
Apprehension test	Anterior inferior labrum (Bankart Lesion)	Patient supine, shoulder at 90° of abduction and externally rotated with elbow at 90° of flexion. Provider slowly and passively externally rotates the arm	Apprehension or pain
Jobe's relocation test	Anterior inferior labrum (Bankart Lesion)	Same as Apprehension Test, but with provider applied posterior force preventing anterior subluxation	Reduced apprehension or pain compared to Apprehension Test, confirmatory
Posterior drawer	Posterior labrum (Reverse Bankart Lesion)	Provider stabilizes scapula while translating head of humerus posteriorly.	High degree of subluxation compared to contralateral side
O'Brien	Superior Labrum Anterior to Posterior (SLAP Tear)	Shoulder at 90° flexion, 20-30° abduction, maximal internal rotation (thumb down). Patient elevates against resistance. Repeated with neutral rotation (thumb up).	Pain when thumb is down but no pain when thumb is up.
Speed's	Biceps (tendinitis)	Elbow slightly flexed, forearm supinated. Patient elevates against resistance	Pain at bicipital groove
Yeargason's	Biceps (tendinitis)	Arm at side, elbow in 90° flexion, forearm pronated. Patient supinates against resistance	Pain at bicipital groove
Neer's	Supraspinatus or biceps (impingement)	Provider stabilizes shoulder while passively flexing the arm	Apprehension or pain
Hawkins-Kennedy	Supraspinatus (impingement)	Shoulder and elbow at 90° flexion with forearm in front of patient. Provider passively internally rotates arm	Apprehension or pain
Scapular winging	Serratus anterior	Patient pushes against wall	Winging of scapula
Cross-body adduction	Acromioclavicular Joint	Beginning with shoulder in 90° elevation, provider passively adducts	Pain

3.8 Sport Specific Considerations

Sideline practitioners at any event, Para sport included, should expect to care for a wide array of injuries including fractures, sprains, strains, cuts, lacerations, and rashes among others. Although the Para athlete provider may tend to a different distribution of acute injuries, as discussed earlier, they will be treating much of the same pathologies seen in non-Para sports. General guidelines for the care of many of these injuries can be found in later portions of this book.

Much of the preceding information was intended to provide the reader insight into the condition-specific considerations they may make when caring for a Para athlete during competition, the following is intended to give an overview of unique characteristics specific to important Para sports. These are considerations that providers may not be familiar with from prior experience at non-Para events and would not be addressed elsewhere in this textbook.

3.8.1 Summer Sports

3.8.1.1 Archery

Shooting sports like Archery have been an important part of the Para sport landscape, dating back to the first exhibition by Dr. Ludwig Guttman. These events are participated by a wide range of classifications using specialized equipment and adaptive devices, which can be sources of injury. Although the risk of injury during shooting events is low, they are considered generally safe sports [86].

Archery athletes compete in wheelchairs or from a standing position and have a wide range of upper extremity impairment (Fig. 3.2). Standing athletes may use a chair or stool for support while participating. Some athletes have full ability to use their bow, while some may require adaptive equipment to hold the bow or draw and release the bowstring. This includes release aids, tabs used to draw the arrow with the mouth, or devices to stabilize the arm used to hold the bow steady. Despite these devices, the sport predominated by overuse type injury of the arm used to draw the bow, mostly of soft tissue structures. While rare, acute injuries may occur and are associated with equipment failure—breakage of the bow, string, or arrow during a shot [86]. Some acute injuries occurred when the bowstring struck the non-drawing arm. Niestroj et al. found that all acute injuries during an event were low-grade [87]. Sideline physicians may expect to care for lacerations, blisters, sprains, and strains.

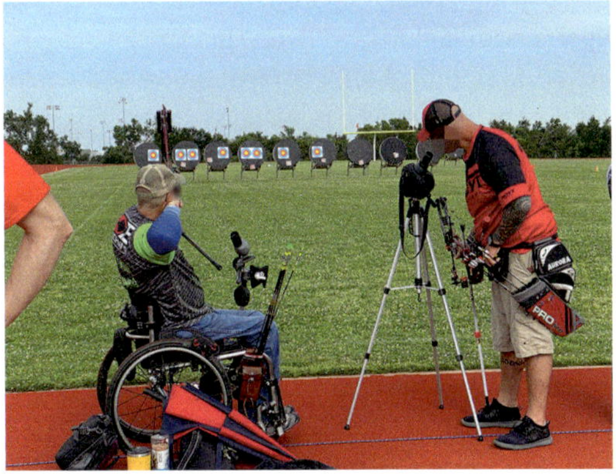

Fig. 3.2 Para Archery athlete

3.8.1.2 Athletics (Track and Field)

Athletics encompass sport activities, such as running, throwing, and jumping, spread over several different competitions. The vast classification scheme of Para sports means that the healthcare team covering Para Athletic events will encounter a swath of impairments and injuries. Epidemiological studies at the 2012 London Paralympic Games found that injury incidence was highest in ambulant track athletes with visual impairment and those with amputation. They also observed that athletes using a wheelchair experienced higher rates of injury during throwing events compared to track events [88].

Athletes competing in wheelchair running events utilize propulsion techniques that rely on the pectoralis, deltoid, triceps, flexor carpi radialis, and rotator cuff muscles. These muscles are likely prone to overuse injuries. However, a lower seat position and wheels positioned toward the back of the chair can reduce the amount of work done by the triceps, deltoid, and pectoralis. A low seat position and wheels toward the middle of the chair will reduce the number of strokes [89]. The repetitive nature of propulsion places the skin of the hands, arm, and axilla at risk of skin breakdown or wounds due to contact with the chair. Consistent skin checks during competition can identify wounds early before progression.

Upper extremity injuries compose a majority of injuries seen in field (throwing) events for athletes using a wheelchair (Fig. 3.3a, b). They compete in their throwing events in a framed chair affixed to the throwing platform. The inability to recruit the lower body into the kinetic chain used to propel an object may contribute to higher rates of upper extremity injury observed in wheelchair field athletes [90]. The biomechanics of overhead throwers, both with and without impairment, place higher relative force on the elbow. Differential diagnoses for associated injuries

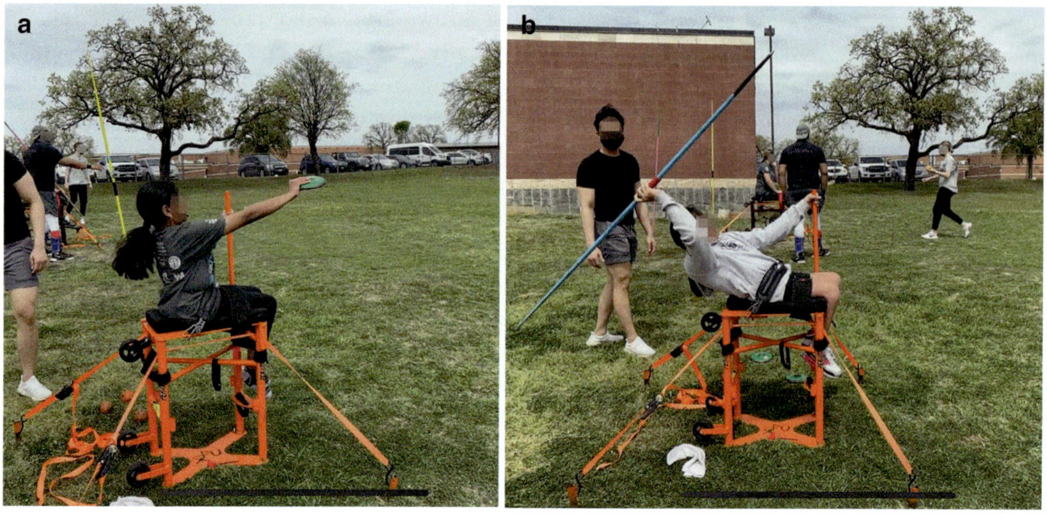

Fig. 3.3 Throwing sports in wheelchair athletes: Para discus (**a**) and Para Javelin (**b**)

should not differ between the groups and include tendon, ligament, nerve, muscle, and bone pathology. Kinematic analysis of javelin throwers revealed that the greatest angular speed occurred in the hand and may suggest a higher risk of hand injuries in throwing athletes [91].

Management of any resultant injury in the Para Athletics competitor can mirror athletes without impairment and will mostly consist of conservative management. Pre-competition warm up and stretching should be emphasized, especially in the upper extremity of throwing athletes. Since these events occur exclusively outdoors, the risk of heat-associated illness should be continually assessed at an event and athlete level. Appropriate risk mitigation includes the availability of adequate fresh water, cooling towels, misting fans, and ice-water immersion for cases of heat stroke.

3.8.1.3 Boccia

Boccia is a precision sport where athletes attempt to land a leather ball as close as possible to another reference ball (the "jack"). Athletes typically throw the ball, but those with more severe impairment use the assistance of a "pointer" attached to their mouth, head, or arm to push their ball down a ramp [92]. At the 2012 Paralympics in London, boccia had the highest rate of acute injury (91% of total boccia injury) [16]. However, it is generally considered a low-risk sport [93]. Recent research found that prolonged boccia matches lead to trapezius fatigue [94] and can result in a higher prevalence of overuse injuries. A biomechanical study by Tsai et al. revealed that boccia players stabilize themselves by increasing the anterior inclination of their wheelchair seat, but this produced more elbow movement [95]. For throwing boccia athletes, this may predispose them to pathology at this joint.

3.8.1.4 Cycling

Para and adaptive cycling make use of a wide variety of cycle designs to meet the demands of the athlete. Those with lower extremity impaired muscle power may use hand-powered cycles and those with visual impairment will ride tandem cycles with sighted cyclists. Handcycles may be set up to optimize athlete positioning and stroke efficiency but must be done on an athlete-specific basis [96]. Cycles, like wheelchairs, interface with the athlete in specific locations and predispose to injury at those locations. These are noted to be between the shoe and pedal, the pelvis and saddle, and the hands and handlebar. Neuropathies may occur at these locations including Morton's neuroma, perineal, and ulnar neuropathies.

Road cycling accidents are associated with lacerations, hematomas, fractures, and head injuries [97]. Para cyclists are subject to the same injuries. During the 2016 Rio Paralympic Games,

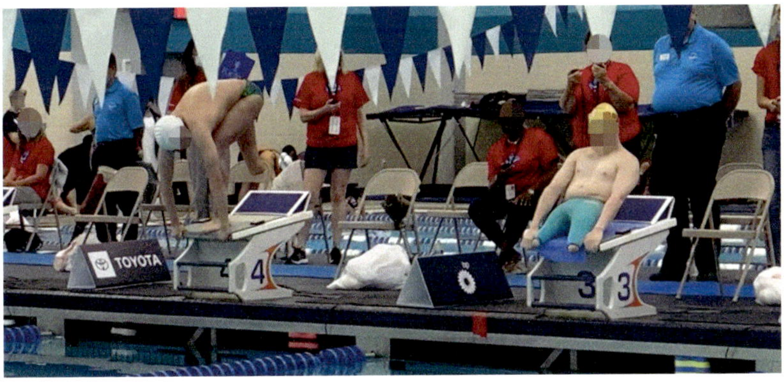

Fig. 3.4 Para swimming

a rider tragically died after experiencing a head injury during a crash in a competition [84]. The emerging importance of concussions and traumatic brain injury in Para sports will be discussed later in the chapter.

3.8.1.5 Swimming

Competition in Para swimming does not permit the use of prosthetics or orthotics (Fig.3.4). Athletes with visual impairment are allowed to have an individual serving as a "tapper" on each side of the pool to tap them with a pole on either their head or upper back to indicate the athlete is approaching the end of the pool. Despite this, athletes with visual impairment may still be prone to injury from jamming fingers into the lane line, bumping their limbs into the lane line or others, or even diving into the wrong lane where another athlete is swimming.

In an injury epidemiology and injury prevention study surveying Para swimmers of a wide spectrum of medical conditions and impairments on the US national team, the shoulder was the most common body part injured, which is similarly seen in swimmers without disabilities. Chronic injuries were more common than acute ones. This study also recognized the need for improvements in injury prevention programs for Para swimmers that are customized to each athlete's unique needs [24].

3.8.1.6 Wheelchair Basketball

Wheelchair Basketball is one of the most popular Para sports, particularly in the United States (Fig. 3.5). The organization of athletes into teams of 5 is unique. Rather than having separate classifications for athletes of varied functional levels, teams are composed of players with a spectrum of functional levels. Each athlete is placed into a category based on their "volume of action"—or ability to voluntarily move and stabilize in multiple planes. Each category has an associated numeric value between 1 and 4.5, and teams must be composed of athletes whose categories do not exceed 14 points [79]. For a sideline provider, this means that they must ensure they have an adequate history of individual athletes to help guide care, rather than relying on a

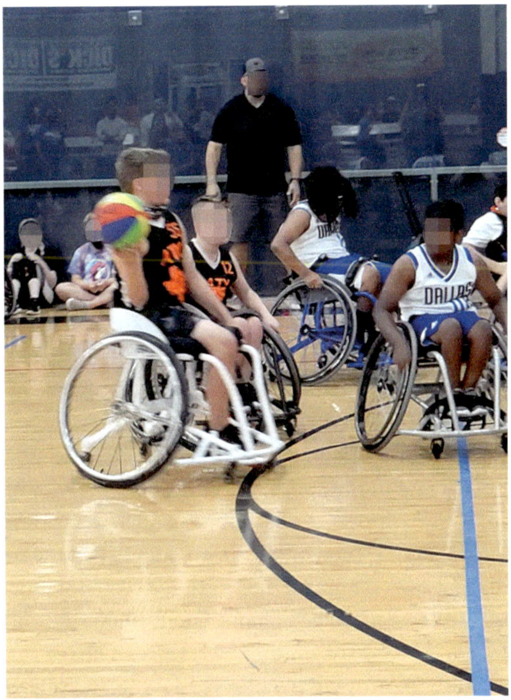

Fig. 3.5 Wheelchair basketball

classification system to clue them into the athlete medical condition(s).

Exclusively competed in wheelchairs, the same considerations discussed in sect. 3.6 apply to this sport. Wheelchair basketball athletes perform repetitive overhead activities in addition to propelling their equipment. This predisposes them to more overuse and impingement-type injuries, especially involving the rotator cuff, acromion, and glenohumeral joint. Physical exam may reveal positive Neer's or Hawkins–Kennedy Tests (see Table 3.3) and gross instability of the shoulder [79]. While these are typically chronic injuries and acute exacerbations are likely during competition, other pathologies like fracture and dislocation must always be included in the differential for these athletes.

3.8.1.7 Wheelchair Rugby

The documentary *Murderball* introduced much of the world to the Para sport of wheelchair rugby. This co-ed team sport requires athletes to have both upper and lower limb impairments and teams are composed of a mix of various impairment classifications. The competition requires a speciality wheelchair with highly cambered (angled) wheels that are fast and can withstand the contact of the sport [98, 99]. Many of the athletes have spinal cord injuries, whose considerations have previously been described. The high-energy nature of the sport and forceful contact between wheelchairs contribute to an increased risk of traumatic injury. Otherwise, overuse injuries will be observed with the highest frequency in the upper extremity, and the risks associated with wheelchair use apply to these athletes.

3.8.1.8 Wheelchair Tennis

Wheelchair tennis is gaining popularity among adaptive sports (Fig. 3.6). It does not require a sport-specific wheelchair, can be recreationally played amongst people with and without impairment, and has easy to follow rules—so the barrier to entry for a person to participate is low. As a competitive Para sport, athletes do not always have to use a wheelchair to qualify with Minimum Impairment Criteria. To qualify for classification, athletes, without a wheelchair, would be unable to run to the degree required for the sport's performance. This means that athletes will have a wide range of mobility disorders like traumatic brain injury, stroke, spinal cord injury (SCI), cerebral palsy (CP), limb deficiency, multiple sclerosis, spinal ataxia, and nerve injury [100].

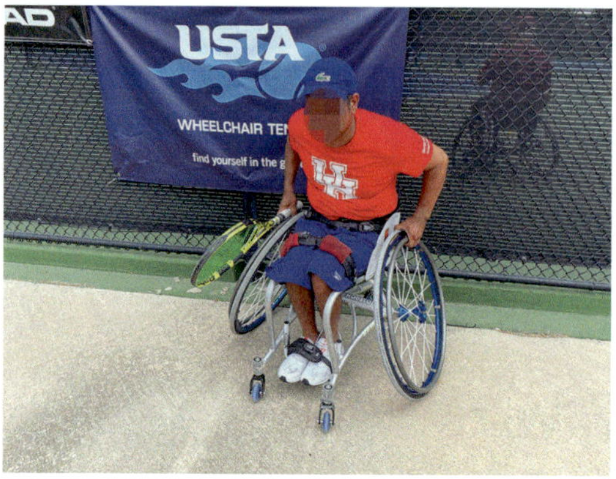

Fig. 3.6 Wheelchair Tennis

During a match, players are allowed two breaks, one between each set, for bathroom relief. Practitioners must encourage their athletes, especially those with SCI, to utilize this time so that they may reduce the risk of bladder and bowel distension, both of which may precipitate autonomic dysreflexia (AD). Additionally, the International Tennis Federation (ITF) has rules regarding how athletes can access care. At any time, should an athlete have an acute medical need, such as AD, they may be evaluated. Otherwise, they may request a medical evaluation at set breaks and are limited to 3 minutes of treatment unless it is reasonable to allot more time to medical personnel. However, providers may intervene at any time if they believe an athlete is having an acute event [101]. It is advised that any provider should be familiar with each competitor's medical conditions in order to identify risks the athlete cannot. For instance, since athletes with SCI may have impaired temperature sensation, a provider may be the first and most important line of defense against heat illness.

Wheelchair tennis follows similar injury incidence patterns as other wheelchair sports identified prior—increased rates of chronic injury to the upper extremity, most notably pathologies of the acromion and supraspinatus. However, it should be noted that they are not at increased risk of injury compared to athletes without impairment [100].

3.8.2 Winter Sports

As reviewed earlier, the rate of injury during winter sports is much higher than in summer sports. Generally speaking, many of the same considerations for various impairments that apply to summer sports also apply to winter sports. Similar patterns of injury have also been noted, like a predominance of upper extremity injury in athletes using seating systems for sports, such as sit skis.

Ambient temperature is an obvious difference between summer and winter sports, but one that calls for extra consideration in athletes with impairments who may have reduced temperature sensation and impaired thermoregulation. Many conditions can result in this functional impairment, but spinal cord injury (SCI) is the most representative of the risk. We previously discussed that athletes with high spinal injuries may retain heat while exercising in the cold. However, if improperly clothed, they will be at risk of complications from cold extremities. Reduced temperature sensation may delay athlete identification of warning signs of frostbite [102].

Winter sport team physicians should establish vigilant monitoring for non-sensory signs and symptoms of frostbite including changes in skin color (red in early stages and white in late stages) and the presence of blisters. In the event that frostbite is identified in an athlete, the affected body part should be protected from further injury. Rewarming should occur in a controlled setting, when possible, in a 40–42° C solution with an added antibacterial agent for 10–15 minutes until complete thawing. If rewarming occurs in the field, transfer to a higher level of care should be planned [103].

3.8.2.1 Alpine Skiing

Para skiing competition is split into two main competition categories: sitting (Fig. 3.7) and standing. Injury patterns follow similar patterns to summer sports. Seated athletes, such as those in a sit ski, are more likely to experience upper extremity injuries. Sit skiers must also be monitored for skin ulcers and nerve entrapment related to their equipment, much the same as wheelchair athletes. Stand skiers are exposed to the risk of fracture and ligamentous injury, which is also observed in skiers without impairment [102].

There are a number of equipment variations for both stand and sit Para skiers. Sit skis are made of a seat in a metal frame that is attached to a suspension system and either one (mono ski) or two (bi ski) skis. Mono skis are maneuvered with handheld outriggers, which resemble short forearm crutches with ski tips held by the athlete. Bi skis may be maneuvered with either handheld outriggers or fixed outriggers. Outriggers may be fixed in place to a sit ski for use by an athlete who

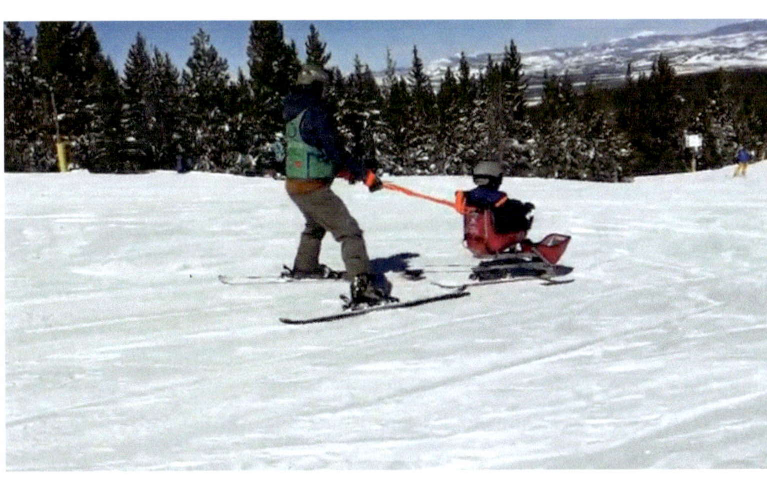

Fig. 3.7 Sit skiing

may not be able to safely use their upper extremities for maneuvering and instead relies mostly on truncal motion to move their skis.

Stand skiers may compete on one or two skis with or without handheld outriggers. These athletes often have limb deficiencies requiring prostheses. Whether transfemoral or transtibial, the prosthesis must ensure a center of gravity over the ankle [102, 104]. As with other prosthetic devices, practitioners must pay close attention to the stump–socket interface as a potential location for injury. Stand skiers with other impairments, such as abnormal muscle tone, may have other adaptations to their equipment, such as devices to hold ski tips together or to prevent them from crisscrossing, depending on the athlete's impairment. Equipment is specialized toward the athlete's needs to ensure safety and optimal performance.

3.8.2.2 Para Snowboarding

Para snowboarding debuted in the 2014 Sochi Winter Games. It has the highest injury incidence rate of any winter sport, which is attributed to loss of control, technique, and technical difficulties. Athletes with lower limb deficiency rely on a combination of prostheses and orthotics to interface with the snowboard. There is no sit-ski equivalent for Paralympic snowboarding events.

During the 2018 Pyeongchang Games, snowboarding exhibited a high proportion of acute traumatic injuries. An epidemiological study revealed several moderate to severe injuries: a reported anterior cruciate injury, an ankle ligament injury concurrent with facial fractures, and a shoulder dislocation. The study noted that the high incidence of injury may be because the sport is relatively new and lacks proper guidance for injury prevention [17].

3.8.2.3 Sled Hockey

Sled Hockey became an official Paralympic Sport in 1994 but was first developed in Sweden during the 1960s. Athletes participating in this sport at the competitive and Elite levels must have an impairment that would prevent them from participating in competitive sports alongside athletes without impairment. Sled hockey participants will thus have a wide array of medical condition(s) and functional impairment levels. Teams consist of five players and one goalie [105].

Participants in Sled Hockey are seated in a sled equipped with two skating blades. Athletes utilized two shortened hockey sticks equipped for both propulsion and shooting a puck. If an athlete's functional level limits their propulsion, they may be propelled from the back by a designated "pusher" [105]. Both athletes and pushers are susceptible to injury during play. Use of the sled predisposes athletes to a higher risk of skin ulcers and tears, just like in wheelchair athletes. Like this population, sledge hockey players also experience a large proportion of upper extremity and shoulder injuries. The use of hockey sticks for both propulsion and puck manipulation places greater stress on the hands and wrist and may contribute to overuse injuries and tendinitis [105].

Sled hockey is a high energy contact sport. During the 2002 Salt Lake Paralympic Games, sled hockey reported the highest incidence of injury. Acute injuries are common during these events, especially when players intentionally collide during a "check." Aside from the obvious risk of contusion, fracture, and laceration, these impacts can predispose sledge hockey athletes to higher rates of concussion. Continued refinement of safety equipment has led to decreased acute injury incidence, a trend which will hopefully continue [105].

3.9 Conclusion

Managing the health and injury of the Para athlete during training and competition may seem like a daunting task given the breadth of medical conditions and impairments a clinician may encounter. In this chapter, we have covered the most pertinent considerations related to an athlete's medical conditions and impairments, sport, and equipment that may impact a sideline practitioner's approach to the athlete. Although evaluation and treatment of athletes without disabilities may apply to Para athletes, this may require customization to each Para athlete's individual medical conditions and impairments.

Factbox 3.1

To appear alongside 3.4 Incidence.

Expected Injury Exercise

- For an elite level Summer Para sport event with 200 athletes over 10 days, a practitioner can expect to address approximately 20–25 injuries
- About 13–16 injuries will be acute or acute on chronic, while 7–9 injuries will be chronic overuse injuries
- May address 4 shoulder complaints, 2 hand and wrist complaints, and 2 foot and ankle complaints

Factbox 3.2

To appear alongside 3.6 Wheelchair in Para Sporty.

The Wheelchair

- Terms to know:
  - Axle—a metal rod that traverses between the center/hub of each main wheel; the position of the axle together with the center of gravity determines weight distribution in a wheelchair
  - Pushrim—portion of wheel athlete uses to propel
  - Dump—the angle of the seat cushion relative to the back rest in the sagittal plane
  - Camber—the angle of the wheels relative to the frame in the coronal plane
  - Frame—metal framework/skeleton of the wheelchair
  - Casters—smaller wheels that may be on the wheelchair (either in front or rear) for added stability
- Anti-tippers—smaller wheel(s) that may be on the wheelchair (most commonly in the rear) for added stability and to prevent tipping
- Key Angles and Positioning:
- The elbow should be in 60–80° of flexion (corresponding to elbow angle of 100–120°) when the hand is at the top of pushrim
  - A dump of 5°—increasing this may redistribute the center of gravity and force, leading to ulcers
  - The axle is placed immediately posterior to the center of mass of the athlete and wheelchair combined
- Signs of a well-fitted chair:
  - The chair moves with the athletes when they rotate or twist
  - The seat does not fit the athlete loosely
  - 2–3″ between the chair and posterior knee
  - Shoulders even

References

1. Schültke E. Ludwig Guttmann: emerging concept of rehabilitation after spinal cord injury. J Hist Neurosci. 2001;10:300–7. https://doi.org/10.1076/jhin.10.3.300.9090.
2. Guttmann L. Sport and recreation for the mentally and physically handicapped. R Soc Health J. 1973;93:208–12. https://doi.org/10.1177/146642407309300413.
3. Rome 1960. In: Int. Paralympic Comm. https://www.paralympic.org/rome-1960. Accessed 16 Aug 2022.
4. Tokyo 2020 Medal standings. In: Int. Paralympic Comm. https://www.paralympic.org/tokyo-2020/results/medalstandings. Accessed 16 Aug 2022.
5. Disability Language Style Guide | National Center on Disability and Journalism. https://ncdj.org/style-guide/. Accessed 16 Aug 2022.
6. International Paralympic Comittee. IPC guide to para and IPC terminology. 2021. https://www.paralympic.org/sites/default/files/2021-01/IPC%20Guide%20to%20Para%20and%20IPC%20Terminology_0.pdf. Accessed 16 Aug 2022
7. International Paralympic Comittee. Athlete Classification Code. 2015. https://www.paralympic.org/sites/default/files/document/151218123255973_2015_12_17+Classification+Code_FINAL.pdf. Accessed 16 Aug 2022.
8. History of Classification. In: Int. Paralympic Comm. https://www.paralympic.org/classification/history. Accessed 16 Aug 2022.

9. International Paralymipic Comittee (2016) International Standard for Eligible Impairments. https://www.paralympic.org/sites/default/files/document/161007092455456_Sec+ii+chapter+1_3_2_subchapter+1_International+Standard+for+Eligible+Impairments.pdf. Accessed 17 Aug 2022.
10. IPC Classification—Paralympic Categories & How to Qualify. In: Int. Paralympic Comm. https://www.paralympic.org/classification. Accessed 17 Aug 2022.
11. Para Archery Classification—USA Archery. https://www.usarchery.org/participate/adaptive-archery/para-archery-classification. Accessed 17 Aug 2022.
12. World Para Athletics. Classification rules and regulations. 2018. https://www.paralympic.org/sites/default/files/document/180305152713114_2017_12_20++WPA+Classification+Rules+and+Regulations_Edition+2018+online+version+.pdf. Accessed 17 Aug 2022.
13. Lexicon Decoder About – Parasport Classification – LEXI. https://lexi.global/about/. Accessed 17 Aug 2022.
14. Hogarth L, Payton C, Nicholson V, Spathis J, Tweedy S, Connick M, Beckman E, Van de Vliet P, Burkett B. Classifying motor coordination impairment in Para swimmers with brain injury. J Sci Med Sport. 2019;22:526–31. https://doi.org/10.1016/j.jsams.2018.11.015.
15. Derman W, Runciman P, Jordaan E, Blauwet C, Webborn N, Lexell J, van de Vliet P, Tuakli-Wosornu Y, Kissick J, Stomphorst J. High precompetition injury rate dominates the injury profile at the Rio 2016 summer paralympic games: a prospective cohort study of 51 198 athlete days. Br J Sports Med. 2018;52(1):24–31.
16. Willick SE, Webborn N, Emery C, Blauwet CA, Pit-Grosheide P, Stomphorst J, Vliet PV de, Marques NAP, Martinez-Ferrer JO, Jordaan E, Derman W, Schwellnus M (2013) The epidemiology of injuries at the London 2012 Paralympic Games. Br J Sports Med 47:426–432. doi: https://doi.org/10.1136/bjsports-2013-092374.
17. Derman W, Runciman P, Jordaan E, Schwellnus M, Blauwet C, Webborn N, Lexell J, Vliet P van de, Kissick J, Stomphorst J, Lee Y-H, Kim K-S (2020) High incidence of injuries at the Pyeongchang 2018 Paralympic winter games: a prospective cohort study of 6804 athlete days. Br J Sports Med 54:38–43. doi: https://doi.org/10.1136/bjsports-2018-100170.
18. Pinheiro LSP, Ocarino JM, Madaleno FO, Verhagen E, de Mello MT, Albuquerque MR, Andrade AGP, da Mata CP, Pinto RZ, Silva A, Resende RA. Prevalence and incidence of injuries in para athletes: a systematic review with meta-analysis and GRADE recommendations. Br J Sports Med. 2021;55:1357–65. https://doi.org/10.1136/bjsports-2020-102823.
19. Webborn AD, Turner HM. The aetiology of shoulder pain in elite Paralympic wheelchair athletes—the shoulder or cervical spine? 5th Paralympic Scientific Congress. Sydney: International Paralympic Committee; 2000.
20. Weiler R, Blauwet C, Clarke D, Dalton K, Derman W, Fagher K, Gouttebarge V, Kissick J, Lee K, Lexell J, de Vliet PV, Verhagen E, Webborn N, Virgile A, Ahmed OH. Infographic. The first position statement of the Concussion in Para Sport Group. Br J Sports Med. 2022;56:417–8. https://doi.org/10.1136/bjsports-2021-104530.
21. Fagher K, Dahlström Ö, Jacobsson J, Timpka T, Lexell J. Prevalence of sports-related injuries and illnesses in paralympic athletes. PM R. 2020;12:271–80. https://doi.org/10.1002/pmrj.12211.
22. Burnham R, Newell E, Steadward R. Sports medicine for the physically disabled: The Canadian Team Experience at the 1988 Seoul Paralympic Games. Clin J Sport Med. 1991;1:193–6.
23. Ramey L, Hayano T, Blatz D, Gedman M, Blauwet C. A comparison of self-reported unmet healthcare needs among adaptive and able-bodied athletes. PM R. 2020;12:36–42. https://doi.org/10.1002/pmrj.12202.
24. Salerno J, Tow S, Regan E, Bendziewicz S, McMillan M, Harrington S. Injury and injury prevention in United States para swimming: a mixed-methods approach. Int J Sports Phys Ther. 2022;17:293–306. https://doi.org/10.26603/001c.31173.
25. Macdougall H, O'Halloran P, Shields N, Sherry E. Comparing the Well-Being of Para and Olympic Sport Athletes: A Systematic Review. Adapt Phys Act Q. 2015;32:256–76. https://doi.org/10.1123/APAQ.2014-0168.
26. Piatt J, Kang S, Wells MS, Nagata S, Hoffman J, Taylor J. Changing identity through sport: the Paralympic sport club experience among adolescents with mobility impairments. Disabil Health J. 2018;11:262–6. https://doi.org/10.1016/j.dhjo.2017.10.007.
27. Marin-Urquiza A, Ferreira JP, Van Biesen D. Athletic identity and self-esteem among active and retired Paralympic athletes. Eur J Sport Sci. 2018;18:861–71. https://doi.org/10.1080/17461391.2018.1462854.
28. National Spinal Cord Injury Statisical Center. Traumatic spinal cord injury facts and figures at a glance. 2022. https://www.nscisc.uab.edu/public/Facts%20and%20Figures%202023%20-%20Final.pdf. Accessed 16 Aug 2022.
29. Ditor DS, Latimer AE, Ginis KAM, Arbour KP, McCartney N, Hicks AL. Maintenance of exercise participation in individuals with spinal cord injury: effects on quality of life, stress and pain. Spinal Cord. 2003;41:446–50. https://doi.org/10.1038/sj.sc.3101487.
30. Cowan H, Lakra C, Desai M. Autonomic dysreflexia in spinal cord injury. BMJ. 2020;371:m3596. https://doi.org/10.1136/bmj.m3596.
31. Krassioukov A, Stillman M, Beck LA. A primary care provider's guide to autonomic dysfunction following spinal cord injury. Top Spinal Cord Inj

Rehabil. 2020;26:123–7. https://doi.org/10.46292/sci2602-123.
32. Bhambani et al. Autonomic dysreflexia and boosting: lessons from an athlete survey. 2022. https://www.paralympic.org/sites/default/files/document/120131183408508_Thompson_Autonomic_Dysreflexia_and_Boosting.pdf. Accessed 19 Aug 2022.
33. Mazzeo F, Santamaria S, Iavarone A. "Boosting" in Paralympic athletes with spinal cord injury: doping without drugs. Funct Neurol. 2015;30:91–8. https://doi.org/10.11138/FNeur/2015.30.2.091.
34. Blauwet CA, Benjamin-Laing H, Stomphorst J, Van de Vliet P, Pit-Grosheide P, Willick SE. Testing for boosting at the Paralympic games: policies, results and future directions. Br J Sports Med. 2013;47:832–7. https://doi.org/10.1136/bjsports-2012-092103.
35. Price MJ, Trbovich M. Chapter 50: Thermoregulation following spinal cord injury. In: Romanovsky AA, editor. Handbook of clinical neurology. Elsevier; 2018. p. 799–820.
36. Kareen Velez (2017) Impaired thermoregulation. In: PMR KnowledgeNow. https://now.aapmr.org/impaired-thermoregulation/. Accessed 28 Oct 2022.
37. Grossmann F, Flueck JL, Perret C, Meeusen R, Roelands B. The thermoregulatory and thermal responses of individuals with a spinal cord injury during exercise, acclimation and by using cooling strategies—a systematic review. Front Physiol. 2021;12:636997.
38. Griggs KE, Stephenson BT, Price MJ, Goosey-Tolfrey VL. Heat-related issues and practical applications for Paralympic athletes at Tokyo 2020. Temp Multidiscip Biomed J. 2019;7:37–57. https://doi.org/10.1080/23328940.2019.1617030.
39. Howe AS, Boden BP. Heat-related illness in athletes. Am J Sports Med. 2007;35:1384–95. https://doi.org/10.1177/0363546507305013.
40. Hosokawa Y, Adami PE, Stephenson BT, Blauwet C, Bermon S, Webborn N, Racinais S, Derman W, Goosey-Tolfrey VL. Prehospital management of exertional heat stroke at sports competitions for Paralympic athletes. Br J Sports Med. 2022;56:599–604. https://doi.org/10.1136/bjsports-2021-104786.
41. Claydon VE, Steeves JD, Krassioukov A. Orthostatic hypotension following spinal cord injury: understanding clinical pathophysiology. Spinal Cord. 2006;44:341–51. https://doi.org/10.1038/sj.sc.3101855.
42. Beutler A, Carey P. Adaptive sports medicine. Chapter 5: Medical considerations in adaptive sports. In: De Luigi AJ, editor. Medical considerations in adaptive sports. Cham: Springer International Publishing; 2018. p. 59–69.
43. De Luigi AJ. Adaptive sports medicine: a clinical guide. Cham: Springer International Publishing; 2018.
44. Eriksson M, Bartonek Å, Pontén E, Gutierrez-Farewik EM. Gait dynamics in the wide spectrum of children with arthrogryposis: a descriptive study. BMC Musculoskelet Disord. 2015;16:384. https://doi.org/10.1186/s12891-015-0834-5.
45. Ágústsson A, Sveinsson Þ, Rodby-Bousquet E. The effect of asymmetrical limited hip flexion on seating posture, scoliosis and windswept hip distortion. Res Dev Disabil. 2017;71:18–23. https://doi.org/10.1016/j.ridd.2017.09.019.
46. De Luigi AJ. Technology and biomechanics of adaptive sports prostheses. In: De Luigi AJ, editor. Adaptive sports medicine: a clinical guide. Cham: Springer International Publishing; 2018. p. 35–47.
47. Wolf SI, Alimusaj M, Fradet L, Siegel J, Braatz F. Pressure characteristics at the stump/socket interface in transtibial amputees using an adaptive prosthetic foot. Clin Biomech. 2009;24:860–5. https://doi.org/10.1016/j.clinbiomech.2009.08.007.
48. Nutter DL. Considerations for coaching athletes with prosthetic limbs for transtibial and transfemoral amputations. Strength Cond J. 2019;41:1–8. https://doi.org/10.1519/SSC.0000000000000463.
49. Cancio JM, Eskridge S, Shannon K, Orr A, Mazzone B, Farrokhi S. Development of overuse musculoskeletal conditions after combat-related upper limb amputation: a retrospective cohort study. J Hand Ther. 2021; https://doi.org/10.1016/j.jht.2021.05.003.
50. Burkett B. Contribution of sports science to performance: swimming. In: Handbook of sports medicine and science: training and coaching the paralympic athlete. 1st ed. Wiley; 2017. p. 199–215.
51. World Para Swimming Classification & Categories - SB9, SM8. In: Int. Paralympic Comm. https://www.paralympic.org/swimming/classification. Accessed 30 Oct 2022.
52. White SC, Gilchrist LA, Wilk BE. Asymmetric limb loading with true or simulated leg-length differences. Clin Orthop Relat Res. 2004;421:287–92. https://doi.org/10.1097/01.blo.0000119460.33630.6d.
53. Golightly YM, Allen KD, Helmick CG, Renner JB, Jordan JM. Symptoms of the knee and hip in individuals with and without limb length inequality. Osteoarthr Cartil. 2009;17:596–600. https://doi.org/10.1016/j.joca.2008.11.005.
54. Forlino A, Marini JC. Osteogenesis imperfecta. Lancet. 2016;387:1657–71. https://doi.org/10.1016/S0140-6736(15)00728-X.
55. Jagannathan J, Dumont AS, Prevedello DM, Shaffrey CI, Jane JA. Cervical spine injuries in pediatric athletes: mechanisms and management. Neurosurg Focus. 2006;21:1–5. https://doi.org/10.3171/foc.2006.21.4.7.
56. Sheean G, McGuire JR. Spastic hypertonia and movement disorders: pathophysiology, clinical presentation, and quantification. PM R. 2009;1:827–33. https://doi.org/10.1016/j.pmrj.2009.08.002.
57. Diener H-C, Dichgans J. Pathophysiology of cerebellar ataxia. Mov Disord. 1992;7:95–109. https://doi.org/10.1002/mds.870070202.
58. Cardoso F. Athetosis. In: Kompoliti K, Metman LV, editors. Encyclopedia of movement disorders. Oxford: Academic Press; 2010. p. 96–7.

59. Patel DR, Greydanus DE. Sport participation by physically and cognitively challenged young athletes. Pediatr Clin N Am. 2010;57:795–817. https://doi.org/10.1016/j.pcl.2010.03.002.
60. Fagher K, Lexell J. Sports-related injuries in athletes with disabilities. Scand J Med Sci Sports. 2014;24:e320–31. https://doi.org/10.1111/sms.12175.
61. Steele KM, DeMers MS, Schwartz MS, Delp SL. Compressive tibiofemoral force during crouch gait. Gait Posture. 2012;35:556–60. https://doi.org/10.1016/j.gaitpost.2011.11.023.
62. Sutherland DH, Davids JR. Common gait abnormalities of the knee in cerebral palsy. Clin Orthop. 1993;288:139–47.
63. Runciman P, Derman W. The athlete with cerebral palsy. Aspetar Sports Med J. 2008;142–47
64. Grobler L, Derman W, Blauwet C, Chetty S, Webborn N, Pluim B. Pain management in athletes with impairment: a narrative review of management strategies. Clin J Sport Med. 2018;28(5):457–72. https://doi.org/10.1097/JSM.0000000000000600.
65. Romito JW, Turner ER, Rosener JA, Coldiron L, Udipi A, Nohrn L, Tausiani J, Romito BT. Baclofen therapeutics, toxicity, and withdrawal: a narrative review. SAGE Open Med. 2021;9:20503121211022196. https://doi.org/10.1177/20503121211022197.
66. Pavone P, Gulizia C, Le Pira A, Greco F, Parisi P, Di Cara G, Falsaperla R, Lubrano R, Minardi C, Spalice A, Ruggieri M. Cerebral palsy and epilepsy in children: clinical perspectives on a common comorbidity. Children. 2020;8:16. https://doi.org/10.3390/children8010016.
67. Griepp DW, Kim DJ, Ganz M, Dolphin EJ, Sotudeh N, Burekhovich SA, Naziri Q. The effects of antiepileptic drugs on bone health: a systematic review. Epilepsy Res. 2021;173:106619. https://doi.org/10.1016/j.eplepsyres.2021.106619.
68. Mus-Peters CTR, Huisstede BMA, Noten S, Hitters MWMGC, van der Slot WMA, van den Berg-Emons Rita JG. Low bone mineral density in ambulatory persons with cerebral palsy? A systematic review. Disabil Rehabil. 2019;41:2392–402. https://doi.org/10.1080/09638288.2018.1470261.
69. Mei C, Reilly S, Reddihough D, Mensah F, Morgan A. Motor speech impairment, activity, and participation in children with cerebral palsy. Int J Speech Lang Pathol. 2014;16:427–35. https://doi.org/10.3109/17549507.2014.917439.
70. Reid SM, Meehan EM, Arnup SJ, Reddihough DS. Intellectual disability in cerebral palsy: a population-based retrospective study. Dev Med Child Neurol. 2018;60:687–94. https://doi.org/10.1111/dmcn.13773.
71. Magno e Silva M, Winckler C, Costa e Silva A, Bilzon J, Duarte E. Sports injuries in paralympic track and field athletes with visual impairment. Med Sci Sports Exerc. 2012;45(5):908–13. https://doi.org/10.1249/MSS.0b013e31827f06f3.
72. British Blind Sport. Visually impaired friendly athletics. 2015. https://britishblindsport.org.uk/uploads/athletics-resource-pdf-version.pdf?v=1690813949. Accessed 23 Aug 2022.
73. Special Olympics. Special Olympics and paralympics comparison fact-sheet. 2018. https://media.specialolympics.org/resources/brand-awareness-and-communication/marketing/Special-Olympics-and-Paralympics-Comparison-Fact-Sheet-2018.pdf. Accessed 23 Aug 2022.
74. Bull MJ, Trotter T, Santoro SL, Christensen C, Grout RW, The Council On Genetics. Health supervision for children and adolescents with down syndrome. Pediatrics. 2022;149:e2022057010. https://doi.org/10.1542/peds.2022-057010.
75. Birrer RB. The special olympics athlete: evaluation and clearance for participation. Clin Pediatr (Phila). 2004;43:777–82. https://doi.org/10.1177/000992280404300901.
76. Lexell J, Lovén G, Fagher K. Incidence of sports-related concussion in elite para athletes—a 52-week prospective study. Brain Inj. 2021;35:971–7. https://doi.org/10.1080/02699052.2021.1942551.
77. Cooper RA, De Luigi AJ. Adaptive sports technology and biomechanics: wheelchairs. PM R. 2014;6:S31–9. https://doi.org/10.1016/j.pmrj.2014.05.020.
78. Klenck C, Gebke K. Practical management: common medical problems in disabled athletes. Clin J Sport Med. 2007;17:55–60. https://doi.org/10.1097/JSM.0b013e3180302587.
79. Mathur R, Martone P, De Luigi AJ. Wheelchair basketball. In: De Luigi AJ, editor. Adaptive sports medicine: a clinical guide. Cham: Springer International Publishing; 2018. p. 123–34.
80. Pillemer R. Examination for specific conditions of the shoulder. In: Pillemer R, editor. Handbook of upper extremity examination: a practical guide. Cham: Springer International Publishing; 2022. p. 187–210.
81. Fairbairn JR, Bliven KCH. Incidence of shoulder injury in Elite wheelchair athletes differ between sports: a critically appraised topic. J Sport Rehabil. 2019;28:294–8. https://doi.org/10.1123/jsr.2017-0360.
82. Burnham RS, May L, Nelson E, Steadward R, Reid DC. Shoulder pain in wheelchair athletes. The role of muscle imbalance. Am J Sports Med. 1993;21:238–42. https://doi.org/10.1177/036354659302100213.
83. Burnham RS, Steadward RD. Upper extremity peripheral nerve entrapments among wheelchair athletes: prevalence, location, and risk factors. Arch Phys Med Rehabil. 1994;75:519–24.
84. Osmotherly PG, Thompson E, Rivett DA, Haskins R, Snodgrass SJ. Injuries, practices and perceptions of Australian wheelchair sports participants. Disabil Health J. 2021;14:101044. https://doi.org/10.1016/j.dhjo.2020.101044.
85. Wilroy J, Hibberd E. Evaluation of a shoulder injury prevention program in wheelchair basketball. J Sport

Rehabil. 2018;27:554–9. https://doi.org/10.1123/jsr.2017-0011.
86. Chen Y-T, Mordus D. Shooting sports (archery, air rifle, trapshooting). In: De Luigi AJ, editor. Adaptive sports medicine: a clinical guide. Cham: Springer International Publishing; 2018. p. 313–22.
87. Niestroj CK, Schöffl V, Küpper T. Acute and overuse injuries in elite archers. J Sports Med Phys Fitness. 2018;58:1063–70. https://doi.org/10.23736/S0022-4707.17.07828-8.
88. Blauwet CA, Cushman D, Emery C, Willick SE, Webborn N, Derman W, Schwellnus M, Stomphorst J, Van de Vliet P. Risk of injuries in paralympic track and field differs by impairment and event discipline: a prospective cohort study at the London 2012 Paralympic Games. Am J Sports Med. 2016;44:1455–62. https://doi.org/10.1177/0363546516629949.
89. Mâsse LC, Lamontagne M, O'Riain MD. Biomechanical analysis of wheelchair propulsion for various seating positions. J Rehabil Res Dev. 1992;29:12–28. https://doi.org/10.1682/jrrd.1992.07.0012.
90. Fisher M. Adaptive sports medicine in the para athlete. 2021. https://www.childrensmercy.org/contentassets/b68a0d38a67741193a6568524f83f25/adaptive-sports-medicine-in-the-para-athlete.pdf. Accessed 10 Aug 2022.
91. Chow JW, Kuenster AF, Lim Y. Kinematic analysis of javelin throw performed by wheelchair athletes of different functional classes. J Sports Sci Med. 2003;2:36–46.
92. The Sport. In: USA Boccia. https://usaboccia.org/about/the-sport/. Accessed 23 Aug 2022.
93. Auriemma M, De Luigi AJ. Adaptive throwing sports: discus, javelin, shot put, and boccia. In: De Luigi AJ, editor. Adaptive sports medicine: a clinical guide. Cham: Springer International Publishing; 2018. p. 301–12.
94. Fong D, Yam K Y, Chu V, Cheung R, Chan KC. Upper limb muscle fatigue during prolonged Boccia games with underarm throwing technique. Sports Biomech Int Soc Biomech Sports. 2012;11:441–51. https://doi.org/10.1080/14763141.2012.699977.
95. Tsai Y-S, Yu Y-C, Huang P-C, Cheng H-YK. Seat surface inclination may affect postural stability during Boccia ball throwing in children with cerebral palsy. Res Dev Disabil. 2014;35:3568–73. https://doi.org/10.1016/j.ridd.2014.08.033.
96. Burkett B, Mellifont R. Sport science and coaching in paralympic cycling. Int J Sports Sci Coach. 2008;3:95–103. https://doi.org/10.1260/174795408784089360.
97. Rooney D, Sarriegui I, Heron N. 'As easy as riding a bike': a systematic review of injuries and illness in road cycling. BMJ Open Sport Exerc Med. 2020;6:e000840. https://doi.org/10.1136/bmjsem-2020-000840.
98. About the Sport—WWR. https://worldwheelchair.rugby/about-the-sport/. Accessed 24 Aug 2022.
99. Irwin DM, Zillen MK, De Luigi AJ. Wheelchair Rugby. In: De Luigi AJ, editor. Adaptive sports medicine: a clinical guide. Cham: Springer International Publishing; 2018. p. 135–47.
100. Wheelchair Tennis and Para-table Tennis | SpringerLink. https://link.springer.com/chapter/10.1007/978-3-319-56568-2_19. Accessed 30 Oct 2022.
101. Tennis Rules and Regulations | ITF. https://www.itftennis.com/en/about-us/governance/rules-and-regulations/. Accessed 31 Oct 2022.
102. Juriga BJ, Yang YS, De Luigi AJ. Adaptive Alpine skiing and para-snowboarding. In: De Luigi AJ, editor. Adaptive sports medicine: a clinical Guide. Cham: Springer International Publishing; 2018. p. 251–99.
103. Murphy JV, Banwell PE, Roberts AHN, McGrouther DA. Frostbite: pathogenesis and treatment. J Trauma Acute Care Surg. 2000;48:171.
104. International Paralympic Committee. Alpine skiing equipment rules and regulations. 2016. https://www.paralympic.org/sites/default/files/document/160805114925874_2016_08_03_IPCAS_EquipmentRulebook_final_0.pdf. Accessed 24 Aug 2022.
105. Ice Sled Hockey (Sledge Hockey Outside the United States) | SpringerLink. https://link.springer.com/chapter/10.1007/978-3-319-56568-2_22. Accessed 31 Oct 2022.

4 Special Olympians

Aaron Rubin

The practice of Sports Medicine requires knowledge of injuries, illness, environmental conditions, and mechanisms of trauma for athletes. The practitioner must understand the stresses of the sports activity and the preparation and underlying condition of the athlete.

Athletes participating in the Special Olympics have similar needs and issues as athletes in all sports and athletic activities. There are some key differences that will help the clinician provide appropriate care in a culturally sensitive manner and prepare for problems more specific in this population of athletes.

Special Olympics is an international movement active in over 170 countries with over five million athletes and supported by a million coaches, staff, and volunteers. There are over 100,000 competitions per year covering over 30 sports as well as other activities to improve the lives of the participants.

The Special Olympics motto, attributed to its founder Eunice Kennedy Shriver is **"Let me win. But if I cannot win, let me be brave in the attempt."**

A. Rubin (✉)
Family and Sports Medicine,
Fontana, CA, USA

Kaiser Permanente Bernard J Tyson School of Medicine, Pasadena, USA

Special Olympics Southern California,
Long Beach, USA
e-mail: Aaron.l.rubin@kp.org

Shriver's sister, Rosemary, was intellectually disabled and they participated in various sports activities together. This led to "Camp Shriver" in 1962 when young people with intellectual disabilities were invited to their homes to participate in sports activities and eventually to the first international games in Chicago, IL, in 1968.

What sets these athletes apart is the presence of an intellectual disability (Intelligence Quotient below 70–75) or a significant developmental limitation in two or more adaptive areas which are skills such as conceptual skills, social skills, or practical skills. As a group, these are referred to as **Intellectual and Developmental Disabilities (IDD)** (See Table 4.1) [1, 2].

Table 4.1 Adaptive behaviors and potential skills deficiencies in IDD

Adaptive area	Potential skills deficiency
Conceptual	Memory, language, reading, writing, math reasoning, acquisition of practical knowledge, problem-solving, judgment in novel situations
Social	Awareness of others' thoughts, feelings, and experiences; empathy; interpersonal communication skills; ability to develop friendships; social judgment
Practical	Self-care; job responsibilities; money management; recreation, self-management of behavior, school and work task organization

Adapted [3, 4]

S. Rocha Piedade et al. (eds.), *Sideline Management in Sports*,
https://doi.org/10.1007/978-3-031-33867-0_4

It is estimated that 1–3% of the population has some level of intellectual disabilities. This would mean up to 200 million worldwide and about 6.5 million persons in the United States. In addition, there may be inequities ranging from a prevalence of 16.41 per 1000 persons in low-income countries to 9.21 per 1000 persons in high-income countries. This demonstrates a potential health equity deficiency for those with IDD.

Often there is not a specific diagnosed condition for the IDD. Those with mild IDD (IQ < 50) are less likely to have a specific diagnosis than those with more severe IDD (IQ > 50).

4.1 Underlying or Associated Diagnoses

Down syndrome is the most common genetic chromosomal disorder, which is most often due to an extra Chromosome 21 (trisomy 21) but can also be due to a gene translocation, a mosaic chromosomal pattern. It is the most common chromosomal condition diagnosed in the United States, occurring in about 1 in every 700 babies. About 6000 babies are born with Down syndrome annually in the United States [5].

About 8% of children with Down syndrome have epilepsy, 50% have congenital heart defects, and about 2% may have atlantoaxial instability. There is also an association with hearing and vision disabilities, obesity, type 1 diabetes, depression, anxiety, and Alzheimer's disease, all of which could complicate sideline and athlete care. In addition, hematologic disorders, hypothyroidism, and sleep apnea are more frequent and may need to be considered in athlete evaluation for sports participation [6].

Fragile-X syndrome (FXS) is an X-linked genetic disorder that is a developmental delay and cognitive and adaptive behavior skills decline after early childhood. Up to 67% of males with FXS meet the criteria for an autism spectrum disorder (ASD) diagnosis and 20% develop seizures. They often have neurobehavioral disorders, including ADHD, anxiety, and intellectual disability [7].

Autism Spectrum Disorder (ASD) is a condition of unknown cause that has diagnostic criteria in the Diagnostic and Statistical Manual of Mental Disorders Fifth editions, Text Revision (DSM5TR). There is a variable disability to this disorder, hence the term "spectrum." The diagnosis requires deficits in social communication, restricted, repetitive patterns of behavior, and impaired function (social, academic, daily routines) that have been present from early developmental periods and are not explained by other causes of intellectual disability [8, 9].

Other diagnoses associated with IDD and Special Olympics athletes include, but are not limited to:

Apert Syndrome is a genetic disease in which the skull bone seams close earlier than normal.

Williams Syndrome, which is caused by the deletion of genetic material from a region of chromosome 7.

Fetal Alcohol Syndrome is a disorder that occurs due to the mother's use of alcohol during pregnancy.

Prader-Willi Syndrome occurs due to partial deletions on chromosome 15.

Phenylketonuria (PKU) is an inherited disorder caused by the inability to process phenylalanine. Children born in US hospitals are tested for PKU and if treated early and consistently develop normally.

Cerebral Palsy is caused by abnormalities in the brain that control muscle movement. Many may also have problems with intellectual disability, seizures, vision, hearing and speech along with scoliosis, osteopenia, and joint contractures.

4.2 Do NOT use the "R-word"

The term "mental retardation" is no longer considered appropriate. In 2013, Diagnostic and Statistical Manual 5 (DSM-5) replaced the term with "intellectual disability or intellectual developmental disorder." The Federal Register of the United States made a similar change in 2013 after the passage of Rosa's Law in 2010 due to the pejorative nature of the "R-word" or "R Slur." The "R-word" should not be used as a description for Special Olympics Athletes or in general for those with IDD [10, 11].

4.3 Organization and Relationships

Special Olympics International (SOI) is based in Washington, DC, USA. SOI has a relationship with the International Olympic Committee (IOC) to officially recognize SOI as a representative of the interests of athletes with intellectual disabilities that allows the use of the term "Special Olympics" and protects the word "Olympics" from unauthorized use or exploitation. SOI is prohibited from using the Olympic 5-ring logo, anthem, or motto.

The United States Olympic Committee (USOC) has a similar agreement with SOI to protect and allow the use of the word "Olympics." There are also formal relationships with National Olympic Committees, international sports federations, and national and international sports governing bodies. As a non-governmental organization (NGO) with the United Nations, SOI has the responsibility to work with nations throughout the world to develop sports training and competitions for persons with intellectual disabilities.

SOI is a not-for-profit corporation that licenses and accredits programs around the world. These Accredited Programs organize and conduct Special Olympics training and competition programs throughout their respective areas. Most competitions are locally organized and supervised. Larger events, such as the Special Olympics USA Games or Special Olympics World Games (SOWG) winter and summer games, are organized under a Games Operating Committee (GOC). SOWG occurs every 2 years alternating between winter and summer games. All events need medical expertise to allow for safe participation by the athletes, volunteers, and spectators when planning these events. One may be working with various leadership groups when participating in a larger event [12].

4.4 Paralympics

A frequent point of confusion when discussing disabled athletes is the differences between the Special Olympics and the Paralympics. The IOC recognizes both. Special Olympics athletes have intellectual disabilities and Paralympics physical disabilities. Other differences are noted in Table 4.2.

Table 4.2 Comparing Special Olympics and Paralympics

	Special Olympics Special Olympics International (SOI)	Paralympics International Paralympic Committee (IPC)
Age of participants	8 and older, not including Young Athletes programs	Generally, 18 and older
Selection	Every person with an intellectual disability who is at least eight years of age is eligible to participate in Special Olympics	Qualifier competitions
Philosophy	Sports to help participants fulfill their potential Inclusive	Make an inclusive world through Para Sport Elite, competitive athletes at higher levels participate in World Championships and Paralympic games
Disability	Intellectual and Developmental disability (onset before age 18) Some may have physical disabilities as well	Must have an eligible impairment. Physical (impaired muscle power, range of motion, limb deficiency or length difference, short stature, hypertonia, ataxia, athetosis) Visual Intellectual
Types of competition	Local, regional, national, international	Local, regional, national, international
Countries represented	200 (2019)	163 (2021)

Table 4.2 (continued)

	Special Olympics Special Olympics International (SOI)	Paralympics International Paralympic Committee (IPC)
Frequency of international games	Every 2 years alternating summer and winter in a location independent of the Olympic Games	Every 2 years alternating summer and winter Since 1988 have been following the Olympic Games in the same location
Number of sports	32	28
First international competition	Summer 1968 Chicago, IL, USA	1960 Rome, Italy
Headquarters	Washington, DC, USA	Bonn, Germany
Website	https://www.specialolympics.org	https://www.paralympic.org/ipc

Adapted [13]

4.5 Eligibility

Any person with an intellectual disability at least 8 years old is eligible to participate. There is no maximum age limit. There is also a "Young Athletes" program for children from age two to seven.

The person should be identified as having an intellectual disability by an agency or professional or a closely related developmental disability.

All participating athletes must be medically cleared to participate and undergo a physical evaluation by a licensed medical professional. MedFest is the organized pre-participation physical program designed by SOI with specific guidance on the contents of the exam and clearance.

There is also a Special Olympics Unified Sports® program that encourages participation with students with and without intellectual disabilities together. It is estimated that 1.4 million people worldwide participate in Unified Sports [14].

4.6 Special Olympic Sports

Official summer sports include Aquatics (Swimming) Golf, Athletics, Handball, Basketball, Judo, Badminton, Gymnastics Artistic, Gymnastics Rhythmic, Bocce Powerlifting, Bowling, Roller Skating, Cycling, Sailing Equestrian Softball, Football (Soccer) Table Tennis, Tennis, and Volleyball.

Official winter sports include Alpine Skiing, Short Track Speed Skating, Cross-Country Skiing, Snowboarding, Figure Skating Snowshoeing, and Floor Hockey.

Other Recognized sports include Cricket, Kayaking, Floorball, and Flag Football.

4.7 Divisioning

Special Olympics thrives to keep competitions level fair and exciting for all participants. Athletes with IDD have various levels of ability and to keep their competition level they are evaluated in a procedure called "divisioning." Athletes are evaluated based on age, gender, time, score, or skills to best match them by age and ability to allow for level competition.

4.8 Physician's Role in Special Olympics

As with any sports activity and organization, there are many potential roles for physicians and other medical providers. Just as a team, the physician will take multiple roles to oversee the safety and well-being of the athletes. A physician working with Special Olympics may choose responsibilities beyond the sideline care of athletes.

Advisory roles to local Special Olympics leadership may include evaluating current risks and safety for athletes including, but not limited to, environmental concerns, training, nutrition, hydration, injury prevention, and prevention of infectious diseases.

The Special Olympics Healthy Athletes® program began in 1997 and provides free medical screenings at competitions and stand-alone events. Physicians play a prominent role in MedFest which provides preparticipation evaluations for athletes and must be done before athletes participate in Special Olympics and needs to be repeated every 3 years.

In addition to MedFest, other Healthy Athletes® disciplines include

- Special Olympics Lions Clubs International Opening Eyes (vision/eye health)
- Healthy Hearing (audiology)
- Special Smiles (dentistry)
- Health Promotion (prevention and nutrition)
- Strong Minds (emotional health)
- FUNfitness (physical therapy)
- Fit Feet (podiatry) [15]

4.9 Sideline and Event Care

Sideline care plans should be in place for all events. For practice and training at the minimum, coaches or some other designee should have some basic first-aid skills. If available, physicians, athletic trainers, nurses, emergency medical technicians, and others trained in first aid for athletes are desirable. This may not be available due to the large number of events that occur daily in Special Olympics.

As events get larger with more athletes participating, medical care should also be elevated. These events may be local or regional competitions. Statewide, national, or worldwide games require careful planning with the local jurisdictions, hospitals, emergency services, and games organizing committee (GOC). Medical care should be integrated into the plans for the event and requires the creation of emergency action plans (EAP) as well as communication plans and operations within the Incident Command System (ICS) or other organizing planning systems.

An Incident Command System (ICS) is an organizational process to distribute planning of events (or incidents). It is based on emergency management but is a good method of ensuring that all needs for an event are covered. The overall event should have a clear chain of command leadership and planning. At the top of ICS is the Incident Commander who is in charge overall. They have a Command Staff including a Safety Officer (to keep the activities safe and secure), a Public Information Officer (to screen and provide communications to the team and public), Liaison Officers (to interact with other groups), and Content experts (to provide information to the Incident Commander). The General Staff includes leaders in areas of Operations (getting stuff done), Planning (looking forward during an incident to do further planning), Logistics (getting the supplies needed to operate), and Finance (tracking costs and funding).

An **Emergency Action Plan (EAP)** should be written for each sporting venue and any locations where the athlete will be during the event. It should reflect the needs of the athletes including any special medical needs that may arise. This includes transportation, check-in, meals, housing (if an athlete is staying overnight), opening and closing ceremonies, and social events, such as dances or recreational activities. The EAP needs to include care of the spectator, which is often delegated to local emergency or venue services. If no plans are made, it would be unethical to not provide emergent care at a venue.

The EAP should include specifics about location and access to the venue, internal directions, communications plans (including radio channels and etiquette), confirmation of cell phone service, security escorts for responders, support for teammates and family members, and documentation and reporting systems.

In addition, the medical staff should have plans for the treatment of minor illnesses and injuries. Most of these can be provided at the venue with more serious conditions either being transported by Emergency Medical System (EMS) to local emergency rooms. Problems not requiring EMS care, but needing observation or more advanced care, can be brought to a Main Medical Tent or in some large events, such as World Games to a specially established "Poly Clinic" staffed for urgent care.

Planning for medical care at a Special Olympics event can start from the baseline of other sporting competitions with additional plans to accommodate for medical conditions more likely in these athletes.

Medical supplies should reflect the need for care of musculoskeletal problems commonly seen in sporting events and consider the increased possibility of medical conditions not frequently seen in other athletic competitions.

4.10 Medical Supplies

Other medical supply considerations should be evaluated based on the event and location (See Table 4.3). Wheelchairs may be needed to transport those with isolated injuries off the field of play to the medical tent. In swimming events, there should be trained lifeguards with spine boards to move someone out of the water. Crutches could be helpful to allow an injured athlete some mobility as needed (Table 4.3).

Table 4.3 Medical supplies

Sideline/venue first aid kit
Item
Scissors
Flashlight
Gloves (S, L, XL)
Sunscreen (small)
Sanitizer (small)
Eyewash/saline irrigation
Bandages
Gauze pads 4 × 4
Antibiotic ointment
Skin lubricant
Tape (1½ cloth athletic)
Bulky gauze wraps 4 in.
Tampon, sanitary napkins
Triangular bandages

Event medical kit
Diagnostic and advanced equipment
Pulse oximeter
Glucometer
BP cuff/stethoscope
Scissors
Flashlight
Gloves (various sizes)
Facemask/personal protective equipment
Sunscreen
Sanitizer
Eyewash/saline irrigation
Oto-ophthalmoscope
[a]Medication kit (optional)
Acetaminophen, Ibuprofen, epi-pen or epinephrine with syringe, antacid, antihistamine[a]
[a]Trauma kit (tourniquet, compressive bandage, wound packing)[a]
[a]Suture kit with suture, anesthetic, syringes, and needles[a]
Automated external defibrillator (AED)
Sharps disposal container
Wound care
Bandages
Gauze pads 4 × 4
Nonstick dressing pads
Antibiotic ointment
Skin lubricant
Wound closure strips ½ × 4
Tincture benzoin amps
Tape (1½ cloth athletic and stretch tapes)
Elastic wrap
6 in.
4 in.
2 in.
Bulky gauze wraps 4 in.
Tongue blades
Absorbent wound pads
Tampon, sanitary napkins
SAM splints, cardboard splints or other splinting systems
General supplies
Blanket
Mylar blankets
Waterproof protective pads
Paper towels
Disinfectant wipes
Trash bags
Biohazard bags
Duct tape
Ice bags/freezer bags
Emesis bags
Instant cold pack
Muscle rub (icy hot)
Clipboard

Created by Aaron Rubin

[a]Medications and suturing decisions must be made by a medical authority and may be subject to local medical and pharmacy regulation

One should also consider the environmental conditions. If in a hot or warm environment, adequate planning for emergent cooling should include access to ice, ice chests, water, cooling towels, and a tank or pool for emergent cooling. In a cold environment, there could be an increased need for blankets and warming stations in the venues and medical tents.

Some of the underlying conditions may predispose athletes to injuries, such as cerebral palsy, Down syndrome, and other conditions.

Individuals with cerebral palsy may have osteopenia predisposing to fractures and joint contractures predisposing to joint, tendon, and muscle injuries.

Down syndrome is associated with atlantoaxial instability which could predispose athletes to cervical spine injuries, even though screened for risk of this problem by history and exam at MedFest. Screening is done by history, physical, and when appropriate evaluation by a specialist with or without radiographic evaluation. Sports activities may be limited to these individuals, but diligence by sideline medical personnel is important.

4.11 Common Medical issues in Special Olympics

Heart and other cardiovascular problems may be seen with many of the underlying medical conditions that affect the Special Olympics Athlete. The medical plan should include rapid response to unconscious or downed athletes or those with symptoms of cardiac issues. Staff should be trained in cardiopulmonary resuscitation. Automated external defibrillators (AEDs) should be readily available. Many venues have public access AEDs available, but medical planning must include knowing these locations and confirming their availability during the event. Owning, borrowing, or leasing dedicated AEDs for events with ready access to all venues is highly recommended.

Head injuries (mild traumatic brain injuries, concussions) are particularly difficult to evaluate in this cohort of athletes. The primary concern should be assuring that the injury is NOT a life-threatening situation such as a subdural hematoma, epidural hematoma, intracranial bleed, or increased intracranial pressure. All athletes should have had a preparticipation evaluation through the MedFest program, but these do not routinely include baseline concussion testing such as SCAT5 (Sport Concussion Assessment Tool Fifth Edition) [16, 17].

SCAT5 includes cognitive testing as well as a Rapid Neurological Screen that includes a "cervical exam, athlete's speech, ability to read, balance, gait, visual tracking and finger to nose coordination," all of which may be problematic in individuals with IDD.

It is important that any suspected head injury is rapidly evaluated by a provider experienced in the evaluation of head injuries with a low threshold for transportation to the appropriate medical facility for further evaluation observation and possible imaging.

Heat Illness should always be considered at sporting events in warm climates. Due to many of the medications taken by Special Olympics Athletes, there may be an increased risk of heart illness. Planning should include prevention through education, cooling stations, and close field-side monitoring of the athletes. The medical team must be prepared to act swiftly to prevent permanent damage or death due to heat illness including plans for temperature monitoring and rapid cooling of the athletes. Monitoring of weather conditions by local measurement of heat, humidity, and heat index is important. At large games such as the SOWG held in Los Angeles in 2015, a meteorologist was part of the staff to help forecast potential days of high heat stress and communicate with the athletes and teams or move higher risk events to alternate times (such as morning or evening when not as hot) or days.

Seizures are seen more often in Special Olympics than in most sports competitions. The primary initial goal is to prevent further injury to the athlete while the seizure is occurring. Well-meaning bystanders may try to intervene with the seizing athletes by trying to force something in their mouth. It is generally best to move any objects that could harm the athletes away from them, gently provide airway support, place the athletes on their side when possible, and activate the emergency action plan. Medical staff should obtain history from family members, coaches, or teammates to try to determine if these seizures are common. Not all seizures require transportation to higher levels of care unless a new onset of a previously seizure-free person, prolonged seizure, or prolonged postictal state. One should also consider transportation if associated with a head injury or other trauma or heat exposure.

The medical team should be prepared to treat prolonged seizures or status epilepticus. This is often complicated by the need to use controlled substances for the initial treatment of these seizures. There are numerous regulations regarding the handling and use of these controlled substances, and one should be familiar with the local rules. There are also numerous regulations regarding the transport and maintenance of these medications.

Initial emergent treatment could include intramuscular midazolam 10 mg, intravenous lorazepam 4 mg, or rectal or intranasal diazepam 0.2 mg per kilogram body weight [18].

Diabetes mellitus is more common in individuals with IDD. The medical team should consider monitoring blood sugar with a glucometer and treating hypoglycemia with glucose gel or some other source of readily available carbohydrates.

Emotional and behavioral problems may occur with many of the underlying conditions that cause IDD. The staff, coaches, parents, guardians, and other athletes set the mood, much as with all sporting events. Athletes at all levels are competitive and get emotional. Clear rules and officiating with even enforcement help minimize conflict. The medical team should be prepared to aid staff as needed with behavioral problems. Pre-event planning with behavioral health and IDD specialists and including these problems in emergency action plans is helpful. Use of medications should be carefully considered with appropriate training and supervision and should follow applicable local medical and pharmacy regulations.

4.12 Conclusions

Medical care for athletes with intellectual and developmental disabilities and Special Olympic events is well within the scope of physicians with an interest in sports medicine with limited additional training. As always, good training, proper planning, adequate supplies and partnering with experts in the field help keep the athletes and participants safe.

References

1. Holder M. The Special Olympics healthy athletes experience. Curr Sports Med Rep. 2015;14(3):165–70. https://doi.org/10.1249/JSR.0000000000000158.
2. Seidenberg PH, Eggers JL. Mass screenings at mass participation events. Curr Sports Med Rep. 2015;14(3):176–81. https://doi.org/10.1249/JSR.0000000000000164.
3. Patel DR, Cabral MD, Ho A, Merrick J. A clinical primer on intellectual disability. Transl Pediatr. 2020;9(Suppl. 1):S23–35. https://doi.org/10.21037/tp.2020.02.02. https://www.psychiatry.org/File%20Library/Psychiatrists/Practice/DSM/APA_DSM-5-Intellectual-Disability.pdf (accessed 7/29/2022)
4. Patel DR, Apple R, Kanungo S, Akkal A. Narrative review of intellectual disability: definitions, evaluations and principles of treatment. Pediatr Med. 2018;1:11. https://doi.org/10.21037/pm.2018.12.02.
5. Centers for Disease Control and Prevention. Facts about Down syndrome. https://www.cdc.gov/ncbddd/birthdefects/downsyndrome.html (accessed August 13, 2022).
6. Antonarakis SE, Skotko BG, Rafii MS, Strydom A, Pape SE, Bianchi DW, Sherman SL, Reeves RH. Down syndrome. Nat Rev Dis Primers. 2020;6(1):9. https://doi.org/10.1038/s41572-019-0143-7.
7. Van Esch H. Fragile X syndrome: Clinical features and diagnosis in children and adolescents. In: Firth HV, Voigt RG, editors. UpToDate. https://www.uptodate.com/contents/fragile-x-syndrome-clinical-features-and-diagnosis-in-children-and-adolescents?search=fragile%20x%20syndrom&source=search_result&selectedTitle=1~49&usage_type=default&display_rank=1 (accessed August 13, 2022).
8. Centers for Disease Control and Prevention Diagnostic Criteria for 299.00 Autism Spectrum Disorder https://www.cdc.gov/ncbddd/autism/hcp-dsm.html (accessed August 13, 2022).
9. American Psychiatric Association. Autism spectrum disorder, 2013. https://www.psychiatry.org/File%20Library/Psychiatrists/Practice/DSM/APA_DSM-5-Autism-Spectrum-Disorder.pdf (accessed August 13, 2022).
10. American Psychiatric Association. Intellectual disability, 2013. https://www.psychiatry.org/File%20Library/Psychiatrists/Practice/DSM/APA_DSM-5-Intellectual-Disability.pdf (accessed August 13, 2022).

11. Change in terminology: "Mental Retardation" to "Intellectual Disability" Federal Register/Vol. 78, No. 148/Thursday, August 1, 2013/Rules and Regulations. p. 46499 https://www.federalregister.gov/d/2013-18552 (accessed August 13, 2022).
12. Special Olympics Official General Rules. https://dotorg.brightspotcdn.com/ef/76/6da131bc4d8ba82cb5ff40de975f/amended-general-rules-v2.pdf (accessed August 13, 2022).
13. Special Olympics vs Paralympics. https://dcp.ucla.edu/special-olympics-vs-paralympics (accessed August 13, 2022).
14. Special Olympics. Unified sports, 2022. https://www.specialolympics.org/what-we-do/sports/unified-sports (accessed on August 13, 2022).
15. Special Olympics. Healthy athletes, 2022. https://www.specialolympics.org/what-we-do/inclusive-health/healthy-athletes (accessed on August 13, 2022).
16. Echemendia RJ, Meeuwisse W, McCrory P, et al. The Sport Concussion Assessment Tool 5th Edition (SCAT5): Background and rationale. Brit J Sports Med. 2017;51:848–50. https://bjsm.bmj.com/content/51/11/848?ijkey=c0d58aaf196b2e158e6900335b4ff573fbe9a1ea&keytype2=tf_ipsecsha
17. Harmon KG, Clugston JR, Dec K, et al. American Medical Society for Sports Medicine position statement on concussion in sport. Brit J Sports Med. 2019;53:213–25. https://bjsm.bmj.com/content/53/4/213.long
18. Drislane FW. Convulsive status epilepticus in adults: management. In: Garcia P, Edlow JA, Rabinstein AA, editors. UpToDate. https://www.uptodate.com/contents/convulsive-status-epilepticus-in-adults-management?search=treating%20seizure%20emergency&source=search_result&selectedTitle=2~150&usage_type=default&display_rank=2 (accessed on August 13, 2022).

Vegan Athletes

5

Special Considerations for the Vegan Athlete

António Pedro Mendes, Francisco Pereira, and Vítor Hugo Teixeira

5.1 Introduction

A growing interest in vegetarian (including vegan) diets, not only due to sustainability, health, or animal welfare reasons but also due to some allegations of performance enhancement in the athletic population [1], has led to an increase in research around this topic. Although there are no absolute data, it is estimated that the prevalence of vegetarians in sport is growing. Seven % of athletes competing in the Commonwealth Games in Delhi were vegetarian and 1% were vegan [2]. Unpublished data indicate about 5% of Portuguese Crossfit® athletes ($n = 1007$) practice some type of vegetarian diet, with 2.4% lacto-ovo-vegetarians, 0.9% ovo-vegetarians, and 1.2% vegetarians.

A. P. Mendes (✉)
Physical Performance Unit, Sporting Clube de Portugal, Estrada da Malhada de Meias, Alcochete, Portugal

F. Pereira
Medical Department, UAE Football Association, Dubai, United Arab Emirates

V. H. Teixeira
Research Centre in Physical Activity, Health and Leisure, CIAFEL, Faculty of Sport, University of Porto, Porto, Portugal

Laboratory for Integrative and Translational Research in Population Health (ITR), Porto, Portugal

Faculty of Nutrition and Food Sciences, FCNAUP, University of Porto, Porto, Portugal

Futebol Clube do Porto, Porto, Portugal

Although some possible benefits of adopting vegetarian diets have been described, the results are controversial [3]. A meta-analysis of observational studies points out that vegetarian diets reduced the risk of mortality from ischemic heart disease by 25% and the incidence of cancer by 8%, with no impact on total mortality, cardiovascular mortality, and cancer mortality [4]. On the other hand, vegetarian and vegan diets are associated with lower bone mineral density, and vegans have a higher fracture risk than omnivores [5].

According to a systematic review, a vegetarian diet is characterized by a lower intake of energy, protein, saturated and monounsaturated fats, some vitamins (B12, B3, B2, and D), and minerals (iron, zinc, calcium, selenium, iodine, and potassium), by an increased intake of carbohydrates and fiber and polyunsaturated fat [6]. Considering this and other similar information from other authors [3, 5], we have designed a figure summarizing the potential risk of increased or decreased intake of specific nutrients (Fig. 5.1).

It is still unclear whether adopting a vegetarian diet interferes with sports performance. Scientific research has yet failed to show the robust difference in physical performance between diets. A review indicates that it is potentially advantageous for endurance performance and potentially disadvantageous for strength performance [7].

S. Rocha Piedade et al. (eds.), *Sideline Management in Sports*,
https://doi.org/10.1007/978-3-031-33867-0_5

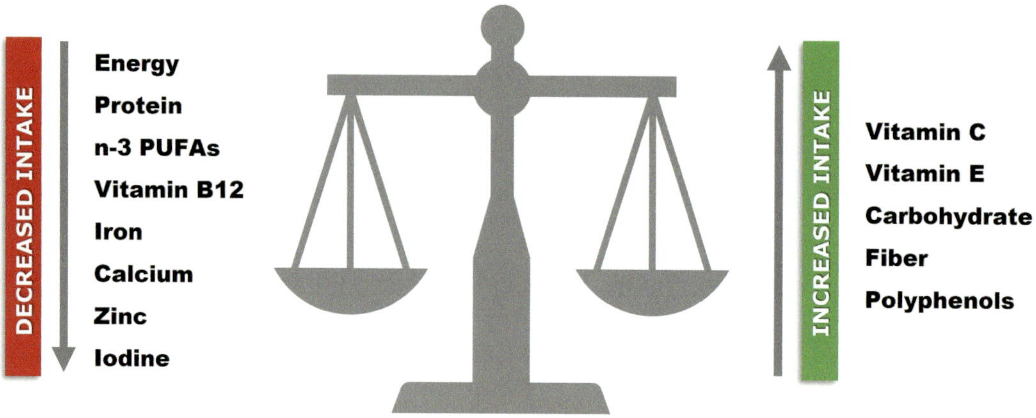

Fig. 5.1 Potential risk of increased or decreased nutrients intake in vegan diets

In this chapter, we discuss the nutritional specifications and recommendations for those adopting (or who are prone to adopt) a vegan dietary pattern.

5.2 Energy

For most athletes, a well-planned diet is expected to provide sufficient energy to achieve energy balance. However, data suggest that a chronically state of energy deficiency is common, namely in athletes participating in endurance, weight-making, and aesthetic sports (e.g., dancing, gymnastics, combat sports) [8].

When it comes to vegan athletes, this issue is likely to be compounded even further due to the high fiber and low energy density of plant-based diets, resulting in early satiation and reduced appetite, ultimately leading to a lower energy intake to support energy expenditure from training [9]. Although these factors might be helpful for weight loss purposes, some athletes can find it difficult to obtain an adequate energy balance, particularly during high-volume training phases or, for example, in the context of hectic travel schedules [10]. This might explain the fact that vegans tend to consume less energy than omnivores, which is likely to be exacerbated by a poorly constructed diet [11, 12]. As a result, athletes who do not meet their respective energy requirements may experience performance and/or recovery impairments. Health consequences such as weight loss, low bone mass, chronic fatigue, and illness can also occur and lead to time off from training and competition [8, 10].

When an increase in energy intake is necessary, increasing feeding frequency, limiting fiber-rich foods and increasing the consumption of energy-dense foods, such as oils, nuts and seeds, is helpful to ensure energetic goals are met [13, 14]. In this sense, the knowledge and capability to plan and compose a diet, especially with major food restrictions, allow dietitians to tailor energy and nutrient requirements for performance while impacting health [15, 16].

5.3 Protein

The adequacy of dietary protein in individuals pursuing a vegan diet has long been controversial, based on the extent of its restrictions, even though there is little evidence showing that the protein requirements of omnivorous athletes are any different from vegan athletes [17]. The latter, however, appear to consume less protein than their vegetarian and omnivorous counterparts, which suggests that a vegan diet may require special considerations, especially when it comes to the quality and quantity of the protein consumed [18, 19].

Most animal-based proteins, such as milk, eggs, meat, poultry, and fish, are typically considered complete protein sources, as they contain all the essential amino acids [20]. Plant proteins, on the contrary, are generally deficient in one or more specific amino acids, namely essential amino acids, such as leucine, which appear to be the primary trigger for muscle protein synthesis and play an important role in promoting recovery and adaptation to exercise [21]. Furthermore, plant-based proteins present a lower digestibility and a higher splanchnic extraction [22].

Increasing daily protein intake to compensate for either a specific amino acid deficiency or the lower essential amino acid content should, theoretically, improve the post-prandial protein synthetic response [23]. However, this increase may not always be feasible when it comes to plant-based foods, because their lower protein density would significantly increase both the total energetic content and volume of food that would need to be consumed [24]. From this perspective, supplementing with plant-based proteins might be interesting, particularly if achieving sufficient protein through wholefoods turns out to be difficult or inconvenient with the added benefit of having a high digestibility (>90%) [25].

An alternative strategy to increase the anabolic potential of a plant-based protein could be mixing complementary protein types and/or sources to provide a complete, or at least a more balanced profile, of all essential amino acids [26]. For example, lysine is often limiting in grain proteins, but those are good sources of methionine. On the other hand, legumes are often rich in lysine but are poor in methionine. Combining these two foods would secure the requirements for both types of essential amino acids [27]. Combining complementary plant-based proteins is an easier strategy to implement than eating more of the same protein because it lowers the amount of protein needed to reach an optimal amino acid profile [28]. This illustrates that a well-balanced and planned vegan diet can satisfactorily supply the protein needs of most athletes, securing long-term adequacy.

5.4 n-3 Fatty Acids

Dietary n-3 polyunsaturated fatty acids (PUFAs) have been proposed to be advantageous for athletes due to important health and performance implications. This claim is predicated on the fact that they exert anti-inflammatory properties, which change the functional capacity of the muscle by modifying the fluidity and permeability of the cell membrane [29]. This ability has been shown to play a role in improving training adaptation, exercise recovery, and subsequent performance across different athletic populations [29].

The most beneficial n-3 fatty acids, eicosapentaenoic acid (EPA) and docosahexaenoic acid (DHA), are mainly obtained from marine-sourced fats in the diet [30]. Thus, by excluding fish and other seafood, the intake of these fatty acids is virtually absent in vegan diets, which explains the lower serum levels comparing to omnivores [11].

Recommendations for plant-based foods containing the most prevalent omega-3 fatty acid in plants—alpha-linolenic acid (ALA)—do also appear. Nevertheless, in humans, this fatty acid can only be converted to EPA and DHA at ~8% and 0.5% efficiency, respectively [31]. This inefficient conversion rate is partly attributed to the amount of n-6 PUFAs in the diet, commonly found in vegetable oils like sunflower, corn, and safflower oils which limits EPA and DHA formation [30].

In order to optimize the conversion of ALA to EPA and DHA, it is advised to limit the intake of omega-6 containing oils and margarines and regularly include good sources of ALA in the diet such as flax seeds, walnuts, and chia seeds [27, 32]. Supplements that may raise both blood EPA and DHA levels can also be considered [33]. This may help to improve health, concurrently with any performance-enhancing effect that augmented n-3 PUFAs diets can offer to athletes.

5.5 Iron

Iron status is of particular importance for athletes due to the effects of increased physical activity on iron homeostasis [34]. Iron-deficiency anemia is caused by the insufficient iron consumption or absorption, leading to symptoms like tiredness and fatigue, weakness, and reduced exercise tolerance. Iron deficiency without anemia has also been shown to reduce endurance capacity, increase energy expenditure, and impair adaptation to endurance exercise [35].

The increased iron loss in some sports is well known, mainly due to gastrointestinal bleeding, heavy sweating, hemolysis, and, in women, menstruation [34]. Indeed, research into the iron status of vegan individuals suggests that women have lower iron stores than men [36, 37].

Adopting a vegan diet does not necessarily imply a low iron intake, given the inclusion of iron-rich foods, such as legumes, integral cereals, nuts, and leafy green vegetables. In fact, they generally contain as much total iron as omnivore diets [18]. But concerns over iron status are usually based on the bioavailability of iron from plant-based foods rather than the amount of total iron present in the diet itself [38]. Actually, vegetarian and vegan have lower ferritin levels compared to omnivorous adults [39].

The only source of iron in the vegan diet is found in the non-heme form, which is less bioavailable than the heme form found in animal products [40]. Moreover, vegan diets commonly contain high amounts of dietary compounds that reduce the amount of absorbed iron, such as polyphenols (found in coffee, tea, cocoa), phytates (present in whole grains and legumes), and calcium (found in some vegetables) [25]. Because vitamin C is the main enhancing factor for non-heme iron absorption, this inhibitory effect could be improved by the parallel consumption of vitamin C-rich foods [22, 25].

Vegan athletes are, therefore, advised to achieve iron sufficiency by selecting wholefood iron sources, reducing the ingestion of inhibitor-containing ingredients when eating iron-rich meals, and, concurrently, consuming vitamin C-containing foods to enhance absorption [25]. If these strategies are not enough to normalize iron stores, supplementation needs must be considered [39].

5.6 Calcium

Calcium plays an important role in many cellular processes, as an adequate intake is necessary for nerve transmission, blood clotting, vitamin D metabolism, muscle stimulation, and maintaining bone structure [41]. It is present in a wide range of foods, most notably dairy products (milk, cheese, yogurt), and despite being also found in appreciable amounts in plant-based sources, data indicate that vegans consume less calcium than omnivores and vegetarians [42].

When in a state of deficiency, the body vigorously defends serum calcium concentrations through the demineralization of bone, which, in turn, leads to a reduction in bone mass over time [43]. In fact, vegan individuals with a low calcium intake have been shown to have a higher risk of bone fractures, which reflects its role in the maintenance of skeletal health during exercise [6, 44].

Athletes that follow a vegan diet are advised to consume calcium-rich sources in sufficient amounts to achieve the 1000 mg/day recommendation [41]. Vegetables like broccoli and kale or calcium-fortified soy, fruit juices, and some grains are also widely available as they represent a readily absorbable form of this nutrient [25]. It should be noticed, however, that green vegetables such as spinach, chard, and arugula contain oxalate, which may limit calcium bioavailability [45]. Thus, vegans should prioritize plant sources with low oxalate levels when designing calcium-rich diets [25].

Because of the variety of plant foods that are naturally good sources of calcium, as well as the growing number of fortified products, it is increasingly easier for vegans to meet calcium requirements, as long as they are given appropriate information and guidance [6].

5.7 Vitamin B12

Vitamin B12, also known as cobalamin, is essential for normal nervous system function and DNA synthesis. Insufficient levels can lead to morphological changes in blood cells and the development of hematological and neurological symptoms [25]. It is synthesized from anaerobic microorganisms in the rumen of cattle and sheep [46]. Humans typically consume preformed cobalamin from animal products, which are the only source of this vitamin in the diet (e.g., dairy, poultry, and meat) [46]. Contrarily, no plant food has ever been shown to contain vitamin B12 consistently unless it has been contaminated, for example, by manure. Being the consumption of animal foods absent in vegans, its introduction is essential, either through supplements or fortified foods [32].

When there is no intake, vitamin B12 body stores last longer than any other essential nutrient [46]. However, signs of deficiency have been detected in adults within 2 years of beginning a vegan diet, suggesting it is important for vegan athletes to use reliable sources of vitamin B12 regularly regardless of the duration of the diet [47, 48]. Fortified cereals or nutritional yeast are some examples of vitamin B12 sources, and their consumption may be useful in preventing deficiency, overcoming the frequent ideological barriers to supplementation. Nevertheless, supplements have been recognized as efficient in restoring vitamin B12 blood concentration, preferably when using high bioavailability forms like methylcobalamin [49, 50].

5.8 Zinc

Zinc is an essential micronutrient, extensively involved in cell growth, repair and protein, and metabolism [51]. Its relevance in numerous biological processes suggests that it warrants special attention when evaluating the nutritional adequacy of vegan diets for athletes [52].

Animal products, particularly meat and dairy, are the main sources of this mineral, as they provide 50–70% of total zinc intake in the omnivore diet [18]. Thus, excluding the above-referred foods may be the one of the reasons for the frequent zinc deficiencies found in vegan athletes (3). However, zinc intake among vegans can be suboptimal not only due to the exclusion of animal products but also due to bioavailability issues [53]. As seen with iron, this mineral is widely spread in plant-based foods (e.g., legumes, whole grains, nuts, seeds, and soy), but its absorption may also be impaired by phytate—a potent zinc inhibitor [54]. Exercise itself can also contribute to zinc deficiency by increasing sweat loss and zinc redistribution between plasma and erythrocytes [54].

In order to satisfy zinc needs, athletes should look to consume foods like pumpkin seeds, hemp, nuts, beans, and other grains. Adopting processing methods like leavening bread, fermenting, and sprouting nuts and grains can also reduce phytate levels and increase zinc bioavailability [55].

The Institute of Medicine has, therefore, suggested that vegans/vegetarians might need to consume up to 50% more zinc than nonvegetarians owing to its poor bioavailability [56].

The knowledge about dietary factors that inhibit zinc absorption is essential when designing strategies to improve bioavailability in vulnerable individuals [51]. If for some reason, this is not achievable, supplementation should be considered.

5.9 The Special Cases for Creatine and Beta-Alanine

Creatine supplementation in sports has been a topic of research for the last decades, and results confirm it as one of the most interesting dietary supplements to be used, not only in assisting performance enhancement but also in recovery [57].

Although muscle creatine stores are not fully saturated in individuals who are not supplementing, vegan athletes are particularly prone to have lower levels [58, 59]. Since creatine is only found in animal products, vegan individuals depend totally on endogenous synthesis, which may be below optimal levels [25].

Data regarding an increased potential for creatine supplementation benefit in vegetarian or vegan athletes is controversial, although it seems that vegan athletes may achieve higher levels of creatine and phosphocreatine after supplementation compared to omnivores [60]. The only study using athletes was performed by Burke et al., although recreational level individuals were enrolled. This study found an ergogenic effect of creatine during resistance training and suggested that vegetarian athletes might be more responsive to supplementation [58].

Creatine has also been particularly studied for its impact on brain function, which is crucial, through different pathways, for athletic performance. Although brain creatine content is similar between omnivorous and vegetarians [61], the latter appear to benefit more from creatine supplementation, with a greater memory and intelligence enhancement [62, 63].

Beta-alanine is a nonproteinogenic amino acid which combines with histidine to form carnosine, an important acid buffer. Beta-alanine supplementation has been shown to improve performance in exercises lasting from 30 s to 10 min [64]. Since carnosine is abundant in beef and other animal sources [65], dietary choices can influence carnosine levels in the long term. In line with this, vegetarians have been found to have a lower carnosine content of 26% in gastrocnemius compared to omnivores [66]. This leads to a theoretical advantage of using beta-alanine in the vegan population, although unfortunately there are no published articles comparing beta-alanine supplementation on performance enhancement in vegetarians.

5.10 Conclusion

Vegan diets seem to be a valid option for athletes, if an adequate dietary planning is performed. Individuals adopting this dietary pattern seem to have a lower energy intake, as well as protein, n-3 PUFAs, iron, zinc, calcium, and vitamin B12, as well as some absorption issues in some of them. On the other hand, vegan diets tend to be richer in antioxidant substances (such as vitamin C and E), fiber, and carbohydrate. Nonetheless, an adequate selection of foods and dietary supplements allows achieving the needs of athletes, while providing important nutrients for performance enhancement. Further research focused on athletic populations is needed, leading to a clarification of some of the queries still remaining.

References

1. Rosenfeld DL. Why some choose the vegetarian option: are all ethical motivations the same? Motiv Emot. 2019;43:400–11.
2. Pelly FE, Burkhart SJ. Dietary regimens of athletes competing at the Delhi 2010 Commonwealth Games. Int J Sport Nutr Exerc Metab. 2014;24(1):28–36. https://doi.org/10.1123/ijsnem.2013-0023.
3. Devrim-Lanpir A, Hill L, Knechtle B. Efficacy of popular diets applied by endurance athletes on sports performance: beneficial or detrimental? A narrative review. Nutrients. 2021;13(2):491. https://doi.org/10.3390/nu13020491.
4. Dinu M, Abbate R, Gensini GF, Casini A, Sofi F. Vegetarian, vegan diets and multiple health outcomes: a systematic review with meta-analysis of observational studies. Crit Rev Food Sci Nutr. 2017;57(17):3640–9. https://doi.org/10.1080/10408398.2016.1138447.
5. Iguacel I, Miguel-Berges ML, Gómez-Bruton A, Moreno LA, Julián C. Veganism, vegetarianism, bone mineral density, and fracture risk: a systematic review and meta-analysis. Nutr Rev. 2019;77(1):1–18. https://doi.org/10.1093/nutrit/nuy045.
6. Bakaloudi DR, Halloran A, Rippin HL, Oikonomidou AC, Dardavesis TI, Williams J, Wickramasinghe K, Breda J, Chourdakis M. Intake and adequacy of the vegan diet. A systematic review of the evidence. Clin Nutr. 2021;40(5):3503–21. https://doi.org/10.1016/j.clnu.2020.11.035.
7. Pohl A, Schünemann F, Bersiner K, Gehlert S. The impact of vegan and vegetarian diets on physical performance and molecular signaling in skeletal muscle. Nutrients. 2021;13(11):3884. https://doi.org/10.3390/nu13113884.
8. Loucks AB. Energy balance and body composition in sports and exercise. J Sports Sci. 2004;22(1):1–14.
9. Wirnitzer K. Vegan diet in sports and exercise—health benefits and advantages to athletes and physically active people: a narrative review. Int J Sports Exerc Med. 2020;6:65. https://doi.org/10.23937/2469-5718/1510165.
10. Potgieter S. Sport nutrition: a review of the latest guidelines for exercise and sport nutrition from the American College of Sport Nutrition, the International Olympic Committee and the International Society for Sports Nutrition. S Afr J Clin Nutr. 2013;26(1):6–16.
11. Clarys P, Deliens T, Huybrechts I, Deriemaeker P, Vanaelst B, De Keyzer W, et al. Comparison of nutritional quality of the vegan, vegetarian, semi-vegetarian, pesco-vegetarian and omnivorous diet. Nutrients. 2014;6(3):1318–32.
12. Bratland-Sanda S, Sundgot-Borgen J. Eating disorders in athletes: overview of prevalence, risk factors and recommendations for prevention and treatment. Eur J Sport Sci. 2013;13(5):499–508.
13. La Bounty PM, Campbell BI, Wilson J, Galvan E, Berardi J, Kleiner SM, et al. International Society of Sports Nutrition position stand: meal frequency. J Int Soc Sports Nutr. 2011;8:4–4.
14. Drewnowski A, Almiron-Roig E, Marmonier C, Lluch A. Dietary energy density and body weight: is there a relationship? Nutr Rev. 2004;62(11):403.
15. Durkalec-Michalski K, Domagalski A, Główka N, Kamińska J, Szymczak D, Podgórski T. Effect of a

four-week vegan diet on performance, training efficiency and blood biochemical indices in crossfit-trained participants. Nutrients. 2022;14(4):894. https://doi.org/10.3390/nu14040894.
16. Barnard ND, Goldman DM, Loomis JF, Kahleova H, Levin SM, Neabore S, Batts TC. Plant-based diets for cardiovascular safety and performance in endurance sports. Nutrients. 2019;11:130.
17. Vitale K, Hueglin S. Update on vegetarian and vegan athletes: a review. J Phys Fitness Sports Med. 2021;2021(10):1–11. https://doi.org/10.7600/jpfsm.10.1.
18. Venderley A, Campbell W. Vegetarian diets. Sports Med. 2006;36(4):293–305.
19. Phillips SM. The impact of protein quality on the promotion of resistance exercise- induced changes in muscle mass. Nutr Metab. 2016;13(1):1–9.
20. Bradbury KE, Tong TYN, Key TJ. Dietary intake of high-protein foods and other major foods in meat-eaters, poultry-eaters, fish-eaters, vegetarians, and vegans in UK biobank. Nutrients. 2017;9:1317.
21. Columbus DA, Fiorotto ML, Davis TA. Leucine is a major regulator of muscle protein synthesis in neonates. Amino Acids. 2015;47(2):259–70. https://doi.org/10.1007/s00726-014-1866-0.
22. Desbrow B, Burd NA, Tarnopolsky M, Moore DR, Elliott-Sale KJ. Nutrition for special populations: young, female, and masters athletes. Int J Sport Nutr Exerc Metab. 2019;29(2):220–7. https://doi.org/10.1123/ijsnem.2018-0269.
23. Trommelen J, Holwerda AM, Pinckaers PJM, Van Loon LJC. Comprehensive assessment of post-prandial protein handling by the application of intrinsically labelled protein in vivo in human subjects. Proc Nutr Soc. 2021;80(2):221–9.
24. Pinckaers PJM, Trommelen J, Snijders T, van Loon LJC. The anabolic response to plant-based protein ingestion. Sports Med. 2021;51(Suppl. 1):59–74. https://doi.org/10.1007/s40279-021-01540-8.
25. Rogerson D. Vegan diets: practical advice for athletes and exercisers. J Int Soc Sports Nutr. 2017;14:36. https://doi.org/10.1186/s12970-017-0192-9.
26. Berning J. The vegetarian athlete. In: Maughan RJ, editor. Nutrition in sport. Oxford: Blackwell Science; 2000. p. 442–56.
27. Phillips F. Vegetarian nutrition. Nutr Bull. 2005;30(2):132–67.
28. Woolf PJ, Fu LL, Basu A. vProtein: identifying optimal amino acid complements from plant-based foods. PLoS One. 2011;6(4):e18836. https://doi.org/10.1371/journal.pone.0018836.
29. Philpott JD, Witard OC, Galloway SDR. Applications of omega-3 polyunsaturated fatty acid supplementation for sport performance. Res Sports Med. 2019;27(2):219–37. https://doi.org/10.1080/15438627.2018.1550401.
30. Lane KE, Wilson M, Hellon TG, Davies IG. Bioavailability and conversion of plant based sources of omega-3 fatty acids—a scoping review to update supplementation options for vegetarians and vegans. Crit Rev Food Sci Nutr. 2021;2021(62):1–16. https://doi.org/10.1080/10408398.2021.1880364.
31. Williams CM, Burdge G. Long-chain n-3 PUFA: plant vs. marine sources. Proc Nutr Soc. 2006;65(1):42–50. https://doi.org/10.1079/pns2005473.
32. Craig WJ. Health effects of vegan diets. Am J Clin Nutr. 2009;89(5):1627S–33S.
33. Conquer JA, Holub BJ. Supplementation with an algae source of docosahexaenoic acid increases (n-3) fatty acid status and alters selected risk factors for heart disease in vegetarian subjects. J Nutr. 1996;126(12):3032.
34. Clénin G, Cordes M, Huber A, Schumacher YO, Noack P, Scales J, Kriemler S. Iron deficiency in sports—definition, influence on performance and therapy. Swiss Med Wkly. 2015;145:w14196. https://doi.org/10.4414/smw.2015.14196.
35. Burden RJ, Morton K, Richards T, Whyte GP, Pedlar CR. Is iron treatment beneficial in iron- deficient but non-anaemic (IDNA) endurance athletes? A systematic review and meta-analysis. Br J Sports Med. 2015;49(21):1389–97.
36. Borrione P, Grasso L, Quaranta F, et al. Vegetarian diet and athletes. Sportmed Präventivmed. 2009;39:20–4. https://doi.org/10.1007/s12534-009-0017-y.
37. Waldmann A, Koschizke JW, Leitzmann C, Hahn A. Dietary iron intake and iron status of German female vegans: results of the German vegan study. Ann Nutr Metab. 2004;48(2):103.
38. Longo DL, Camaschella C. Iron-deficiency anemia. N Engl J Med. 2015;372(19):1832–43.
39. Hunt JR. Bioavailability of iron, zinc, and other trace minerals from vegetarian diets. Am J Clin Nutr. 2003;78(Suppl. 3):633S–9S.
40. Haider LM, Schwingshackl L, Hoffmann G, Ekmekcioglu C. The effect of vegetarian diets on iron status in adults: a systematic review and meta-analysis. Crit Rev Food Sci Nutr. 2018;58(8):1359–74. https://doi.org/10.1080/10408398.2016.1259210. Epub 2017 Jul 5
41. Ross AC, Taylor CL, Yaktine AL, Del Valle HB, Institute of Medicine (US), editors. Committee to review dietary reference intakes for vitamin D and calcium. Washington (DC): National Academies Press (US); 2011.
42. Davey GK, Spencer EA, Appleby PN, Allen NE, Knox KH, Key TJ. EPIC–Oxford: lifestyle characteristics and nutrient intakes in a cohort of 33 883 meat-eaters and 31 546 non-meat eaters in the UK. Public Health Nutr. 2003;6(3):259–68.
43. Weaver CM. Nutrition and bone health. Oral Dis. 2017;23(4):412–5. https://doi.org/10.1111/odi.12515.
44. Ho-Pham L, Nguyen N, Nguyen T. Effect of vegetarian diets on bone mineral density: a Bayesian meta-analysis. Am J Clin Nutr. 2009;90(4):943.
45. Heaney RP, Weaver CM, Fitzsimmons ML, Recker RR. Calcium absorptive consistency. J Bone Miner Res. 1990;5(11):1139–42.
46. Truswell AS. Vitamin B12. Nutr Diet. 2007;64(s4):S120–5.

47. Crane MG, Register UD, Lukens RH, Gregory R. Cobalamin (CBL) studies on two total vegetarian (vegan) families. Vegetarian Nutr. 1998;2:87–92.
48. Donaldson MS. Metabolic vitamin B(12) status on a mostly raw vegan diet with follow-up using tablets, nutritional yeast, or probiotic supplements. Ann Nutr Metab. 2000;44(5–6):229–34.
49. VanDusseldorp M, Schneede J, Refsum H, Ueland PM, Thomas CM, deBoer E, vanStaveren WA. Risk of persistent cobalamin deficiency in adolescents fed a macrobiotic diet in early life. Am J Clin Nutr. 1999;69:664–71.
50. Pawlak R, Babatunde SELT. The prevalence of cobalamin deficiency among vegetarians assessed by serum vitamin B12: a review of literature. Eur J Clin Nutr. 2016;70(7):866.
51. Lönnerdal B. Dietary factors influencing zinc absorption. J Nutr. 2000;130(Suppl. 5S):1378S–83S. https://doi.org/10.1093/jn/130.5.1378S.
52. Foster M, Chu A, Petocz P, Samman S. Effect of vegetarian diets on zinc status: a systematic review and meta-analysis of studies in humans. J Sci Food Agric. 2013;93(10):2362–71. https://doi.org/10.1002/jsfa.6179.
53. Micheletti A, Rossi R, Rufini S. Zinc status in athletes: relation to diet and exercise. Sports Med. 2001;31(8):577–82. https://doi.org/10.2165/00007256-200131080-00002.
54. Hunt J. Moving toward a plant- based diet: are iron and zinc at risk? Nutr Rev. 2002;60(5):127–34.
55. Fuhrman J, Ferreri DM. Fueling the vegetarian (vegan) athlete. Curr Sports Med Rep. 2010;9(4):233–41.
56. Institute of Medicine (US). Panel on micronutrients. Dietary reference intakes for vitamin A, vitamin K, arsenic, boron, chromium, Copper, iodine, iron, manganese, molybdenum, nickel, silicon, vanadium, and zinc. Washington, DC: National Academies Press (US); 2001.
57. Hall M, Manetta E, Tupper K. Creatine supplementation: an update. Curr Sports Med Rep. 2021;20(7):338–44. https://doi.org/10.1249/JSR.0000000000000863.
58. Burke DG, Chilibeck PD, Parise G, Candow DG, Mahoney D, Tarnopolsky M. Effect of creatine and weight training on muscle creatine and performance in vegetarians. Med Sci Sports Exerc. 2003;35:1946–55.
59. Brosnan ME, Brosnan JT. The role of dietary creatine. Amino Acids. 2016;48:1785–91.
60. Kaviani M, Shaw K, Chilibeck PD. Benefits of creatine supplementation for vegetarians compared to omnivorous athletes: a systematic review. Int J Environ Res Public Health. 2020;17(9):3041. https://doi.org/10.3390/ijerph17093041.
61. Solis MY, Artioli GG, Otaduy MCG, Leite CDC, Arruda W, Veiga RR, Gualano B. Effect of age, diet, and tissue type on PCr response to creatine supplementation. J Appl Physiol (1985). 2017;123(2):407–14. https://doi.org/10.1152/japplphysiol.00248.2017.
62. Benton D, Donohoe R. The influence of creatine supplementation on the cognitive functioning of vegetarians and omnivores. Br J Nutr. 2011;105(7):1100–5. https://doi.org/10.1017/S0007114510004733.
63. Rae C, Digney AL, McEwan SR, Bates TC. Oral creatine monohydrate supplementation improves brain performance: a double-blind, placebo-controlled, cross-over trial. Proc Biol Sci. 2003;270(1529):2147–50. https://doi.org/10.1098/rspb.2003.2492.
64. Saunders B, Elliott-Sale K, Artioli GG, Swinton PA, Dolan E, Roschel H, Sale C, Gualano B. β-alanine supplementation to improve exercise capacity and performance: a systematic review and meta-analysis. Br J Sports Med. 2017;51(8):658–69. https://doi.org/10.1136/bjsports-2016-096396.
65. Wu G. Important roles of dietary taurine, creatine, carnosine, anserine and 4-hydroxyproline in human nutrition and health. Amino Acids. 2020;52(3):329–60. https://doi.org/10.1007/s00726-020-02823-6.
66. Everaert I, Mooyaart A, Baguet A, Zutinic A, Baelde H, Achten E, Taes Y, De Heer E, Derave W. Vegetarianism, female gender and increasing age, but not CNDP1 genotype, are associated with reduced muscle carnosine levels in humans. Amino Acids. 2011;40(4):1221–9. https://doi.org/10.1007/s00726-010-0749-2.

Part II

Evaluation and Management of Sports Trauma/Injury

Initial Assessment of the Injured Athlete

6

Sérgio Rocha Piedade, Alban Pinaroli, Ivan Córcoles Martínez, André Pedrinelli, and Daniel Miranda Ferreira

6.1 Introduction

Dreams and challenges drive athletes to push their body's limits to achieve better results and sports performance. Although it could be exciting for the athletes, in some circumstances, this condition may create a scenario for injuries during training or competition. In sports practice, traumatic injuries are prevalent, but clinical disorders could also affect the athlete's health.

Sports differ according to the rules, the field of play, indoors or outdoors, sports modality, age of participants, recreative or competitive experience, physical demand, and competition level. In addition, the mechanism and energy of trauma in a particular anatomical location could cause specific sports injuries.

Moreover, sports injuries may differ in severity according to the involved anatomical site, mechanism of injury, and trauma energy. Thus, the sports medicine physician should pay careful attention to the head, neck, chest, and abdominal and musculoskeletal injuries and also to the athlete's previous health conditions (syncope, hypoglycemia, epilepsy, and heart problems.)

In sports, medical assistance is generally carried out outside the hospital, and fortunately, most of the times, it involves minor clinical complaints and/or orthopedic problems, acute or chronic ones. However, the sports physician should be well-prepared to manage major clinical events that can also occur in training or competitions. At the same time, environmental conditions such as hot or cold temperatures could expose the athlete's physical and mental distress resulting in systemic disorders such as dehydration, hypothermia, exertional heat stroke, and the overwhelming condition of sudden cardiac arrest.

This chapter explores the assessment and initial treatment of some specific indoor and outdoor sports injuries and clinical conditions in athletes, such as facial injuries, knockout event, syncope, upper and lower limb injuries, water events, and red flags.

S. R. Piedade (✉)
Exercise and Sports Medicine, Department of Orthopedics, Rheumatology, and Traumatology, University of Campinas, UNICAMP, Campinas, SP, Brazil
e-mail: piedade@unicamp.br

A. Pinaroli
Medipôle de Savoie, Chambéry, France

I. C. Martínez
Private Practice at Hospital Viamed Monegal, Tarragona, Spain

A. Pedrinelli
Department of Orthopedics, University of São Paulo—USP, São Paulo, Brazil

D. M. Ferreira
Department of Radiology, University of Campinas—UNICAMP, Campinas, SP, Brazil

São Leopoldo Mandic, Faculty of Medicine, Campinas, SP, Brazil

S. Rocha Piedade et al. (eds.), *Sideline Management in Sports*,
https://doi.org/10.1007/978-3-031-33867-0_6

6.2 Medical Bag

Even though the medical bag could have a standard arrangement with the same drugs, braces, and immobilizers, the sports physician should establish their medical planning according to the sports modality event, sports-related injuries, field of play, weather conditions, and athlete's health condition and medical history (Fig. 6.1). Therefore, it is essential to define competencies, know the operational flow, and register the necessary contacts for emergencies/needs for a good working plan. Also, the size and composition of the delegation are relevant to guide the quantity and type of drugs and materials needed as well as the duration of the trip and competition [1, 2].

These points will allow the sports medicine physician to have equipment suitable for working conditions and sufficiently equipped to treat and stabilize an injured athlete before transferring to an ambulance or hospital. In clinical practice, it implies the use of three types of medical bags: the individual bag (for immediate use), the bag/suitcase itself (immediate use at the edge of the field), and a locker room/center of training [1].

6.3 Sports Trauma Injuries

6.3.1 Head And Facial Trauma

The physician should be aware that high-kinetic facial trauma may cause substantial soft tissue and bone injury and, consequently, airway obstruction. Therefore, in severe facial injuries, the initial assessment begins by assessing the athlete's airway, breathing, circulation, neurological status, and careful attention to stabilization of the cervical spine. Therefore, the initial assessment of the injured athlete is critical for the physician to analyze the need of transferring the athlete to a hospital for intensive care. In more severe trauma injuries, the ABCDE trauma protocol plays an important role to organize this initial approach, reducing time interval to definitive care and minimizing the risk of undiscovered injuries [3] (Table 6.1).

Table 6.1 ABCDE trauma protocol

ABCDE trauma protocol	
A	Airway maintenance with cervical spine protection
B	Breathing and ventilation
C	Circulation with hemorrhage control
D	Disability (neurologic assessment)
E	Exposure and environment

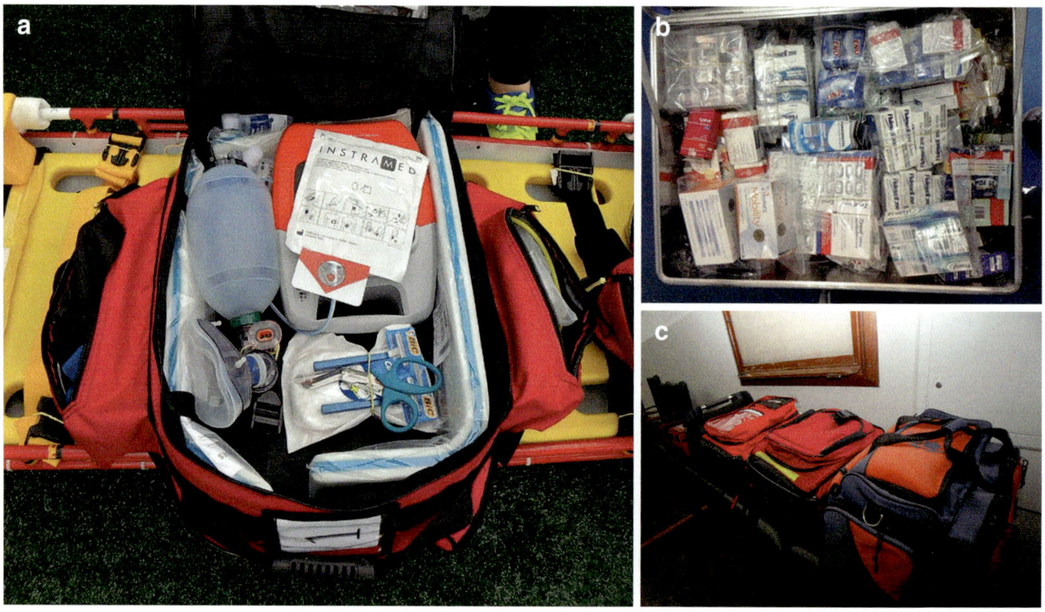

Fig. 6.1 Medical sports bags showing event medical kit (**a**), medical supplies (**b**), and examples of medical bags (**c**)

Although head and facial traumas are more prevalent in contact sports, they could happen in any sport and involve different mechanisms and energy of trauma [4]. Due to the similarity of the mechanism of sports trauma to the face, head, and cervical spine, the sports medicine physician should manage facial injuries with closer attention and careful assessment of the head and cervical spine status [5, 6]. In the initial evaluation of an injured athlete that had suffered a head or facial trauma, the sports medicine physician should be aware of the athlete's level of consciousness, briefing, and mental status. It is important to state that only the medical staff is authorized to move the injured athlete.

In most reported cases, the facial injury refers to minor skin abrasions and mild bleeding that are well-controlled by direct pressure and ice, followed by the athlete returning to the field of play. On the other hand, in combat sports, significant injuries result from blows (such as uppercuts, punches, and countercoups) and kicking to the head and face that could cause skin abrasions, facial cuts, contusions, and even facial bone fractures [7–10].

Under these circumstances, the physician should carefully assess the facial cuts and their localization, by gently palpating the facial bone with both hands to rule out any loss of bone integrity, abnormal mobility, severe local pain, and tenderness or bone cracking [11].

This clinical evaluation will help decide whether it is necessary to remove the fighter or athlete from the competition to avoid additional injuries and major complications. Figure 6.2 shows the danger zones related to facial cuts.

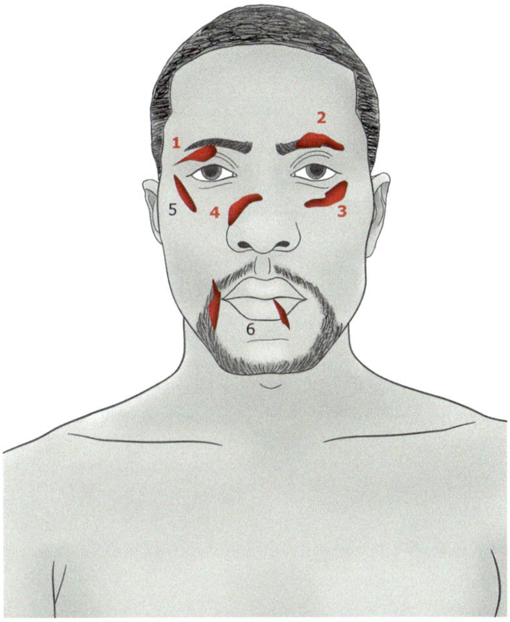

Fig. 6.2 Areas 1, 2, 3, and 4 showing facial cuts near the eye's medial aspect and the nose's bridge are binding sites because the injury can extend into the lacrimal tear duct. (Source: Mariana Percario Piedade)

Facial Cut Areas and Their Clinical Implications

- **1** (upper eyelid) **is a danger zone** because it can endanger the tarsal plate.
- **2 and 3** (supraorbital and infraorbital nerves) near the nasal lacrimal duct are considered **dangerous zones, and the fight should be stopped.**
- **4** (bridge of the nose) **assessment for an underlying open nasal fracture or injury to the boney orbit is mandatory.**
- **5 does not endanger vision, nor damage significant underlying structures** and rarely lead to long-term disability.
- **6** (vertical cuts) through the vermillion lip borders potentialize further tearing (precise sutures prevent future disfigurement).

Facial cuts near the medial aspect of the eye (orbit) and the bridge of the nose are critical because they can extend into the lacrimal tear duct, close to the surface. Therefore, only an expert should carry out the sutures because a deep suture could tie-off this duct and require further extensive reconstruction.

6.3.2 Eye Injury

6.3.2.1 Sports-Related Eye Injuries

Sports-related trauma remains a prevalent cause of ocular trauma, particularly in male adolescent athletes. Ocular trauma may result in the pathology of the ocular surface, adnexa, extraocular muscles, orbital walls, and eye and optic nerve. The sports medicine physician should be

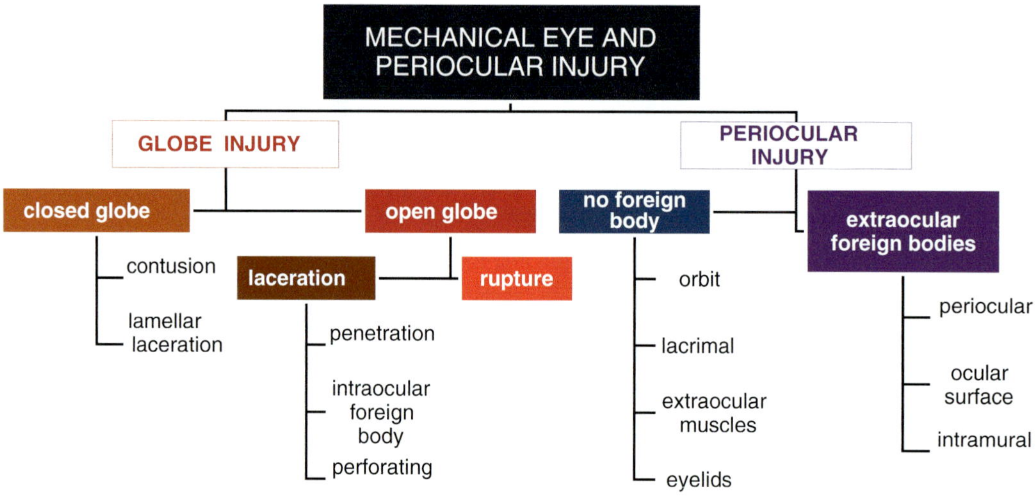

Fig. 6.3 A modified Birmingham Eye Trauma Terminology (BETT) classification [15]

able to identify important clinical signs and symptoms that can lead to lifelong ocular sequelae and the type of mechanical eye and periocular injury (Fig. 6.3) [12–14].

Eye Trauma Assessment

Visual acuity and fields, pupil symmetry and reflex, conjunctiva, cornea, and eyelids should be examined. Search for a foreign body and anterior chamber bleeding should be given special attention. It is important to determine whether a patient with ocular trauma can be reassured or requires immediate referral for further investigation and surgical repair (Table 6.2) [14].

Table 6.2 Red flags for ocular trauma requiring urgent referral to an ophthalmologist

Clinical signs and symptoms	Careful assessment to confirm the diagnosis
No or poor red reflex	Vitreous hemorrhage, retinal detachment
Relative afferent pupillary defect	Compromised optic nerve function by an orbital apex fracture and/or retrobulbar hemorrhage
Reduced vision	Corneal infection, hyphema, lens dislocation, vitreous hemorrhage, retinal detachment, optic nerve injury
Hypopyon	Endophthalmitis
Peaked, abnormally shaped pupil (corectopia) pointing toward the corneoscleral wound	Penetrating eye injury (iris prolapse) **in the case of a suspected penetrating injury, caution against measuring intraocular pressure**
Limbal whitening and large corneal epithelial defect	Limbal ischemia
Subconjunctival hemorrhage with conjunctival flap	Lamellar laceration or foreign body
Diplopia and proptosis	Medial orbital wall or inferior orbital floor blowout fracture
Proptosis/increased intraocular pressure	Retrobulbar hemorrhage **intraocular pressure—in case of preexisting glaucoma**

Adapted from Heath Jeffery RC, Dobes J, Chen FK (2022) Eye injuries: Understanding ocular trauma. Aust J Gen Pract 51:476–482

6.3.2.2 Ear Injuries

Even though ear injuries are not common in sports, these injuries could result in some vital function impairment to the athlete, such as hearing and balance [16, 17]. Therefore, the sports medicine physician should be prepared to manage these injuries, making a careful clinical evaluation and avoiding damage.

Ear Lacerations and Auricular Hematomas

These injuries result from dull and recurrent trauma on the ear's thin skin and subcutaneous tissue. Ear lacerations and auricular hematoma are commonly seen in combat sports, such as wrestling, judo, boxing, jiu-Jitsu, and water polo [17]. Lacerations bigger than 3 cm will probably need a graft to close the wound, while smaller than 2 cm could be repaired primarily.

In the case of an auricular hematoma, the main athlete's complaints are tenderness, swelling, pressure, and local pain. Early drainage performed within one or two days remains the best strategy for treatment [17, 18]. Even though returning to play can be immediate, the athlete should be advised to wear protective gear. In chronic cases, the ear may remind a cauliflower, the so-called cauliflower ear, resulting from the new fibrous cartilage and necrosis [18].

Otitis Externa

It results from an inflammatory or infectious process of the external auditory canal secondary to a cerumen disruption, water, high environmental temperature, or foreign objects, such as earplugs [17, 18]. The main complaints are discharged otalgia, and drainage from the ear (otorrhea) varies from gray to green in color. External hygiene and prescription of topical antibiotics, analgesics, and corticosteroids are the therapeutic approach. In most cases, the pathogens are covered by fluoroquinolones and steroids. The athlete should be away from the sports practice until the end of treatment that, in general, lasts 1 week.

6.4 Managing an Unconscious Athlete: Knockout X Syncope

Although semantically related, knockout and syncope are different clinical conditions.

6.5 Knockout

Facial and head trauma could make an athlete fall asleep or unconscious because of twisting or pulling the brain stem during the blow, while the rest of the brain shifts out of place—it breaks the brain circuits and shuts down parts of the brain—a knockout. Although knockout is commonly related to boxing, kickboxing, Muay thai, mixed martial arts, and karate, it could also occur in any sports involving facial or head trauma.

When a fighter suffers a knockout, it is essential to identify the primary mechanism of the knockout, such as the accumulation of blows, fatigue, or one solid punch on the head or body, and if there was a second one, such as the head hitting the canvas or ropes during the fighter falls.

The first measure is to certify how clear the airway is (tongue or turf, or any material is not preventing a clear airway) and whether the athlete is breathing spontaneously. In sports where the athlete wears a helmet, it should not be removed until a C injury is ruled out because its remotion could cause undesirable and deleterious movements to C spine. While mouthpieces could be removed when preventing the athlete's breathing, the helmet could be helpful to control C spine stabilization; then, an oral-pharyngeal airway or bag-valve mask is applied to offer oxygen.

In outdoor sports, an unconscious athlete should be removed from the field, immobilizing their C spine with a cervical collar and body stabilized in a rigid board, while in a ringside, the fighter's awaking and level of consciousness should be reassured before removing them to a private room for a complete evaluation.

6.6 Syncope in Athlete

Syncope is a transient loss of consciousness secondary to cerebral hypoperfusion and is followed by whole and spontaneous recovery. Although the leading cause of syncope in athletes is not related to cardiac etiology, an underlying cardiac disorder, metabolic disorders, ischemic events, or seizures should be ruled out. In clinical practice, it is essential to have close attention to the athlete's complaint of dizziness and weakness because it may present a presyncope that almost always could precede a loss of consciousness.

6.6.1 Classifying Syncope in an Athlete

The main point is to identify in which conditions the syncope occurred, such as non-related to exercise, post-exertional, or during physical exercise.

The non-related-to-exercise syncope is usually the most common presentation in more than 85% of cases, and involves a vasovagal mechanism triggered by changing from sitting to standing or could be related to distress such as fear and anxiety. In this type of syncope, the athlete may complain of dizziness, diaphoresis, warmth, nausea, or epigastric pain. Another point to consider is the **situational syncope** in which clinical conditions involving dehydration and reduced intravascular volume may result in orthostatic hypotension, manifested by many prodrome features similar to vasovagal syncope but without loss of consciousness.

The post-exertional syncope occurs mainly when an intense physical exercise is stopped abruptly, which results in postexercise hypotension. It occurs because the lower limb muscles pumping breaks, resulting in a reduced cardiac venous return and output. It is followed by an acute myocardial activity that could activate the cardiac depressor reflex that promotes bradycardia, and hypotension, termed the Bezold–Jarisch reflex—cardioprotective action, vasodilating the coronary arteries.

The syncope during physical exercise should be considered *a clinical event of high suspicion of structural heart disease*. Therefore, it raises more concerns about the athlete's health, such as an underlying heart disease that could precede a sudden cardiac arrest. Moreover, other cardiac disorders such as hypertrophic myocardiopathy, cardiac arrhythmias, myopathy, anomalous coronary artery, long QT syndrome, or Brugada syndrome should be carefully screened to be ruled out.

6.6.2 Assessing the Syncope in an Athlete

The assessment starts by defining the situations and timeline of how the syncope occurred. A patient's comprehensive history and physical exam are essential to decision-making for the best clinical approach. To rule out potential red flags often related to a cardiac disorder, the physician should always pay attention to the patient's symptoms and complaints, such as chest pain, diaphoresis, and shortness of breath.

Moreover, how the athlete recovers from the syncope could help to identify a specific disease. For example, an athlete presenting a myoclonic jerking associated with or not bladder or bowel incontinence may suggest a seizure. Besides that, the patient's social history is essential to assess the use of illicit recreational drugs or any other substance to enhance sports performance.

6.6.3 Heat Exhaustion and Heat Stroke

High environmental temperatures are an adverse condition to practice sports and vigorous physical activity, directly affecting athletes' sports performance and health. In the summer, endurance sports make athletes work close to their physical and mental body limits, predisposing them to heat exhaustion or even heat stroke.

Heat exhaustion may occur when the athlete's body temperature is normal or elevated but inferior to 40 °C. It is clinically manifested by fatigue, nausea and vomiting, shortness of breath, dizziness or syncope, and no mental distress. In comparison, heat stroke takes place when the athlete's body temperature rises to 40 °C or higher. It is more commonly reported in endurance sports associated with prolonged exposure to sun or heat during an athlete's vigorous physical exertion, particularly in the summer.

Initially, the athlete's skin becomes red, hot, dry or slightly moist, followed by headache, mental confusion, delirium, seizures, nausea and vomiting, and increased breathing and heart rate. Therefore, a sports medicine physician must be aware of heat stroke's initial symptoms because the persistence of this clinical picture causes rapid organ dysfunction, damaging the brain, heart, kidneys, and muscles and, in more severe cases, may evolute into a coma.

The immediate treatment focuses on cooling the overheated athlete, removing the excess of their clothes, applying ice packs and/or immerging them into cold water in a shower or bath, and using sponges and towels moistened with cold water on the head, neck, and arms, and groin. It is also vital to support airways, breathing, and circulation and prepare the athlete for hospital transfer in severe cases.

6.6.4 Water Sports Injuries

Diving and open-water marathons were the sports of highest illness incidence in Rio de Janeiro Olympic Games [19]. In swimming, most injuries are due to overuse in diving due to the impact on the surface of the water, which is more frequent in training than in competition. Most swimming injuries are strains and inflammatory conditions and can be treated with a nonsteroidal anti-inflammatory. Only between 1–7% of injuries in swimming are fractures or dislocations and between 3–10% in diving [20].

6.6.4.1 Open-Water Swimming

Injuries and illnesses related to open-water swimming result from the same factors as swimming pool swimming but are also related to the environments where it is practiced (lakes, oceans, rivers) like effects of cold-water immersion and barotrauma.

(a) Cold-Water Immersion

Cooling in water occurs 3–5 times faster due to the higher thermal conductivity. As the temperature decreases, cardiorespiratory, cognitive, and muscular functions also decrease.

If hypothermia has been established, we must [21–23]:

1. Dry swimmers and put dry clothes on.
2. Shivering may be protective if there are mild or moderate.
3. Avoid immediate warm baths and shower postrace.
4. Limit race distances in colder water. Measure the water temperature 2 h before de start and at one-hour intervals during the race. If water temperature is less than 16 °C, the race will be stopped.
5. Drink warm drinks and monitor rectal temperature for an hour postrace.

(b) Barotrauma

Barotrauma is the most common morbidity associated with recreational scuba diving, and it can occur during ascent or descent due to an ineffective balance of pressures [24, 25].

6.6.4.2 Descent

During the descent, injuries in the middle ear, inner ear, and paranasal sinus are commonly seen. Middle ear barotrauma or "ear squeeze" consists of pain, vertigo, tinnitus, and conducting hearing loss and can break the tympanic membrane. The treatment consists of topic nasal and systemic decongestants and abstinence from diving until recovery. In tympanic membrane perforations, a referral to an otolaryngologist specialist is appropriate.

Inner ear barotrauma may be a consequence of a too-vigorous Valsalva with consequent impairment of cochlear and vestibular function. Symptoms are like the middle ear with pain, vertigo, tinnitus, and conducting hearing loss. Inner ear barotrauma is treated with bed rest, elevating the head of the bed and avoiding maneuvers like Valsalva.

Sinus barotrauma is divers' second most common disease and affects frontal and maxillary sinuses. Pain over the sinus, headache, and epistaxis are the predominant symptoms.

6.6.4.3 Ascent

When the diver returns to the surface, inhaled air expands. If the diver does not ascend correctly, then that air can go to the tissues (pulmonary barotrauma, mediastinal or subcutaneous emphysema, and air embolism). An air embolism is the most severe form of pulmonary barotrauma. Bursting alveoli release air bubbles through the pulmonary vein and enter the systemic circulation, causing a seizure, loss of consciousness, disorientation, or stroke-like symptoms with hemisensory or motor deficits [24, 25].

Treatment in Cases of Barotrauma

- Get the swimmer out of the water as soon as possible.
- Advanced life support.
- Administrate:
  - Oxygen.
  - Saline solution and avoid glucose solution to minimize the risk of worsening cerebral edema.

- Corticosteroids and anticoagulants have not been shown to be efficacious.
- The fast evacuation to the hyperbaric camera can reduce the neurologic sequelae and improve survival.

6.6.5 Sudden Cardiac Death

The etiology of this sudden death in open-water swimmers is unknown; there are several theories, one of which is immersion pulmonary edema. A higher proportion of left ventricular hypertrophy has been found in triathletes that died during open-water swimming [26]. Another theory would be an Autonomic Conflict between the autonomic sympathetic system (tachycardia) which is activated by water temperature, exercise, and the stress of competition, while the parasympathetic (bradycardia) is activated by the face immersion and breath holding (diving response). It would produce fatal cardiac arrhythmia [21]. Therefore, every swimmer must be observed closely during the race or training to be fastly attended to in case of struggling or losing consciousness, being rescued from being promptly assessed, treated, or even stabilized by the emergency team before transferring to the hospital.

FINA has published a guide of open-water swimming safety regulations to minimize risks in the organization of races [23].

6.7 Upper Limb Injury

In sports, injuries to the upper limbs are frequent and may indistinctly affect professional and amateur athletes. The type and pattern of injuries are closely related to the sport's biomechanics, intensity, and physical demands involved in training and competition. Shoulder injuries are the most prevalent, followed by elbow and wrist. Each sport has a particular DNA that involves a complex and physically demanding activity, intensity, and, consequently, specific sports-related injury.

From the biomechanical point of view, sports involving throwing, pitching, and swimming impose high physical demands on the shoulder and elbow. This mechanical stress on these joints may cause acute injuries and, if not treated properly and promptly, may become chronic.

In equestrian sports, the reported injuries in the shoulder, forearm, hand, and fingers are bruises and fractures mainly due to the horse's kick. While in the golfer, a frequently reported injury is lateral or medial epicondylitis (50%), which results from repetitive stress impacting the valgus or varus on the elbow joint during training or competition. In martial arts, an armlock or hammerlock may result in elbow ligament injury or dislocation.

In Lacrosse, the athletes have contact and simultaneously demand throwing and catching a ball during running, jumping, cutting, and having a crosse when leading to both on-and-off platform movements that stress the upper limb's muscles, ligaments, and bones to injury. Moreover, in sports practice, injury mechanisms involving falls are common in any sport.

In Judo, the throwing (nage-waza) and control (katame-waza) techniques may expose the upper limb to injury (Figs. 6.4 and 6.5). A strategy commonly adopted by a fighter when defending from a nague-waza technique is, during the fall, instinctively try to place their hand on the ground to absorb the impact and prevent the opponent's score, supporting their body weight and transferring the trauma energy to the upper limb. According to the trauma level and the upper limb position (outstretched hand or flexed elbow), a contusion, sprain, fracture, or even a joint dislocation could result. Another injury condition is an armlock applied on the elbow (katame-waza) because it may cause ligament strain or dislocation.

Therefore, the sports medicine physician must keep his eyes open to the particularities of each sports modality. Most sports upper limb injuries are generally restricted to contusions and joint sprains, presenting minor soft tissue damage and allowing the athlete to return to the field after a quick medical assessment. However, the sports trauma energy is not uniform; consequently, more critical bone and soft tissue injuries may occur.

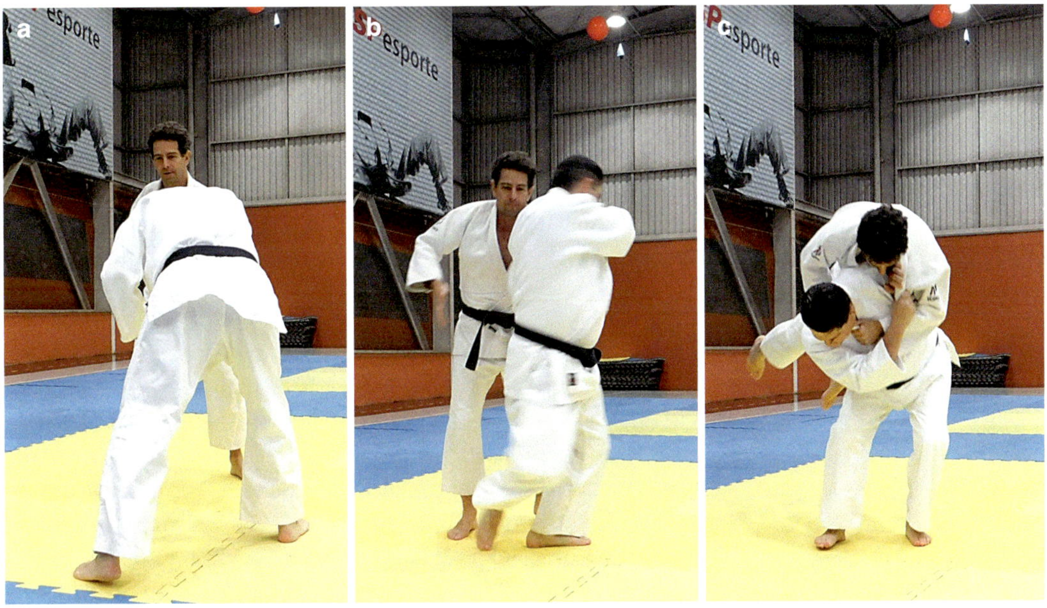

Fig. 6.4 Sequence of Morote Seoi Nage application technique. (Source: Sérgio Rocha Piedade)

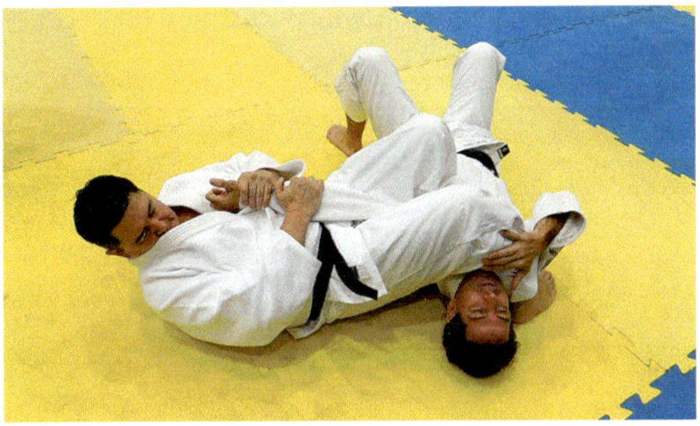

Fig. 6.5 Juji gatame technique (Source: Sérgio Rocha Piedade)

6.7.1 Initial Clinical Assessment of Upper Limb Sports Trauma

When evaluating upper limb trauma, the sports physician must pay close attention to how the trauma mechanism occurred because it can help identify a possible injury diagnosis. The physician should inspect the affected limb and search for any sign of tenderness area, limb deformity, edema, ecchymosis, superficial skin lesions, or cut-blunt wounds with significant tissue damage. The physician should also palpate the upper limb site related to the athlete's complaints because it may elicit pain and help identify bone crepitus, edema, or collection (hematoma).

In sports trauma, the physician should perform the initial assessment of the athlete's injury, and as soon as possible, the athlete should be removed from the field of play. This procedure is necessary to avoid public manifestation or interference and offer the best conditions for the physician to treat the injured athlete.

Carefully evaluate the upper limb with close to indirect signs of a fracture or joint dislocation, such as edema, deformity, ecchymosis, joint movement restriction or inability, and crepitus on palpation. Another important aspect, particularly for physicians, is knowledge of the athlete's injury history, surgeries, and complaints reported to this new trauma, which can help identify new injuries or even a reinjury.

Joint mobility should be evaluated as well as movement limitation and pain. Moreover, it is important to emphasize that the clinical evaluation must be done in a comparative way between the right and left upper limbs. Bone deformity shoulder is realigned with gentle traction maneuvers and immobilized for athlete comfort, and in case of suspicion of fracture, joint dislocation radiological evaluation should be carried out.

6.7.2 Radiological Assessment of Upper Limb Injuries in Athletes Following Sports Trauma

Figures 6.6, 6.7 and 6.8 present clinical cases of athlete's sports trauma, their history, clinical complaints, and radiological assessment.

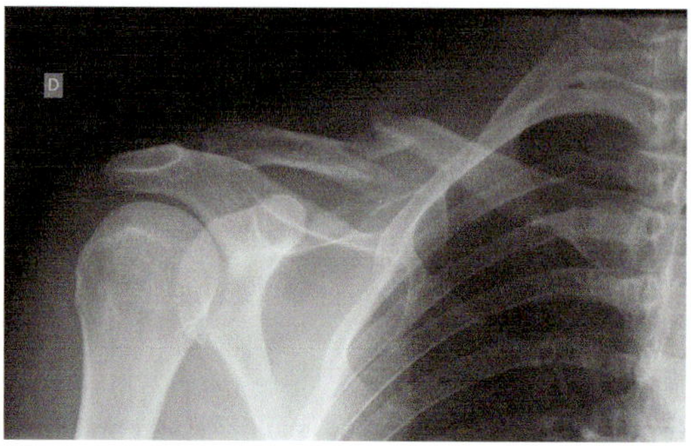

Fig. 6.6 Fracture of the middle third of the clavicle bone in a Judo fighter

Case 1

During judo training, a fighter fell onto the lateral shoulder and immediately reported pain in his shoulder and an inability to move his arm. At palpation of his shoulder, edema, tenderness, and crepitus were identified on the right clavicle topography. An X-ray assessment confirmed the diagnosis of a fracture of the right clavicle (Fig. 6.6).

Case 2

A 24-year-old basketball player complained of wrist pain after falling on his outstretched right hand during a match. He reported that he could not return to play due to the pain. The physical examination showed swelling and tenderness in the anatomical snuff box. The clinical suspicious was a scaphoid fracture and an X-ray exam was performed, but it was inconclusive. Due to the important athlete's complaint, an MRI was carried out, the scaphoid fracture diagnosis was confirmed, and adequate treatment was performed (Fig. 6.7).

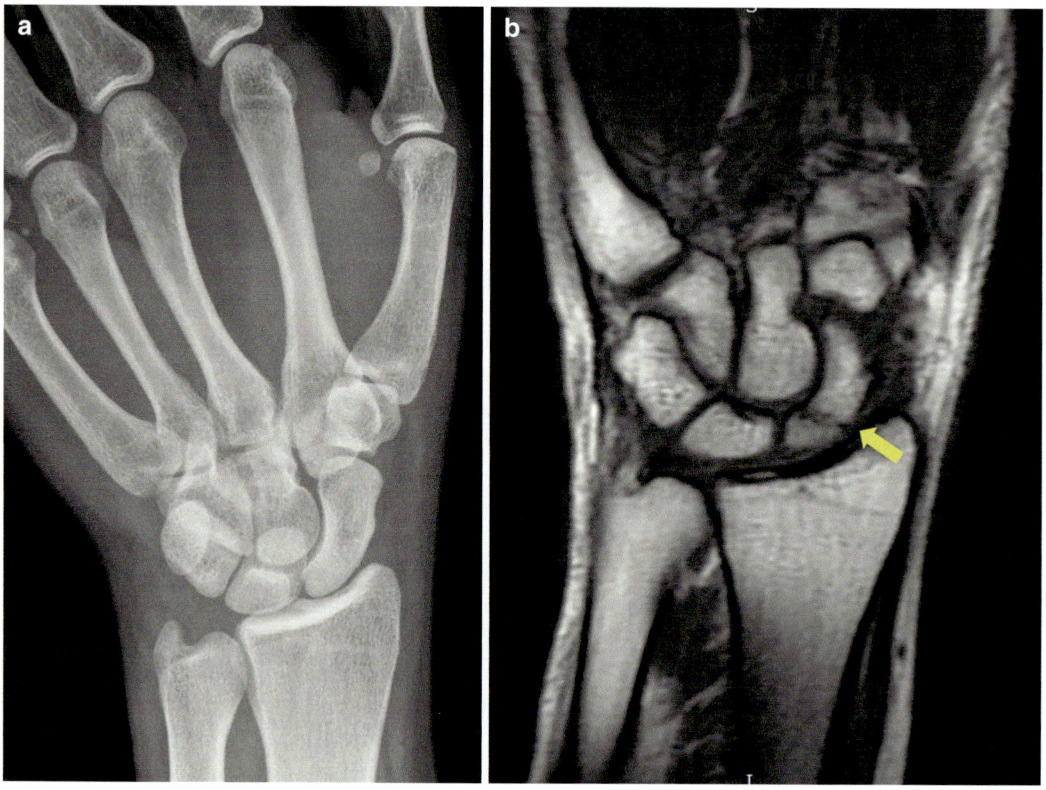

Fig. 6.7 Inconclusive X-ray for bone injury (**a**) and MRI (**b**) showing a fracture of the proximal third of the scaphoid bone in a basketball player

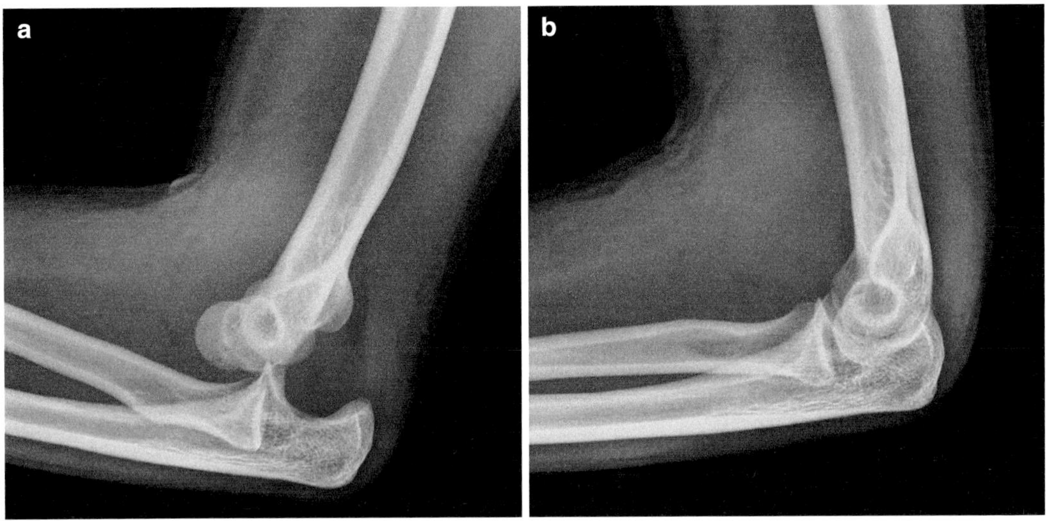

Fig. 6.8 An X-ray profile view evaluation of the dislocated elbow (**a**) and after elbow dislocation reduction (**b**) in a Judo fighter

Case 3

During a judo competition, a 30-year-old judo fighter heroically resisted an armlock on his right elbow to win the fight. However, this heroism caused an elbow dislocation. He was removed from the competition area. The physical exam identified a deformity and incapability to move the elbow. An X-ray evaluation was performed before (A) and after the elbow reduction (B) to confirm the joint reduction (Fig. 6.8).

6.7.3 Lower Limb Injuries and Sport

An injury is a physical complaint experienced by a player during a competition that requires medical attention or time loss [27]. The frequency and type of injuries are various, depending on the involved sport [28–30].

The difference between collective and individual sports is almost due to the risk of contact injury [27, 31]. Contacts are rare during individual sports such as gymnastics, athleticism, and tennis but possible, for example, in short track or frequent during fighting sports (MMA, karate, judo, etc.). Nevertheless, even in collective sports, most injuries are noncontact [27, 32]. Low and repeated impact sports, such as long-distance running, are exposed to the risk of recurrent tendinous tears and stress fractures [33].

Injuries occurring during mechanical sports are high-velocity traumatisms and are frequently severe. Deep wounds and vascular lesions are possible in a bullfight. The occurrence and severity of the injury, depending on gender and age, are controversial in literature [27, 28, 30–35] and will not be detailed here.

Repartition of lower limb injuries is difficult and hereby depends on the type of sport. Anyway, thigh muscular and tendinous lesions are most frequent before ankle ligament and knee ligament tears [27, 28, 31, 32, 36, 37].

6.7.4 Management of the Lower Limb-Injured Athlete

Hopefully, most injuries are considered minor or moderate [27]. But the management of the different injuries is different and sometimes requires medical gestures such as suture, strapping or immobilization, dislocation reduction, or vascular lesion compression. But in most cases, the principal challenge is to know if and/or convince an athlete to stop competition/game. The physician's role is also to evaluate the need and emergency for specific care to address the athlete for adapted management (rest, physiotherapy, imaging, and need for a medical doctor or surgeon).

6.7.5 Superficial Lesions and Bruises

Superficial lacerations and skin abrasions need most of the time only superficial care with cleaning and a pad, but sometimes sutures or staples are necessary when bleeding. Games or competitions can generally go on.

Local ice application treats hematoma or contusion, and competition is rarely stopped. Deep and voluminous hematomas are very painful, and ultrasonography is recommended a few days later to adapt treatment (almost medical, rarely surgical with drainage).

6.7.6 Tendinous and Muscular Lesions

Muscular tears are frequent [27, 28, 31, 32, 34, 38], especially for hamstrings and adductors, less for calf muscles, well known by athletes (Fig. 6.9). Immediate rest at the end of the game with local ice application is recommended. A rapid medical assessment is necessary, and imaging is helpful (US or MRI) to choose the best medical treatment (aspiration, PRP injection, physiotherapy ++, rarely surgical muscular hematoma drainage). Return to sports is generally possible a few weeks later.

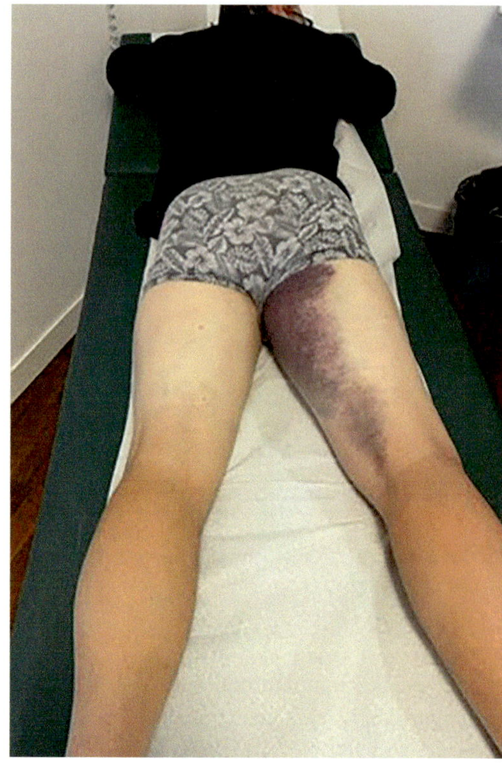

Fig. 6.9 Male, 40 years old, hamstrings proximal avulsion during a football game

Thigh tendon avulsions (proximal hamstrings, biceps tendon, and rectus femoris) are not common but early diagnosis is easier before the hematoma. Rapid imaging (X-ray, US, and/or MRI) is mandatory to help the surgical decision, ideally before 3 weeks but better 10 days post-trauma. Surgical bony reinsertion needs prolonged immobilization and long rehabilitation before return to sports.

Tendinous ruptures (Achilles tendon, quadriceps tendon, or patellar ligament) are easily diagnosed on field with complete inability. Initial rest and immobilization are recommended, and surgical management is needed a few days after trauma, mostly without imaging. Long rehabilitation and delayed return to sports are the rule.

6.7.7 Ankle Ligament Lesions

Ankle ligament tears are very frequent in majority of sports [27, 31, 32, 37, 38] (except downhill skiing) [36]. Pursuit of competition is sometimes possible, in the case of benign lesions, with strapping. When gravity criteria exist, the end of the game is necessary. A strap or splint is useful, and a rapid medical assessment is recommended with imaging (X-rays and US, rarely MRI). Rest and physiotherapy are usually sufficient with return to sports within 10 to 45 days.

Orthopedic treatment with a cast is commonly used for children and syndesmosis lesions. In general, surgical treatment is rare, but it could be necessary in cases of multiple ligament lesions and major laxity, as well as in fifth metatarsal avulsion. Immobilization during 45 days is common in these cases with delayed RTS for three months.

6.7.8 Knee Ligament Lesions

Knee ligament tears are frequent lower limb injuries in all sports [27, 31, 32, 36–38]. This joint is particularly exposed in contacts and falls, and the majority of traumas are hopefully simple contusions that will not stop competition. This joint is also vulnerable to noncontact and contact torsions with potential ligament and/or meniscal lesions. Figure 6.10 shows one possible mechanism of anterior cruciate ligament (ACL) injury when two rugby players disputing the ball. Crack, immediate instability, effusion, or blockage is gravity criteria. Immediate testing is often very informative for collateral and cruciate ligaments. Immediate rest, ice, and splint immobilization are necessary. A rapid medical assessment is needed, and imaging, especially MRI, is mandatory mainly. Medical treatment with physiotherapy is sufficient when benign collateral ligament tears occur, with return to sports within 3 to 6 weeks.

Treatment of cruciate ligaments, multiple ligament injuries, and meniscal tears is mostly surgical for athletes. Return to sports is delayed, depending on the lesions and their treatment (3 to 6 weeks for meniscectomy but three months after a meniscal suture) and depending on the sport and the age (pivot sport 6 to 7 months commonly but 12 months at minimum for children after ACL reconstruction). Return to sports is sometimes impossible at the same level, especially when multiple ligament injuries.

6.7.9 Fractures and Dislocations

Traumatic fractures are brutal, with immediate inability and severe pain (Fig. 6.11). They can occur during direct contact or fall or while a torsion mechanism [36].

Diagnosis is generally easy with painful palpation and hematoma, sometimes limb deformity, and rarely an opened fracture. The athlete has to end the game/competition. Rapid immobilization is necessary with ice (a pad when opened), and the patient is transferred as soon as possible to the hospital for X-rays and medical or surgical management. Toes fractures are generally simply immobilized for 3–6 weeks, and return to sport is achieved after healing. Displaced fractures are generally operated on for fixation, except for children for who orthopedic treatment is often preferred.

Immobilization and rest are as long as the bony healing, and return to sports is generally between 2 and 6 months. Recurrent fracture risk exists mainly for children in cases of tibia or femur shaft fractures during 12 months. Fixation materials such as screws, plates, or nails can be annoying during sports, and their removal is generally made after 12–18 months. Risk of refracture after material removal exists during 1 or 2 months.

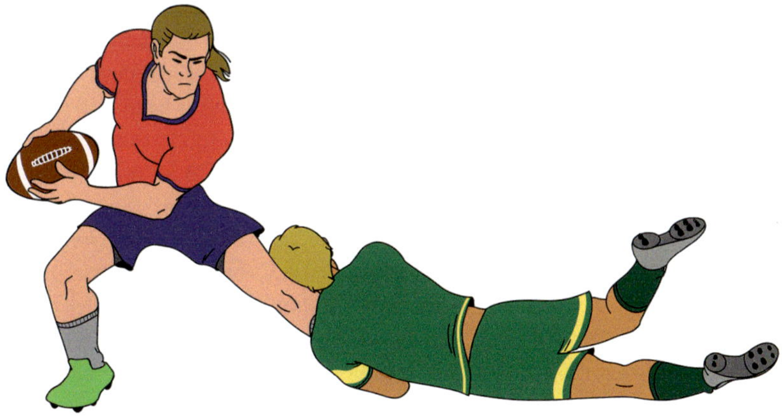

Fig. 6.10 Possible mechanism of ACL rupture (knee valgus stress and external rotation) in the left knee of a rugby player during a game. (Source: Mariana Percario Piedade)

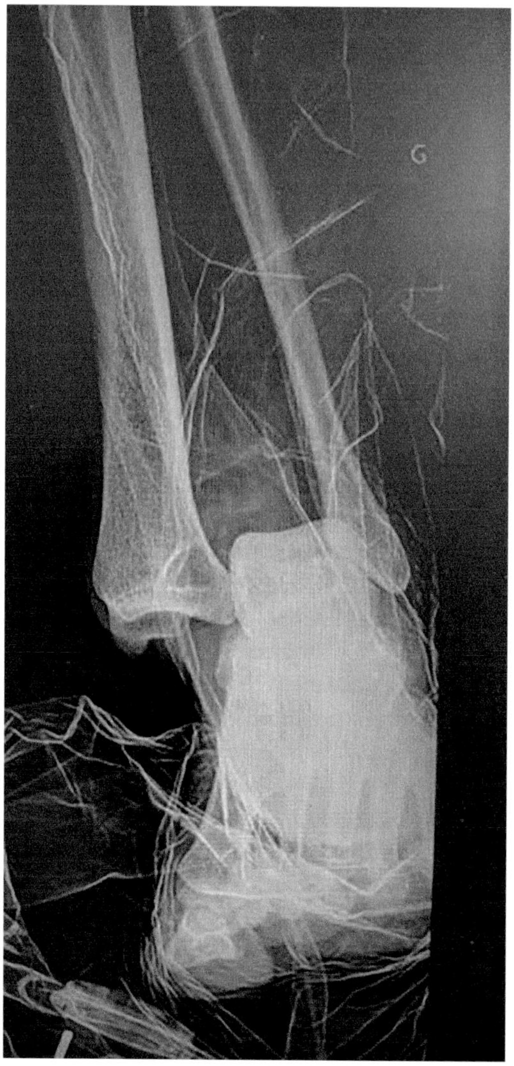

Fig. 6.11 Male, 30 years old, ankle dislocation during karate fight

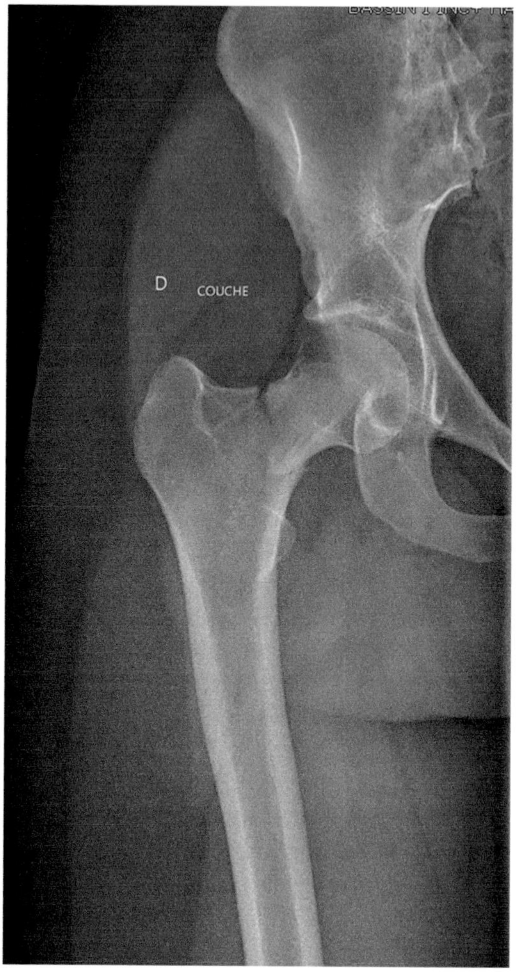

Fig. 6.12 Female, 23 years old, femoral neck displaced stress fracture during long-distance running

Patella and toe dislocations are relatively common; diagnosis is clear, and immediate reduction is relatively easy and can probably be done by any physician, before imaging and medical assessment a few hours or days later. Although forefoot, ankle, knee, and hip dislocations are rare during falls (3), they could occur due to severe contact traumas or high-velocity crashes (mechanical sports). Immediate reduction is not recommended (except for medical doctors when tarso-tibial dislocations). Immediate transfer to hospital is the rule with most adequate immobilization. Reduction under anesthesia should be done in the emergency room after an X-rays assessment. Fractures or severe ligamentous lesions, rarely vascular or neurological lesions, are associated, and surgical repair is often purposed. Immobilization, rehabilitation, and return to sports (when possible) are very long.

Stress fractures are particular cases more frequent in repeated impact sports [29], such as long-distance running and trails [33]. Metatarsal or calcaneus stress fractures are well known, but femoral condyle, tibial plateau, tibial shaft, and femoral neck stress fractures also exist (Fig. 6.12). Immediate severe pain during a long run with an inability can focus on this diagnosis. Radiographs are often poor, and MRI or CT scan can be necessary. A bone scan can be indicated when the diagnosis is challenging (sesamoid forefoot bone). Medical treatment with prolonged rest (45 days–3 months) is classical, and surgical treatment is exceptional with the fixation of displaced fracture or sesamoid bone resection.

6.7.10 Deep Wounds

Deep wounds potentially associated with vascular injuries are extremely rare. Bullfighting in certain countries requires the presence of a vascular surgeon and an operative room inside the arena for extremely urgent care.

6.7.11 Prevention of Athlete Injury

Prevention is probably the most challenging factor in avoiding or reducing injuries during sports [27].

Specific training with daily exercise (gestures, positions [34], and rehabilitation are ideally adapted to each athlete for his sport, his position in the team (defensive/offensive lines), the particularity of his efforts (endurance/explosivity), and depending on gender and age [27, 28, 31–33, 37–39].

Analysis of large sports injury series permitted an evolution of sports rules, materials, and equipment [36]. Some rules are made to protect the athlete himself:

- Length and width of ski boards, height and strength of fixations, rigidity and flexion of boots in downhill skiing [36].
- Airbags in motorcycle suits, boots, and knee braces for motocross (but carbon fiber prohibited to avoid deep wounds in case of breakage).
- Friction coefficient for grounds and/or shoes in handball and basketball.
- Landing mats in gymnastic, tatamis for fighting sports.

Other rules are made to protect other athletes during collective sports:

- Metallic articulated knee braces are prohibited.
- Crampon length is limited in football, soccer, rugby, etc.

Most injuries are considered minor or moderate, but some are serious and may have other long-term consequences. When the injury is not so important, the challenge is to convince the athlete to stop the game, sometimes confronting the staff, to avoid a more critical lesion. Management in an emergency is a big deal, and the following adapted medical treatment has to restore function with perfect healing to prevent recurrent injury and establish an effective physical and mental well-being for the athlete and his ability to return to sport and return to play. In this way, injury prevention is also a big challenge.

Take-Home Message

- The medical bag should be tailored to the sports modality and specific sports-related injuries and adverse environmental conditions related to sports practice.
- Syncope during physical exercise should be considered a clinical event of high suspicion of structural heart disease.
- ABCDE trauma protocol systematizes the approach to the severe sports injury and minimizes the occurrence of undiscovered injuries.
- Facial cuts near the medial aspect of the eye (orbit) and the bridge of the nose are critical because they can extend into the lacrimal tear duct, close to the surface.
- The physician should be prepared to identify when an ocular injury requires immediate referral for further investigation or surgical repair.
- Cooling in water 3–5 times faster.
- The knowledge of sports dynamics, careful physical evaluation, and adequate radiological play an essential role in minimizing the risk of undiscovered injuries.

Acknowledgments The authors thank Mariana Percario Piedade for preparing the figures.

References

1. Joseph SR. Traveling management. In: Rocha Piedade S, Imhoff AB, Clatworthy M, Cohen M, Espregueira-Mendes J, editors. Sports medicine physician. Cham: Springer International Publishing; 2019. p. 471–80.
2. Kaeding CC, Borchers J. Issues for the traveling team physician. J Knee Surg. 2016;29:364–9.
3. Sundstrøm T, Grände PO, Luoto T, Rosenlund C, Undén J, Wester KG. Management of severe traumatic brain injury: evidence, tricks, and pitfalls. Springer International Publishing; 2020.
4. Black AM, Eliason PH, Patton DA, Emery CA. Epidemiology of facial injuries in sport. Clin Sports Med. 2017;36:237–55.
5. Rahman SA, Chandrasala S. When to suspect head injury or cervical spine injury in maxillofacial trauma? Dent Res J (Isfahan). 2014;11:336–44.
6. Bhamra J, Morar Y, Khan W, Deep K, Hammer A. Cervical spine immobilization in sports related injuries: review of current guidelines and a case study of an injured athlete. Open Orthop J. 2012;6:548–52.
7. Farrington T, Onambele-Pearson G, Taylor RL, Earl P, Winwood K. A review of facial protective equipment use in sport and the impact on injury incidence. Br J Oral Maxillofac Surg. 2012;50:233–8.
8. Piccininni P, Clough A, Padilla R, Piccininni G. Dental and orofacial injuries. Clin Sports Med. 2017;36:369–405.
9. Marston AP, O'Brien EK, Hamilton GS 3rd. Nasal injuries in sports. Clin Sports Med. 2017;36:337–53.
10. Piedade SR, Carvalho LM, Mendes LA, Possedente M, Ferreira DM. Facial trauma. In: Rocha Piedade S, Imhoff AB, Clatworthy M, Cohen M, Espregueira-Mendes J, editors. Sports medicine physician. Cham: Springer International Publishing; 2019. p. 261–73.
11. Estwanik JJ. Ringside medicine BT. In: Rocha Piedade S, Imhoff AB, Clatworthy M, Cohen M, Espregueira-Mendes J, editors. The sports medicine physician. Cham: Springer International Publishing; 2019. p. 497–514.
12. Haring RS, Sheffield ID, Canner JK, Schneider EB. Epidemiology of sports-related eye injuries in the United States. JAMA Ophthalmol. 2016;134:1382–90.
13. Patel V, Pakravan P, Mehra D, Watane A, Yannuzzi NA, Sridhar J. Trends in sports-related ocular trauma in United States Emergency Departments from 2010 to 2019: multi-center cross-sectional study. Semin Ophthalmol. 2023;38(4):333–7.
14. Heath Jeffery RC, Dobes J, Chen FK. Eye injuries: understanding ocular trauma. Aust J Gen Pract. 2022;51:476–82.
15. Kuhn F, Morris R, Witherspoon CD. Birmingham Eye Trauma Terminology (BETT): terminology and classification of mechanical eye injuries. Ophthalmol Clin N Am. 2002;15:139–43.
16. Hirose Y, Shikino K, Ikusaka M. Surfer's ear and external auditory canal exostoses. QJM. 2016;109:759.
17. Osetinsky LM, Hamilton GS 3rd, Carlson ML. Sport Injuries of the Ear and Temporal Bone. Clin Sports Med. 2017;36:315–35.
18. Eagles K, Fralich L, Stevenson JH. Ear trauma. Clin Sports Med. 2013;32:303–16.
19. Soligard T, Steffen K, Palmer D, et al. Sports injury and illness incidence in the Rio de Janeiro 2016 Olympic summer games: a prospective study of 11274 athletes from 207 countries. Br J Sports Med. 2017;51:1265–71.
20. Boltz AJ, Robison HJ, Morris SN, D'Alonzo BA, Collins CL, Chandran A. Epidemiology of Injuries in National Collegiate Athletic Association men's swimming and diving: 2014–2015 through 2018–2019. J Athl Train. 2021;56:719–26.
21. Shattock MJ, Tipton MJ. "Autonomic conflict": a different way to die during cold water immersion? J Physiol. 2012;590:3219–30.
22. Chamberlain M, Marshall AN, Keeler S. Open water swimming: medical and water quality considerations. Curr Sports Med Rep. 2019;18:121–8.
23. FINA. Open water swimming guide. Lausanne: Fédération Internationale de Natation; 2022.
24. Buzzacott PL. The epidemiology of injury in scuba diving. Med Sport Sci. 2012;58:57–79.
25. Burkett JG, Nahas SJ. Diving headache. Curr Pain Headache Rep. 2019;23:46.
26. Moon RE, Martina SD, Peacher DF, Kraus WE. Deaths in triathletes: immersion pulmonary oedema as a possible cause. BMJ Open Sport Exerc Med. 2016;2:e000146.
27. Anderson DS, Cathcart J, Wilson I, Hides J, Leung F, Kerr D. Lower limb MSK injuries among school-aged rugby and football players: a systematic review. BMJ Open Sport Exerc Med. 2020;6:e000806.
28. Ishøi L, Krommes K, Husted RS, Juhl CB, Thorborg K. Diagnosis, prevention and treatment of common lower extremity muscle injuries in sport—grading the evidence: a statement paper commissioned by the Danish Society of Sports Physical Therapy (DSSF). Br J Sports Med. 2020;54:528–37.
29. Khan M, Madden K, Burrus MT, Rogowski JP, Stotts J, Samani MJ, Sikka R, Bedi A. Epidemiology and impact on performance of lower extremity stress injuries in professional basketball players. Sports Health. 2018;10:169–74.
30. Kim HC, Park KJ. Injuries in male and female elite aquatic sports athletes: an 8-year prospective, epidemiological study. J Sports Sci Med. 2020;19:390–6.
31. Martín-Guzón I, Muñoz A, Lorenzo-Calvo J, Muriarte D, Marquina M, de la Rubia A. Injury prevalence of the lower limbs in handball players: a systematic review. Int J Environ Res Public Health. 2021; https://doi.org/10.3390/ijerph19010332.
32. Hess MC, Swedler DI, Collins CS, Ponce BA, Brabston EW. Descriptive epidemiology of injuries

in professional ultimate frisbee athletes. J Athl Train. 2020;55:195–204.
33. Francis P, Whatman C, Sheerin K, Hume P, Johnson MI. The proportion of lower limb running injuries by gender, anatomical location and specific pathology: a systematic review. J Sports Sci Med. 2019;18: 21–31.
34. Bezuglov E, Talibov O, Butovskiy M, et al. The prevalence of non-contact muscle injuries of the lower limb in professional soccer players who perform Salah regularly: a retrospective cohort study. J Orthop Surg Res. 2020;15:440.
35. Foss KDB, Thomas S, Khoury JC, Myer GD, Hewett TE. A school-based neuromuscular training program and sport-related injury incidence: a prospective randomized controlled clinical trial. J Athl Train. 2018;53:20–8.
36. Davey A, Endres NK, Johnson RJ, Shealy JE. Alpine skiing injuries. Sports. Health. 2019;11:18–26.
37. Taylor JB, Ford KR, Nguyen A-D, Terry LN, Hegedus EJ. Prevention of lower extremity injuries in basketball: a systematic review and meta-analysis. Sports Health. 2015;7:392–8.
38. Herman K, Barton C, Malliaras P, Morrissey D. The effectiveness of neuromuscular warm-up strategies, that require no additional equipment, for preventing lower limb injuries during sports participation: a systematic review. BMC Med. 2012;10:75.
39. Ha S, Jeong HS, Park S-K, Lee SY. Can neurocognitive function predict lower extremity injuries in male collegiate athletes? Int J Environ Res Public Health. 2020; https://doi.org/10.3390/ijerph17239061.

Shoulder and Elbow

7

Lukas N. Muench, Sebastian Siebenlist, and Andreas B. Imhoff

7.1 Introduction

The most common sports-related injuries of the shoulder and elbow joint are chronic injuries that result from overuse (e.g., rotator cuff tendinopathy, posterosuperior impingement, long head of the biceps pathology, acromioclavicular joint arthropathy, and flexor or extensor tendinopathy), which are generally treated away from the competition field. However, there are some acute shoulder and elbow injuries that require immediate on-field or sideline management, including dislocations and fractures, as well as acromioclavicular joint (ACJ) separations. These injuries are mainly observed in contact sports (e.g., American football, rugby, ice hockey, and soccer) and can have a significant impact on the athlete's career given the prolonged absence from play [1].

In general, the sideline physician should follow a structured algorithm for a complete evaluation of the athlete in the setting of an acute injury to minimize the risk of missing a more severe or life-threatening injury to the head or thorax. Obvious deformities or neurovascular damage should be seen as red flag signs, where the athlete may require urgent transfer to the emergency room. Severely dislocated fractures may be provisionally stabilized before removing the player from the field, and dislocations may undergo a reduction attempt. If the decision is made to remove the player from the competition, a more thorough physical evaluation should be performed in a controlled environment (e.g., locker room) [1].

7.2 Shoulder Injuries

The most common shoulder injuries requiring immediate on-field or sideline management comprise glenohumeral dislocations, ACJ separations, and fractures of the clavicle, proximal humerus, or scapula. In the setting of acute trauma, the examination of the shoulder can be very challenging due to significant pain. A detailed evaluation of the trauma mechanism may assist in making the correct diagnosis.

7.2.1 Glenohumeral Dislocation

The shoulder is the most commonly dislocated joint in athletes, accounting for approximately half of all sports-related dislocations [2]. The unique anatomy of the glenohumeral joint is characterized by a complex interaction of dynamic and static stabilizers in an attempt to compensate for its very little intrinsic osseous stability [3]. Although allowing for the largest

L. N. Muench · S. Siebenlist · A. B. Imhoff (✉)
Department of Sports Orthopaedics, Technical University of Munich, Munich, Germany
e-mail: lukas.muench@tum.de; sebastian.siebenlist@tum.de; imhoff@tum.de

S. Rocha Piedade et al. (eds.), *Sideline Management in Sports*,
https://doi.org/10.1007/978-3-031-33867-0_7

range of motion of any joint in the human body, these anatomic features explain why glenohumeral dislocations and subsequent recurrent shoulder instability are so frequently encountered [4]. Over 95% of glenohumeral dislocations occur in an anteroinferior direction, while posterior and inferior (*luxatio erecta*) dislocations are only observed in 5% and < 1% of cases, respectively [5, 6].

The underlying mechanism for an anterior shoulder dislocation usually involves a combination of forward elevation, abduction, and external rotation of the shoulder. A posterior dislocation usually results from a posterior directed force with the shoulder in a flexed, adducted, and internally rotated position, usually occurring during the fall on the outstretched arm. A *luxatio erecta* can be caused by a forced hyperabduction to the abducted arm with the acromion acting as a fulcrum, consequently levering the humeral head out of the glenohumeral joint in an inferior direction, or by a direct blow to the fully abducted arm [1, 5].

Clinically, athletes with an anterior dislocation present with holding the affected shoulder in an adducted cradle-like position. There may be an obvious visual deformity of the shoulder with a more prominent acromion and a flattened appearance inferiorly. Palpation of the humeral head in the axilla may also be a clinical sign. In the setting of a posterior dislocation, the patient usually holds the arm in an internally rotated and adducted position close to the side, while the humeral head may be palpated posteriorly. A *luxatio erecta* shows a distinctive clinical presentation, as the arm is in a hyperabducted and locked position over the patient's head. The elbow is flexed, while the forearm is pronated, resting on the top of the patient's head. Generally, the assessment of axillary nerve function should be performed by evaluating deltoid contraction and sensory testing of the lateral proximal arm [2, 5, 7, 8].

Once diagnosed, immediate treatment of a dislocated shoulder is critical. In the absence of any red flag signs (neurovascular injury, concomitant humeral head or clavicle fractures, and cervical spine injury), an immediate on-field or sideline reduction attempt should be performed. This holds the advantage of an easier reduction prior to the onset of muscle spasms and patient apprehension [1, 8]. Consequently, in clinical practice, many reductions are performed without prior radiographic imaging. Interestingly, Shuster et al. [9] reported that prereduction radiographs were of no additional value if physicians were certain of dislocation by physical examination. In contrast, a traumatic dislocation, such as a sports injury, is considered a criterion for the necessity of prereduction radiographs according to the Quebec Decision Rule [10]. However, in the absence of a clear consensus or treatment algorithm for sideline management of shoulder dislocations, the physician should consider the performance of prereduction radiographs in the presence of local tenderness, crepitus, and ecchymosis, or signs of neurovascular injury (Fig. 7.1) [8, 11].

Various reduction methods have been described in the literature without one technique being proven to be superior to others. Although an immediate reduction is recommended, the athlete should first be moved off the competition field. Reduction maneuvers should be performed in the locker room away from spectators to minimize distraction. For an anterior dislocation, the traction–countertraction, chair, or Milch methods are feasible maneuvers, most of them using some form of axial traction with simultaneous external rotation and abduction. In the setting of a posterior dislocation, the arm is flexed to 90° and adducted in internal rotation to disengage the humeral head from the glenoid rim, while an assistant pulls countertraction with a sheet around the athlete's torso in a supine position. This is followed by applying a gentle anterior force with external rotation. In the case of a *luxatio erecta*, traction should be applied in a superior and lateral direction with the arm in hyperabduction, while an assistant provides countertraction. Subsequently, an upward force is applied to the humeral head while the arm is taken into adduction. Both posterior and inferior dislocations may require adequate sedation to be successful. A post-reduction neurologic assessment is mandatory with a focus on axillary nerve function. If the reduction attempt remains unsuccessful, the athlete should be sent to the emergency department

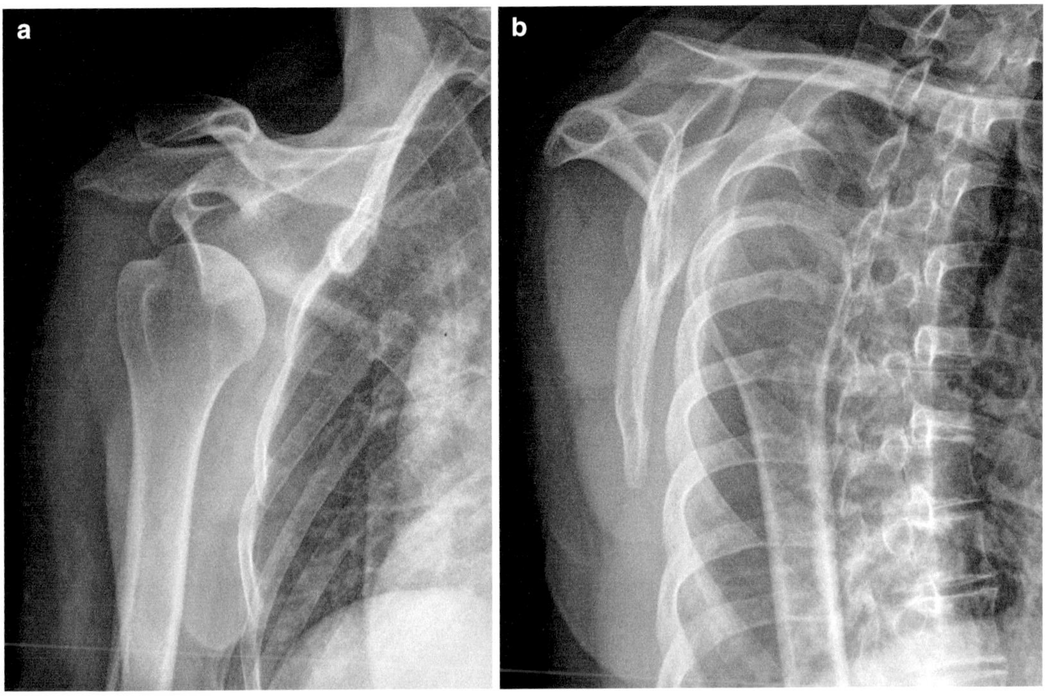

Fig. 7.1 Anteroposterior (**a**) and y-view (**b**) radiograph of an anteroinferior dislocation of the right shoulder of a 32-year-old athlete, without a concomitant fracture of the humeral head or glenoid

for radiographic imaging and reduction under sufficient sedation/analgesia [1, 2, 5].

Following successful reduction, the affected shoulder should be immobilized in a sling and the patient should undergo radiographic imaging as soon as possible to confirm joint congruency and assess concomitant fractures of the glenoid or proximal humerus (Fig. 7.2). Adequate analgesia should be provided using NSAIDs and cryotherapy.

7.2.2 Acromioclavicular Joint Injuries

ACJ injuries are most commonly caused by a direct fall on the superolateral aspect of the shoulder with the arm in an adducted position. Consequently, these injuries are mainly observed in contact and collision sports. An indirect injury may occur by falling on the outstretched arm, causing the humeral head to translocate superiorly and drive the humeral head into the acromion.

The athlete may present with local tenderness and/or ecchymosis over the ACJ and a visual deformity depending on the severity of the injury. In case of a high-grade injury, prominence of the distal clavicle may be observed due to drooping of the shoulder. Specific provocative tests for the assessment of ACJ pathology (e.g., cross-arm adduction test and O'Brien test) may not be tolerated by the athlete in the acute setting and may be considered negligible during the sideline management of these injuries.

Generally, reduction attempts of the ACJ are unsuccessful and not necessary except in the rare case of an open fracture dislocation or impending open dislocation. The athlete should be moved off the competition field with the affected shoulder placed in a sling for comfort. Radiographic imaging (bilateral Zanca view or Panorama view) should be performed to classify the severity of the injury according to Rockwood et al. and rule out concomitant fractures of the clavicle and coracoid (Fig. 7.2). Depending on the severity of the injury, conservative (I–IIIa) or operative (IIIb–VI) treatment may be recommended [1] (Fig. 7.3).

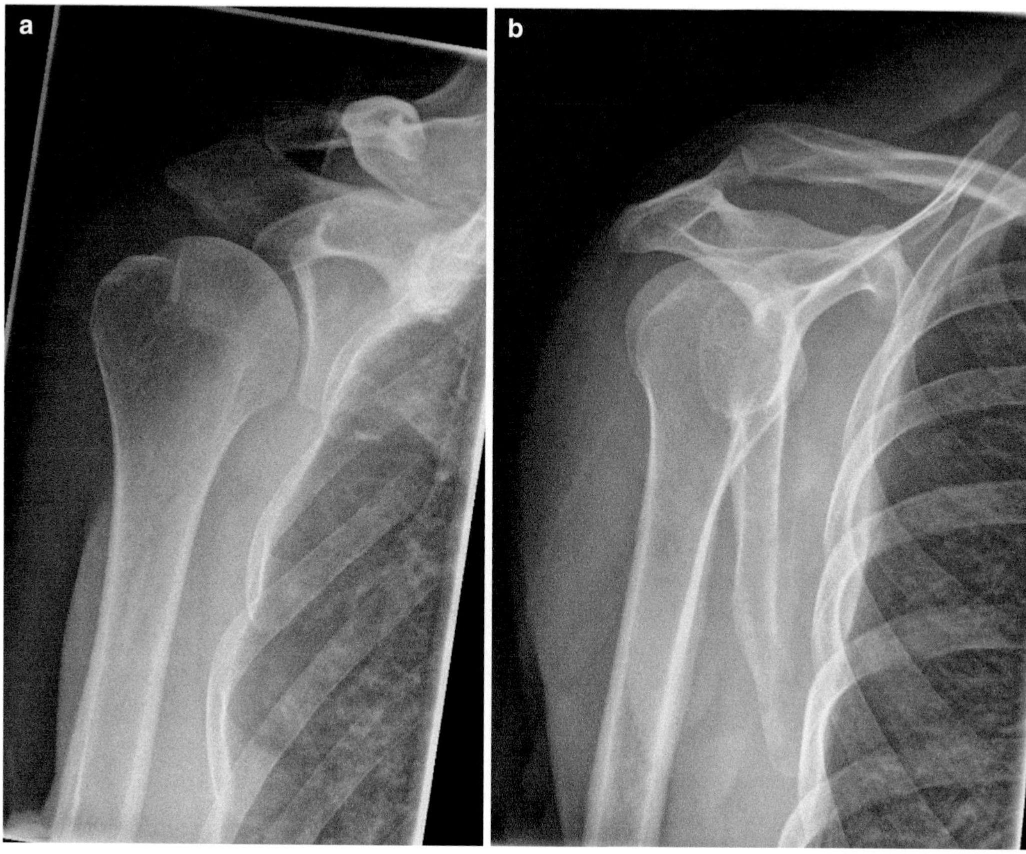

Fig. 7.2 Anteroposterior (**a**) and y-view (**b**) radiograph of the same 32-year-old athlete's right shoulder after successful reduction. Joint congruency is confirmed without signs of a concomitant fracture

7.2.3 Fractures of the Shoulder Girdle

The most commonly fractured bone of the shoulder girdle is the clavicle, accounting for around 35% of all fractures, with the middle third (80%) being the most frequent site of injury. The usual mechanism of injury involves a direct fall on the shoulder or a direct blow to the clavicle, while a fall of the outstretched arm is less frequently observed. Athletes typically present with localized tenderness, swelling, and crepitus over the clavicle with or without a visual deformity. An exacerbation of pain may be provoked during cross-body adduction of the arm. If the physical examination reveals tenting of the skin, a reduction in the fracture is recommended to reduce the risk of skin necrosis and/or perforation. Involvement of the brachial plexus or subclavian artery is a potential complication. The athlete should be moved off the field, and the affected shoulder should be immobilized in a sling. Subsequently, a referral for radiographic imaging and evaluation by a specialist should be initiated [7, 12, 13].

Other fractures of the shoulder include those of the glenoid, proximal humerus, tuberosities, and scapula, which are usually the result of a direct fall or impact. Fractures of the glenoid are often associated with glenohumeral dislocations. The clinical presentation typically shows localized tenderness, swelling, and crepitus and pain during active and passive range of motion. Fractures of the tuberosities often result in dysfunction of the rotator cuff. Fractures of the scapular body indicate a high-energy trauma and should raise awareness of other significant associated injuries (e.g., pneumothorax and neurovascular injuries) [12, 14].

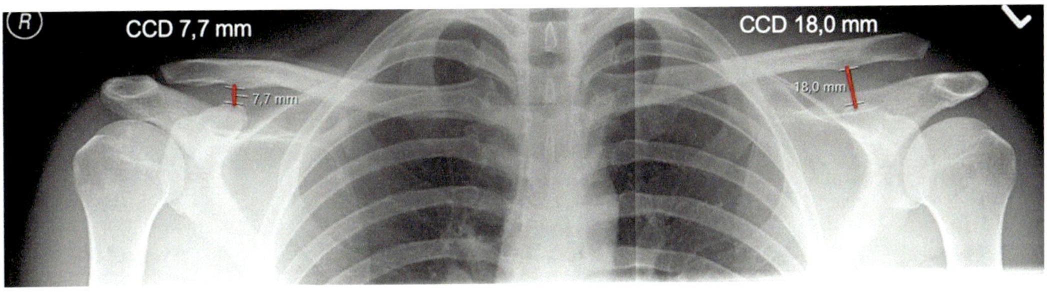

Fig. 7.3 Male athlete with ACJ instability of the left shoulder. Compared to the unaffected right side, the coracoclavicular distance (CCD; *red line*) of the left shoulder is increased by 134%, resulting in a grade V injury, according to Rockwood et al.

In general, sideline management of closed fractures is focused on preventing the injury from becoming an open fracture and minimizing the risk of neurovascular damage due to displaced bone ends. In case of a severely unstable fracture, a reduction attempt may be performed by gently applying longitudinal traction for improved alignment and protection of surrounding soft tissues. A post-reduction neurovascular assessment is mandatory, and any change in neurovascular status requires immediate transfer to an emergency room. Immobilization of the fractured bone and adjacent joints using a sling is recommended, while cryotherapy and NSAIDs may help reduce swelling and facilitate early treatment of fractures requiring surgery after radiographic imaging has been performed [12, 15].

7.3 Elbow Injuries

The most common acute elbow injuries athletes may suffer during play include soft tissue contusions due to direct trauma and acute rupture of the collateral ligaments or distal biceps or triceps tendon. However, these injuries usually do not necessitate specialized on-field or sideline management. In contrast, more severe injuries, such as dislocations or fractures of the elbow, require immediate sideline treatment to minimize the risk of future complications [1].

7.3.1 Dislocation

The elbow is the second most commonly dislocated joint in adult athletes while being even the most commonly dislocated joint in the pediatric population. Simple dislocations present as a dissociation of the ulnohumeral joint without a concomitant fracture. In contrast, complex dislocations are associated with fractures of the radial head/neck or coronoid and bony avulsions of the medial or lateral epicondyle [16]. The vast majority of elbow dislocations are caused by a fall on the outstretched hand combined with elbow supination and valgus stress [1, 16]. In around 90% of cases, the elbow is dislocated in a posterolateral direction [2]. A dislocation occurs after a ring of soft tissue restraints, including the lateral collateral ligament, anterior capsule, and medial collateral ligament, have sequentially been disrupted, with progressive translation from stable to perched and finally a complete dislocation [17]. An incidence of 0.38 per 100,000 athletic exposures has been reported in high school athletes [5].

Athletes clinically demonstrate an obvious deformity and swelling, with the elbow often held in a varus position with simultaneous fore-

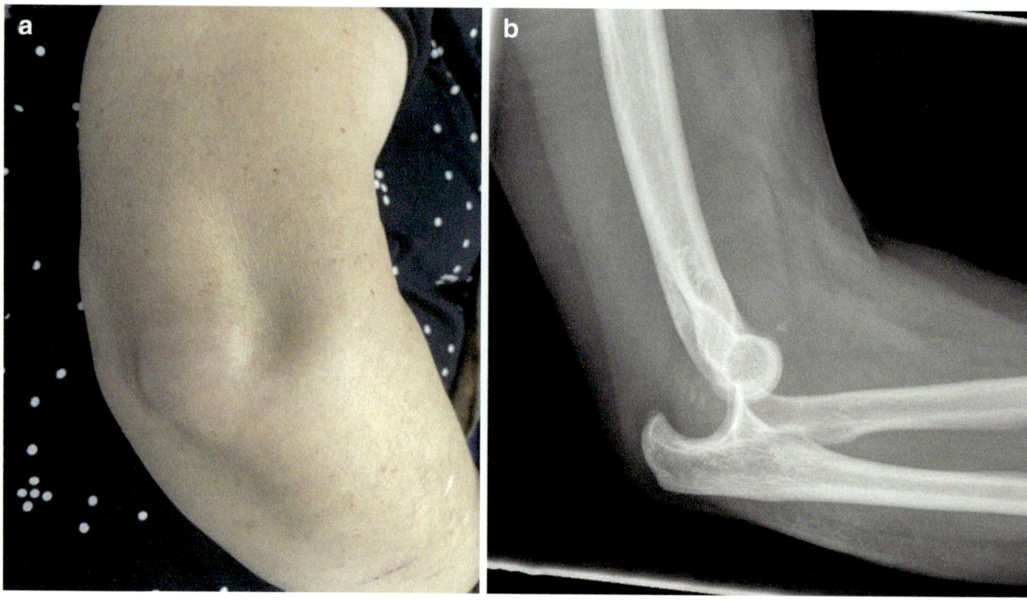

Fig. 7.4 Clinical (**a**) and radiographic (**b**) presentation of a female athlete with a posterolateral dislocation of the right elbow

arm supination (Fig. 7.4). Quick assessment for the integrity of neurovascular structures is critical, as there is potential for injuries to the ulnar (most frequently involved) and median nerves, as well as the brachial artery. This should be followed by palpation of the medial and lateral epicondyle to assess for concomitant fractures. A physical examination should also include an evaluation of the shoulder, forearm, and wrist for associated injuries [1, 5, 16].

Once a complex elbow fracture–dislocation has been clinically excluded, an immediate reduction attempt should be initiated. Several reduction methods have been proposed in the literature, which are all based on traction/countertraction maneuvers. Of note, an elbow dislocation often requires conscious sedation to ensure enough relaxation for an atraumatic reduction. Thus, the athlete should first be removed from competition and escorted to the training room, where the decision for a reduction attempt should be made individually. If there is any concern for a major bony injury of the distal humerus or proximal radius, a sideline reduction attempt is not recommended unless there is severe acute neurovascular compromise. Generally, rapid transfer to an emergency room is safest where adequate sedation can be administered and reduction can be performed under radiographic visualization [1, 2, 16].

In the case of the most frequently encountered simple posterolateral dislocation, the reduction is achieved by applying hyper-supination and valgus stress, as this maneuver re-creates the injury mechanism and disengages the coronoid from the distal humerus. As soon as shifting of the elbow is observed, longitudinal traction is performed with varus stress and simultaneous pronation.

After successful reduction, the elbow should be immobilized in 90° of flexion with the forearm in pronation using a splint. Following reduction, reevaluation of the neurovascular status is mandatory, as worsening or loss of neurologic function may be an indication for urgent surgical exploration to rule out nerve entrapment. Subsequently, radiographic imaging should be performed to ensure joint congruency and assess for concomitant fractures of the radial head or coronoid (Fig. 7.5) [1, 2, 16].

7.3.2 Fractures

Elbow fractures comprise any fracture of the proximal radius or ulna and distal humerus. The

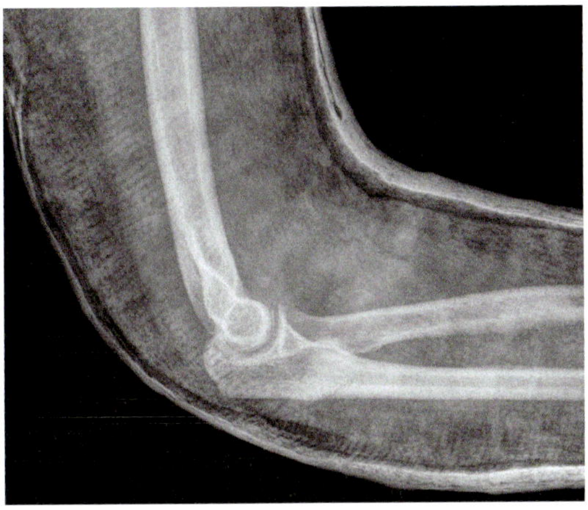

Fig. 7.5 Radiographic control after successful reduction in the female athlete's posterolateral dislocation of the right elbow with joint congruency and absence of concomitant fractures. The elbow is immobilized in a splint

most common injury mechanism is a fall of the outstretched arm. However, they can also be a result of direct trauma (e.g., collision sports) or hit (e.g., baseball and hockey) to the elbow. These fractures can either occur as an isolated injury or in the setting of an elbow dislocation. Pediatric and adolescent athletes require special consideration, given the high risk of physeal fractures in the case of open growth plates [1, 12, 18].

Clinically, the athlete may present with localized tenderness and significant swelling over the respective bony prominence of the elbow (e.g., radial head, medial or lateral epicondyle, and olecranon), and crepitus may also be observed depending on the fracture site. Active and passive range of motion is usually very painful and limited. A careful assessment of distal neurovascular function is mandatory. A visual deformity suggesting an unstable and displaced fracture requires prompt reduction and early referral to a specialized surgeon. Any change in neurovascular status requires immediate surgical intervention. In general, the athlete should be moved off the competition field, immobilized in a sling or splint, and transferred for radiographic imaging [1, 12].

Take-Home Message

- Dislocations and fractures of the shoulder or elbow require immediate on-field or sideline management. In the absence of any red flag signs like neurovascular injury or concomitant fractures, a sideline reduction attempt of a dislocated shoulder or elbow should be performed. A post-reduction neurovascular assessment is mandatory. If the reduction attempt remains unsuccessful, the athlete should urgently be sent to the emergency department for radiographic imaging and reduction under sufficient sedation/analgesia. Following successful reduction, the affected joint should be immobilized using a sling or splint and radiographic imaging should be performed as soon as possible to confirm joint congruency and assess concomitant fractures.
- Sideline management of closed fractures is focused on preventing the injury from becoming an open fracture and minimizing the risk of neurovascular damage due to displaced bone ends. In case of severe displacement, a reduction attempt may be performed for improved alignment and protection of surrounding soft tissues. Again, post-reduction neurovascular assessment is mandatory and any change in neurovascular status requires immediate transfer. Immobilization of the fractured bone and adjacent joints using a sling is recommended, while cryotherapy and NSAIDs may help reduce swelling and facilitate early treatment of fractures requiring surgery after radiographic imaging has been performed.

Fact Box 7.1: Mechanism and Clinical Presentation of Shoulder Dislocation

- Anterior dislocation due to a combination of forward elevation, abduction, and external rotation.
- Posterior dislocation due to a posterior directed force with the shoulder in a flexed, adducted, and internally rotated position.
- *Luxatio erecta* due to a forced hyperabduction to the abducted arm or a direct blow to the fully abducted arm.
- Anterior dislocation presents with the shoulder in an adducted cradle-like position and palpation of the humeral head in the axilla.
- Posterior dislocation presents with the arm in an internally rotated and adducted position close to the side, while the humeral head may be palpated posteriorly.
- *Luxatio erecta* presents with the arm in a hyperabducted and locked position over the patient's head.

Fact Box 7.2: Elbow Dislocation

- Fall on the outstretched hand combined with elbow supination and valgus stress.
- In around 90% of cases dislocation in a posterolateral direction.
- Clinical presentation with the elbow in a varus position and forearm supination.
- Reduction maneuver includes applying gentle hyper-supination and valgus stress, followed by longitudinal traction with varus stress and simultaneous pronation.
- Subsequently, the elbow should be immobilized in 90° of flexion with the forearm in pronation using a splint.
- Radiographic imaging to ensure joint congruency and assess for concomitant fractures.

References

1. Carr JB 2nd, Chicklo B, Altchek DW, Dines JS. On-field management of shoulder and elbow injuries in baseball athletes. Curr Rev Musculoskelet Med. 2019;12:67–71.
2. Skelley NW, McCormick JJ, Smith MV. In-game management of common joint dislocations. Sports Health. 2014;6:246–55.
3. Wilk KE, Arrigo CA, Andrews JR. Current concepts: the stabilizing structures of the glenohumeral joint. J Orthop Sports Phys Ther. 1997;25:364–79.
4. Muench LN, Imhoff AB. The unstable shoulder: what soft tissue, bony anatomy and biomechanics can teach us. Knee Surg Sports Traumatol Arthrosc. 2021;29:3899–901.
5. Schupp CM, Rand SE, Hanson TW, Lee BM, Jafarnia K, Jia Y, et al. Sideline management of joint dislocations. Curr Sports Med Rep. 2016;15:140–53.
6. Walton J, Paxinos A, Tzannes A, Callanan M, Hayes K, Murrell GA. The unstable shoulder in the adolescent Athlete. Am J Sports Med. 2002;30:758–67.
7. Hudson VJ. Evaluation, diagnosis, and treatment of shoulder injuries in athletes. Clin Sports Med. 2010;29:19–32.
8. Norte GE, West A, Gnacinski M, van der Meijden OA, Millett PJ. On-field management of the acute anterior glenohumeral dislocation. Phys Sportsmed. 2011;39:151–62.
9. Shuster M, Abu-Laban RB, Boyd J. Prereduction radiographs in clinically evident anterior shoulder dislocation. Am J Emerg Med. 1999;17:653–8.
10. Emond M, Le Sage N, Lavoie A, Moore L. Refinement of the Quebec decision rule for radiography in shoulder dislocation. CJEM. 2009;11:36–43.
11. Gould SJ, Cardone DA, Munyak J, Underwood PJ, Gould SA. Sideline coverage: when to get radiographs? A review of clinical decision tools. Sports Health. 2014;6:274–8.
12. Hutchinson M, Tansey J. Sideline management of fractures. Curr Sports Med Rep. 2003;2:125–35.
13. Quillen DM, Wuchner M, Hatch RL. Acute shoulder injuries. Am Fam Physician. 2004;70:1947–54.
14. McKoy BE, Bensen CV, Hartsock LA. Fractures about the shoulder: conservative management. Orthop Clin North Am. 2000;31:205–16.
15. Wascher DC, Bulthuis L. Extremity trauma: field management of sports injuries. Curr Rev Musculoskelet Med. 2014;7:387–93.
16. Parsons BO, Ramsey ML. Acute elbow dislocations in athletes. Clin Sports Med. 2010;29:599–609.
17. O'Driscoll SW, Jupiter JB, King GJ, Hotchkiss RN, Morrey BF. The unstable elbow. Instr Course Lect. 2001;50:89–102.
18. Redler LH, Dines JS. Elbow trauma in the athlete. Hand Clin. 2015;31:663–81.

Hand and Wrist

8

Carlos Henrique Fernandes,
João Baptista Gomes dos Santos,
and Rodrigo Guerra Sabongi

8.1 Wrist Injuries

8.1.1 Bone and Joint Injuries

Wrist injuries can cause the joint capsule, ligaments, and bones damage in isolation or combination. A thorough history and physical examination are highly recommended, and radiographic evaluation aids in diagnosis. Sometimes, computerized tomography (CT) can be helpful for a better understanding of injury patterns. Magnetic resonance imaging (MRI) can be solicited for detecting ligamentous injuries and occult fractures.

Distal radioulnar joint (DRUJ) instability

Sports requiring repeated pronation/supination, radial/ulnar deviation, and axial loading of the forearm and wrist can lead to DRUJ instability and triangular fibrocartilage complex carpus (TFCC) injuries. There is contact only about 20% between the sigmoid notch of the distal radius and the head of the ulna. The primary stabilizer of the DRUJ is the TFCC. Most traumatic TFCC tears result from an acute rotational injury to the forearm, a combined axial load, or a fall on the pronated outstretched hand. The evaluation of distal radioulnar joint instability can be difficult, and examination in comparison with the contralateral side is helpful. Athletes may present with ulnar-sided wrist pain and report clicking and abnormal movements. There may be swelling over the ulnar side of the wrist, and a dorsal prominence of the ulna head can be observed. Subluxation of the ulna head is typically detected with supination/pronation. Increased dorsopalmar translation of the radius on the ulna during the ballottement test is evidence of DRUJ instability. The examiner grasps the radius and the carpus firmly while translating the distal ulna in the dorsal and palmar directions within the sigmoid notch using the thumb and index finger of the other hand (Fig. 8.1a). The swimming pool test is positive if ulnocarpal pain is provoked when the athlete pushes his hands to stand up. It is important to make true lateral radiographs of the wrist with the forearm to evaluate the bone position of the distal radioulnar joint. Bilateral computed tomography (CT) scans of the distal radioulnar joint are indicated when there is suspicion of instability. Magnetic resonance imaging (MRI) is indicated for the evaluation of TFCC tears and soft-tissue structures about the wrist. Diagnostic arthroscopy is sensitive for identifying ulnocarpal ligament injuries, traumatic TFCC tears or degeneration, and chondromalacia. Nonsurgical treatment is indicated for TFCC tears in the absence of DRUJ instability. Activity modification and rest are many times enough because the fovea and peripheral TFCC are well vascularized and have good healing potential.

C. H. Fernandes (✉) · J. B. G. dos Santos
R. G. Sabongi
Department of Orthopedic Surgery, Escola Paulista de Medicina-Universidade Federal de São Paulo, São Paulo, SP, Brazil

S. Rocha Piedade et al. (eds.), *Sideline Management in Sports*,
https://doi.org/10.1007/978-3-031-33867-0_8

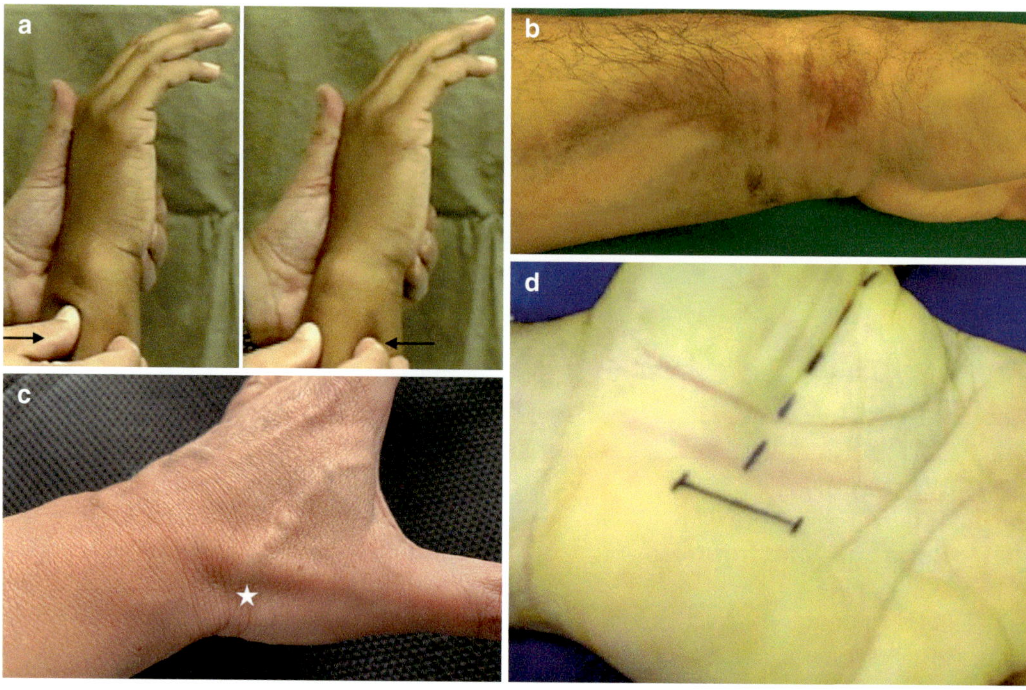

Fig. 8.1 (**a**) Ballottement test. The ulna head is dislocated in dorsal and palmar directions according to the direction of the forces applied by the examiner (black arrows). (**b**) The observation of ecchymosis and swelling on the wrist and distal forearm are common after a distal radius fracture. (**c**) The wrist snuffbox (star) is triangularly shaped, the medial border is the tendon of the extensor pollicis longus, the lateral border is the tendons of the extensor pollicis brevis and abductor pollicis longus, the proximal border is the styloid process of the radius, and the floor is the scaphoid bone. (**d**) Hook of hamate fracture causes pain on the ulnar side of the palm (black line)

Immobilization in neutral pronation–supination is often adequate to treat DRUJ instability caused by TFCC injury if the athlete refuses the surgery. The TFCC and radioulnar ligaments can be repaired arthroscopically or as an open procedure. The success of the treatment is the early recognition and treatment.

8.1.1.1 Distal Radius Fractures

Distal radius fractures are most common after high-energy accidents, a falling from standing height onto an outstretched hand, or hyperflexion. Less than 10% of distal radius fractures occur due to athletic injury [1]. There is a painful range of wrist motion and swelling with ecchymosis. It can be hard to move or use the hand and wrist (Fig. 8.1b). X-rays of the wrist in posterior–anterior and lateral projection need to be performed. The nonoperative management is often selected for patients with extra-articular simple fractures or articular congruity without less than 2 mm step-off and minimum displacement. However, even in cases in which nonoperative treatment is warranted, athletes should anticipate 6–8 weeks of immobilization. The immobilization consists of a period of 4–6 weeks with a short splinting or casting. The operative management is indicated for intra-articular fractures or those with instability characteristics. Open reduction and internal osteosynthesis have demonstrated better short-term outcomes for managing displaced fractures. The injury to the scapholunate ligament is frequently associated with a fracture of the distal radius of the type with compression articular [2]. Patients with untreated instability associated with distal radius fracture have more pain and more restrictions in performing daily activities. The treatment of one-stage surgery is better indicated. Non-contact sports permit return to sport quickly after internal fixation, whereas clinical and radiographic evidence of healing is necessary for high-impact sports practice.

8.1.1.2 Perilunate Injuries

Wrist perilunate fractures and dislocations are severe carpal disruptions around the lunate bone and can present with numerous combinations of fractures, dislocations, and/or complete or partial ligament injuries. They usually occur due to high-energy trauma such as falls with the hand extended occurring in sports of contact, affecting mainly young males. Despite the seriousness of perilunate injuries, diagnostic failure ranges from 7% to 40% and may be related to the experience of the assistant physician [3]. The mechanism most commonly described is a fall on the outstretched hand with the wrist in extension, ulnar deviation, and intercarpal supination. This can cause a wide spectrum of injuries, from minor SL sprains to complete perilunate dislocations.

Scapholunate dissociation (SLD) is the most frequent carpal instability, and the diagnosis is often delayed. On inspection, there may be minimal or no changes in the appearance of the wrist. An acute scapholunate ligament lesion is suspected if there are pain in the dorsal wrist (scapholunate joint), swelling, and ecchymosis. Range of motion is usually limited, and there is a weakness in grasp. Radiographic evaluation includes contralateral wrist radiographs for comparison. On the PA view can be sought a scapholunate diastasis, named as "Terry Thomas sign" and the scaphoid ring sign caused by flexion of the scaphoid. The early diagnosis can be performed by measuring the radiolunate index (RLI) on the lateral view [4]. The RLI is the ratio V to D, where V is the distance between the most volar point of the distal radius and the most volar point of the distal lunate, and D is the distance between the most dorsal point of distal radius and the most dorsal point of the distal lunate (Table 8.1). MRI may be useful to better understand the injury. Arthroscopy is considered the gold standard procedure. The injury is considered acute if it has occurred within 6 weeks of presentation. Surgical repair in the acute phase is generally successful and can prevent degenerative changes and chronic wrist pain. Referral to a hand surgery specialist should be considered.

Table 8.1 Interval of the RLI for each of the diagnoses

Diagnoses	RLI
Without changes	1136 ± 0,172
Scapholunate dissociation	1907 ± 0,428
Trans-scaphoid perilunate fracture	0,743 ± 0,099
Lunate dislocation	0,47 ± 0,086

Athletes with perilunate fracture–dislocations often present with intense symptoms such as decreased range of motion, swelling, pain, and a palpable deformity of the wrist. As a consequence of carpal bone dislocation, median nerve compression may cause acute carpal tunnel syndrome. Symptoms of paresthesias of the palmar surface of the first three digits can be present. Assessment of the motor function of the hand can be limited secondary to pain. The clinical assessment of the patient is generally complemented by a radiographic examination on the initial assessment. The main difficulty in recognizing these injuries is because there is an alteration in the position of the lunate bone to the articular surface of the distal end of the radius. Initial management involves an emergent closed reduction in the dislocation and sedation is frequently necessary for a successful reduction. The maneuver for reduction can be difficult and require the application of traction to the arm, with the hand suspended as a form of countertraction. Once closed reduction is obtained, splint immobilization is required. Surgical definitive management is indicated for ligamentous repair/reconstructions and reductions and fixations of the associated fractures. The missed injuries can be treated with salvage procedures, such as proximal row carpectomy, and partial or total wrist fusions.

8.1.1.3 Carpus Bone Fractures

The scaphoid bone is the most commonly fractured bone of the carpus in young and active individuals. The mechanisms of trauma described during sports practice are a falling on an outstretched hand, a collision of the wrist against an obstacle, or a direct blow against an adversary. The management of scaphoid fractures in athlete presents the difficulty of making an accurate, early diagnosis, and the need for an early return to play. Scaphoid fractures lead to mild symptoms, such as pain on the radial side of the wrist, which leads to a limited range of motion, but, in general, the outward signs of trauma may be subtle. Physical examination starts with a visual inspection, and there is no visible deformity. A positive test is pain and tenderness when pressure is exerted on the anatomical snuffbox (Fig. 8.1c). Another positive test is pain and tenderness when pressure is exerted on the scaphoid tuberosity at the proximal wrist crease with the opposite hand. A longitudinal pressure down the thumb is performed in a scaphoid axial compression test. A positive test is the reproduction of pain.

Plain radiographs should be obtained. When the radiographs do not confirm the scaphoid fractures on the injury day, the wrist may be cast and radiographs repeated in 10–14 days to be safe. Prompt diagnosis of scaphoid fractures in elite athletes is important to minimize time away from the sport and any complications that can arise from a delayed diagnosis. If the suspicion is great or the period of immobilization interferes with sport or training, a CT scan can be used to assist with a fast diagnosis. MRI is very sensitive to diagnosing scaphoid fractures, and when an MRI is negative, the athlete can safely return to play without a period of immobilization. Early diagnosis and appropriate treatment are important to avoid the risk of delayed union and nonunion with later consequences of avascular necrosis, arthritis, and carpal collapse. Treatment of a scaphoid fracture depends on many factors, including age, activity level, symptom intensity, localization, and presence of arthritis and/or collapse. Acute, non-displaced fractures of the scaphoid waist can be treated by short-arm cast immobilization and thumb immobilization does not affect union rates according to more recent data, with a high rate of union [5]. Short-arm cast immobilization is much less unwieldy for the athlete; however, this treatment entails 6–12 weeks. There is a current trend in orthopedic practice to treat non-displaced or minimally displaced fractures with early open reduction and internal fixation instead of cast immobilization. The results of clinical trials suggest that CT-confirmed non-displaced scaphoid waist fractures heal with 6 weeks of immobilization [5]. A study demonstrated that non-displaced middle third scaphoid fractures can be effectively immobilized for competition in football players with a short-arm custom-made SILASTIC cast. In a series of 14 patients treated, 12 patients went on to union, with one nonunion occurring in a proximal pole fracture and one nonunion occurring after a delay in diagnosis [6]. The nonsurgical treatment of scaphoid fractures is not free of complications, despite the good levels of bone union. The time of immobilization causes muscular atrophy and a decrease in strength, leading to an increase in the degree of joint stiffness of the wrist, which in turn requires a longer rehabilitation time. Minimally invasive techniques may reduce surgical trauma and improve athletes' care and recovery [7]. Rettig and Kollias [8] recommend more aggressive treatment in cases of non-dislocated fractures, especially in athletes. The percutaneous fixation technique with a compression screw for the treatment of waste and proximal scaphoid fractures has allowed early active mobility of the wrist with a low rate of complications and earlier return to sports practice. The use of arthroscopy during the internal fixation provides a full examination of the articular surface in the radiocarpal joint and the midcarpal joint and of the quality of reduction in the scaphoid fracture. We believe that it has been a good alternative to prolonged plaster cast use. If the fracture is in the proximal third or if the fracture is at all displaced, screw or pins would be placed in surgery. Surgical access to the scaphoid can be via a dorsal or volar approach. The choice is based on the anatomical localization of the fracture. The volar approach is used for waist and distal pole fractures. The dorsal approach is preferred for waist or proximal pole fractures. If a scaphoid fracture is untreated, there is a high risk of chronic pain with associated reduced range of motion and grip strength.

Trapezoid fractures are very uncommon, accounting for less than 1% of all wrist fractures. The trapezoid bone has a very stable position within the wrist, forming a relatively immobile joint with the second metacarpal base distally. Very strong ligaments also connect it to the trapezium, capitate, and scaphoid. Trapezoid fractures occur when a strong bending or axial force is applied to the second metacarpal base. Fractures of the trapezoid bone usually have a good clinical outcome. A non-displaced fracture can be treated with cast immobilization for 4 weeks [9].

Hamate fractures are commonly divided into hook fractures and body fractures and represent only 2–4% of all carpal bone fractures. They are quite common in athletes and may be divided into direct and indirect injuries. The direct injury occurs by acute impingement on the hamate hook caused by striking the palm on a solid object, such as a racquet, bat, or club, by falling on the palm, or by a crush injury to the hand. Tenderness directly over the hook is always present, and grip strength is typically weak. Ulnar nerve paresthesia or weakness and mild carpal tunnel syndrome are frequently present. Flexor tendon rupture may occur in a few athletes. The indirect injury refers to shearing fractures of the hamate hook base by flexor tendons contracting forcefully as they move in the ulnar direction during a power grip. The athletes complain of pain and tenderness on the ulnar side of the palm (Fig. 8.1d). The fracture can be diagnosed on a carpal tunnel view and an oblique roentgenogram of the wrist supinated. CT scan is the best imaging technique for demonstrating this fracture. The remotion of the fracture fragment permits the patients to return to their regular occupational and athletic pursuits [10].

8.1.2 Tendon Injuries

Avulsion fractures involving the extensor carpi radialis longus and avulsion fractures of the extensor carpi radialis brevis have been previously reported. The open reduction and internal fixation permit the patient to heal uneventfully and return to full painless activity [11].

The repetitive gliding of tendons of the dorsal compartments, beneath the sheath, during long training times can be involved in the pathogenetic process of wrist tenosynovitis. It often results from the abnormal kinematics of a tendon associated with a patient's anatomical determinants. The tenosynovitis of the first dorsal compartment of the wrist is more common in women than men and is called de Quervain. It results from resisted gliding of the abductor pollicis longus and the extensor pollicis brevis tendons in the fibro-osseous canal. Athletes with de Quervain's tenosynovitis have pain in the wrist or thumb aggravated by movement and/or while gripping or hitting, with a racquet, bat, or club. Diagnosis may be made on physical examination. Swelling at the thumb base and over the radial styloid can be observed (Fig. 8.2a). The Finkelstein test is performed by having patients make a fist with the thumb folded inside the fist and then moving their hand downward; if the motion triggers pain, the condition is confirmed (Fig. 8.2b). An X-ray is indicated to rule out bony abnormalities. The ultrasound is a reliable and sensitive method for detecting de Quervain, demonstrating accessory compartments, tendon thickening, effusion, ganglion, and paratendinitis. The initial treatment consists of splinting and corticosteroid injections, and if no progress is seen, surgical release of the compartment might be indicated.

The extensor carpi ulnaris (ECU) tendon passes through the sixth extensor compartment and is maintained within a bony groove on the dorsal surface of the ulna by a retinaculum. It provides a variable contribution to wrist flexion and extension depending on forearm position, and this variation impacts its function and relative stability. The sports-related ECU pathology includes tenosynovitis of the tendon sheath, tendinopathy, tendon disruption, and tendon instability. These conditions can occur in isolation or combined and have been most frequently reported in sports such as tennis, golf, and certain high-impact contact sports. A full clinical and radiological assessment is necessary, and there are many other causes of ulnar-sided wrist pain and are mandatory to exclude coexistent

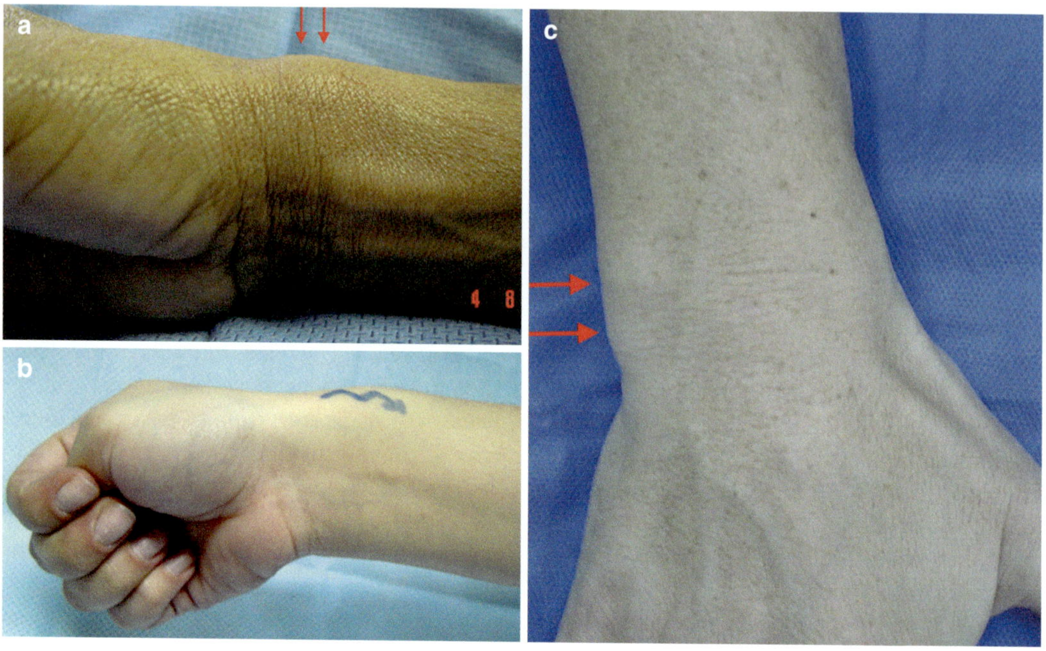

Fig. 8.2 (**a**) De Quervain tenosynovitis causing swelling on the topography of the radial styloid (first dorsal compartment). (**b**) The Finkelstein test. The motion triggers wrist pain. (**c**) Tenosynovitis of the ECU causing swelling on the topography of the ulna head (red arrows).

injuries in the triangular fibrocartilage complex (TFCC), lunotriquetral ligament, distal radioulnar joint, or ulnar styloid. Swelling over the ulnar head can be observed (Fig. 8.2c). The treatment is based on the distinction between stable and unstable conditions. The stable condition usually responds to nonoperative, rest, and splint. The intratendinous injection of corticosteroids needs to be avoided because of the risk of subsequent rupture. The surgical treatment may be indicated in cases of acute traumatic injuries and cases of chronic subluxation combined with tendinopathy [12].

8.2 Hand Injuries

8.2.1 Bone and Joint Injuries

8.2.1.1 Metacarpal Fractures

The metacarpal bones present a head, neck, shaft, and base. The II–V metacarpal bones are connected proximally by interosseous ligaments and distally by the deep transverse metacarpal ligament, which maintains the stability of the metacarpal arch [13]. The fractures can be subdivided into four anatomic regions, base, neck, shaft, and head. Not all metacarpal fractures present deformities. Metacarpal and phalangeal fractures are among the most common skeletal injuries in the general population, accounting for 10% of all fractures and 1% of emergency department visits in the United States [14]. Common fracture patterns exist secondary to the relative anatomy and deforming forces on susceptible areas of the bone. Torsion, compression, shear, bending, and tension can all result in specific fracture patterns [15]. During physical activity, metacarpal fractures sustained from a direct blow, fall, or crush occur most, especially in contact sports [16]. Although the number of injuries sustained is higher during practice, the injury rate is higher during competitive games. This is because more time is spent at practice as opposed to games, but competition typically increases the intensity level [17]. Fractures of the metacarpals or phalanges can significantly affect an athlete's training program, season, or career, depending on the timing and severity of the injury [18].

The metacarpal base is articulated with the carpal bones. The carpometacarpal (CMC) joints of the ring and small finger metacarpal bases allow a larger degree of motion; for this reason, more displacement can be permitted in fractures of the ulnar metacarpals because the deformity can more easily be compensated [18]. In general, the injury results from an axial load to the hand with the wrist in flexion and the elbow in extension. Metacarpal base fractures are frequently associated with CMC dislocations. The most common injury is the intra-articular base of the small finger metacarpal fractures because the action of the extensor carpi ulnaris causes the proximal and ulnar displacement of the metacarpal base. The physical examination consists of observing the presence of edema, ecchymosis, and a deformity centered on the ulnar side of the dorsum of the hand (Fig. 8.3a). To avoid a missed diagnosis on standard radiographs, a 30° pronated lateral view permits visualization of the small and ring finger CMC joints. As with other intra-articular fractures, surgical fixation to restore the articular surface is recommended to prevent post-traumatic arthritis.

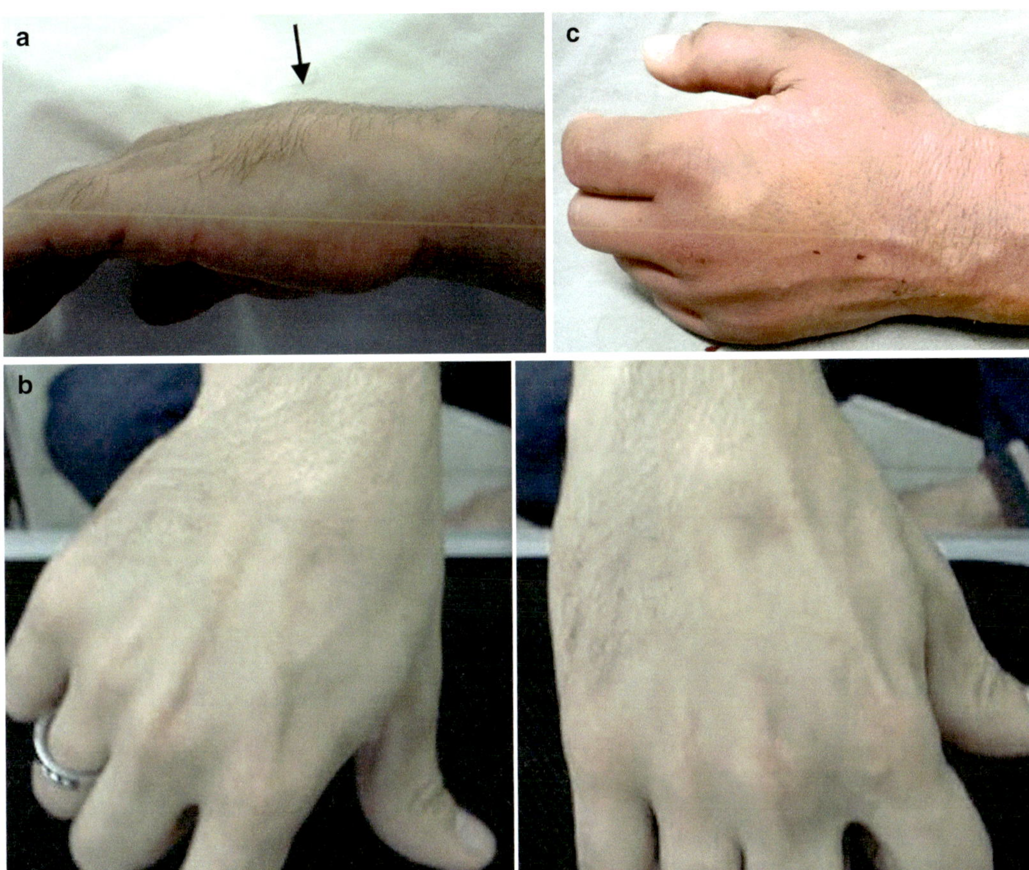

Fig. 8.3 (**a**) Deformity centered on the ulnar side of the dorsum of the hand in a metacarpal base fracture associated with CMC dislocation. (**b**) The different positions of the extensor tendon to carpal boss in consequence of the wrist deviations. (**c**) A swelling and ecchymosis in the thumb consequence of Bennett's fracture. (**d**) Swelling, ecchymosis, and index finger overlapping. (**e**) A missing knuckle of the left fourth metacarpal in a fist position. (**f**) Swelling and ecchymosis in consequence of a metacarpal head fracture. (**g**) An impossibility to extend the ring finger because of an extensor tendon injury after a "fight bite." (**h**) The extensor tendon of the index and long fingers typically deviates in the radial direction during the flexion of the MCP joint. (**i**) A valgus stress test in a thumb ulnar collateral ligament injury

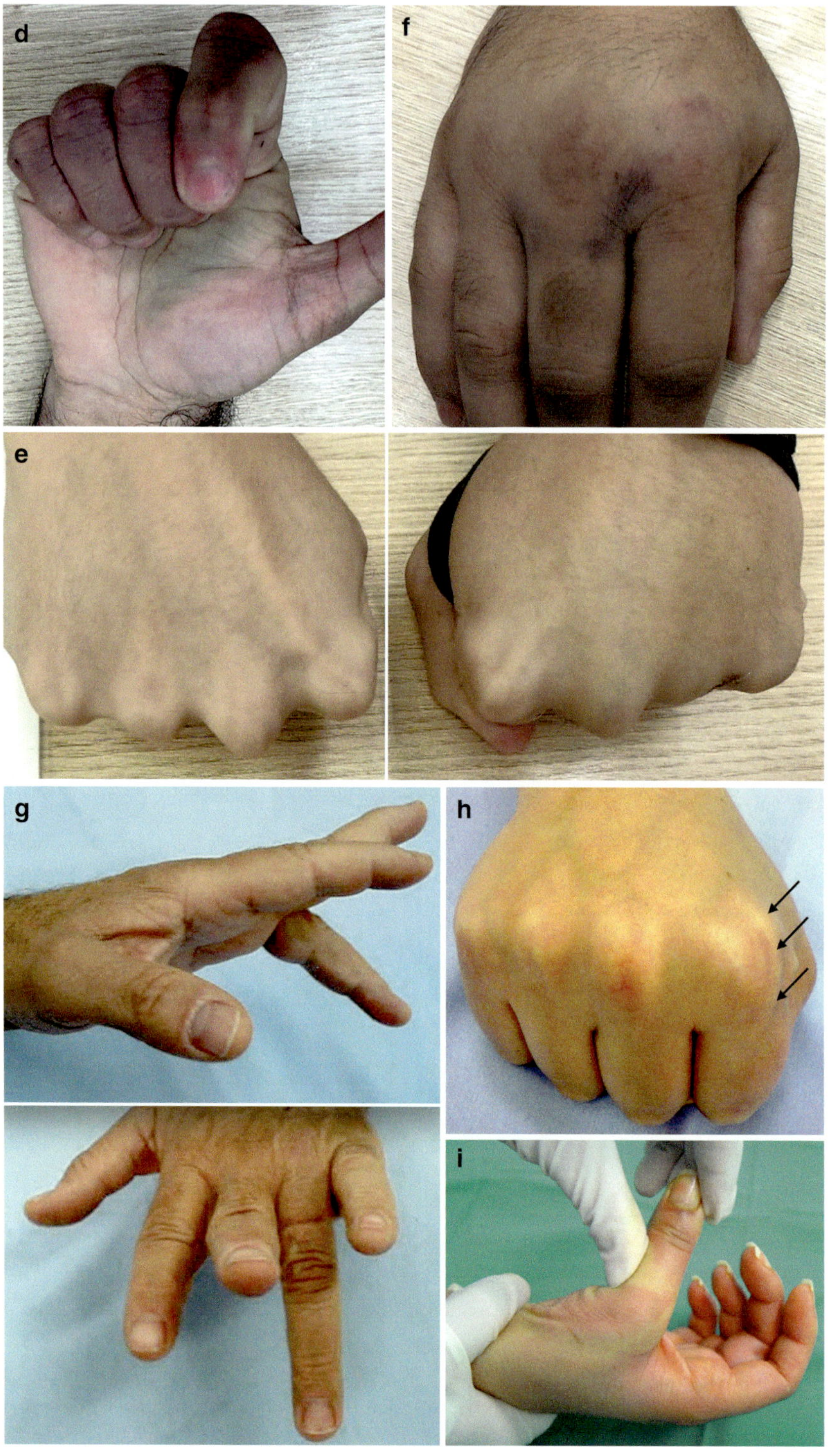

Fig. 8.3 (continued)

As a consequence of violent trauma, dorsal and palmar ligament lesions can occur, causing instability of the CMC joint without fracture–dislocation. The repeated trauma to the unstable CMC joints creates periarticular hypertrophic bone spurs with concomitant articular subluxation and degenerative changes so-called carpal boss. Usually, the second and third metacarpals are affected. There is a formation of a small hard and firm mass on the dorsal aspect of the wrist that is more visible on the volar flexion of the wrist. Sometimes, the mass resembles a ganglion cyst due to its location on the wrist and its rounded external appearance. The wrist's movement in radial deviation and ulnar deviation can cause a snap, due to the movement of the index finger extensor over the carpal boss (Fig. 8.3b). Radiographs are best conducted using the "carpal boss view," a lateral projection of the wrist with flexion and supination of 30–40° and ulnar deviation of 20–30°. Computed tomography can be useful for the evaluation of bone deformity. The technetium bone scan is helpful when plain radiographs are inconclusive and provides information about the state of underlying CMC joints. Magnetic resonance images may show edema and synovitis at this location. Diminished grip strength, pain, and point tenderness turn the athletes unable to compete. For a symptomatic traumatic carpal boss, selective CMC joint fusion is the indicated surgical treatment [19].

The thumb has a great range of motion, permitting pinch and opposition. The thumb metacarpal has a different position, and it is pronated compared with the rest of the hand. Similar to other joints with a large range of motion, there is little bony stability. Because of the anatomy, injuries involving the thumb's base are common, such as trapezium fracture, CMC dislocation, first metacarpal base fracture, or a fracture–dislocation association. The isolated traumatic dislocation of the first carpometacarpal joint is not common. Pain, deformity, and swelling at the dorsomedial side of the hand are present. The dislocation can be diagnosed on a roentgenogram. The closed reduction needs to be performed and can be done under adequate analgesia. It involves axial traction on the thumb to pull the metacarpal distally, palmar abduction, and pronation while applying external pressure, with the pulp thumb, over the metacarpal base medially to return it to anatomical position. An immobilization is applied after the close reduction. The anatomic restoration after the first reduction needs to be evaluated by radiograph. An open reduction and ligament reconstruction can be necessary in cases of chronic instability.

First metacarpal fractures make up almost 25% of all metacarpal fractures; of these fractures, over 80% involve the base of the first metacarpal. Fractures of the base of the first metacarpal result from bending, rotation, direct blows, indirect forces, or any combination of these forces. Athletes with thumb injuries classically present with pain and loss of function of the thumb. We can observe the thumb's local swelling and volar and dorsal ecchymosis (Fig. 8.3c). Sometimes, the thumb presents an angular deformity and shortening. As initial treatment, to reduce pain and limit swelling, the physician team can perform a temporary immobilization with splints, and the judicious use of ice packs can provide some comfort.

Radiographs are routinely used in anteroposterior, oblique, and lateral views. A true AP view of the thumb requires that the hand be placed in pronation so that the dorsum of the thumb lies against the radiographic plate (Robert's view). A true lateral TM joint (Bett's view) is where the sesamoids of the thumb MP joint overlap. Computed tomography (CT) can be helpful, particularly when assessing intra-articular fractures. Regardless of the type of injury, the well-established principles of stable anatomic reduction and early functional motion are the keystones of treatment.

Edward H. Bennett was the first author to describe the fracture of the volar, ulnar portion of the thumb metacarpal base in 1882. From this early account, this fracture pattern now carries his name. With these fractures, the small proximal and ulnar fragment of the first metacarpal continues to articulate with the trapezium via the volar ligament. The distal aspect of the metacarpal is supinated and dislocated radially by the adductor pollicis brevis, whereas the abductor pollicis longus, inserted on a radial tubercle of the base, pulls the shaft fragment in a dorsal, radial, and proximal direction. The abductor pollicis longus also imparts some supination to the shaft of the thumb metacarpal. This muscular action results in a dislocation of the first carpometacarpal joint. Closed reduction and percutaneous fixation with intermetacarpal Kirschner wires can be used. The K-wires are positioned approximately 2 cm apart, through the first metacarpal with a 90° angle and also through the second metacarpal. Another technique is to use a Kirschner wire through the metacarpal across the joint and into the trapezium. Subsequently, to prevent shortening and adduction of the thumb, another K-wire with a diameter of 1.5–2 mm is inserted between the metacarpal diaphysis of the thumb and the index finger. When the proximal fragment is too big, we preferred to fix the fracture with a percutaneous cannulated screw [20].

Isolated metacarpal shaft fractures of the long and ring fingers tend to be stable, and opposite index and little finger metacarpals are more susceptible to shortening. In a normal flexed hand, the fingertips should align and point toward the scaphoid tubercle on the radial volar aspect of the wrist. Mild rotation in the metacarpal can lead to significant finger overlapping when the patient makes a fist (Fig. 8.3d). A degree of dorsal angulation can be acceptable and depends on the metacarpal involved, with no greater than 10° tolerated in the index, and up to 30° in the small finger. The limit of the shortening is 2 mm. Cast immobilization is usually the best treatment for fractures with acceptable alignment and generally should not exceed 3–4 weeks. The collateral ligaments of the metacarpophalangeal (MCP) joint are at maximum length and tension in flexion and lax in extension. The MCP joint can be immobilized in 70° to 90° of flexion to avoid contractures of the collateral ligaments. Despite immobilization, the athletes are encouraged to mobilize the non-injured digits and joints, including the elbow and shoulder. The possibility of an athlete being allowed to play with an orthosis or cast depends on the sport, position, level of play, and, ultimately, the play rules. For unstable or rotated fractures, surgical treatment is indicated. The treatment with Kirchner wires is of relatively easy application with minimal damage to soft tissue. The disadvantage is a lack of stability, which requires a period of postoperative immobilization. More common complications following percutaneous fixation, such as stiffness and pin-track infection, may be associated. Fracture fixation with plates and screws may provide immediate stability while granting anatomic reduction. Although an open reduction and internal fixation may cause potential soft tissue damage, the benefit of a stable construct may overcome these disadvantages [21].

The fifth metacarpal neck fracture is the most common metacarpal neck fracture. It occurs because the neck comprises the weakest area of the bone, and the injury mechanism usually punches a firm object. The fifth metacarpal neck fractures appear to be far more commonly seen in fist-fighting between individuals with little or no knowledge of boxing. Boxers with good technique rarely incur this particular type of hand injury. Boxer's fractures typically present with pain, swelling, and hematoma. A finger deformity, such as a missing knuckle, can be observed when the athlete makes a fist position (Fig. 8.3e). Diagnosis is confirmed by radiography to display the fracture and its angulations. The management of the boxer's fracture is still a matter of debate. The rate of angulation is acceptable up to 70°. The reduction in angulated fractures of less than 70° seems not of value for the range of motion (ROM) of the fifth MCP joint [22]. Injuries occurring during the off-season and at lower levels of competition are more likely to be managed nonoperatively. Considering that these patients tend to remain active and may be less compliant with activity restrictions while healing, particularly in the younger population, weekly follow-up for up to 3 weeks may be necessary [23]. The surgical treatment can be indicated in the presence of severe displacement or rotational deformity. The use of intramedullary fixation of the metacarpal neck and shaft fractures using headless compression screws is an option resulting in excellent clinical outcomes [22].

There have been reports of metacarpal stress fractures in the dominant hand of racquet-playing athletes, such as golfers, batters, or tennis players. These injuries are managed similarly to lower extremity stress fractures and are primarily treated by rest, activity modification, and immobilization [24].

Fractures of the metacarpal heads are relatively uncommon. Trauma caused by a direct blow or torsional, valgus, or varus stress can cause rupture of the collateral ligaments or avulsion fractures of the metacarpal head. The metacarpal head of the index finger is most commonly involved. Compression fracture of the metacarpal head has been described in association with subsequent avascular necrosis.

8.2.1.2 Metacarpophalangeal Joints

Traumatic injuries of the metacarpophalangeal joints are common, especially in the fourth and fifth metacarpals. The injury usually results from a forceful impact with a clenched fist. The spectrum of injuries varies from simple skin laceration to closed sagittal band injury, extensor tendon rupture, dorsal capsule rupture, metacarpal fractures, and carpometacarpal joint injuries. The clenched fist "fight bite" injuries are more common in nonathletes during street fights. When the patient presents with a skin laceration, prompt treatment is necessary to prevent potential complications associated with these injuries. The number of débridements is performed as necessary. If an extensor tendon lesion occurs, the athlete is unable to extend the finger from the flexed position (Fig. 8.3g). The closed sagittal band injury often results in symptoms ranging from metacarpophalangeal joint pain, swelling, and/or tenderness over the dorsum of the MCP joint to subluxation or dislocation of the extensor digitorum communis tendon with flexion of the MCP joint (Fig. 8.3h). Some acute injuries in nonathletes can be managed nonsurgically with extension splints for the metacarpophalangeal joint. The treatment of this lesion in athletes is a direct repair of the disrupted extensor hood, without the need for tendon augmentation [25].

Dorsal dislocation of the metacarpophalangeal (MCP) joint is usually caused by a sudden force eliciting hyperextension of the joint. The dislocation may be anatomically reduced by simple manual maneuvers, flexing the wrist, and applying distal traction with gentle force in the phalangeal base. Uncommonly, the volar plate becomes entrapped between the metacarpal head and the proximal phalanx. Surgical reduction requires returning this structure to its original location to obtain a stable reduction through a full range of motion.

The most common lesion on the thumb is called skier's thumb. It occurs as a cause of opening the fingers as much as they can, so the thumb lies in maximum adduction and is liable to suffer a sprain of the ulnar collateral ligament (UCL). The UCL lesion can be associated with injury to the joint capsule, the volar plate, and the adductor aponeurosis. Athletes present with pain and swelling at the thumb MCP joint. Complete ligament injuries are differentiated from mild sprains through a careful valgus stress test. If 35° of joint angulation was noted on valgus stress of the flexed MCP joint or if instability of the injured thumb exceeded stability of the uninjured thumb by at least 15°, we should suspect a complete ulnar collateral ligament injury (Fig. 8.3i). On-plain X-ray can show a non-displaced avulsion fracture. Treatment of non-displaced avulsion fractures and partial tears of UCL entails 4 weeks of immobilization in a thumb-spica splint or cast. Unstable injuries, however, require operative intervention to repair or reconstruct the UCL. The "Stener lesion" is when the aponeurosis of the adductor policies is interposed between the ligament and its insertion on the proximal phalanx. Magnetic resonance imaging (MRI) can provide the presence of the interposed tissue and is therefore an indication for surgical treatment. Distal avulsions of the base of the metacarpal can be repaired back to bone using suture anchors. After surgery, athletes involved in contact sports should be cast for four weeks with an additional two weeks of splinting.

8.3 Fingers Injuries

8.3.1 Skin Lesions

Calluses are the most common hand and wrist lesions in combat sports athletes. Sometimes, they are associated with finger joint pain and deformities. The hands and fingers have much contact time with the opponent and are used to

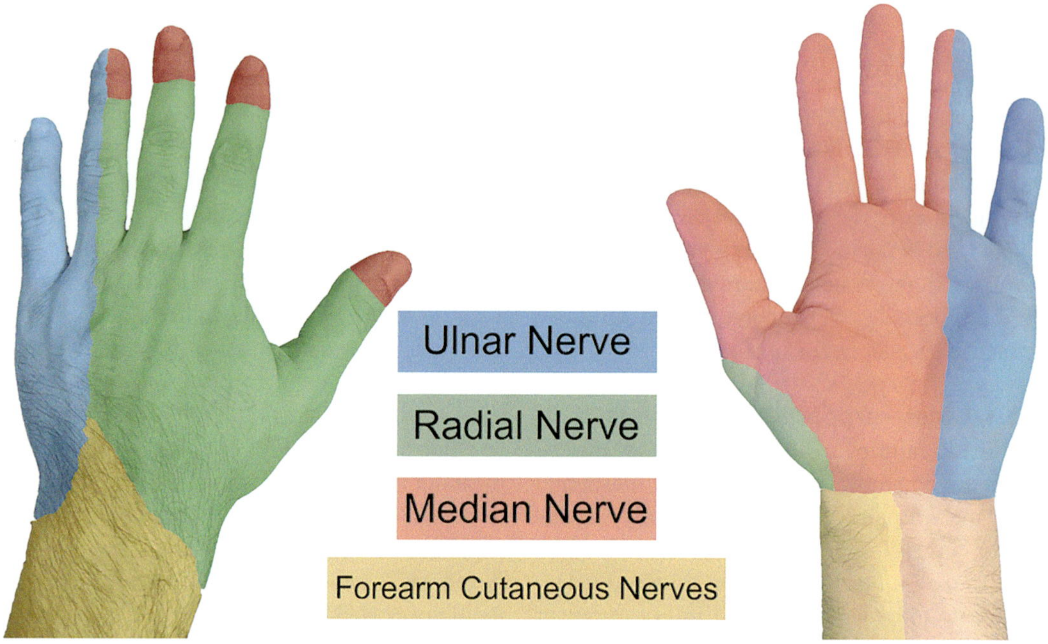

Fig. 8.4 Sensory supply of the hand

grasp the opponent's clothing and body to maintain control, increasing the potential for injury. No specific treatment is necessary [26].

Skin hand injuries can happen in a multitude of sports scenarios. Superficial burns can happen in athletes due to falling on the outstretched hand. It can range from scratches to small cuts and perforations. Open injuries and lacerations of the hand must be assessed with care to determine the extent of the injury. Even small wounds may be associated with important underlying tendon or nerve disruptions. Even simple injuries can lead to scar retraction. Initial treatment must be focused on cleaning the injured area with soap and water and cover with a clean cloth. This first approach is fundamental to remove infected debris and reduce the risk of infection. Avoid removing blisters at the sideline because it can lead to pain and increase the risk of infection [27]. Sensory evaluation is fundamental for identifying nerve injuries in the hand and digits. At the sideline, sensibility can be primarily tested by a light touch off and object or the tip of the finger of the examiner on the suspected denervated area. Understanding the specific nerve anatomy is mandatory to properly suspect a nerve injury and examine its autonomous zone. Figure 8.4 represents the trajectory and innervation of the main sensory nerves of the hand.

8.3.1.1 Frostbite

Frostbite is a special type of injury in winter sports that can start superficially and cause extreme damage to hand tissues. It can lead to long-term irreversible damage if not identified and managed properly. Although medical personnel's main focus should be preventing frostbite injuries to winter sports activities, they should also be trained to recognize and manage this event promptly. Early recognition and initial treatment are crucial to prevent further damage. The first signs of cold injury may be a sensation of numbness and/or tingling. The athlete may refer to clumsy movements and difficulty handling equipment. Appearance is variable and can be misleading. Edema and blistering can only form after rewarming and changes in color cannot occur. After prompt recognition, the patient must be taken urgently to shelter. In site, rewarming is not ideal since freeze–thaw–freeze cycles can lead to further damage. Gloves, rings, and other garments must be removed since swelling can rapidly occur. Oral hydration with preferred warm fluid is warranted. Rewarming strategies must be applied as soon as the injury is identified and a safe shelter is achieved. Placing the hand in another person's armpit or groin can be attempted for up to 10 min as the first measures. Avoid applying dry heat (heat guns and heat pads) or rubbing, which can cause further tissue damage. Ideally, the hand must be immersed in water at 37 °C to 39 °C. If a thermometer is unavailable, medical personnel or the unaffected limb should be placed first for at least 30 s to ensure that the water is not too hot since the affected hand will have impaired sensation. Following rewarming, the hand must be air-dried and covered with a non-circumferential dry dressing. Rubbing or debridement of blisters should not be performed. Elevate the hand to minimize swelling and transfer the patient immediately for specialized care [28].

8.3.2 Nail Bed Injuries

Acute nail bed injuries may be present on a fingertip trauma and are frequently associated with direct trauma in sports activities. Although very common, they are frequently mismanaged and prone to chronic pain and deformities if not treated accordingly. Understanding the anatomy and physiology of the nail complex is key to adequately managing nail bed injuries. The perionychium is composed of multiple structures such as hyponychium, paronychium, eponychium, nail bed, nail fold, and nail plate (Fig. 8.5a). Nail growth is mainly provided by the germinal matrix situated inside the nail fold and extends just distal to the eponychium, forming in some fingers a white arch named lunula. The sterile matrix adds a thin layer of cells that keeps the nail adherent to the nail bed and is situated under the nail plate, from the lunula to the hyponychium. Different types of trauma can result in specific injuries to those structures. A wider area of compression (crush injuries) causes an exploding-type injury that can result in subungual hematoma, stellate-type laceration of the sterile matrix, and/or tuft fractures of the distal phalanx and cause excruciating pain (Fig. 8.5b). The treatment is still controversial. Some advocate for hematoma drainage by perforating the nail plate with an 18-gauge needle, ophthalmic cautery, or even with a heated paperclip. Sharp objects compressing the nail bed usually cause splitting laceration. Initial evaluation of the nail bed injury is essential to guide proper treatment [29]. The specific structures must be analyzed to define adequate surgical intervention. Generally, the anesthetic block is performed to allow thorough examination and effective cleansing of the wound. If the nail plate is avulsed or is unstable, it must be cleaned and preserved for future reconstruction. The original nail plate is an excellent biological protection for repair and must be preserved if in good conditions. Most are tuft fractures that are quite stable after nail bed repair. However, some fractures can occur more proximally, can be unstable, lead to secondary nail deformity, and must be treated with proper fixation [30].

8.3.3 Bone and Articular Injuries

8.3.3.1 Phalanx Fractures

The phalanx fractures can be divided into three anatomic regions, a head(condylar), a shaft, and a base. Regarding the type of fracture, transverse fractures tend to occur from a trauma to a clenched fist, whereas oblique or spiral fractures can occur during a twisting injury. Extra-articular fractures with minimal displacement can safely be treated with buddy taping because the adjacent finger can act as a protective splint, especially in the border digits. Protective splints can be applied to permit an early return to play. Clinical consolidation rarely requires more than three weeks of immobilization because of internal stability. Fractures of the proximal and middle phalanx can be unstable or assume that the typical deformity with apex volar angulation can be managed with closed reduction and percutaneous fixation with K-wires or intramedullary screws or open reduction and fixation with plates. Fracture–dislocations of the proximal interphalangeal joint can be problematic as they can result in stiffness,

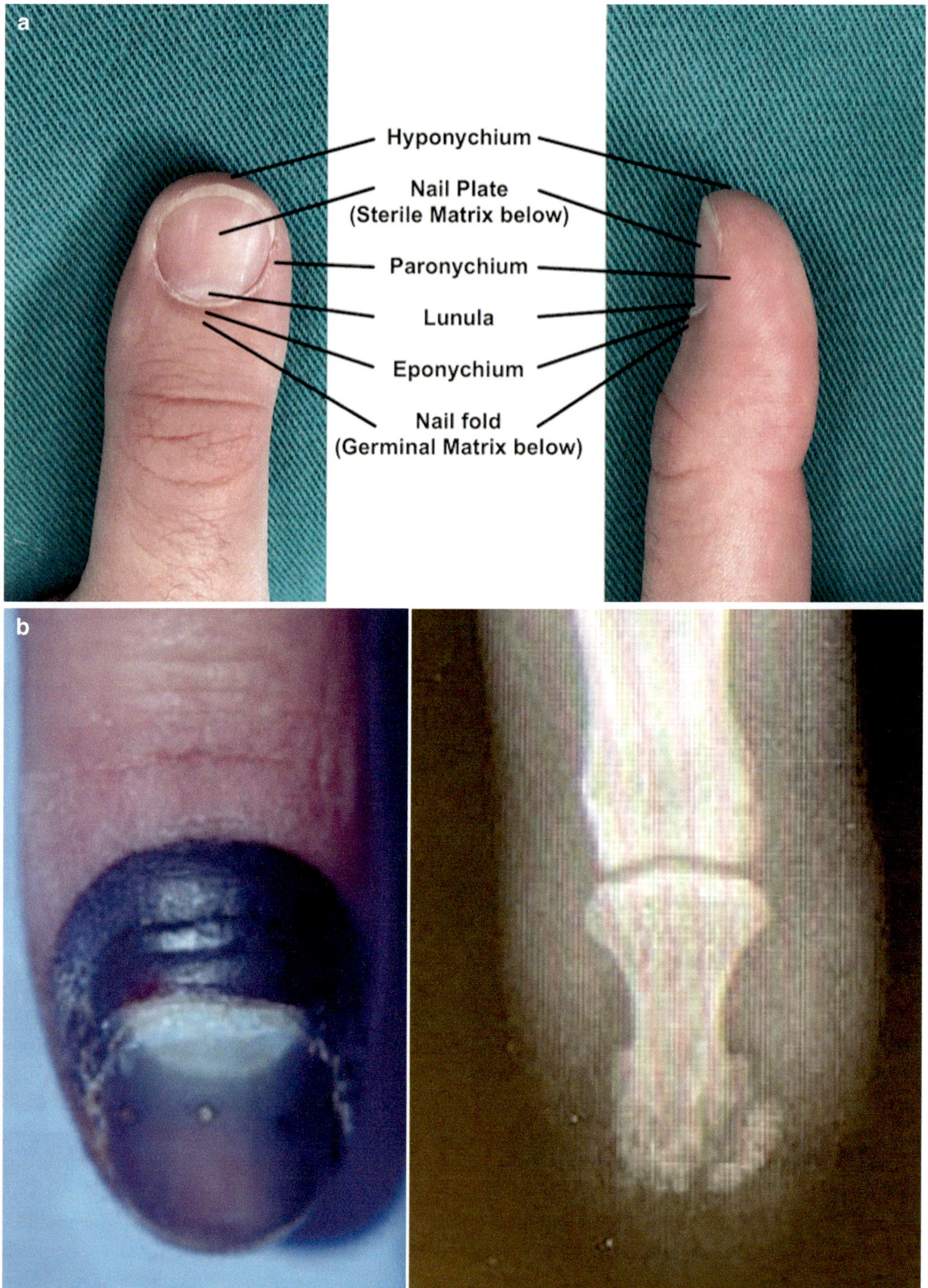

Fig. 8.5 (**a**) Nail anatomy. (**b**) Subungual hematoma and tuft fractures of the distal phalanx

pain, and secondary osteoarthritis. Characteristics of the articular fracture of the middle phalanx that are thought to indicate a benefit of operative treatment are subluxation of the joint, greater than 2-mm articular step-off, and more than 40% of articular surface involvement (Fig. 8.6a). A lack of reduction can lead to pseudo-clawing and extensor lag. Surgical treatment is indicated for fractures that involve more than 40% PIPJ surface, open injuries, irreducible dislocations, or those that require more than 30° flexion to reduce the fragment [31].

Sprains and dislocations of fingers are very common in sports practice. Finger sprains represent incomplete lesions of the capsular and ligament layers without loss of joint congruence. It results from a direct axial impact or contact during the fight. According to the direction of the forces and the energy expended, one or more structures of the PIP joint can be injured to varying degrees, including the collateral ligaments and central slip for the extensor mechanism. At least two must be completely ruptured to cause dislocation. Dislocations involve a complete breakdown in the joint structure. Finger dislocations result in functional disability and dorsal deformity in 90% of cases. Often, the finger dislocation is reduced immediately after the injury.

Digital collateral ligament strains are common due to excessive torsion in certain grip positions. Once strained, the collateral ligaments often return to their same level of tension and stability. The sprains cause persistent pain associated with local swelling, and there may be lateral laxity in case of a complete rupture of the collateral ligament (Fig. 8.6b). Partial rupture will cause joints to become voluminous due to capsuloligamentous scarring that may persist for several months associated with joint stiffness. A hyperextension injury at the proximal interphalangeal joint (PIP) of the long fingers is the cause of full or partial volar plate (VP) rupture with or without avulsion fracture. The VP is a fibrocartilaginous structure that forms the floor of the PIP, which has a ligamentous origin on the proximal phalanx and insertion onto the middle phalanx. During a physical examination, we can observe swelling, tenderness, or deformity and assessment of the patient actively flexing and extending the finger. Passive stability of PIP is assessed by applying valgus and varus stress in extension and 30° of flexion. Plain anteroposterior (AP) and lateral X-rays of the finger are often sufficient for the diagnosis. At fractures that involve less than 30–40% PIPJ surface and are reducible in less than 30° flexion, an extension-blocking immobili-

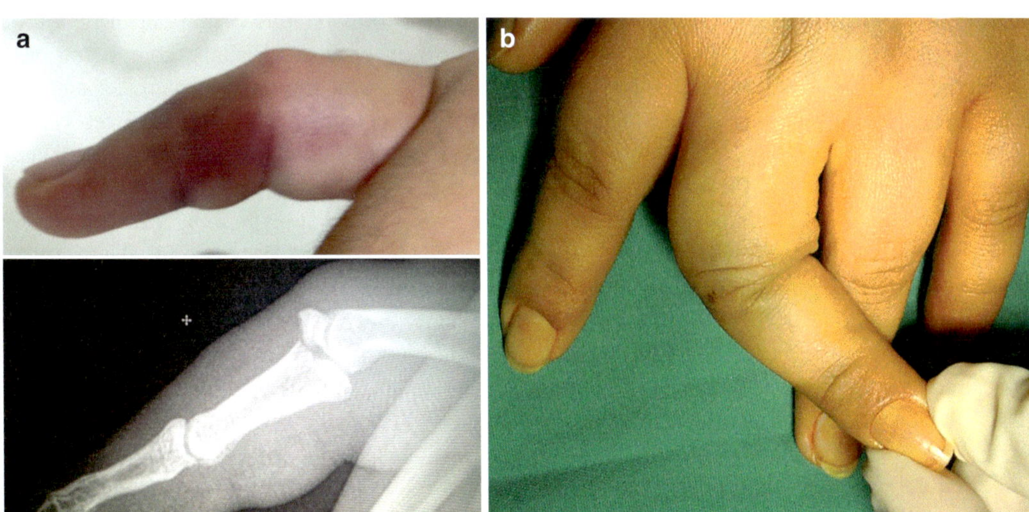

Fig. 8.6 (**a**) Articular fracture of the middle phalanx. Clinic and radiology. (**b**) A stress test in a long finger collateral ligament injury

zation, maintaining the PIPJ in 20° to 30° flexion, is applied during four weeks. Buddy taping to adjacent digits can help support the injured collaterals, prevent the offending position, and allow early motion. The joint may remain swollen for several months, impairing athletic activity. Chronic collateral ligament injury and subsequent IP joint instability lead to early IP joint OA with swelling and fixed flexion at the PIP joint [32].

8.3.4 Tendon Injuries

8.3.4.1 Pulley Ruptures

Pulley ruptures of flexor tendons can often be felt as pop with pain at the time of injury. The athlete will present with pain and swelling over the volar surface of the finger. Bowstringing of the tendon can be observed if the A2 or A4 pulley is completely ruptured. On MRI, a ruptured pulley can result in volar displacement of the tendon from the underlying phalanges by greater than 2 mm. Conservative treatment is often adequate for two weeks in a volar splint, followed by pulley protection with tape or thermoplastic splints. Sporting activities need to be suspended for 8 weeks. Surgical reconstruction indicates multiple pulley injuries.

Boutonniere Deformity

Injuries to the central slip of the extensor mechanism at the PIP can be opened or closed. In acute cases of central slip rupturing and the triangular ligament is injured, the athlete cannot actively extend the PIP joint, but the PIP can be passively extended. Radiographs are indicated to rule out some fractures. Nonsurgical treatment with splinting of the PIP joint in full extension for 6 weeks is indicated (Fig. 8.7a). The DIP joint is left free, and active flexion-extension movements are desired. It is recommended nigh splinting for an additional 6 weeks after treatment.

The non-treatment can cause a boutonniere deformity, defined as a flexion deformity at the PIP joint with a hyperextension deformity at the DIP joint (Fig. 8.7b). Surgical options for chronic boutonniere deformities include various procedures for reconstructing the lateral bands [33].

Baseball Finger

The fingertip is a common site of injuries in athletes. Injury of the extensor tendon, or intra-articular fractures at the base of the distal phalanx, leads to a flexion deformity of the distal interphalangeal joint (DIPJ). It is common in sporting practices and referred to as mallet, baseball, or drop finger. The mechanism of injury is when an extended finger receives a sudden axial load to the finger, causing forced flexion of the DIP joint. It is common in sports where the athlete has contact with a ball, such as baseball, volleyball, and rugby. All fingers can be affected, but the dominant hand's most frequently involved digits are on the ulnar side. The closed injury of the terminal extensor tendon can be stretching or avulsion of the tendon insertion with or without a bone fragment from the distal phalanx. Open injuries such as lacerations, abrasions, or crushes are less frequent. The loss of extensor force at the DIP joint, leaving only the action applied by the flexor digitorum profundus tendon, causes the "drop" of the fingertip. The appearance of the deformity is immediate, and the diagnosis is easy (Fig. 8.7c) The findings on a DIPJ radiograph in lateral view divide the lesions into four types according to Albertoni's classification: (A) pure tendon lesion without fracture; (B) bone avulsion lesion; (C) lesion associated with fracture of the dorsal region of the base of the distal phalanx, comprising one-third or more of the articular surface; and (D) epiphyseal detachment in children. Each type is divided into two subtypes. In types A and B, subtype 1 is characterized by a flexion deformity of less than 30° and subtype 2, by a flexion deformity greater than or equal to 30°. Deformities greater than 30° indicate injury to the retinacular ligaments and capsular structures in types A2 and B2. Type C is subdivided into C1, congruent joint (stable), and C2, sub-dislocated or dislocated joint (unstable). Type D is subdivided into D1, epiphyseal detachment (Salter and Harris lesion type 1), and D2, fracture detachment (Salter and Harris type 3). Each type has a specific treatment. Nonsurgical treatment has been the gold standard for types A1, B1, C1, and D. Only the DIP joint needs to be immobilized in

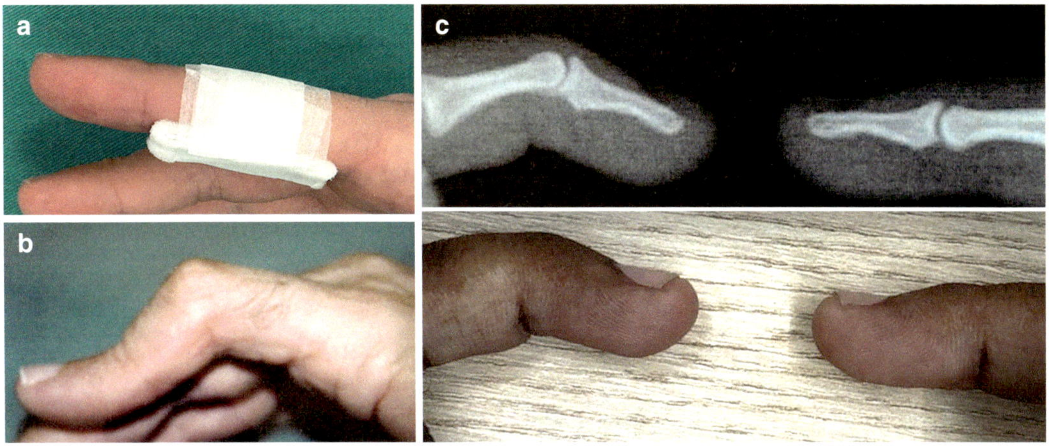

Fig. 8.7 (**a**) Splinting of the PIP joint in full extension. (**b**) Typical Boutonniere deformity. (**c**) Radiological clinical characteristics of a baseball finger on the left side

full extension (types C1 and D) or slight hyperextension (types A1 and B1). Continuous immobilization is maintained for 4 (types B1, C1, and D) to 8 (A1) weeks, followed by nighttime splint use for four weeks. During the treatment period, the DIP joint cannot be flexed during cleaning or splint removal. If this occurs, a full-length period of immobilization is recommended. Surgical treatment is reserved for open injuries, types C2, B2, and C2, or patients who fail to comply with the conservative treatment. Generally, K-wires are used to fix the DIP in extension. The athlete needs to be advised that an extensor lag is common after surgical and nonsurgical treatments, but with excellent clinical outcomes In general, the return to sport is permitted after 8–12 weeks of treatment [34].

Jersey Finger

The flexor digitorum profundus tendon (FDP) is responsible for flexing the DIP joint. Closed injury of FDP occurs as the result of forcible hyperextension of the DIP joint while the FDP is in maximal contraction. It is called the jersey finger because the most common mechanism is when an athlete grasps the jersey of an adversary player It can occur in any finger, but the ring finger is the most affected. There are swelling, ecchymosis, and loss of active IFD joint in the affected finger. In acute cases, tendon reattachment surgery is the gold standard treatment [35].

References

1. Lawson GM, Hajducka C, McQueen MM. Sports fractures of the distal radius–epidemiology and outcome. Injury. 1995;26(1):33–6.
2. Gradl G, Neuhaus V, Fuchsberger T, Guitton TG, Prommersberger KJ, Ring D, Science of Variation Group. Radiographic diagnosis of scapholunate dissociation among intra-articular fractures of the distal radius: interobserver reliability. J Hand Surg Am. 2013;38(9):1685–90.
3. Tanure AA, de Andrade FR, Rezende LGRA, Cagnolati AF, Mandarano-Filho LG, Mazzer N. Diagnostic Failure Rate in Detecting Perilunate Carpal Fractures and Dislocations Using Plain Wrist X-Rays. Rev Bras Ortop (Sao Paulo). 2021;56(3):340–5.
4. Pinto FNZ, Fernandes CH, Dos Santos JBG. The Radiolunate Index: a retrospective radiographic analysis of a new diagnostic measurement for perilunate injuries. J Hand Surg Eur. 2022;47(6):660–1.
5. Bulstra AEJ, Crijns TJ, Janssen SJ, Buijze GA, Ring D, Jaarsma RL, Kerkhoffs GMMJ, Obdeijn MC, Doornberg JN, Science of Variation Group. Factors associated with surgeon recommendation for additional cast immobilization of a CT-verified nondisplaced scaphoid waist fracture. Arch Orthop Trauma Surg. 2021;141(11):2011–8.
6. Riester JN, Baker BE, Mosher JF, Lowe D. A review of scaphoid fracture healing in competitive athletes. Am J Sports Med. 1985;13(3):159–61.
7. Severo AL, Cattani R, Schmid FN, Cavalheiro HL, Castro Neto DN, Lemos MB. Percutaneous treatment for waist and proximal pole scaphoid fractures. Rev Bras Ortop. 2018;53(3):267–75.
8. Rettig AC, Kollias SC. Internal fixation of acute stable scaphoid fractures in the athlete. Am J Sports Med. 1996;24(2):182–6.

9. Ribeiro LM, Botton MA. Isolated Trapezoid Fracture in a Boxer. Am J Case Rep. 2019;20:790–3.
10. Fernandes CH, Meirelles LM, Faloppa F, Albertoni WM. Fracture of the hook of the hamate in a boccie player: case report. Braz J Sports Med. 1998;4(1):18–9.
11. Breeze SW, Ouellette T, Mays MM. Isolated avulsion fracture of the extensor carpi radialis brevis insertion due to a boxer's injury. Orthopedics. 2009;32(3):210.
12. Campbell D, Campbell R, O'Connor P, Hawkes R. Sports-related extensor carpi ulnaris pathology: a review of functional anatomy, sports injury and management. Br J Sports Med. 2013;47(17):1105–11.
13. al-Quattan MM, Robertson GA. An anatomic study of the deep transverse metacarpal ligament. J Anat. 1993;182:443–6.
14. Immerman I, Livermore MS, Szabo RM. Use of emergency department services for hand, wrist, and forearm fractures in the United States in 2008. J Surg Orthop Adv. 2014;23(2):98–104.
15. Court-Brown CM, Wood AM, Aitken S. The epidemiology of acute sports-related fractures in adults. Injury. 2008;39(12):1365–72.
16. Rettig AC, Ryan R, Shelbourne KD, et al. Metacarpal fractures in the athlete. Am J Sports Med. 1989;17(4):567–72.
17. Singletary S, Freeland AE, Jarrett CA. Metacarpal fractures in athletes: treatment, rehabilitation, and safe early return to play. J Hand Ther. 2003;16(2):171–9.
18. Cotterell IH, Richard MJ. Metacarpal and phalangeal fractures in athletes. Clin Sports Med. 2015;34(1):69–98.
19. Melone CP Jr, Polatsch DB, Beldner S. Disabling hand injuries in boxing: boxer's knuckle and traumatic carpal boss. Clin Sports Med. 2009;28(4):609–21.
20. Fernandes CH, Faloppa F, Santos JBG, Raduan Neto, J. First Metacarpal fractures. In: Gregoire Chick. (Org.). Acute and chronic finger injuries in ball sports. 1st ed. Springer, 2013, pp. 14–28.
21. Fernandes CH, Sabongi RG . Fracture after Prior Kirschner's wire fixation. In: Michael W. Neumeister; Michael Sauerbier. (Org.). Problems in hand surgery: solutions to recover function. 1st ed. New York: Thieme, vol. 1, 2020, pp. 156–159.
22. Tosti R, Ilyas AM, Mellema JJ, Guitton TG, Ring D, Science of Variation Group. Interobserver variability in the treatment of little finger metacarpal neck fractures. J Hand Surg Am. 2014;39(9):1722–7.
23. Piedade, S.R., Ferreira, D.M., Cristante, A.F., Ikemoto, R.Y., Fernandes, C.H. (2021). Judo, Karate, and Taekwondo. In: Rocha Piedade, S., Neyret, P., Espregueira-Mendes, J., Cohen, M., Hutchinson, M.R. (eds) Specific Sports-Related Injuries. Springer. pp 315–28
24. Waninger KN, Lombardo J. Stress fracture of index metacarpal in an adolescent tennis player. Clin J Sports Med. 1995;5:63–6.
25. Kleinhenz BP, Adams BD. Closed Sagittal band injury of the metacarpophalangeal joint. J Am Acad Orthop Surg. 2015;23(7):415–23.
26. Oliveira Miranda CD, Fernandes CH, Meirelles LM, Ejnisman B, Cohen M, Faloppa F. Prevalence of upper extremity musculoskeletal injuries and symptoms in Brazilian Jiu-Jitsu athletes. Clin Surg. 2019;4:2339.
27. Brölmann FE, Ubbink DT, Nelson EA, Munte K, Van Der Horst CMAM, Vermeulen H. Evidence-based decisions for local and systemic wound care. Br J Surg. 2012;99(9):1172–83.
28. Handford C, Thomas O, Imray CHE. Frostbite. Emerg Med Clin North Am. 2017;35(2):281–99.
29. Brown RE. Acute nail bed injuries. Hand Clin. 2002;18(4):561–75.
30. Mastey RD, Weiss APC, Akelman E. Primary care of hand and wrist athletic injuries. Clin Sports Med. 1997;16(4):705–24.
31. Elfar J, Mann T. Fracture-dislocations of the proximal interphalangeal joint. J Am Acad Orthop Surg. 2013;21(2):88–98.
32. Pattni A, Jones M, Gujral S. Volar Plate Avulsion Injury. Eplasty. 2016;16:ic22.
33. Fox PM, Chang J. Treating the Proximal Interphalangeal Joint in Swan Neck and Boutonniere Deformities. Hand Clin. 2018;34(2):167–76.
34. Almeida VAS, Fernandes CH, Santos JBGD, Schwarz-Fernandes FA, Faloppa F, Albertoni WM. Evaluation of interobserver agreement in Albertoni's classification for mallet finger. Rev Bras Ortop. 2017;53(1):2–9.
35. Goodson A, Morgan M, Rajeswaran G, Lee J, Katsarma E. Current management of Jersey finger in rugby players: case series and literature review. Hand Surg. 2010;15(2):103–7.

9 Hip and Groin

Sideline Evaluation and Management of Hip and Groin Injuries

Corey R. Dwyer and Marc R. Safran

Hip injuries in sports are being recognized with increasing frequency. Part of this is the result of increased awareness of hip injuries in sports, part is the result of better physical examination of the hip that has evolved as we have become aware of newer pathologies about the hip and part is the result of advanced imaging techniques.

With knowledge of asking the pertinent questions and an appropriate focused physical, the team physician can generate a differential diagnosis and initiate treatment. This chapter will evaluate emergent entities, such as a hip dislocation, as well as osseous and soft tissue injuries one is likely to evaluate on the sideline. Due to the nature of the hip as a constrained joint with thick surrounding soft tissue envelop, radiographs are important as part of the initial evaluation. Discussion of treatment provides context for these injuries.

9.1 Hip Dislocation

Although sports-related hip dislocations are uncommon, this is an important injury to identify and respond quickly. Time to reduction of dislocation correlates with the risk of developing avascular necrosis in addition to post-traumatic arthritis [1–3]. Sahin et al. describe that time to reduction and associated injuries were the most important factors for a patient's prognosis following a hip dislocation [4]. If an athlete were to experience a dislocation, it is usually a posterior hip dislocation, that is to say, the femoral head dislocates posteriorly from, and relative to, the acetabulum. To sustain a posterior hip dislocation, the hip and knee are typically flexed, and the hip may be adducted as well. This can occur in sports like football and rugby, when an athlete is getting tackled and lands on the knee while the hip and knee are flexed.

9.1.1 Evaluation

Hip dislocations must be recognized and treated quickly. The athlete may present with the lower extremity shortened and internally rotated, often with the hip mildly flexed. For anterior dislocations, the hip may be externally rotated. Following inspection, palpation may identify a prominent femoral head, or fullness in the buttock region for posterior dislocations. The patient usually reports pain with subtle range of motion, including just log rolling the extremity. Due to the proximity of the sciatic nerve as well as the nature of the high-energy injury, a thorough neurovascular examination should be performed.

Radiographs including an anteroposterior (AP) view of the pelvis demonstrates the femoral

C. R. Dwyer · M. R. Safran (✉)
Stanford University, Stanford, CA, USA
e-mail: msafran@stanford.edu

S. Rocha Piedade et al. (eds.), *Sideline Management in Sports*,
https://doi.org/10.1007/978-3-031-33867-0_9

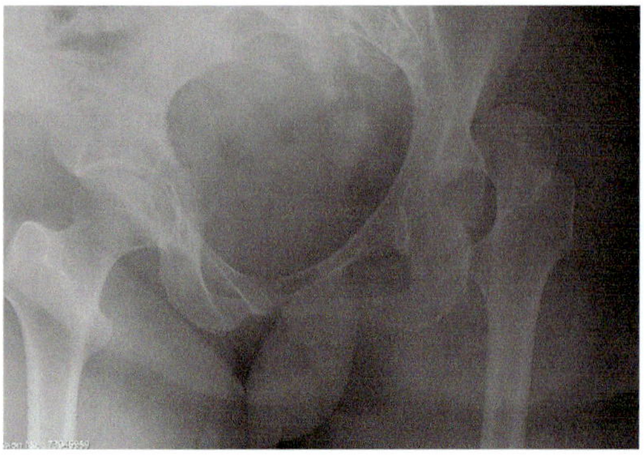

Fig. 9.1 AP Pelvis radiograph of a woman with a left hip posterior dislocation. Note the femoral head is not within the acetabulum, is proximal to the acetabulum, and the lesser trochanter seen more prominently relative to the contralateral hip

head not concentrically located within the acetabulum (with the head usually located proximal to the socket), asymmetry in size of the femoral heads, as well as lesser trochanter seen more prominently relative to the contralateral hip (Fig. 9.1). Orthogonal images should be obtained for better characterization of the dislocation and potential associated fractures. A key to this injury is have an action plan that can safely remove the player from the sideline and into a higher level of care that will have imaging and provide a form of anesthesia.

9.1.2 Treatment

Reduction should be performed in an urgent manner. Anesthesia allowing for muscle relaxation should be utilized to limit further cartilage damage, though an attempt on the sideline or locker room, before muscle spasms set in, may be attempted. This can be performed if adequate sedation and relaxation can be achieved. In most cases, this should be performed at a nearby hospital's emergency room for potential airway management and further imaging.

The Allis maneuver can be performed with the patient being supine, while the provider applies traction in line with the deformity while also gently internally and externally rotating the extremity while an assistant provides countertraction, stabilizing the pelvis (Fig. 9.2). This is performed with the assistant firmly placing his or her hands over the athlete's anterior superior iliac spine [5].

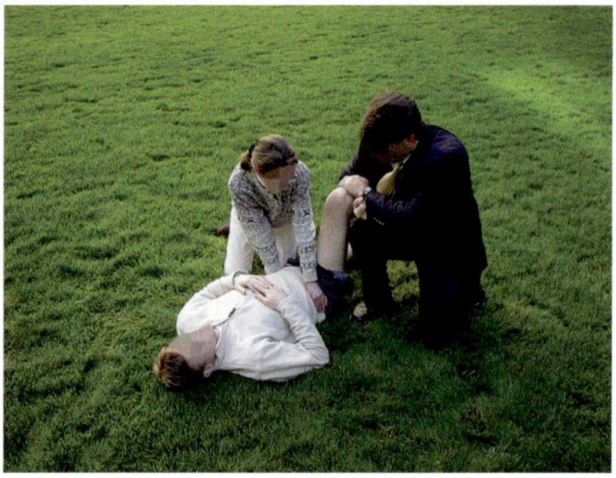

Fig. 9.2 The Allis maneuver. This is performed while the patient is supine. The assistant stabilizes the pelvis, while the provider applies longitudinal traction in line with the femur while also gently internally and externally rotating the extremity

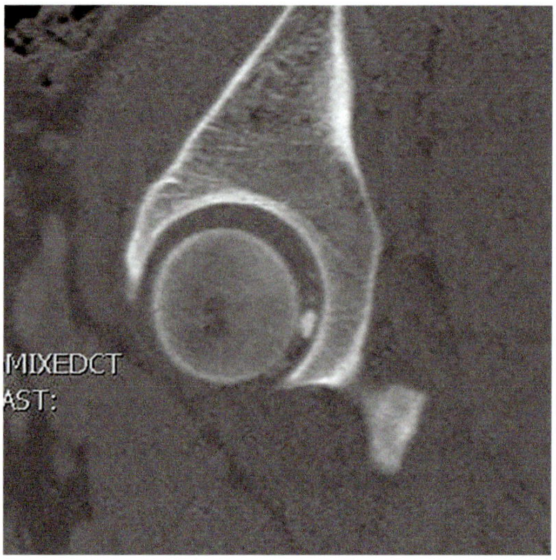

Fig. 9.3 CT scan post reduction of a left hip demonstrating non-concentric reduction and a loose body between the femoral head and the acetabulum

After reduction is performed, repeat radiographs should confirm concentric reduction. Additionally, a computed tomography (CT) scan should be performed to confirm a complete and concentric reduction. Thin-cut CT scans can identify intra-articular bodies as well as other intra-articular injuries (Fig. 9.3) [6].

Hip subluxation must also be considered in athletes with acute onset hip pain. If the patient has pain with log roll, but appears to be reduced on radiographs, higher level imaging should be performed. Subluxation may only be seen on CT or MRI. It is important to have a high level of suspicion for hip subluxation.

A pillow providing slight abduction in addition to a knee immobilizer may be beneficial to limit immediate recurrence of a dislocation. MRI can help demonstrate labral tears, chondral pathologies, and soft-tissue interposition. If there is nonconcentric reduction after a hip instability event, an MRI should be performed to evaluate soft tissue obstruction [7].

For non-concentric reduction without an acetabular fracture, surgical intervention in the form of hip arthroscopy may be indicated to remove any loose bodies or soft tissue obstruction to full reduction. There is no consensus as to whether capsular or labral repair is indicated at the time of early hip arthroscopy for non-concentric reduction after a first-time hip dislocation. The concern about early hip arthroscopy is the potential risk of increasing the likelihood of AVN as the blood supply to the femoral head may have been affected by the dislocation and adding traction and/or intra-articular pressure from fluid for hip arthroscopy to potentially compromised blood supply. There is the additional concern about extravasation of fluid from the hip joint when operating on a patient with an acute dislocation. However, Ilizaliturri's review did not find this as a complication of hip arthroscopy in 17 patients following traumatic posterior hip dislocation [8]. Bartlett et al., however, has notably described a case of cardiopulmonary arrest secondary to intraabdominal extravasation while undergoing hip arthroscopy. However, the hip underwent arthroscopy following an open reduction and internal fixation of a both-column fracture pattern [9].

There is debate in regard to weightbearing following a simple hip dislocation (without fracture). Protected weightbearing for at least 6 weeks with gradual return to activity is suggested to allow for soft tissue recovery, including the articular cartilage [7]. Details for rehabilitation after this injury are still controversial.

Some athletes may be predisposed to hip instability events. Athletes with femoroacetabular impingement in addition to acetabular retroversion with decreased posterior coverage may be at increased risk of posterior instability events [10, 11].

Following an instability event, an MRI should be performed at 3 months to evaluate for possible osteonecrosis [7].

9.2 Hip Pointer

A hip pointer is common in contact athletes, especially those that do not wear pads to protect their pelvis at the waist. A direct blow or impact to the iliac crest and surrounding tissues can lead to a hip pointer. Contact athletes including those who participate in football, rugby, and hockey can be predisposed to this injury [12]. Theories have been proposed as to whether this iliac crest and adjacent tissue contusion is secondary to bleeding of subperiosteal edema or compression of the abductor muscles along the ilium [13].

9.2.1 Evaluation

Upon inspection, especially after an hour or more from injury, swelling can be visualized over the iliac crest. Most commonly, athletes will have discomfort and tenderness to palpation over the iliac crest. One may have severe pain in the area with movement and can be with running, as well as while coughing or sneezing or even doing a sit up [13].

9.2.2 Treatment

Much of the treatment for a hip pointer includes symptomatic pain relief. Compression and ice help reduce further bleeding and swelling through vasoconstriction. For pain control, avoid nonsteroidal anti-inflammatories and aspirin in the first 24–48 h as they are platelet inhibitors and thus may increase the bleeding and further hematoma formation. Acetaminophen-based drugs are therefore preferred [14].

However, some athletes will attempt to return to play the same day as the injury. A combination of local anesthetic and corticosteroid may be placed in the area of maximal tenderness to aid the athlete in returning to play in some situations. A study in rugby players has found an injection with anesthetic is helpful in early return to play [15]. Additional padding can also be beneficial for return to play. For more severe hip pointers, some athletes have pain with weightbearing, and as such may require crutches until the athlete can comfortably walk without a limp. A study in hockey players demonstrated that rehabilitation focusing on hip abductors is important prior to returning to competition [14].

9.3 Pelvic Avulsions

9.3.1 Osseous Avulsions

Growth plates about the hip tend to close later, on average, compared to other physes and may be as late as 25 years of age. Thus teenage athletes, and those into their 20s, are susceptible to physeal injuries about the pelvis Apophyseal injuries can occur with quick, forceful, eccentric contraction causing the musculotendinous unit to create an avulsion fracture. The cartilaginous growth plate fails under tension rather than other structures in the musculotendinous unit itself, as the physis is the weakest link in the musculoskeletal system. Teenage athletes, and those into their 20s, are strong enough to generate the force to sustain some of these pelvic avulsions. Therefore, the team physician should especially be aware of the possibility of these injuries in athletes under 25 years of age.

9.3.1.1 Anterior Superior Iliac Spine (ASIS) Avulsion

Both the sartorius and the tensor fascia lata originate from the ASIS. It is however the sartorius that is responsible for these fractures. As the sartorius is a hip flexor and rotator, this avulsion injury is associated with kicking, jumping, sprinting, or running. The secondary ossification of the ASIS closes approximately at age 16 for females and 18 for males [16].

Evaluation

Athletes may report a pop during the athletic activity, and report pain over the anterior pelvis. The athlete may avoid placing full weight on the affected lower extremity. Upon examination, there can be ecchymosis or swelling overlying the ASIS. There will be tenderness over the ASIS. Resisted hip flexion can be painful and weak, when compared to the contralateral leg. Radiographs should be obtained including anterior posterior (AP) views of the pelvis in addition to orthogonal images including a cross-table lateral view (Fig. 9.4). Displacement is also secondary to the integrity of the inguinal ligament. The avulsion may be confused with an anterior inferior iliac spine avulsion due to its displacement inferior and initial lateral relative location. CT scans with three-dimensional reconstructions can better help characterize the fracture fragment.

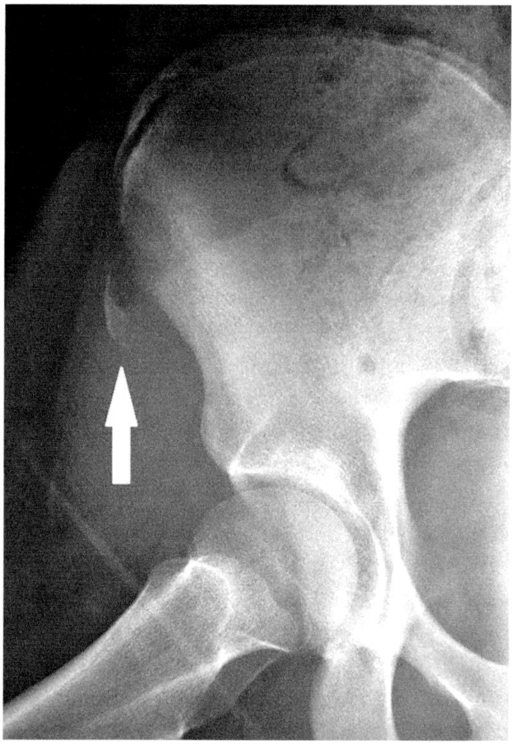

Fig. 9.4 AP Pelvis radiograph demonstrating a displaced Anterior Superior Iliac Spine (ASIS) Avulsion fracture. Arrow pointing to the displaced ASIS

Treatment

After confirmation of the diagnosis, management includes protected weightbearing, rest, and analgesics. There can be progression of weightbearing with the assistive of crutches over the course of 6 weeks, with most athletes typically returning to sport by 3 months.

Surgical indications are limited and should be only for those who have displacement greater than 3 cm or those suffering from compression of the lateral femoral cutaneous nerve [17].

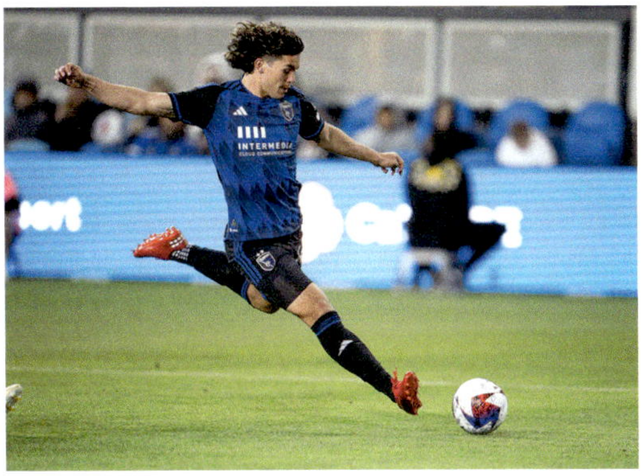

Fig. 9.5 Classic position that may result in an Anterior Inferior Iliac Spine Avulsion—the hip extended and knee flexed such as with kicking a ball is a common mechanism

9.3.1.2 Anterior Inferior Iliac Spine (AIIS) Avulsion

Avulsion fractures of the AIIS are secondary to the direct head of the rectus femoris. An eccentric force created from movements including sprinting or kicking can cause such an injury. Compared to ASIS avulsions, AIIS injuries are more so related to ball-related sports, kicking against resistance. The hip extended and knee flexed meeting resistance by kicking a ball is a common mechanism (Fig. 9.5) [18]. Median closure of the AIIS secondary ossification center is 16.3 years for males and 14.5 years for females [16].

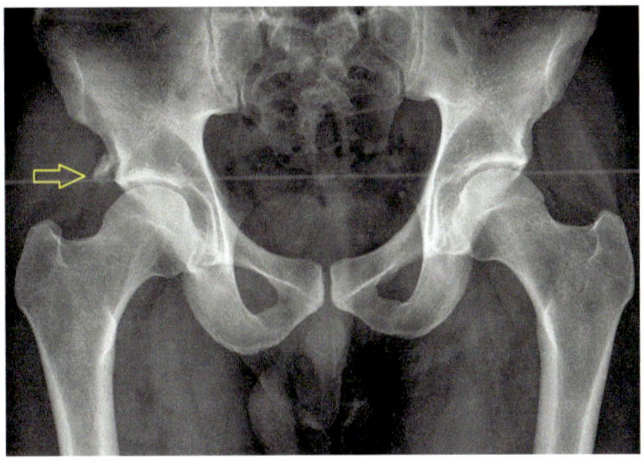

Fig. 9.6 AP Pelvis radiograph demonstrating a displaced Anterior Inferior Iliac Spine (AIIS) Avulsion fracture of the right hip. Often these fractures may not be as displaced or radiographically apparent

Evaluation

An athlete with an AIIS avulsion may have similar symptoms to those who sustain an ASIS avulsion. One may describe a pop with the potential for ecchymosis and swelling. Tenderness can be elicited over the AIIS. However, an athlete may have pain with resisted hip flexion, knee extension, and straight leg raise.

Radiographs should also be obtained including an AP of the pelvis with orthogonal images of the hip (Fig. 9.6). There may be minimal displacement on radiographs, so the suspicion of injury should be elevated when evaluating these athletes. If radiographs are unremarkable, more advanced imaging, such as CT or MRI will reveal the avulsion fracture of the AIIS.

Treatment

Treatment for this avulsion injury is usually nonoperative treatment, but there has been recent interest in fixing the AIIS due to the potential for AIIS subspinous impingement when older from a distally displaced AIIS fragment (Fig. 9.7). However, the standard of treatment continues to be progressive weightbearing with the assistance of crutches, analgesia, ice, and rest from sport. Positioning the hip flexed for the first 2 weeks may be included. Operative indications remain reserved for displacement over 2 cm and in cases of painful non-unions though there have been reports of associated heterotopic bone formation if early surgery is undertaken [19].

9.3.1.3 Ischial Tuberosity Avulsion

The ischial tuberosity is the site of attachment for long head of the biceps femoris, semimembranosus, semitendinosus, and part of the adductor magnus.

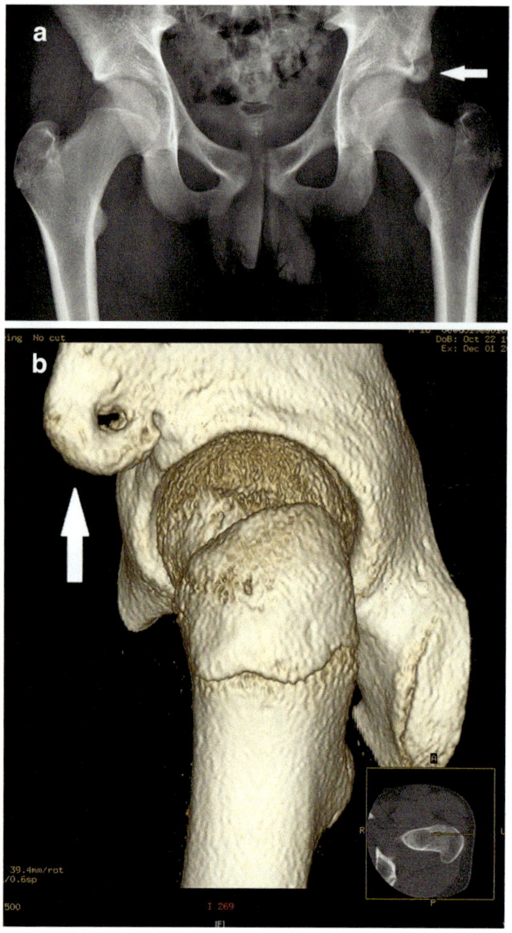

Fig. 9.7 Residuals of an old, healed AIIS Avulsion Fracture. (**a**) is a plain AP Pelvis radiograph demonstrating the prominence of the malunited AIIS, while (**b**) is a 3D reconstruction of the same patient demonstrating the anterior and inferior displacement of the malunited AIIS fragment

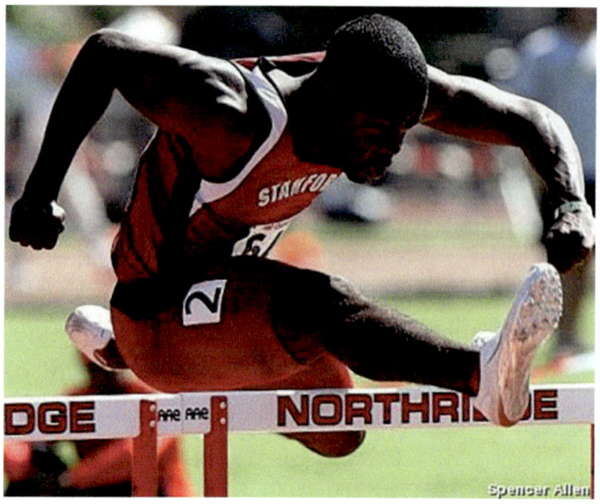

Fig. 9.8 Photograph of a sprinter demonstrating the classic position that may result in an ischial tuberosity avulsion fracture. The right hip flexed and knee extended, or so called hurdler's position

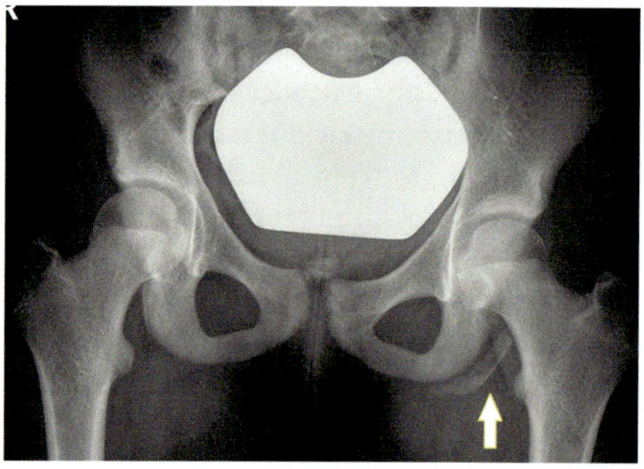

Fig. 9.9 AP Pelvis radiograph with a solid arrow pointing to the acute, displaced left ischial tuberosity avulsion fracture

Avulsion fractures can occur with the combination of knee extension and hip flexion, such as when kicking, performing hurdles, or sprinting (Fig. 9.8) [20]. Studies have found there is a higher prevalence of these injuries among soccer players and gymnasts [21]. Mitchell et al. has attempted to classify these avulsion fractures by ossification stage, displacement, and tendon attachment [22].

Evaluation

Similar to previously mentioned avulsion fractures, patients may feel a pop at the onset of injury and have tenderness to palpation over the location. Swelling and ecchymosis is more common through the posterior thigh with this injury. Movements that put the hamstrings on tension can reproduce discomfort—contraction of the hamstrings (resisted knee flexion) and stretching of the hamstring (hip flexed and knee extended). Radiographs including an AP of the pelvis should be obtained by higher level imaging including CT or MRI may be necessary to make an accurate diagnosis as displacement may not always be obvious (Fig. 9.9) [23].

Treatment

Rest, analgesia, and protected weightbearing are recommended. Conservative treatment can be pursued for patients with less than 15 mm of displacement. Early operative intervention should be considered when displacement is above this threshold [24]. Bracing may be helpful in maintaining knee flexion and hip extension in conservative management. Athletes may need postoperative bracing ranging from 6 to 12 weeks postoperatively as well [23].

9.3.1.4 Iliac Crest Avulsion

The mechanism of iliac crest avulsions can occur through sudden twisting or lateral flexion resulting in a pull from the abdominal muscles inserting onto the crest in addition to contraction of the tensor fascia lata [23]. Other mechanisms can include a direct blow or a sudden pivot.

Parvaresh and colleagues have suggested that the iliac crest on review of CT scans may close between 16 and 23.9 years and 15.8 and 25.8 years of age, for males and females, respectively [16].

Evaluation

Athletes can describe pain and have tenderness over the iliac crest. Movements associated with the trunk including bending or rotation as well as hip abduction can cause pain. Ecchymosis can be present over the crest as well. Imaging including X-rays can demonstrate fracture. However, it may be difficult to discern given the secondary ossification appears between 13 and 15 years old. Thus, an AP Pelvis radiograph showing both iliac crests can be helpful to identify these fractures (Fig. 9.10). MRI may also be useful to diagnose these injuries.

Treatment

Similar to other avulsion injuries, this can be managed with similar conservative management for the vast majority. However, there can be a discussion to potentially drain the hematoma for pain relief. Patient may bear weight at 2 weeks and return to play at 4 weeks [25]. Surgical intervention can be performed on those with displacement greater than 3 cm [26].

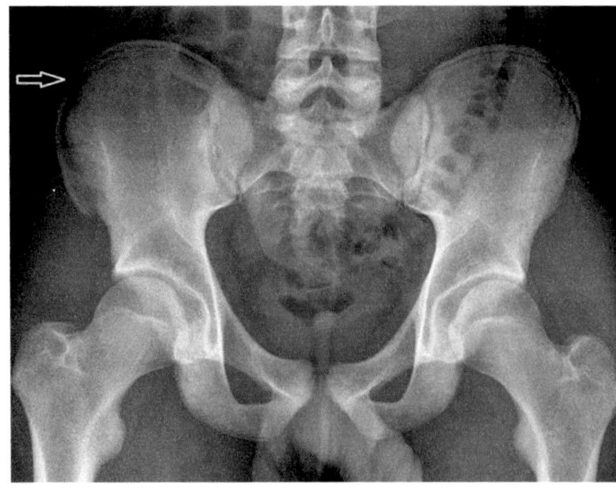

Fig. 9.10 AP Pelvis radiograph with the arrow outline pointing to the iliac crest avulsion fracture in an 18-year-old collegiate basketball player. These injuries may be missed if the radiographs do not include all of the pelvis including the iliac crests

9.3.1.5 Lesser Trochanteric Avulsions

The iliopsoas inserts onto the lesser trochanter, causing proximal displacement in this fracture pattern. A portion of the metaphysis has even been described with the apophyseal fragment and proximal femur [27]. Although this fracture is quite uncommon, Ruffing and colleagues found this fracture pattern demonstrated a peak incidence at the age of 14 in boys [28]. Median closure for males is 14.1 years of age while 12.6 years of age for females [16].

Evaluation

Athletes complain of anterior pelvic or groin pain with this injury. The hip may be held in mild adduction and internal rotation, and the patient may be unable to flex the hip when seated. Radiographs including AP of the pelvis and orthogonal images of the hip and femur should be obtained. Again, this can demonstrate medial and proximal displacement due to the insertion of the iliopsoas attachment to the fragment (Fig. 9.11).

Treatment

Fernbach and Wilkonson were able to show that patients with lesser trochanteric avulsion fractures can do quite well treated nonoperatively. Athletes did well despite some persistent radiographic abnormalities [27].

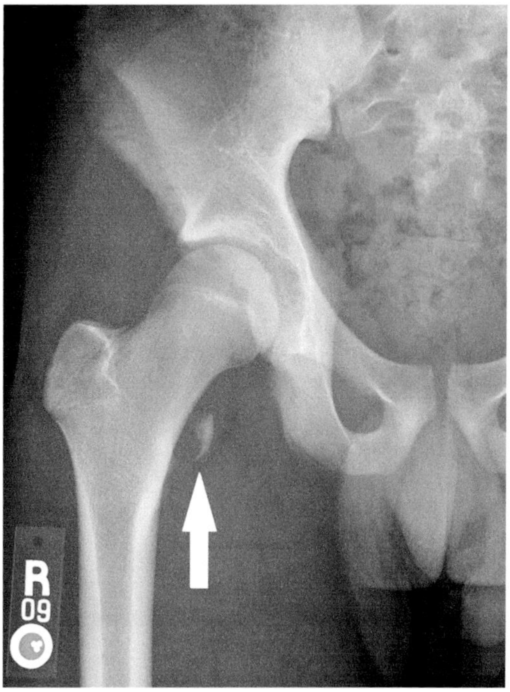

Fig. 9.11 An AP radiograph of the right hip in a 15-year-old soccer player demonstrating the lesser trochanteric avulsion fracture (solid arrow)

Symptoms can be treated with gradual return to sport when healing is present, which may be up to 12 weeks [29]. Surgical intervention has been discussed for those with symptomatic non-union who are having the inability to return to sport as well as displacement greater than 2 cm [30].

9.3.2 Musculotendinous Injuries

9.3.2.1 Proximal Hamstring Avulsion

Hamstring injuries are quite common in athletes, though avulsions from the proximal attachment are less common and managed differently than midthigh injuries. The hamstring muscles include the biceps femoris, semitendinosus, and semimembranosus. The long head of the biceps and tendons of the remaining two muscles original from the ischial tuberosity. Proximal avulsions are likely secondary to eccentric contraction as the knee is extended with the hip flexed.

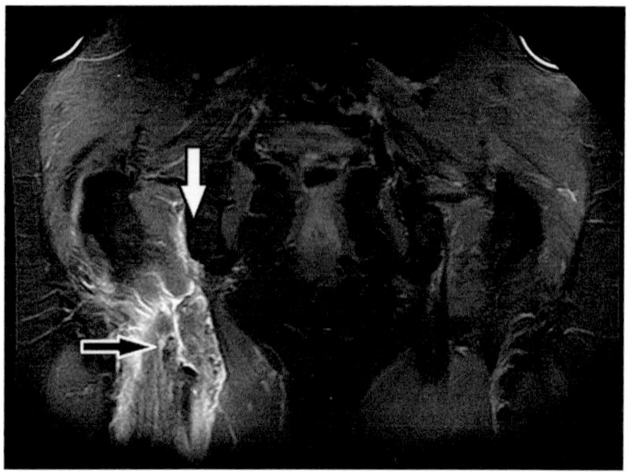

Fig. 9.12 Coronal MRI of a 22-year-old female lacrosse player demonstrating an acute hamstring avulsion. The Black arrow (with white outline) points to the proximal aspect of the hamstring tendon displaced 6 cm, while the solid white arrow points to the ischial origin of where the tendon should be attached

Evaluation

Athletes describe a sharp, acute pain in the posterior aspect of the thigh, while some also describe a pop [31]. Furthermore, they can have discomfort with sitting in addition to walking.

Inspection may not demonstrate ecchymosis immediately. Ecchymosis may develop overtime throughout the posterior aspect of the thigh. There can be tenderness to palpation at the insertion. A defect may also be noted. Range of motion of both the hip and knee should be obtained.

The athlete should then be placed prone. Prone strength testing should be performed at 90°, 45°, and 15°. Pain and weakness compared to the contralateral limb may be appreciated. If there are symptoms only 15°, it may suggest a mild tear with one-tendon involvement. In contrast, a moderate or two-tendon tear may be present if pain and weakness occur at only 15° and 45°. Two or three tendon involvement may exist when there are symptoms throughout 90°, 45°, and 15°. A thorough assessment of sciatic nerve function should be performed.

Plain radiographs should be obtained to help rule out a bony avulsion fracture of the ischial tuberosity. Ultrasound can be performed to assess the muscle and tendons, including surrounding edema [32].

MRI should be obtained to help further determine location, number of tendon involvement, and retraction (Fig. 9.12). Cohen and colleagues have provided an MRI scoring system for hamstring injuries based on age, number of muscles involved, location, insertion involvement, cross-section percentage of the injury, retraction, and length of involvement on T2 [33].

Treatment

The number of tendons involved and amount of retraction help determine operative versus nonoperative treatment. For one or two tendon tears with retraction less than 2 cm, nonoperative management has demonstrated good success. A focus on rehabilitation with adjuncts for analgesia has been described. Both corticosteroid and platelet-rich plasma injections have previously been investigated.

Operative intervention is recommended for 3 tendon tears as well as 2 tendon involvement with 2 cm or greater of retraction [34]. Surgical intervention includes tendon repair followed by bracing and rehabilitation.

9.3.2.2 Adductor Injury

The adductors of the hip include the adductor longus, adductor magnus, adductor brevis, gracilis, obturator externus, and pectineus. The most commonly injured adductor is the adductor longus [35]. This injury can be common in hockey, soccer, and football.

Evaluation

An adductor strain can cause tenderness to palpation over the muscle belly or over the origin of the pubis. It can also cause pain with resisted adduction or passive abduction. Adduction strength is tested with the patient supine and hips in neutral flexion – extension, as well as with the hips and knees in flexion. Adductor strains can be classified into one of three degrees. A first-degree strain is minimal loss of motion and strength. A second-degree strain demonstrates compromised strength. Lastly, a third-degree strain demonstrates complete disruption that causes a loss of muscle function [36]. Radiographs of the pelvis and hip should be obtained. An MRI will help better characterize edema and hemorrhage (Fig. 9.13).

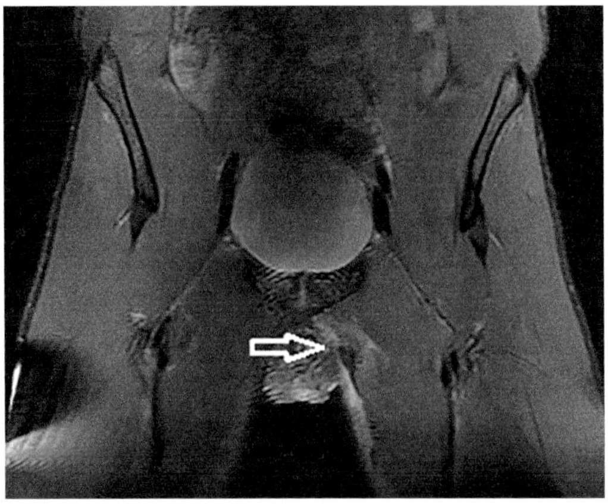

Fig. 9.13 An MRI of the pelvis demonstrating a 2 cm retracted acute adductor longus tendon avulsion in a male professional soccer player. The arrow points to the retracted avulsed tendon end

Treatment

In large, nonoperative management is the mainstay for this injury, regardless of the degree of injury. Gentle stretching and passive treatment can begin immediately followed by focusing on progressive eccentric resistance [37].

9.3.2.3 Athletic Pubalgia/Core Muscle Injury

Core muscle injury, athletic pubalgia, and sports hernia all refer to pain in the lower abdomen and groin. There is debate in the literature of the etiology of this discomfort. Sports hernia was popularized by Greg Lovell, noting the subtle bulge in the transversalis fascia creating pressure over the sensory nerves, though no true hernia [38]. Athletic pubalgia has been coined by Gilmore and Meyers. Gilmore described this injury as a torn external oblique aponeurosis causing dilatation of the superficial inguinal ring and a torn conjoined tendon [39]. Meyers notes a sports hernia as hyperextension leading to chronic lower abdomen and groin pain. Both the rectus abdominus and adductor longus insert onto the pubis [40]. These muscles act as antagonists and asymmetric co-contraction can lead to injury to the other muscle. Overall, however,

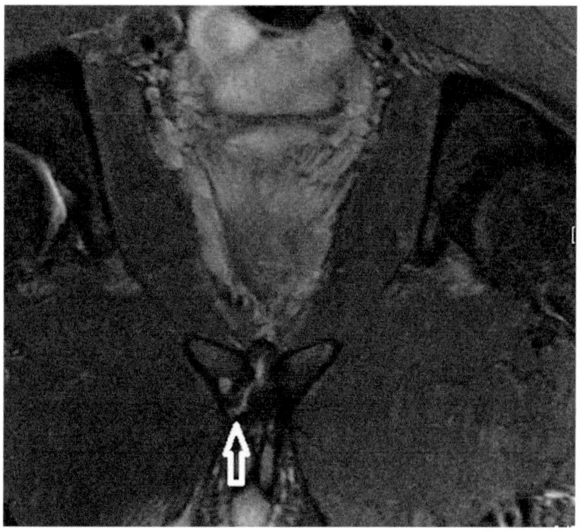

Fig. 9.14 MRI of the Pelvis focused on the pubic symphysis demonstrating a core muscle injury/sports hernia/athletic pubalgia in a 22-year-old professional basketball player. The arrow points to the abnormal cleft at the pubis where there is a tear in the rectus abdominus and adductor aponeurosis while also demonstrating subchondral edema in the pubis at the symphysis

there continues to be debate as to the pathologic etiology.

Evaluation

An athlete may describe insidious onset of deep and diffuse pain within the lower abdomen or groin and upper medial thigh. It is more common in those that kick, cut, and perform explosive twisting that include sports such as American football, soccer, hockey, tennis, and rugby.

A patient should be evaluated in both the standing and supine position. The player may demonstrate tenderness at or above the pubic tubercle, near the rectus insertion, lateral edge of the rectus, or the conjoined tendon/rectus abdominis interface. A resisted sit-up can or a sit-up while palpating the lateral edge of the rectus as it inserts onto the pubis can produce discomfort. Resisted adduction should be performed to determine if the adductor longus is a source of one's pain [41].

Radiographs and CT scans may highlight osseous abnormalities, but MRI is essential. MRI protocols have been established to better visualize tears in the rectus abdominus in addition to the adductor aponeurosis (Fig. 9.14) [42]. Other pathologies such as labral tears, iliopsoas bursitis, and occult fractures may be appreciated. Dynamic ultrasound can allow for visualization of abnormal ballooning of the posterior inguinal wall as the athlete is asked to strain, but this is quite operator dependent [43].

Management

Treatment options may vary based on timing of the injury. For the in-season athlete, a period of rest, typically four weeks in conjunction with closed-chain lower extremity workouts should be attempted. Furthermore, steroid or platelet-rich plasma injections to the rectus abdominus or adductor longus insertions may be helpful to hasten return to play. Athletes unable to return to play due to core muscle injury may require surgery to return to sport. Different techniques have been described with good results and return within 2–12 weeks.

9.3.2.4 Femoroacetabular Impingement (FAI)

Athletes who complain of hip pain should have FAI within the differential. A player may have a rather insidious onset of groin pain though traumatic onset also can precipitate hip symptoms from FAI. This condition is caused by abnormal contact between the femur and the acetabulum that can generate labral and chondral injury. This includes cam or pincer impingement in addition to a combination thereof.

Evaluation

Pain is a predominant feature of this condition. Clohisy demonstrated that 88% of patients had groin pain while 67% had lateral hip pain [44]. Affected individuals may also report their pain with the "C sign," which is when one places a thumb posterior to the hip and the remaining fingers deep into the anterior groin when describing the pain [45]. Pain may be described with certain movements such as running, pivoting, or even walking. When evaluating these athletes on the sideline, it is important to inquire about previous and childhood hip injuries. This should heighten awareness for this injury.

Gait can be assessed while looking for symmetry. A supine exam can allow for assessment of resting rotation and limb length. Palpation can be performed to help rule out previously described avulsion injuries. Range of motion compared to the contralateral limb should be performed. Limited flexion and internal rotation are found in patients with anterior FAI [46].

Flexion-adduction-internal rotation (FADIR) testing is performed by flexing the hip to 90° followed by adduction and internal rotation (Fig. 9.15). This is intended to assess if this reproduces the patient's pain. While not pathognomonic for hip impingement, it is a good test to assess for hip joint pain.

Initial management with history and physical examination should include radiographs to look for other pathology in addition to a crossover sign or a high α angle (Fig. 9.16). MR arthrogram can be utilized with an intra-articular injection. Gadolinium containing contrast may exacerbate one's hip pain [47]. Therefore, our senior author recommends intra-articular local anesthetic instead of dye to aid in diagnosis [48].

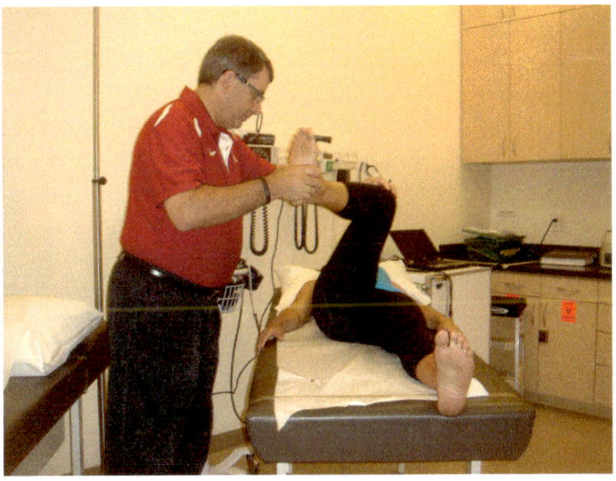

Fig. 9.15 The FADIR test. Also known as the hip impingement test, it is not pathognomonic for hip impingement. The hip is flexed to 90°, adducted and then internally rotated. This often causes pain seen in intra-articular pathology, including hip impingement

Treatment

Initial treatment for athletes with FAI can vary based on timing within the season. Physical therapy with the goal of muscle strengthening including the core, hip flexors, and hip abductors are important aspects to rehabilitation. Activity modification should include avoiding squats if this is an early season injury. NSAIDs may be used as an adjunct but can have side effects including gastrointestinal ulcer, hypertension, renal issues, and bleeding. Studies of NSAIDs in FAI have used other therapies simultaneously, making it difficult to discern NSAIDs' true effect on FAI. Midseason management can also include corticosteroid injection with a complete discussion that there is a high likelihood surgical intervention will be indicated at the conclusion of the

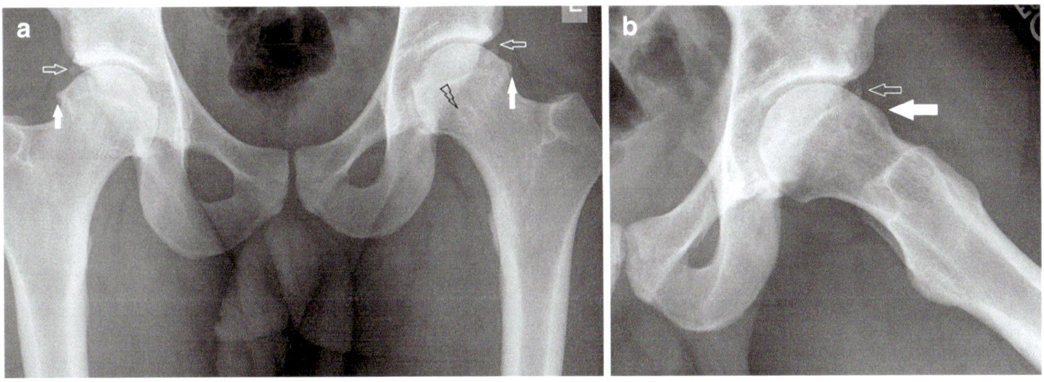

Fig. 9.16 Femoroacetabular Impingement. (**a**) is an AP Pelvis radiograph of a 23-year-old professional (American) football player. The solid arrow points to the femoral head being out of round (the cam lesion), while the black lightning bolt points to a subchondral cyst of the anterior femoral head-neck region. The open arrows point to os acetabuli, of both hips. (**b**) is a lateral radiograph of the same player. Again, the solid arrow points to the cam lesion while the open arrow points to the os acetabulum

season to address the etiology. If surgery is to be considered, return to play may take 4–6 months, and return to optimal pre-injury performance even longer.

9.4 Conclusion

Hip injuries in athletics are being increasingly appreciated in sports medicine. Knowledge of common symptoms and mechanism of injury can clue in a provider to the athlete's injury. An effective physical examination is necessary as imaging can be limited at an event. Provocative maneuvers can help decide return to play and initial management. Advanced imaging and appreciation for the athlete's sport, position, and goals can help establish a treatment plan.

References

1. Hodge DK, Safran MR. Sideline management of common dislocations. Curr Sports Med Rep. 2002;1:149–55.
2. Safran MR, Hodge DK. Sideline management of common dislocations. In: Bull's sports injuries handbook. 2nd ed. New York: McGraw-Hill Professional; 2004.
3. Smith MV, Sekiya JK. Hip instability. Sports Med Arthrosc Rev. 2010;18:108–12.
4. Sahin V, Karakas ES, Aksu S. Traumatic dislocation and fracture dislocation of the hip: a long-term follow-up study. J Trauma. 2003;54:520–9.
5. Epstein HC. Traumatic dislocations of the hip. Clin Orthop Relat Res. 1973;92:116–42.
6. Frick SL, Sims SH. Is computed tomography useful after simple posterior hip dislocation? J Orthop Trauma. 1995;9:388–91.
7. Chona D, Minetos PE, LaPrade CM, Cinque ME, Abrams GE, Sherman SL, Safran MR. Hip dislocation and subluxation in athletes—a systematic review. Am J Sports Med. 2022;50(10):2834–41.
8. Ilizaliturri VM, Gonzalez-Gutierrez B, Gonzalez-Ugalde H, Camacho-Galindo J. Hip arthroscopy after traumatic hip dislocation. Am J Sports Med. 2011;39:50–7.
9. Bartlett CS, DiFelice GS, Buly RL, Quinn TJ, Green DS, Helfet DL. Cardiac arrest as a result of intraabdominal extravasation of fluid during arthroscopic removal of a loose body from the hip joint of a patient with an acetabular fracture. J Orthop Trauma. 1998;12(4):294–9.
10. Mayer SW, Abdo JC, Hill MK, Kestel LA, Pan Z, Novais EN. Femoroacetabular impingement is associated with sports-related posterior hip instability in adolescents: a matched-cohort study. Am J Sports Med. 2016;44(9):2299–303.
11. Novais EN, Ferrer MG, Williams KA, Bixby SD. Acetabular retroversion and decreased posterior coverage are associated with sports-related posterior hip dislocation in adolescents. Clin Orthop Relat Res. 2019;477(5):1101–8.
12. Feeley BT, Powell JW, Muller MS. Hip injuries and labral tears in the national football league. Am J Sports Med. 2008;36(11):2187–95.
13. Blazina ME. The "hip-pointer", a term to describe a specific kind of athletic injury. Calif Med. 1967;106(6):450.
14. LaPrade RF, Wijdicks CA, Griffith CJ. Division I intercollegiate ice hockey team coverage. Br J Sports Med. 2009;43(13):1000–5.
15. Orchard JW, Steet E, Massey A. Long-term safety of using local anesthetic injections in professional rugby league. Am J Sports Med. 2010;38(11):2259–66.
16. Parvaresh KC, Upasani VV, Bomar JD. Secondary ossification center appearance and closure in the pelvis and proximal femur. J Pediatr Orthop. 2018;38(8):418–23.
17. Kautzner J, Trc T, Havlas V. Comparison of conservative against surgical treatment of anterior-superior iliac spine avulsion fractures in children and adolescents. Int Orthop. 2014;38:1495–8.
18. Eberbach H, Hohloch L, Feucht MJ. Operative versus conservative treatment of apophyseal avulsion fractures of the pelvis in the adolescents: a systematical review with meta-analysis of clinical outcome and return to sports. BMC Musculoskelet Disord. 2017;18:1–8.
19. Carr J, Conte E, Rajadhyaksha E, Laroche K, Gwathmey F, Carson E. Operative fixation of an anterior inferior iliac spine apophyseal avulsion fracture nonunion in an adolescent soccer player. JBJS Case Connect. 2017;7(2):e29.
20. Schiller J, DeFroda S, Blood T. Lower extremity avulsion fractures in the pediatric and adolescent athlete. J Am Acad Orthop Surg. 2017;25(4):251–9.
21. Rossi F, Dragoni S. Acute avulsion fractures of the pelvis in adolescent competitive athletes: prevalence, location and sports distribution of 203 cases collected. Skelet Radiol. 2001;30(3):127–31.
22. Mitchell B, Bomar J, Wenger D, Pennock A. Classifying ischial tuberosity avulsion fractures by ossification stage and tendon attachment. J Bone Joint Surg. 2021;103(12):1083–92.
23. Yeager KC, Silva SR, Richter DL. Pelvic avulsion injuries in the adolescent Athlete. Clin Sports Med. 2021;40(2):375–84.
24. Ferlic PW, Sadoghi P, Singer G. Treatment for ischial tuberosity avulsion fractures in adolescent athletes. Knee Surg Sports Traumatol Arthrosc. 2014;22:893–7.
25. Li X, Xu S, Lin X. Results of operative treatment of avulsion fractures of the iliac crest apophysis in adolescents. Injury. 2014;45(4):721–4.

26. Schuett DJ, Bomar JD, Pennock AT. Pelvic apophyseal avulsion fractures: a retrospective review of 228 cases. J Pediatr Orthop. 2015;35(6):617–23.
27. Fernbach SK, Wilkinson RH. Avulsion injuries of the Pelvis. Am J Roentgenol. 1981;137:581–4.
28. Ruffing T, Rückauer T, Bludau F, Hofmann A, Muhm M, Suda AJ. Avulsion fracture of the lesser trochanter in adolescents. Injury. 2018;49(7):1278–81.
29. Tahir T, Manzoor QW, Gul IA, Bhat SA, Kangoo KA. Isolated avulsion fractures of lesser trochanter in adolescents—a case series and brief literature review. J Orthop Case Rep. 2019;9(1):11–4.
30. Khemka A, Raz G, Bosley B, Ludger G, Al Muderis M. Arthroscopically assisted fixation of the lesser trochanter fracture: a case series. J Hip Preserv Surg. 2014;1:27–32.
31. Clanton TO, Coupe KJ. Hamstring strains in athletes: diagnosis and treatment. J Am Acad Orthop Surg. 1998;6(4):237–48.
32. Mariani C, Caldera FE, Kim W. Ultrasound versus magnetic resonance imaging in the diagnosis of an acute hamstring tear. PM R. 2012;4(2):154–5.
33. Cohen SB, Towers JD, Zoga A. Hamstring injuries in professional football players: magnetic resonance imaging correlation with return to play. Sports Health. 2011;3(5):423–30.
34. Cohen S, Bradley J. Acute proximal hamstring rupture. J Am Acad Orthop Surg. 2007;15(6):350–5.
35. Renström P, Peterson L. Groin injuries in athletes. Br J Sports Med. 1980;14(1):30-36. 27.
36. Lynch SA, Renstrom PA. Groin injuries in sport: treatment strategies. Sports Med. 1999;28(2):137–44.
37. Meyers WC, Lanfranco A, Castellanos A. Groin pain in athletes. Curr Sports Med Rep. 2002;1(5):301–5.
38. Garvey JF, Read JW, Turner A. Sportsman hernia: what can we do? Hernia. 2010;14(1):17–25.
39. Diduch DR, Brunt LM. Sports hernia and athletic Pubalgia: diagnosis and treatment. Springer; 2014.
40. Meyers WC, Yoo E, Devon ON, Jain N, Horner M, Luencin C, Zoga A. Understanding "Sports Hernia" (Athletic Pubalgia): the anatomic and pathophysiologic basis for abdominal and groin pain in athletes. Oper Tech Sports Med. 2007;15(4):165–77.
41. Litwin DEM, Sneider EB, McEnaney PM, Busconi BD. Athletic Pubalgia (Sports Hernia). Clin Sports Med. 2011;30(2):417–34.
42. Zoga AC, Kavanagh EC, Omar IM. Athletic pubalgia and the "sports hernia": MR imaging findings. Radiology. 2008;247:797–807.
43. Koulouris G. Imaging review of groin pain in elite athletes: an anatomic approach to imaging findings. Am J Roentgenol. 2008;191:962–72.
44. Clohisy JC, Knaus ER, Hunt DM, Lesher JM, HarrisHayes M, Prather H. Clinical presentation of patients with symptomatic anterior hip impingement. Clin Orthop Relat Res. 2009;467:638–44.
45. Byrd JWT. Physical examination. In: Byrd JWT, editor. Operative hip arthroscopy. 2nd ed. New York: Springer; 2005.
46. Siebenrock KA, Schoeniger R, Ganz R. Anterior femoro- acetabular impingement due to acetabular retroversion. J Bone Joint Surg Am. 2003;85:278–86.
47. Saupe N, Zanetti M, Pfirrmann CW. Pain and other side effects after MR arthrography: prospective evaluation in 1085 patients. Radiology. 2009;250(3):830–8.
48. Botser I, Safran MR. MR imaging of the hip. Magn Reson Imaging Clin N Am. 2009;21:169–82.

Knee Injury: Sideline Management 10

Sarah-Anne Bolton, Philippe Neyret,
João Espregueira-Mendes, and David Parker

10.1 Review of Clinical Presentation and Differential Diagnosis

The knee is a complex joint comprising the tibiofemoral and patellofemoral joints. Stability of the knee is conferred by a combination of static and dynamic factors. Dynamic stabilisers of the knee include any muscles which cross the knee joint. The static factors include the osseous anatomy, the menisci and ligaments. Regarding the osseous anatomy; there is asymmetry of the femoral condyles, with the medial femoral condyle being larger and more distal than the lateral femoral condyle, which is smaller but projects more anteriorly. The tibia has a convex surface laterally and a more concave surface medially. Combined with the asymmetry of the femoral condyles, this results in the femur internally rotating on the tibia as the knee moves from flexion to extension, the so-called screw home mechanism [1].

Separating the femoral condyles is the femoral notch, containing the anterior and posterior cruciate ligaments (ACL/PCL), which resist anterior and posterior translation of the tibia on the femur, respectively. The medial and lateral collateral ligaments (MCL/LCL) control valgus and varus movements, respectively. The medial and lateral menisci are different with regards to their anatomy, resulting in the medial meniscus being more mobile than the lateral.

S.-A. Bolton (✉)
Royal National Orthopaedic Hospital Training Programme, Stanmore, Middlesex, UK
e-mail: sarah.bolton@doctors.org.uk

P. Neyret
Abu Dhabi Reem Hospital, Al Reem Island, Abu Dhabi, United Arab Emirates

J. Espregueira-Mendes
Clínica Espregueira—FIFA Medical Centre of Excellence, Porto, Portugal

Dom Henrique Research Centre, Porto, Portugal

School of Medicine, University of Minho, Braga, Portugal

ICVS/3B's–PT Government Associate Laboratory, Braga/Guimarães, Portugal

3B's Research Group—Biomaterials, Biodegradables and Biomimetics, University of Minho, Headquarters of the European Institute of Excellence on Tissue Engineering and Regenerative Medicine, Barco, Guimarães, Portugal
e-mail: jem@espregueira.com; clinica@espregueira.com

D. Parker
Sydney Orthopaedic Research Institute, Sydney, Australia

The University of Sydney, Camperdown, NSW, Australia

Asia Pacific Knee, Arthroscopy & Sports Medicine Society (APKASS), Sydney, NSW, Australia

International Society for Arthroscopy, Knee Surgery & Orthopaedic Sports Medicine (ISAKOS), San Ramon, CA, USA
e-mail: dparker@sydneyortho.com.au

S. Rocha Piedade et al. (eds.), *Sideline Management in Sports*,
https://doi.org/10.1007/978-3-031-33867-0_10

The knee joint is not surrounded by a great muscle mass, particularly anteriorly, and therefore has minimal protection against direct trauma which, combined with the significant biomechanical stress placed on the knee in many sports, explains why it is so frequently injured [2].

Knee injuries are very common among the athletic population and can present either as an acute injury, or over a longer period of time as a chronic overuse injury. This chapter will focus on acute injuries.

Injuries around the knee can present in a variety of ways such as pain with an inability to bear weight, mechanical symptoms (such as locking or giving way), and swelling (effusion). Pain can be global, localised or more rarely referred to. Injuries around the knee can be divided into fractures/dislocations, injuries to tendon, ligaments, meniscus or cartilage.

In high energy injuries fractures can occur in the medial or lateral tibial plateau, patella, distal femur, tibia or fibula. Dislocations of the patella as well as the knee joint can also occur. The extensor mechanism tendons in the knee, the patella tendon and quadriceps tendon, can also be ruptured.

Ligamentous injuries include full or partial tears of the ACL, PCL, LCL and MCL. MCL and ACL are the most commonly injured ligaments. A multi-ligamentous knee injury is one in which two or more of the following structures are ruptured: ACL/PCL/posterolateral corner (which comprises the LCL/popliteal tendon/popliteofibular ligament)/posteromedial corner (which comprises the posterior oblique ligament, oblique popliteal ligament, semimembranosus tendon, posterior horn of the medial meniscus and capsule). Multi-ligamentous knee injuries are synonymous with knee dislocations due to the fact that many knee dislocations reduce spontaneously, therefore patients with suspected multi-ligamentous injuries should be assumed to have a dislocated knee until proven otherwise [3, 4].

Medial and lateral meniscal pathology can occur in isolation or combined with other injuries; meniscal injury can include tears within the meniscus substance, root avulsions and "ramp" lesions. A ramp lesion is a menisco-capsular separation of the posterior horn of the medial meniscus from the posteromedial capsule [5] most commonly associated with ACL ruptures [6].

Chondral injuries can occur from direct impact to the knee joint, and as a consequence of a patella dislocation resulting in an osteochondral defect (OCD) on the medial patella facet or lateral femoral condyle secondary to a lateral dislocation of the patella.

Take Home Message

- Knee injuries are common in the athletic population and can be either soft tissue injuries or involve fractures or dislocations of the patellofemoral or tibiofemoral joint.

10.2 Discussion of Key Physical Examination Pearls and Findings

Examining the knee in the acute setting can be a challenge but can usually be done effectively with the right knowledge and technique. This section will address key features which help establish whether a patient can return to play or not, and the urgency of possible transfer for further diagnostics and treatment. Tailoring the examination to the clinical situation should be done to accurately assess the injury and determine the most effective acute management.

Understanding the mechanism of injury can aid the physician about the potential injuries sustained; therefore, if not witnessed directly it is important to speak to the player directly or an observer.

A direct blow to the lateral or medial aspect of a knee in extension would raise the suspicion about MCL/LCL injuries, respectively, whereas a non-contact pivoting injury on a planted foot with the knee in flexion is likely to result in an ACL ± meniscal injury. Table 10.1 demonstrates common injury mechanisms with associated injuries and special tests to perform.

Table 10.1 Common injury mechanisms, related injuries, and clinical tests

Mechanism	Injury suspected	Tests
Direct blow medially/laterally	MCL/LCL	Valgus/Varus stress test
Pivoting/twisting injury	ACL ± meniscal injury	Anterior drawer/Lachman test
Fall onto a flexed knee/posterior force to tibia with knee in flexion	PCL	Posterior sag/posterior drawer
High velocity hyperextension injury	Multi-ligament knee injury	ACL/PCL/PLC

Prior to undertaking a focused examination, the team physician needs to first assess whether the mechanism of injury warrants an ATLS (advanced trauma and life support) approach with a primary survey. Assuming that there is an isolated knee injury, the examination follows the same format as most other orthopaedic examinations, i.e. look/feel/move/special tests/neurovascular examination.

10.2.1 Look

For an isolated knee injury, the examination starts with an initial observation by inspecting the overall alignment of the lower limb. Carefully inspect the skin and soft tissues for any bruises or abrasions. If able, with both of the patient's knees at 90°, the uninjured side for the normal attitude of the tibiofemoral joint, then compare to the other side to see whether there is a posterior sag, indicating a potential PCL injury.

Assess whether there is an effusion by initially inspecting and then by palpation; if there is an effusion shortly after the injury this indicates a significant knee injury and the player should not return to play.

10.2.2 Feel

Palpation to identify the anatomical areas of tenderness can help to guide the rest of the examination. Palpation should include the tibial and femoral landmarks, with significant bony tenderness raising the suspicion of a fracture. Tenderness on the medial and lateral joint line may indicate meniscal pathology. Palpate the patella tendon and quadriceps tendon for any tenderness and in full-thickness ruptures a palpable gap may be present. In the case of patella tendon ruptures, the patella will be high riding.

10.2.3 Move

Movement is often limited by pain, but asking a patient to actively move their knee can give valuable insight into the severity and type of injury. Whilst it may be inhibited by pain, asking the patient to perform a straight leg raise is a useful screening tool to assess whether the extensor mechanism is intact. An inability to do this or an extensor lag may represent an injury to the extensor mechanism. Loss of active extension strength is often present in both patella and quadriceps tendon ruptures; however, some patients may still be able to perform extension against gravity if either the medial or lateral retinaculum are intact. Tenderness, localised swelling, and a palpable defect may be present around the superior pole of the patella.

The inability to straighten the knee may also indicate a bucket handle meniscal tear or may simply relate to pain and the presence of a large effusion. If the player has limited movement, difficulty weight bearing, or is developing an effusion then they clearly should not return to the pitch but should be moved to the side line for further focused assessment. Preliminary ligament assessment can occur on the field, but once safely off the pitch the examination can continue to include a more thorough assessment of the ligaments.

10.2.4 Special Tests

10.2.4.1 ACL Injury: Anterior Drawer, Lachman, and Pivot Shift Test

There is wide variation in the reported sensitivities of the anterior drawer test. The relatively low

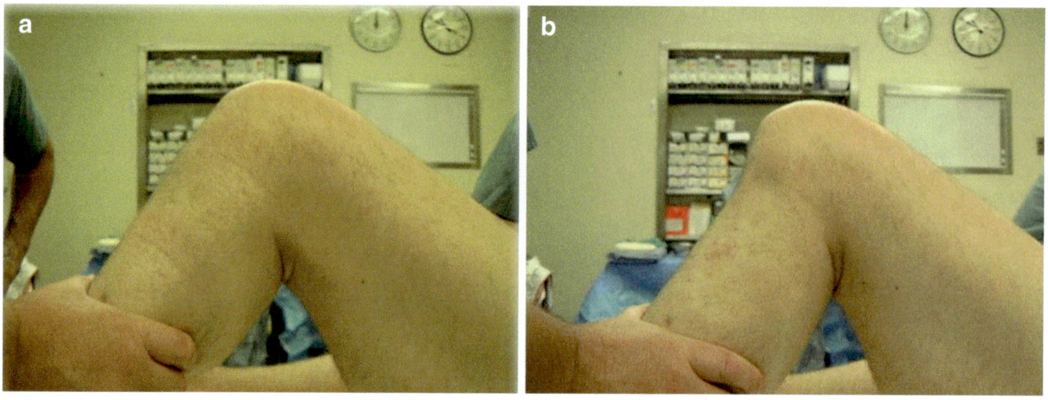

Fig. 10.1 Clinical photo demonstrating the posterior drawer test. In the first image (**a**), the surgeon has brought the tibia forward to a neutral position. In the second image (**b**), the surgeon applies a posterior force, and the tibia subluxes posteriorly; note the posterior position of the tibia in relation to the femur, this is a posterior sag

sensitivity for detecting ACL tears in the acute setting should serve as a caution to examiners not to rule out an acute ACL injury solely on the basis of a negative anterior drawer test. Conversely, the specificity of the test is quite high, and, therefore, a positive anterior drawer would strongly suggest ACL or other intra-articular pathology [7].

The Lachman test is performed with the patient's knee held at approximately 20–30 degrees of flexion, the femur is stabilised with one hand whilst firm pressure is applied to the posterior aspect of the proximal tibia in an attempt to translate it anteriorly. Injured and non-injured knees should be compared, and a positive test indicating disruption of the anterior of cruciate ligament is one in which there is increased anterior translation of the tibia in relation to the femur with a "soft" end point. Sensitivity of the Lachman test has been described as being around 80–99%, with a specificity of 95% [7, 8].

The Lachman test has been shown to be the most sensitive and specific test for the diagnosis of ACL tears, especially in cases of acute injury [7–9]. A pivot shift test at the side of the sports field is not usually possible in the setting of an acutely painful knee and is not required to make the initial provisional diagnosis.

10.2.4.2 PCL Injury: Posterior Sag and Posterior Drawer Test

In the presence of a PCL injury with the knee flexed to approximately 90°, the medial tibial plateau, which normally passively sits anterior to the femoral condyles, will be subluxed posteriorly, when compared to the uninjured side. A small difference compared to the other side would suggest a partial injury, whereas subluxation posterior to the femoral condyles suggests a likely complete injury. In the acute setting, a patient may not be able to flex to 90°, in which case placing both knees at 30° of flexion with support under the distal femur will demonstrate the posterior sag of the injured side (Fig. 10.1a, b).

The posterior drawer test is performed with the knee at approximately 90° of flexion. The examiner has both hands behind the proximal tibia and thumbs on the tibial plateau. Having noted the resting position of the tibia, a posterior force is applied to the proximal tibia. Increased posterior tibial displacement, as compared to the uninvolved side, is indicative of an injury to the PCL [10]. The posterior drawer test is sensitive and specific for a PCL injury [7].

10.2.4.3 Potential Pitfall

A PCL injury can be misinterpreted as an ACL injury if not carefully examined. This relates to posteriorly translation (the posterior sag) of the tibia in a PCL injury, such that when an examiner performs an anterior drawer test the tibia appears to have increased anterior translation, leaving an unsuspecting examiner thinking there is an ACL injury. This misinterpretation can be avoided if the examiner notes the abnormal resting position of the tibia in relation to the femur in a PCL injury, and that there should be a firm end point during an anterior drawer test if the ACL is intact.

10.2.4.4 Collateral Ligament Injury: Varus/Valgus Stress Test

Assessment of the collateral ligaments should be done with the knee in both extension and 30 degrees of flexion, a varus stress examines the lateral collateral ligament and a valgus stress the medial collateral ligament.

MCL injuries are graded as follows: grade I (no valgus laxity), grade II (valgus laxity at 30° of flexion), and grade III (valgus laxity at 0° and 30°). Valgus instability at 30° of flexion is suggestive of a tear in the superficial MCL, whereas valgus instability at full extension, indicates both the superficial MCL and the posteromedial capsule (including the deep MCL) are likely to be torn [11].

An LCL injury if present should prompt an examination of the posterolateral structures as LCL injuries are associated with PLC and PCL injuries.

10.2.4.5 Posterolateral Corner Injury

Posterolateral corner (PLC) injuries are rare injuries that usually occur in the sporting context from a direct blow to the anteromedial knee, causing a varus and hyperextension force. They can less commonly occur in a non-contact from severe hyperextension of the knee. In the acute setting, there will usually be significant pain and the inability to weight bear. Clinical suspicion should be raised from the mechanism of injury, the severity of the symptoms, and the presence of varus laxity in extension on gentle stress testing. Whilst there are many additional tests to more precisely examine the PLC, these are not usually practical in the acute setting, in which clinical suspicion and appropriate subsequent imaging is necessary.

10.2.4.6 Neurovascular Assessment

Assessing the neurovascular status of the limb is essential in significant knee injuries. Here the patient should have their footwear and any protective equipment such as shin pads or leg guards carefully removed, and comparison with the uninjured limb essential. Firstly assess the colour of the feet and feel the temperature. Assessment of capillary refill can be performed by applying pressure to the tip of the hallux, releasing and timing how long it takes for the skin to return to normal, more than 2 s indicates delayed perfusion. An assessment of the pedal pulses should be performed (dorsalis pedis and posterior tibial pulse). If pulses are difficult to palpate, a handheld Doppler can be useful if available. A motor and sensory examination can be quickly done; asking the patient to dorsiflex their ankle/extend the hallux and everting their foot assesses the motor component of the deep and superficial peroneal nerves, respectively. Assessment of the sensory aspect should include testing sensation in the webspace between the hallux and second ray for the deep peroneal nerve and the dorsum of the foot for the superficial peroneal nerve. Assessment of the tibial nerve involves asking the athlete to plantarflex their ankle/toes and testing the sensation on the lateral half of the sole of the foot.

Note: The neurovascular examination should be reperformed after application of a splint or any movement of the limb in a patient with a suspected fracture or dislocation.

The key of the pitch side examination is to identify whether the injury requires an urgent or time critical transfer to an appropriate hospital for definitive care and management. The flow diagram below offers a quick screening tool to aid assessment and examination.

The flow diagram—Quick screening for clinical assessment and examination.

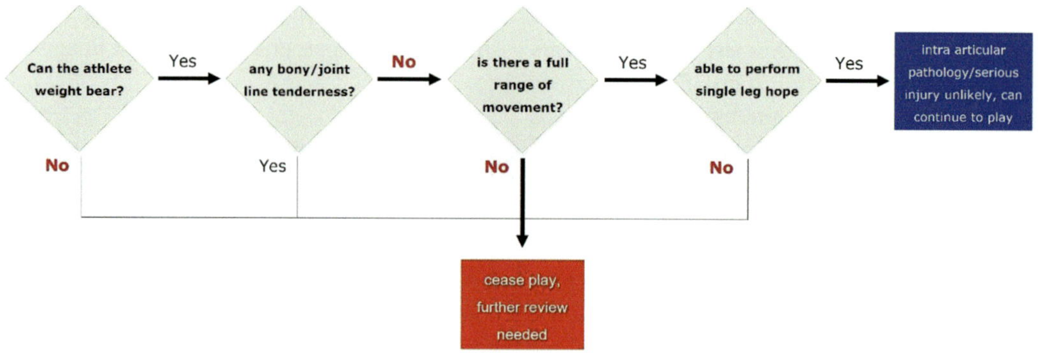

Take Home Message

- An understanding of the mechanism of injury in combination with the examination findings can identify the nature of the injury. Differentiating an injury which requires an urgent transfer vs. non-urgent transfer is crucial and can impact the outcome and management of the injured athlete.

10.3 Indications and Benefits of Additional Testing/ Imaging (Point of Care or Referral)

Improvement and advances in diagnostic imaging is at the forefront of the diagnosis and management of knee injuries as well as the rest of the sports medicine field. Imaging can not only aid diagnosis but can also monitor injury progression and decisions about return to sport.

Conventional X-ray is still the modality of choice in the initial evaluation of any musculoskeletal complaint [12].

The Ottawa Knee Rules were published in 1995 by Stiell et al. [13] as a tool for determining whether to obtain knee radiographs to detect a fracture in the setting of acute knee trauma. The Ottawa rules describe getting a knee radiograph in a patient with knee pain in the presence of one or more of the following variables (as depicted in the table below [13]).

Ottawa Knee Rules

- Age 55 years or older.
- Tenderness at the head of the fibula.
- Isolated tenderness of the patella.
- Inability to flex to 90°.
- Inability to bear weight both immediately and in the ED (four steps).

The Pittsburgh knee rules [14] apply to both children and adults and recommend a knee radiograph in patients less than 12 years of age or over 50 years who present with a fall or blunt trauma. X-rays are also recommended in patients with an inability to take four steps regardless of their age.

The original Pittsburgh knee rules state 100% sensitivity and 79% specificity for detecting a fracture. Both the Ottawa and Pittsburgh rules are often thought of in the same context, however although they demonstrate the same sensitivity, some research suggests the Pittsburgh knee rules offer increased specificity [15].

Radiographs are useful not only to rule out fracture but can also provide a clue to potential ligamentous injuries. A Segond fracture is an avulsion fracture of the anterolateral complex from the lateral tibial plateau, and is thought to be pathognomonic for an ACL injury, although it can also occur in other ligamentous injuries such as a PLC injury [16]. If a Segond fracture is present, an MRI scan is recommended to assess further. Bony avulsions of either cruciate ligament will be seen on plain radiographs, and an avulsion fracture of the proximal fibula, or a fracture of the anteromedial tibial plateau is usually indicative of a PLC injury.

The assessment of the medial and lateral joint spaces on (antero-posterior) AP radiographs can also highlight potential collateral ligament injuries (even in the absence of a dedicated varus or valgus stress X-ray). In cases in which there is significant joint space opening, PLC/PMC injuries should be strongly suspected.

In cases of suspected extensor tendon rupture, the lateral radiograph is most useful. Here avulsion fractures may be present; an avulsion fracture of the superior pole of the patella may be seen in quadriceps tendon ruptures, and an avulsion fracture of the inferior pole of the patella may be seen in patella tendon ruptures.

Whilst these injuries can usually be diagnosed reliably from clinical examination, imaging can be used to confirm the diagnosis. On plain radiographs, patella alta may be observed in complete patella tendon tears. An Insall–Salvati index over 1.2 is indicative of a patella tendon tear [17], although a wide variation exists so the most relevant measure is a comparison to the contralateral knee. Ultrasound is often used to diagnose patellar and quadricep tendon tears. Ultrasound is inexpensive and readily available; however, the accuracy is quite user-dependent, and there is a high reported rate of false-positive results (up to 33%) [18]. MRI scan is more expensive and may be more difficult to access but is the ideal imaging modality for extensor mechanism injury when available.

MRI scans are the higher level imaging modality of choice for soft tissue knee injuries, and the ideal modality to assess for meniscal pathology, injuries to ligaments, tendons, cartilage and muscle. MRI is also very useful to assess for bone marrow oedema, and therefore MRI can detect fractures missed on X-rays (Figs. 10.2 and 10.3).

CT scans allow multiplanar assessment of bony anatomy and is indicated to obtain better definition of any fracture initially detected on plain radiographs. CT can also be used for assessment of arterial and venous vasculature in the form of a CT angiogram. In the presence of an MLKI, a CT angiogram should be performed to rule out vascular pathology which may be present even with the presence of distal pulses. Rate of vascular injuries in MLKI is reported to be up to 18% in some studies [19, 20].

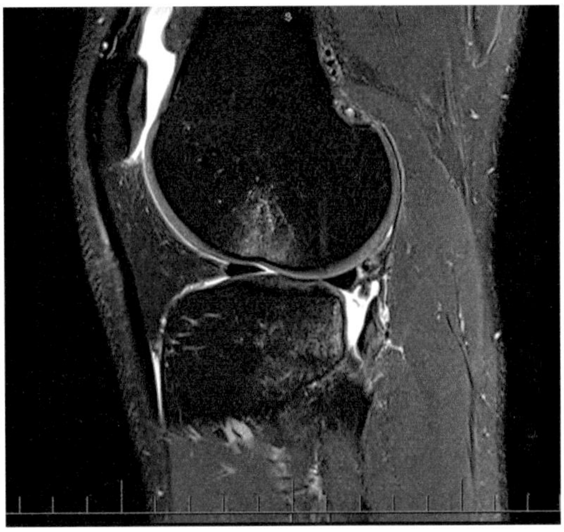

Fig. 10.2 Sagittal MRI sequence demonstrating the pattern of bone bruising/oedema seen in an ACL rupture. Here the pivot shift mechanism causes the tibia to sublux anteriorly, coming into contact with the lateral femoral condyle

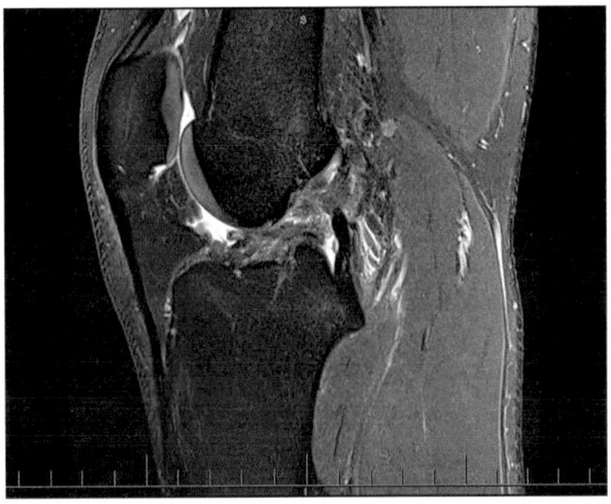

Fig. 10.3 Sagittal MRI sequence demonstrating a mid-substance rupture of the ACL

10.4 Incidence/Prevalence as well as Predisposing Risk Factors of Each Specific Diagnosis

10.4.1 ACL

The ACL and MCL are the two most common injured ligaments in the knee [21, 22]. More than 120,000 ACL injuries occur annually in the United States, most of which are in high school and college students [23]. The incidence of ACL injuries and reconstructions is continuing to rise.

In a systematic review and meta-analysis Gornitzky et al. [23] found an overall incidence of ACL injuries of 0.081 per 1000 exposures in females for all sports combined. The highest risk sport for women were soccer and basketball. Male athletes had a lower overall incidence of ACL injuries with 0.05 per 1000 exposures. For males, the highest risk sports were football and lacrosse.

A recent Canadian population-based study [24] found that the average annual increase in ACL reconstruction (ACLR) incidence was higher among females (1.8% per years) compared to males (0.96% per year). The overall peak incidence and peak incidence among males was observed in 20–29 year age group, whereas peak incidence in females was observed in 10–19 years of age. The number of ACLR in females outnumbers those among males for 10–19 year age group. The incidence of ACLR is increasing, especially among females and among younger cohorts under 20 years of age [24].

Women are 4–6 times more likely to injure their ACL compared to male athletes [25], the reasons for this are multifactorial. Biomechanical studies have demonstrated differences in female landing biomechanics with a predisposition to use quadriceps and gastrocnemius muscles to resist anterior tibial translation, compared to male athletes who recruited the hamstring muscles to stabilise the knee. Female athletes have increased laxity when compared to male athletes and demonstrate higher anterior tibial translation [26]. Furthermore, there are gender differences in the joint kinematics with women demonstrating an increased dynamic lower extremity valgus which also contributes to ACL injury risk in women.

In the professional athletic population ACL injuries are likely to involve other pathology, with up to 67% of ACL injuries involve the MCL complex [22]. With regard to injury mechanism, 70% of ACL injuries are non-contact and 30% are contact injuries [27], with landing or plant-and-cut manoeuvres are the most common sporting tasks responsible for ACL injuries [28] (Fig. 10.4).

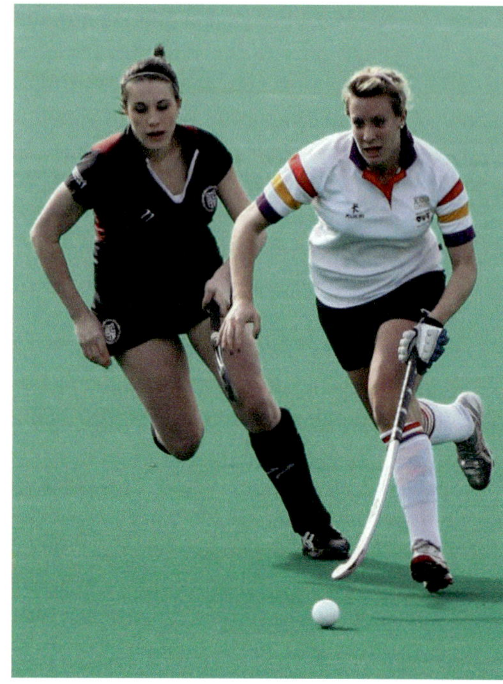

Fig. 10.4 A female field hockey player carrying the ball, demonstrating a plant-and-cut manoeuvre with the knee in valgus

10.4.2 MCL

The MCL is the most common knee injury in high school, collegiate, and professional football players, due to the lateral side of the knee being more exposed to direct contact. Isolated MCL injuries occur as a result of a valgus force to the knee and can occur in a contact or non-contact situation. Rotational mechanisms more commonly result in multiple ligament injuries [29]. Risk factors for MCL injuries include contact sports such as wrestling, hockey, judo, and rugby. Male athletes are at a greater risk than female athletes [30].

10.4.3 LCL

Injuries of the lateral ligaments of the knee are rarer than medial sided lesions and are often part of a multi-ligament injury with concomitant lesions of anterior cruciate ligament (ACL) and/or posterior cruciate ligament (PCL) and the remainder of the posterolateral corner. The PLC is a complex structure consisting of many components, including the LCL, the popliteus tendon, and the popliteofibular ligament [31] as major stabilisers.

10.4.4 Menisci

Meniscus tears occur across all ages, sexes, and activity levels, with a wide variation in tear pattern and treatment [32]. Participation in sport places high loads on the meniscus when athletes cut, jump, squat, change direction, and lift heavy objects [33].

The overall incidence rate of meniscus injury in high school athletes is 5.1 per 100,000 athlete exposures (AEs), with lower risk during practice sessions (3/100,000 AEs) and higher risk during games and competition (12/100,000 AEs) [34].

Non-modifiable risk factors provide important information about individual and population risk, but by definition are not targets for injury prevention. In contrast, modifiable risk factors can be altered to reduce injury risk. Common non-modifiable risk factors for meniscal injury include age, sex, and race. Modifiable risk factors include body mass index (BMI), tobacco use, and participation in sports and occupation [32].

A meta-analysis looking at risk factors for acute meniscal tears found that there is an increased risk if participating in sports such as soccer and rugby. The same meta-analysis found there was minimal evidence for running as a risk factor for acute meniscal tears. A delay more than 12 months between ACL injury and reconstruction surgery, also presented as a risk factor for medial meniscal tears, but there was no evidence of such an association for the lateral meniscus [35].

Tear pattern and aetiology will vary with patient age. Complex degenerative tears are seen more often in the older population, and acute and longitudinal tears are observed more often in younger active populations and athletes. Other patient risk factors for meniscus tears are obesity and participation in competitive sports. Overall, the medial meniscus is more commonly torn; however, lateral meniscal injuries are more commonly associated with in in acute ACL injury, in wrestlers, NFL and NBA athletes. Meniscal root tears are seen more frequently in patients with ACL ruptures and also obese patients. Root tears tend to progress to symptomatic knee osteoarthritis more frequently than non-root tears [32].

10.4.5 Tendon Ruptures: Patella and Quadricep Tendon Ruptures

Extensor mechanism disruptions of the knee can involve the patella or quadriceps tendon.

The incidence of patellar tendon ruptures has been reported to be 0.68 per 100,000 person-years in the general population [36]. Patella tendon ruptures can occur as a result of a sharp or blunt trauma directly to the patella tendon, or more commonly as a result of a forced eccentric contraction. Injury to the extensor mechanism is usually characterised by a sudden contraction of the quadriceps with the knee in flexion and excessive axial loading; therefore, these injuries are seen more commonly in jumping sports, such as basketball and football/soccer [37]. An epidemiological study performed by Garner looking at the demographic characteristics and comorbidities from a review of 726 patient records, found the mean patient age for quadriceps tendon rupture to be 61.0 ± 13.1, and 39.5 ± 12.2 years for patellar tendon ruptures. They also found that of those patients with patella tendon ruptures 95.5% were male and 4.5% were female, in the quadriceps tendon group 91% were males and 9% female [38].

Quadriceps tendon tears are usually seen in older patients compared to patellar tendon tears. A high proportion of quadriceps tendon ruptures occur in patients with pre-existing comorbidities such as diabetes, obesity, rheumatoid arthritis. Healthy patients may also experience quadriceps tendon tears due to forceful eccentric contraction of the muscle [17].

10.4.6 Fractures

Compared to other knee injuries, sports-related fractures of the knee are relatively rare. Fractures around the knee can include tibial plateau fractures, distal femoral fractures, patella fractures, osteochondral fractures following patella dislocation and avulsion fractures. Children and adolescent athletes can present with specific fractures such as avulsion fractures of the tibial spine/ tuberosity, or patella, for example, sleeve fractures, as well as fractures involving the growth plate.

Tibial plateau and distal femoral fractures most commonly result from high velocity or high energy injuries. Some high-speed sports such as downhill skiing or motor cross, and sports with heavy contact, have a higher risk of fracture than other sports [39].

10.4.7 Dislocations: Patella and Knee Dislocation

Patellar dislocations are commonly encountered orthopaedic injuries and account for 3% of all knee injuries [40]. The incidence of lateral patellar dislocation ranges between 2.29 and 23.2 per 100,000 person-years [41, 42]. Patella dislocation is highest among adolescents aged 14–18 years with the annual incidence being similar between male and female patients [42].

The stability of the patellofemoral joint depends on both bony and soft tissue components (Fig. 10.5). It is important to consider not only the mechanical axis and the rotational profile of both the tibia and femur, but also the integrity of the extensor mechanism, as well as other structures such as the medial patellofemoral ligament (MPFL) [43].

Female sex is cited as a risk factor for patellofemoral instability although for isolated patella dislocation; however, a 21-year population-based study found there is no statistically significant difference in the overall or gender-specific annual incidence rate of first-time patellar dislocation [42].

Non-modifiable risk factors for patella dislocation, as described by Dejour include major and minor criteria. The major factors include trochlear dysplasia, patella alta, a laterally placed tubercle, and patellar tilt. Minor factors include the integrity of the MPFL as well as increased

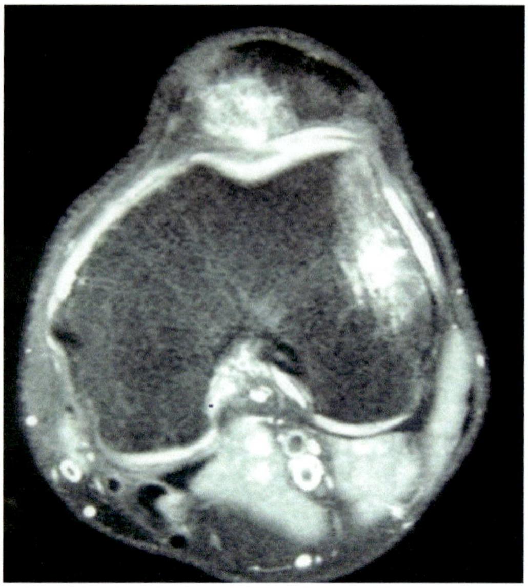

Fig. 10.5 Axial MRI sequence demonstrating the typical pattern of bone bruising seen after a lateral patella dislocation. As the patella dislocates laterally, the medial facet of the patella comes into contact with the lateral femoral condyle resulting in bone oedema as seen below

external femoral or tibial rotation and genu recurvatum or valgum [44].

Although rare an acute traumatic knee (tibiofemoral) dislocation requires prompt assessment, clinical examination and communication to urgently transfer/evacuate the patient to an appropriate health care facility. Multi-ligamentous injuries (MLKI) are rare but devastating injuries; they have a low incidence of around 0.02–0.20% of all orthopaedic injuries [45]; however, this number is likely to be under reported given that many knee dislocations will spontaneously reduce [46]. There is a male preponderance with MLKI with a 4:1 male to female ratio [47]. Obesity is a risk factor and is associated with a higher risk of neurovascular injury and complications [47, 48].

10.4.8 Summary

Risk factors for knee injury is based on the patients age, gender, bony anatomy and sport participation. ACL injuries are common and often involve other intra-articular injuries; there is a higher incidence in female athletes. Injuries to the extensor mechanism are more common in male athletes and often involve jumping sports and the older athlete. Sports which involve dynamic changes of direction increase the risk of meniscal tears. Anatomical variants of bony anatomy such as trochlea dysplasia and patella alta increase the risk of patella dislocation. It is important as a team physician to be aware of the individuals risk factors, as well as those associated to the sport being undertaken.

10.5 Sideline Management Guidelines and Suggestions of the Specific Traumatic Injuries and Clinical Issues in Athletes

10.5.1 Logistics

Knowledge of the local health care facilities should be sought out prior to competition or matches. Knowing the quickest evacuation route for the athlete if they have a serious injury such as a fracture, knee dislocation or MLKI, can be potentially limb saving. Quick and streamlined evaluation and evacuation of these patients to an appropriate health care setting is essential. If possible, the receiving hospital should have the facilities to perform imaging including CT and MRI scans and also have vascular, as well as orthopaedic surgeons on site to appropriately manage the more severe injuries. If present, ambulance services on site should be able to quickly facilitate this.

Specific Equipment for Knee Injuries

Provision List for Match Day/Training

- PPE—gloves/apron.
- Crutches—adjustable.
- Extension brace—universal sizing.
- Stretcher.
- Ice/cool pack.
- Hand-held Doppler.

Injuries Requiring Same Day Transfer and Review

- Ligamentous injury.
- Meniscal injury.
- Reduced patella dislocation.

10.5.2 Ligamentous/Meniscal Injuries

Examining the knee should establish whether the injury allows the player to continue or cease playing. If the athlete is unable to continue competing, then the decision needs to be made whether play needs to cease to allow further support to move the athlete off the pitch/playing arena. In the majority of knee injuries, the player can usually be assisted off the field for further assessment, whereas in the rarer instance of fractures or dislocations a stretcher or motorised cart may be necessary.

Once off the playing field, a more thorough assessment of the injured limb can be performed and a provisional diagnosis and plan for management can be made. Initial splinting of the limb with a simple extension splint (as demonstrated in the picture below) can provide analgesia and also facilitate easier transfer of the patient if unable to bear weight. Provision of crutches if the patient is unable to bear weight will also be useful. Ice can be applied either in the form of a cool pack or a compression cooling device, providing the skin is not broken. Care should be taken to avoid prolonged use which may result in freezer burns. Simple analgesics can be given to assist with pain management as required. After initial management with ice and splint, the patient can be transferred to a local hospital facility if further assessment and management is required urgently (Fig. 10.6). In the case of less urgent injuries that have been adequately managed at the field, arrangements for further outpatient imaging and consultation can be arranged.

A note on extension splints: Whilst useful in the immediate acute setting, these splints should

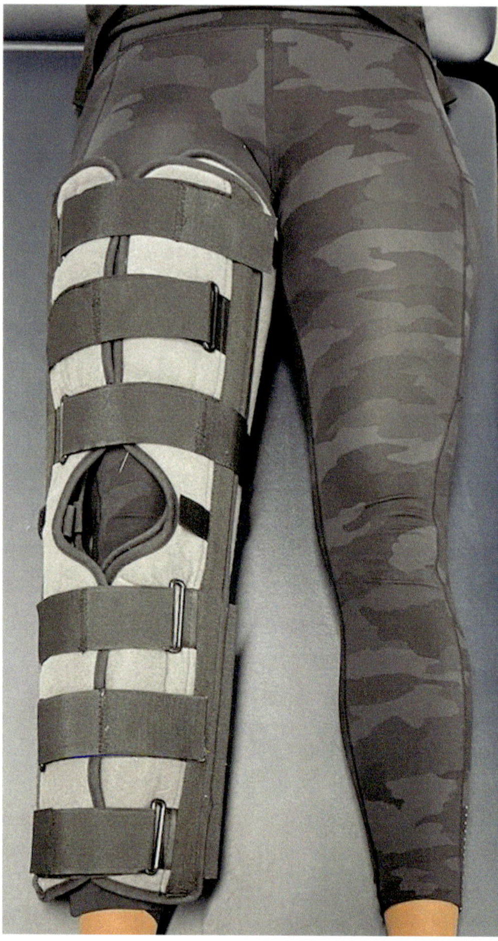

Fig. 10.6 An example of an extension splint

not be used for extended periods of time as this can result in significant knee stiffness. Using the correct support/splint for the injury is essential.

Injuries Requiring Immediate Transfer (Emergent Transfer Without Delay)

- Knee dislocations/multi-ligament knee injuries.
- Irreducible patella dislocation.
- Femoral or long bone fracture.

10.5.3 Fractures

Most fractures around the knee will be as a result of high energy trauma. With this in mind in a high energy injury where a fracture is suspected the patient should be treated according to ATLS principles as there may be other injuries present. After the initial primary survey, examination of the knee should follow the standard protocol. Careful attention should be made during the inspection, examining the skin diligently to assess its integrity is vital; any abrasion overlying a fracture indicates a possible open fracture, which should be treated urgently. Any contamination of a wound should be cleaned with normal saline or sterile water to reduce the potential for infection. Antibiotics should be administered within an hour of injury [49].

A careful assessment of the neurovascular status should be performed and documented. In cases of suspected fracture, or any injury that may require surgery, it is important to keep the patient fasted in case there is a need for sedation or anaesthesia on arrival to the Emergency Department. After the primary survey, the pitch side management of any fractures around the knee include splinting the limb (the neurovascular examination should be repeated after any splint application) and urgent transfer to an appropriate medical centre with Orthopaedic specialists present. In the case of open fractures affecting long bones the patient should be transferred to a centre with both Orthopaedic and plastic surgeons present if possible [49].

10.5.4 Dislocations

In the case of a patella dislocation reduction can be performed in the acute setting by the team physician or first aider (if appropriately trained to do so). There are benefits of early reduction and a low perceived risk of harm associated with the reduction procedure. For a lateral dislocation of the patella, reduction can be attempted by applying an anteromedially based pressure whilst extending the knee. It is unusual not be able to reduce the patella but should this be the case, further attempts should not be carried out and transfer to a medical facility to obtain an X-ray should ensue [50]. Once the patella is reduced, a simple extension splint can be applied, and the patient can be transferred to a local health care facility where radiographs and further imaging should be obtained to confirm reduction and also look for any osteochondral injury. In the case of an irreducible patella, urgent transfer to a hospital with an orthopaedic facility should ensue.

Knee (tibiofemoral) dislocations are a medical emergency. Many knee dislocations spontaneously reduce, however, if the knee is visibly dislocated then the medical team can try to gently reduce this at the side of the pitch with in-line traction to correct the deformity. Early reduction of the joint will take the pressure off the neurovascular structures and overlying soft tissues which can be compromised. The longer the joint remains dislocated, the more muscular contraction and soft tissue swelling ensues resulting in a more difficult reduction. The ultimate pitchside management of a knee dislocation involves immediate transfer to a definitive area of treatment and so reduction attempts should not delay this. Whether the knee is able to be reduced or not a splint will provide support and facilitate the movement of the patient. Careful documentation of the neurovascular status should be performed and handed over to the receiving medical team, including the time of the injury as this may denote the limb ischemia start time. As with any serious knee injury such as a fracture or dislocation, the patient should be kept nil by mouth as sedation or anaesthesia may be required.

10.6 Suggested Prevention Measures that Could be Implemented for Early Recognition of Risk Reduction (Attitude, Rules Modification, Referee Instruction)

10.6.1 Prevention

The ideal treatment for sporting injuries is preventing them in the first place. Preventing knee injuries is a complex and multifactoral mission. Injury prevention includes not only optimising the players individual physical well-being and conditioning and being alert to changes in a player's performance or movement patterns, but also encompasses an awareness of sports field conditions, appropriate safety equipment and playing conditions.

Injury prevention generally focuses on modifiable risk factors: extrinsic factors, such as equipment, playing surface, rule changes and playing time, or intrinsic factors, such as fitness, flexibility and balance. This is based on adult research, but is now supported by studies of sports injury prevention in children and adolescents [51].

Soccer injury prevention programs have been developed by the Federation Internationale de Football Association (FIFA). The FIFA 11 and FIFA 11þ programs combine training in both technique and balance along with neuromuscular training exercises including strengthening and plyometrics with the goal of eliminating injuries [52]. Knee injury prevention has been studied extensively in ACL injury and can reduce up to 25% of injuries with neuromuscular and proprioceptive training. There is less available data regarding prevention of other injuries such as meniscal injury [53]. Regardless, it seems reasonable that preventing even 25% of ACL injuries would also prevent a substantial number of concomitant intra-articular injuries [32].

10.6.2 Screening

Screening athletes prior to the season starting is a useful tool to identify those individuals who may be at risk of injury. Athletes who have had a previous knee injury or those individuals with a family history of an ACL rupture are at increased risk. Careful assessment of sport-specific biomechanics can provide useful information, in female athletes who land in valgus, studies have shown an increased risk of ACL injuries [54]. Focused pre-season athletic testing, and specific programs to correct any deficiencies in strength, balance and technique should be routine practice wherever possible.

10.6.3 Playing Conditions

With regard to pitch conditions and playing surface more ACL injuries occurred on natural grass than on an artificial surface. In a study looking at non-contact ACL injuries in the National Football League over five seasons almost half of all injuries (47.5%) occurred during game-day exposures, despite the fact that the practice versus game-day exposure rate was 5:1. Also more than 95% of ACL injuries occurred on a dry field [55].

Final Chapter Take Home Message

- Knee injuries are common in the athletic population and can be either soft tissue injuries or involve fractures or dislocations of the patellofemoral or tibiofemoral joint.
- An understanding of the injury mechanism in combination with the examination findings is critical to making an accurate timely diagnosis that facilitates expedient management. Differentiating more severe injuries that require urgent attention from those that can be managed in an outpatient setting is particularly important and allows prompt transfer for patients with a dislocated joint or suspected MLKI to an appropriate hospital. Being aware of the local health care facilities and having a transfer protocol will ensure a prompt evacuation of the injured athlete if required. Specific sports will have increased risks for certain knee injuries and therefore this should be factored into pre-season training, warm-up protocols and game-day competition. As well as insight into the sport played, assessing individual players within the team who are at increased risk of injury, as discussed in this chapter, can minimise the risk of injury to the individual by controlling modifiable variables such as proprioceptive strength and conditioning.

References

1. Chhabra A, Elliott CC, Miller MD. Anatomy and biomechanics of the knee. New York, NY: Springer; 2004.
2. Daniel Miranda Ferreira JMML, Cabrera LGG, Sérgio Rocha Piedade PN. Radiological assessment of sports injuries. In: Sérgio Rocha Piedade PN, Espregueira-Mendes J, Cohen M, Hutchinson MR, editors. Specific sports-related injuries. Springer; 2021.
3. Seroyer ST, Musahl V, Harner CD. Management of the acute knee dislocation: the Pittsburgh experience. Injury. 2008;39(7):710–8.
4. Shelbourne KD, Pritchard J, Rettig AC, McCarroll JR, Vanmeter CD. Knee dislocations with intact PCL. Orthop Rev. 1992;21(5):607–8.
5. Strobel MJ. Knee joint—special part. In: Manual of arthroscopic. surgery: Springer; 2002. p. 97–669.
6. Kim SH, Seo HJ, Seo DW, Kim K-I, Lee SH. Analysis of risk factors for ramp lesions associated with anterior cruciate ligament injury. Am J Sports Med. 2020;48(7):1673–81.
7. Malanga GA, Andrus S, Nadler SF, McLean J. Physical examination of the knee: a review of the original test description and scientific validity of common orthopedic tests. Arch Phys Med Rehab. 2003;84(4):592–603.
8. Torg JS, Conrad W, Kalen V. Clinical I diagnosis of anterior cruciate ligament instability in the athlete. Am J Sports Med. 1976;4(2):84–93.
9. Donaldson WF, Warren RF, Wickiewicz T. A comparison of acute anterior cruciate ligament examinations: initial versus examination under anesthesia. Am J Sports Med. 1985;13(1):5–10.
10. Hughston JC. The absent posterior drawer test in some acute posterior cruciate ligament tears of the knee. Am J Sports Med. 1988;16(1):39–43.
11. Fetto JF, Marshall JL. Medial collateral ligament injuries of the knee: a rationale for treatment. Clin Orthop Rel Res. 1978;132:206–18.
12. Ferreira DM, Luiz JMM, Cabrera LGG, Piedade SR. Radiological assessment of sports injuries. In: Specific sports-related injuries. Springer; 2021. p. 509–37.
13. Stiell IG, Greenberg GH, Wells GA, McKnight RD, Cwinn AA, Cacciotti T, et al. Derivation of a decision rule for the use of radiography in acute knee injuries. Ann Emerg Med. 1995;26(4):405–13.
14. Seaberg DC, Jackson R. Clinical decision rule for knee radiographs. Am J Emerg Med. 1994;12(5):541–3.
15. Cheung TC, Tank Y, Breederveld RS, Tuinebreijer WE, de Lange-de Klerk ES, Derksen RJ. Diagnostic accuracy and reproducibility of the Ottawa knee rule vs the pittsburgh decision rule. Am J Emerg Med. 2013;31(4):641–5.
16. Wharton R, Henckel J, Bhattee G, Ball S, Church S. Segond fracture in an adult is not pathognomonic for ACL injury. Knee Surg Sports Traumatol Arthrosc. 2015;23(7):1925–8.

17. Tandogan RN, Terzi E, Gomez-Barrena E, Violante B, Kayaalp A. Extensor mechanism ruptures. EFORT Open Rev. 2022;7(6):384–95.
18. Swamy G, Nanjayan S, Yallappa S, Bishnoi A, Pickering S. Is ultrasound diagnosis reliable in acute extensor tendon injuries of the knee? Acta Orthop Belg. 2012;78(6):764–70.
19. Kim SH, Park Y-B, Kim B-S, Lee D-H, Pujol N. Incidence of associated lesions of multiligament knee injuries: a systematic review and meta-analysis. Orthop J Sports Med. 2021;9(6):23259671211010409.
20. Medina O, Arom GA, Yeranosian MG, Petrigliano FA, McAllister DR. Vascular and nerve injury after knee dislocation: a systematic review. Clin Orthop Rel Res®. 2014;472(9):2621–9.
21. Gianotti SM, Marshall SW, Hume PA, Bunt L. Incidence of anterior cruciate ligament injury and other knee ligament injuries: a national population-based study. J Sci Med Sport. 2009;12(6):622–7.
22. Willinger L, Balendra G, Pai V, Lee J, Mitchell A, Jones M, et al. High incidence of superficial and deep medial collateral ligament injuries in 'isolated' anterior cruciate ligament ruptures: a long overlooked injury. Knee Surg Sports Traumatol Arthrosc. 2022;30(1):167–75.
23. Kaeding CC, Léger-St-Jean B, Magnussen RA. Epidemiology and diagnosis of anterior cruciate ligament injuries. Clin Sports Med. 2017;36(1):1–8.
24. Paudel YR, Sommerfeldt M, Voaklander D. Increasing incidence of anterior cruciate ligament reconstruction: a 17-year population-based study. Knee Surg Sports Traumatol Arthrosc. 2023;31(1):248–55.
25. Arendt EA, Agel J, Dick R. Anterior cruciate ligament injury patterns among collegiate men and women. J Athletic Training. 1999;34(2):86.
26. Huston LJ, Wojtys EM. Neuromuscular performance characteristics in elite female athletes. Am J Sports Med. 1996;24(4):427–36.
27. McNair P, Marshall R, Matheson J. Important features associated with acute anterior cruciate ligament injury. New Zealand Med J. 1990;103(901):537–9.
28. Boden BP, Dean GS, Feagin JA, Garrett WE. Mechanisms of anterior cruciate ligament injury. SLACK Incorporated Thorofare: NJ; 2000. p. 573–8.
29. Encinas-Ullán CA, Rodríguez-Merchán EC. Isolated medial collateral ligament tears: an update on management. EFORT Open Rev. 2018;3(7):398–407.
30. Roach CJ, Haley CA, Cameron KL, Pallis M, Svoboda SJ, Owens BD. The epidemiology of medial collateral ligament sprains in young athletes. Am J Sports Med. 2014;42(5):1103–9.
31. LaPrade RF, Ly TV, Wentorf FA, Engebretsen L. The posterolateral attachments of the knee. Am J Sports Med. 2003;31(6):854–60.
32. Adams BG, Houston MN, Cameron KL. The epidemiology of meniscus injury. Sports Med Arthrosc Rev. 2021;29(3):e24–33.
33. Ruzbarsky J, Maak T, Rodeo S. Meniscal injuries. In: DeLee, Drez, and Miller' s orthopaedic sports medicine: principles and practice. 5th ed. Philadelphia: Elsevier; 2020. p. 1154–60.
34. Mitchell J, Graham W, Best TM, Collins C, Currie DW, Comstock RD, et al. Epidemiology of meniscal injuries in US high school athletes between 2007 and 2013. Knee Surg Sports Traumatol Arthrosc. 2016;24(3):715–22.
35. Snoeker BA, Bakker EW, Kegel CA, Lucas C. Risk factors for meniscal tears: a systematic review including meta-analysis. J Orthop Sports Phys Ther. 2013;43(6):352–67.
36. Clayton RA, Court-Brown CM. The epidemiology of musculoskeletal tendinous and ligamentous injuries. Injury. 2008;39(12):1338–44.
37. Nguyen MT, Hsu WK. Performance-based outcomes following patellar tendon repair in professional athletes. Phys Sports Med. 2020;48(1):110–5.
38. Garner MR, Gausden E, Berkes MB, Nguyen JT, Lorich DG. Extensor mechanism injuries of the knee: demographic characteristics and comorbidities from a review of 726 patient records. JBJS. 2015;97(19):1592–6.
39. Bharam S, Vrahas MS, Fu FH. Knee fractures in the athlete. Orthop Clin. 2002;33(3):565–74.
40. Van Mechelen W, Hlobil H, Kemper HC. Incidence, severity, aetiology and prevention of sports injuries. Sports Med. 1992;14(2):82–99.
41. Waterman BR, Belmont PJ, Owens BD. Patellar dislocation in the United States: role of sex, age, race, and athletic participation. J Knee Surg. 2012;25(01):051–8.
42. Sanders TL, Pareek A, Hewett TE, Stuart MJ, Dahm DL, Krych AJ. Incidence of first-time lateral patellar dislocation: a 21-year population-based study. Sports Health. 2018;10(2):146–51.
43. Bolton S, Bailey M, Wei R, McConnell J. Paediatric injuries around the knee: soft tissue injuries. Injury. 2022;53(2):237–43.
44. Dejour H, Walch G, Nove-Josserand L, Guier C. Factors of patellar instability: an anatomic radiographic study. Knee Surg Sports Traumatol Arthrosc. 1994;2(1):19–26.
45. Howells NR, Brunton LR, Robinson J, Porteus AJ, Eldridge JD, Murray JR. Acute knee dislocation: an evidence based approach to the management of the multiligament injured knee. Injury. 2011;42(11):1198–204.
46. Ng JWG, Myint Y, Ali FM. Management of multiligament knee injuries. EFORT Open Rev. 2020;5(3):145–55.
47. Neri T, Myat D, Beach A, Parker DA. Multiligament knee injury: Injury patterns, outcomes, and gait analysis. Clin Sports Med. 2019;38(2):235–46.
48. Ockuly AC, Imada AO, Richter DL, Treme GP, Wascher DC, Schenck RC. Initial evaluation and classification of knee dislocations. Sports Med Arthrosc Rev. 2020;28(3):87–93.
49. Association BO. BOAST 4: the management of severe open lower limb fractures. Br Orthop Assoc Br Assoc Plast; 2009. p. 1–2.

50. Lord S, Brodell J, Lenhardt H, Dailey M, Cushman J. Implementation of a prehospital patella dislocation reduction protocol. Prehosp Emerg Care. 2020;24(6):800–3.
51. Abernethy L, Bleakley C. A systematic review of strategies to prevent injury in adolescent school sport. Br J Sports Med. 2007;41(10):627–38
52. Stephenson SD, Kocan JW, Vinod AV, Kluczynski MA, Bisson LJ. A comprehensive summary of systematic reviews on sports injury prevention strategies. Orthop J Sports Med. 2021;9(10):23259671211035776.
53. Donnell-Fink LA, Klara K, Collins JE, Yang HY, Goczalk MG, Katz JN, et al. Effectiveness of knee injury and anterior cruciate ligament tear prevention programs: a meta-analysis. PLoS One. 2015;10(12):e0144063.
54. Hewett TE, Myer GD, Ford KR, Heidt RS Jr, Colosimo AJ, McLean SG, et al. Biomechanical measures of neuromuscular control and valgus loading of the knee predict anterior cruciate ligament injury risk in female athletes: a prospective study. Am J Sports Med. 2005;33(4):492–501.
55. Scranton PE Jr, Whitesel JP, Powell JW, Dormer SG, Heidt RS Jr, Losse G, et al. A review of selected noncontact anterior cruciate ligament injuries in the National Football League. Foot Ankle Int. 1997;18(12):772–6.

Leg, Ankle and Foot

11

Raouf Nader Rekik and Pieter D'Hooghe

11.1 Review of Clinical Presentation and Differential Diagnosis

11.1.1 Upper Leg

Considering the anterior part of the thigh, it is important to know the injury mechanism and define the exact location of the pain. Contusions and muscle strains of the quadriceps muscle are common and generally well identifiable [1, 2]. In contusions, a direct blow to the thigh is reported, whereas the quadriceps muscle strains present with an injury mechanism that consists of an acceleration or deceleration (while running or kicking the ball). Sometimes, however, the athlete can have difficulty after the game to remember the exact injury mechanism. Other muscles of the anterior part of the thigh that alternatively could be affected are the Sartorius muscle and the Gracilis muscle.

Quadriceps contusions are frequently encountered in contact and team sports. They can be very painful, depending on the precise injury mechanism. Most athletes are familiar with this condition and will frequently report it as a "dead leg" or a "cork thigh."

The quadriceps muscle strain' injury mechanism presents as an explosive muscle contraction during kicking, sprinting, or jumping or a sudden deceleration effort. The most common location is the distal myotendinous junction of the rectus femoris muscle. The more proximal localization is more difficult to diagnose and presents with a longer rehabilitation process and overall time loss.

Tip

Differentiating a mild contusion from a grade 1 quadriceps muscle strain: A contusion is a contact injury, causing an early swelling and bruising with an immediate onset of pain, improving with mild activity. It is localized laterally or distal in the muscle and associated with a limited range of motion and an obvious tenderness on palpation. In a muscle strain, which is a noncontact injury, the pain onset is delayed after cool-down and aggravated with activity, the bruising may be absent, the palpatory tenderness not always easy to find, and a muscle spasm could be present. It also causes a direct loss of strength.

It is important in the differential diagnosis of anterior thigh pain, to consider the referred pain from the hip, the sacroiliac joint and/or the upper lumbar spine [3]. These conditions can present with an intermittent and variable pain, sometimes

R. N. Rekik (✉)
National Sport Medicine Programme Department, Aspetar—Qatar Orthopaedic and Sports Medicine Hospital, Doha, Qatar
e-mail: Raouf.Rekik@aspetar.com

P. D'Hooghe
Department of Surgery, Aspetar—Qatar Orthopaedic and Sports Medicine Hospital, Doha, Qatar

S. Rocha Piedade et al. (eds.), *Sideline Management in Sports*,
https://doi.org/10.1007/978-3-031-33867-0_11

poorly localized and with no clearly defined aggravating factors. If the pain is bilateral, this finding is in favor of a referred pain from the upper lumbar spine. These conditions can be discovered for the first time on the sideline by a focused medical support.

A stress fracture of the femur is uncommon but important to diagnose and to manage urgently [4]. The occurrence of gradual onset pain not clearly localized in an endurance athlete with progressive aggravation during the activity should raise the initial suspicion. Other features to consider are quadriceps tendinopathy/rupture, nerve entrapment or rare conditions like tumors [5–10].

In the posterior thigh, the most common injuries in popular sports (football, track and field and others) are hamstring muscle strains [11]. They can occur by sprinting or stretching mechanism.

Less common features over the posterior thigh are hamstring muscle contusions, tendinopathies, bursitis, nerve entrapments, vascular conflicts and tumors [10, 12–15]. Referred pain (lumbar spine, sacroiliac joint) should not be overlooked [16].

11.1.2 Lower Leg

Lower leg injuries are common in running and contact sports. The clinical presentation is variable ranging from an athlete that walks to the sideline to report a potential injury (contusion, medial tibial stress syndrome and others) versus an inability to walk (fracture, severe muscle injury and others). Additionally, a deformity or bone protrusion, swelling, skin laceration, bleeding or hematoma can be noticed.

The major symptom is leg pain, frequently reported by team sport athletes or long-distance runners as shin splint, a wrong appellation as nonspecific in terms of anatomy and diagnostic terminology. Other symptoms include swelling, paresthesia, muscle hernia and others.

Two specific complaints frequently present on the sideline. Firstly, the muscle cramps, that present as unvoluntary and painful muscle contractions, commonly related to repetitive muscle contractions/muscle fatigue (altered neuromuscular control), dehydration, electrolyte issues and/or overexertion [17–21]. The presence of scar tissue due to recurrent minor calf injuries can also be a contributor factor. The calf is the most common site of predilection for cramps [22]. Secondly, the delayed onset muscle soreness (DOMS) that generally occurs 24–48 h following resuming physical exercise after a period of rest or doing a high intensity session. This condition is known to resolve spontaneously after a few hours or days but can interfere with sports practice, depending on the athlete's tolerance to muscle pain [23].

The most common lower leg injuries seen on the sideline are abrasions and contusions as well as muscle injuries (Table 11.1) [22]. They cause pain and sometimes difficulty/inability to walk and/or run. Abrasions result from friction against the ground when falling or following a contact with other players or equipment. Similarly, contusions are caused by a direct blow to the lower leg on the bone, the muscle or soft tissues. This results in a bone bruise or a muscle contusion

Table 11.1 Classification of the major leg injuries according to the incidence in sports [22, 27]

Common	Less common	Uncommon Not to be missed
Abrasion	Chronic compartment syndrome (anterior, lateral, deep and superficial posterior)	Achilles tendon rupture
Contusion	Acute fracture	Deep vein thrombosis
Acute muscle injury	Referred pain from spine	Acute compartment syndrome
Stress fracture (medial tibia, anterior tibia)	Stress fracture fibula	Infection
Medial tibial stress syndrome	Vascular causes	Tumors
Achilles midportion tendinopathy	Superficial peroneal nerve entrapment	
Achilles insertional tendinopathy	Proximal tibiofibular subluxation	

(±external bleeding). Muscle injuries are the most common cause of acute calf pain and require direct attention to avoid aggravation of the condition. The musculotendinous junction and the medial head of the gastrocnemius are the most common location of injury. They occur mainly in racquet sports and middle-aged athletes. The association of different muscle strains should always be considered, and it includes the soleus, the plantaris, the tibialis posterior and others. A sudden acceleration or jump is a commonly reported injury mechanism [24–26].

Acute fractures and stress fractures (located over the medial and anterior tibia, fibula) are less frequent but more severe and laborious in terms of management and return to sport. The player will not be able to continue to play and an urgent management and treatment pathway is required. An acute fracture is caused by a high-energy direct or indirect contact. A stress fracture is rarely discovered on the sideline. This could happen when the athlete requests medical attention on the sideline because of pain to receive local anesthetic spray or cream to try to continue to play. Rarely, during the competition and following a jump or change of direction, the stress fracture transforms in a full fracture [28–31].

The medial tibial stress syndrome presents more frequently in running and jumping sports. Generally, the athlete is already known to have such chronic conditions and is allowed to play under antalgic treatment and according to the pain tolerance. The pain is generally localized along the posterior medial border of the tibia, mainly around the lower and mid third tibial junction. A more localized apprehension should however also raise a potential stress fracture suspicion [32].

Another first-presentation-athlete-sideline complaint can be Achilles tendinopathy. It is important to differentiate this feature between midportion and insertional tendinopathy (according to the pain location and swelling) and to eliminate tendon rupture (loss of function following an acute severe blow) and posterior impingement syndrome (repetitive excessive plantar flexion such as in ballet dancers, football players and gymnasts) in the differential diagnosis setup [33, 34].

Peroneal and tibialis posterior tendon ruptures should also not be overlooked [35, 36]. The differential diagnosis consists furthermore of proximal tibiofibular subluxations, acute compartment syndrome, tumors and referred spinal conditions [22]. Additionally, it is important to be aware of some uncommon features that represent medical emergencies such as the acute compartment syndrome. This entity is caused by a trauma with high velocity leading to large bruises on the calf muscles and severe pain, exacerbated by muscle contraction or stretch. Burning or tingling over the skin may be reported as well. The injury mechanism can be from a fall during a motorcycle race, a trauma by a helmet or other equipment as well as a long and extenuating exercise causing muscular rhabdomyolysis [37–39]. Chronic compartment syndromes generally occur in endurance athletes due to repetitive loading such as during marathon running, presenting with symptoms of pain, muscle cramps and even numbness [40, 41].

11.1.3 Ankle

Ankle injuries are more common in running, jumping and pivoting sports. Lateral ligament sprains are the most commonly encountered acute ankle injuries. A combined inversion and plantar flexion injury mechanism is frequently reported after a rapid change in direction or landing after jumping. The location of pain and swelling is a direct indication of the injured ligaments and is most frequently situated on the anterolateral aspect of the ankle. The most commonly affected ligament is the anterior talofibular ligament (ATFL). Other lateral ligaments (calcaneofibular ligament, posterior talofibular ligament) and the medial ligament (deltoid ligament) can also be affected in more severe ankle sprains. The swelling, the bruising and degree of disability are generally related to the injury severity. A precise classification of ankle instability is directly linked to the rehabilitation protocol. Seen on the sideline, if the athlete was playing with a brace or tape before the injury, it might have been that a preexisting instability was already apparent [42, 43].

Tip

Following an acute ankle sprain, the validity and reliability of the manual stress tests (anterior drawer test and talar tilt test) is high when done 4–7 days post injury, but not in the acute phase on the sideline.

Tendinopathies (tibialis posterior, flexor hallucis longus and peroneal) represent a common cause of progressive onset of ankle pain [44]. It causes medial or lateral pain behind the malleolus. Retro malleolar swelling is commonly present in peroneal tendinopathy.

Sinus tarsi syndromes present with poorly localized pain anterior to the lateral malleolus and should not be overlooked [45]. Less common injuries include the medial ligament sprains and syndesmotic injuries (the so-called high ankle sprains). These are normally subject to a more complex and higher velocity injury mechanism. They may also be associated with fractures/avulsions. Surgery can be indicated according to the injury gradation with longer time loss depending on the classification severity [46, 47].

Acute fractures (malleolus, tibial plafond, anterior process of the calcaneum, lateral or posterior process of the talus, os trigonum) are uncommon and not always easy to diagnose. The Ottawa rules can be useful in this case to indicate an X-ray in the emergency setting [48, 49].

Other uncommon injuries include osteochondral lesions of the talus, ankle dislocation (±fracture), tendon rupture or dislocation (tibialis posterior tendon medially, peroneal tendons laterally) and stress fractures [42, 44].

11.1.4 Foot

A common cause of rear foot and inferior heel pain symptomatology is called plantar fasciitis. It causes a gradual onset of pain mostly over the medial aspect of the heel and mainly aggravated by activity. Manual stretching of the plantar fascia may reproduce the pain [50–52]. Another common condition is the fad pad contusion. The fad pad serves at heel strike as a calcaneal shock absorber. The main complaint is a weightbearing-induced heel pain generally over the lateral aspect, which helps in differentiating from the medial aspect pain in plantar fasciitis [53].

The most common diagnostic challenges over the midfoot include navicular stress fracture, metatarsal joint sprain (calcaneonavicular and calcaneocuboid ligaments), extensor and tibialis posterior tendinopathy and plantar fascia strain [53–55].

Over the forefoot, common diagnoses include corns, calluses, first metatarsophalangeal joint sprain (turf toe), onychocryptosis, stress fracture of the metatarsal, Morton's neuroma, subungual hematoma, synovitis of the metatarsophalangeal joints and others [53, 55].

11.2 Discussion of Key Clinical Examination Pearls and Findings

The clinical examination should start with inspection and include furthermore the assessment of the range of motion and motor function, together with targeted palpatory, functional and resistance testing. This should follow a methodological sequence and be repetitive across athletes to allow for a better accuracy and pertinence even in the initial sideline assessment. However, as the time is limited on the sideline, according to the injury mechanism, the symptomatology and the specific athlete situation, we aim to focus more on some components of the clinical examination and anything that proves to be relevant for our decision making [22, 42, 53, 56]

1. Inspection: According to the suspected diagnosis and the condition of the athlete, observation will be performed while the athlete is walking (on toes and heels), standing up and/or lying on the ground (supine and/or prone position). It starts by observing the lower limbs to search for a swelling, a deformity, a bleeding or any other apparent, clinical sign, all the way to the lower limb alignment as well.
2. Active, passive and resisted movements: to measure the range of motion of the joints and the muscles' movement and strength. The

main challenge in this part of the assessment is pain, as it may be exacerbated in conditions such as muscle injuries, tendinopathies, fractures and compartment syndromes.

3. Functional tests: these should be performed while preventing not to aggravate the potential injury. This includes—without limitation—jumping/hopping on the spot or for a distance, squatting and running in a short distance, as well as single leg stance or heel/toe raise and kick simulation. The lunge test is performed to assess the comparative ankle dorsiflexion with the contralateral side.
4. Palpation: It basically looks for the area of maximal tenderness.
   (a) Upper leg: The thigh and particularly the quadriceps and hamstring muscles are palpated to localize specific areas of tenderness, a defect, swelling or muscle thickening while the muscle is either relaxed or contracted. The skin temperature should be compared to the contralateral side.
   (b) Lower leg: To check the soft tissue compartments around the tibia, including the muscles as well (four compartments over the lower leg). It assesses the skin warmth (compared to the contralateral side), the pulses, an eventual swelling/edema or hematoma or crepitus.
      – Tibia and fibula: A focal pain suggests an acute or stress fracture. Medial tibial stress syndrome is suspected in case the pain is diffuse over the posterior medial border of the tibia. A high-grade syndesmotic injury of the ankle may be associated with a fracture of the proximal fibula (Maisonneuve fracture).
      – Muscles (gastrocnemius, plantaris and soleus): These muscles can be subject to strains or ruptures like a tennis leg (plantaris or gastrocnemius medial head partial rupture).
   (c) Ankle and foot: Checking the pulses as well as palpating the malleolus, the lateral and medial ligaments, the talus, the peroneal tendons, the anterior joint line, the dome of the talus, the antero-inferior tibiofibular ligaments, the base of the fifth metatarsal, the metatarsals, the first metatarsophalangeal joint and the sesamoid bone.
5. Special tests: they are performed according to the suspected diagnosis and include without limitation:
   (a) Squeeze test: Squeezing both tibia and fibula around the proximal tibio-fibular joint that causes pain in case of a high-grade ankle syndesmosis injury (so-called high ankle sprain).
   (b) A femoral stress fracture test or fulcrum test: Difficult to realize on the sideline as it needs the athlete to be seated, while performing a pressure on the anterior distal thigh. In case of stress fracture, it may reproduce pain.
   (c) A lower leg stress fracture test: Vibration on the painful location in the bone would exacerbate pain and suspect a stress fracture.
   (d) The Thompson's or Simmonds' test: Squeezing the calf in prone position would cause an ankle plantar flexion. Its absence indicates a complete Achilles tendon or musculotendinous junction tear.
   (e) The modified Thomas test (neurodynamic test): Passive knee flexion/extension in a patient during psoas stretch position may reproduce anterior thigh pain suspecting a referred pain from the lumbar spine.
   (f) The Slump test (neurodynamic test): The athlete is being asked to slump forward at the thoracic and lumbar spine while being seated with the hands behind the back. If no pain is reported, have the patient flex the neck by placing the chin on the chest and then extending one knee as much as possible. This maneuver helps to differentiate between a posterior thigh injury and a referred pain from the lumbar spine.
   (g) Posterior impingement test: Passive maximal plantar flexion of the ankle reproduces the pain of posterior ankle impingement syndrome.

(h) External rotation test: External rotation of the foot and ankle while the leg is in straight position. It causes pain in case of a syndesmotic ankle injury (so-called high ankle sprain).

11.3 Indications and Benefits of Additional Testing/Imaging (Point of Care or Referral)

Sometimes imaging and/or other investigations are required to confirm the suspected sideline diagnosis. X-rays are mostly suitable to confirm acute fractures. They may also be useful to confirm other relevant features like a myositis ossificans, which presents basically as a muscle calcification that can be detected 3–4 weeks after a thigh contusion [57]. However, they have a low sensitivity for stress fractures but can sometimes indicate indirect signs such as a periosteal reaction. Rarely, they show a subtle radiolucent line that requires further investigation by MRI and/or CT scan imaging modalities [22].

When considering thigh pain, radiological investigations are not required at first since the clinical judgment is key. If indicated, ultrasound and MRI scan are helpful to confirm the diagnosis while searching for signs of hematoma or calcification [58, 59].

When considering lower leg pain, MRI scan is the investigation of choice thanks to its capability to assess bony and soft tissue injuries as well as marrow changes and direct correlation with clinical findings [22, 60]. MRI scan of the lower leg can identify a muscle strain with a higher sensibility compared to diagnostic ultrasound [61, 62].

Diagnostic ultrasound is the golden standard for imaging of plantar fasciitis by confirming the swelling and measuring the plantar fascia thickness. MRI is a good alternative as well [50, 53, 63].

As always, in case of referred pain or clinical doubt, imaging is indicated to support the clinical assessment.

Further extended workup can always be indicated and is guided by the clinical assessment and history taking. It includes an EMG/nerve conduction study (peripheral nerve entrapment), an ultrasound venous Doppler (deep venous thrombosis) and blood tests like CBC, erythrocyte sedimentary rate, creatine phosphokinase, D-dimer, urine analysis and others.

11.4 Incidence/Prevalence as Well as Predisposing Injury Risk Factors

The injury incidence varies according to the specificity and type of sports. In long distance runners, a systematic review estimated that the incidence of the most common locations of lower limb injuries was the knee (7.2–50.0%), the lower leg (shin, Achilles tendon, calf and heel) (9.0–32.2%), the foot and toes (5.7–39.3%) and the upper leg (hamstring, thigh and quadriceps) (3.4–38.1%) [64].

In football, a recent systematic review reported that lower limb injuries present with the highest incidence. The authors stated in regards to the main study injury locations that "*The mean incidence per 1000 player hours of exposure with 95% CIs were in descending order: thigh (1.8, 95% CI 1.5 to 2.2,* I^2 *= 91.78); knee (1.2, 95% CI 1.0 to 1.4,* I^2 *= 91.86); ankle (1.1, 95% CI 0.9 to 1.2,* I^2 *= 92.58); hip/groin (0.9, 95% CI 0.7 to 1.0,* I^2 *= 95.32); lower leg/Achilles tendon (0.8, 95% CI 0.6 to 1.0,* I^2 *= 93.01) and foot/toe (0.4, 95% CI 0.3 to 0.5,* I^2 *= 91.4)*" [65].

A systematic review on the epidemiology of ankle injuries reported that ankle sprains are the most common presentation of all ankle injuries, that the ankle was the second most common location in terms of injury incidence and that the ankle injury incidence was higher in team sports and court games [66].

11.4.1 Leg

Muscle strains may occur in the absence or due to an inadequate warming up, a limited knee or ankle range of motion, muscle tightness, weakness or muscle imbalance, fatigue, inadequate training load or recovery and a previous or recurrent muscle injury. The athlete's age and body mass index have been as well reported as an important contributing factor [67–70]. Recent research also suggests that excessive subtalar pronation may overload the calf muscles (gastrocnemius and soleus muscles) as they contract, which could predispose to calf muscle strains [62, 71].

Risk factors for femur stress fractures include training type and load errors, inadequate sport practice surfaces and footwear, leg length discrepancies and excessive foot supination or pronation [72].

Risk factors for medial tibial stress syndrome are reported to be linked to an increase in the traction on the posterior medial border of the tibia and include a female gender, an increased weight and body mass index, a flat foot, a higher navicular drop, a low flexibility, a greater hip external rotation with the hip in flexion, a previous running injury or fatigue as well as an excessive training load, specific shoe design and shoe surface type [73–76].

The Achilles tendon is at higher risk of injury when subject to high loads while running and jumping. Thus, compared to sedentary people, runners have 30 times higher risk of tendinopathy and 15 times higher risk of tendon rupture [77]. Achilles tendinopathy risk factors include important foot supination or pronation, calf muscle weakness, limited calf flexibility and ankle range of motion and the use of the drug ofloxacin [27, 34, 78–80].

11.4.2 Ankle

The most common acute traumatic injury in the world of Sports is the ankle sprain. It represents about 14% of the overall sport related injuries [81]. The risk factors for acute ankle sprains include an increased sport activity intensity, higher foot size and width, higher ankle eversion strength compared to inversion strength and the ratio between dorsiflexion and plantarflexion strength [81].

11.4.3 Foot

The risk factors for plantar fasciitis include a high body mass index, pes planus (flat feet) or pes cavus (high arches), limited ankle dorsiflexion, muscle tightness in the gluteal, hamstring and calf regions, sport activities requiring excessive ankle plantarflexion with the metatarsophalangeal joints in dorsiflexion and an excessive walking in inappropriate shoes [82–87]. When considering fad pad contusion, this condition is known to be caused by a high fall onto the heels or by activities including repetitive heel strike, stops and change of directions [53].

A stress fracture of the navicular bone is one of the most common stress fractures in athletes especially in runners and jumping sports [88]. It occurs more frequently with overload or training errors and limited ankle dorsiflexion [89–91].

Risk factors, linked to a first metatarsophalangeal joint sprain, include the practice on artificial turf with soft flexible footwear, pes planus and limited ankle and metatarsophalangeal range of motion [53, 92, 93].

11.5 Sideline Management Guidelines and Suggestions

11.5.1 Upper Leg

Mild quadriceps contusions will normally allow the athlete to continue his sport activity. In more severe cases, a period of rest will be required for few days to several weeks depending on the clinical symptomatology. Crutches can be helpful to temporary offload the leg. On the sideline and in the course of the first few days, icing for 20 min several times a day (ice packs), compression by a soft bandage and elevation are suggested. To assess the importance of the hematoma, passive knee flexion is a good test to perform 24 h after injury. Further management will then be based upon controlling the hemorrhage, restoring pain-free full range of motion and a tailored rehabilitation protocol. Two potential complications may commonly result from quadriceps contusions, especially if severe or not well managed: the acute compartment syndrome of the thigh and myositis ossificans that both require an individual injury management [37, 57, 94, 95].

In grade 1 distal quadriceps muscle strains, the athlete may be able to continue sports activity and experience pain only after the cooling down phase. Sometimes, local anesthetics or a cooling spray may be requested by the athlete on the sideline, but it is advised to stop the physical activity to avoid aggravation. The initial treatment is similar to the management of quadriceps contusions (rest, ice, compression, elevation). In muscle strains—compared to contusions—the range of motion is normally more preserved, but the loss of strength is more important. Grading a muscle strain is important to arrange for the next steps in the injury management, mainly rehabilitation. Surgery can be indicated in grade 3+ injuries.

Hamstring muscle strains require similar initial treatment on the sideline like the quadriceps muscle strains and the plan consists of rest, ice, compression and elevation, followed by early rehabilitation. In hamstring injuries, the main challenge is the common reinjury risk [96, 97]. Hamstring contusions are less frequent and treated in the same way as quadriceps contusions.

For any other less common injury over the thigh (or sideline suspicion), the key consideration is risk of aggravation. If the athlete is able to continue the activity without direct risk of aggravation, a treatment plan focusing on pain relief is started. Afterwards, a referral for further investigations and management will be put in place.

11.5.2 Lower Leg

Although there remains conflicting evidence on the topic, treatment options for exercise-induced muscle cramps depend on the decision to continue the sport activity or no and incorporate stretching and electrical stimulation sessions. While dehydration can be managed by drinking to thirst, repetitive cramps should be investigated furthermore as they can be linked to an acute compartment syndrome or a rare genetic myopathy [21, 98].

Delayed onset muscle soreness is known to resolve spontaneously. Sideline intervention is based on pain relief by means including nonsteroids anti-inflammatory medication (NSAIDs) and continued activity. The athlete will continue or not and accommodate the activity intensity according to his tolerance to muscle pain [99].

Abrasions, according to their extent, can be quickly managed by local care (see Chap. 6). Generally, the athlete is allowed to continue to practice after a few minutes of local treatment and applying a mildly compressive bandage if indicated. Massage is contraindicated to avoid aggravation and infection due to the potential underlying skin damage. A topical antibiotic ointment can be applied and skin cuts can be sutured during break time or at the end of sports practice. Wound disinfection is essential and should be checked daily afterwards to avoid signs of infection (swelling, redness, pus, inguinal lymph node) and to evaluate the need for adjuvant antibiotherapy.

Contusion management consists of stopping an eventual bleeding and reduction strategies towards effusion. Generally, they allow to continue the sports participation and the decision will depend on the athlete's pain tolerance. When the contusion causes an important muscle damage, the injury will be managed such a muscle strain. In this case, even if the athlete is able to continue, the risk of aggravation towards the importance of the game or competition should be considered through a risk assessment and shared decision-making process.

When a muscle injury is suspected on the sideline, direct rest, icing, compression, elevation and analgesics are started to reduce pain and swelling. Crutches may be useful in case of temporary difficulty to bear weight. Heel pads can be used over both feet to off-load the calf muscles. Early stretching or massage are contraindicated within the first 48 h after injury to avoid aggravation. Immobilization will be short in time according to the grading, location and severity of the injury and will be followed by an early rehabilitation protocol. During this rehabilitation, platelet-rich plasma injections and stem cell therapies have been suggested and require further investigation in dose and use prior to implementation [62, 71].

When an acute or stress fracture is suspected, bracing (preferably pneumatic bracing) will be applied. A bone reduction is indicated in case of deformity while checking the neurovascular status regularly before and after manual reduction. Open fractures require an aggressive wound irrigation and local care and require emergency orthopedic care.

On the sideline, the main goal in treating medial tibial stress syndrome is symptoms relief if the sportsman decides to continue his sport activity. Treatment includes pain killers, icing or local anesthetics. Tapping could help by controlling foot pronation. Rest is important when the pain persists, however, doing other activities not triggering the pain, like swimming, can keep the person active. Regarding further treatment in the office, extracorporeal shockwave therapy (ESWT) showed promising results as well as targeting for risk factors, using special shoes wear and orthotics, but actual evidence does not support any single available treatment [100, 101].

Achilles tendinopathy, seen on the sideline, will be managed according to the history, intensity of pain and risk of rupture. The frequency and intensity of tendon load will be adjusted and reduced. Medication such as analgesics could help as well as many modalities that were suggested to manage tendinopathies. However, physiotherapy with eccentric exercises holds a place of choice. In case of total or partial rupture of the Achilles tendon, the sportsman will stop the sport activity, crutches will be used as well as a boot moon if available or taping and he will be referred for imaging and decision regarding the conservative or surgical treatment.

Less common conditions such as vascular causes, nerve entrapments, acute compartment syndrome, referred pain and tumors will be referred for further investigation and management. The initial treatment on the sideline will be mainly symptoms based. Some conditions (e.g., acute compartment syndrome) represent a medical emergency which requires an urgent treatment before the occurrence of late signs of permanent muscle and tissue damage such as paralysis and numbness. Its treatment is surgical (fasciotomy) [94]. Important to note that chronic compartment syndrome in running sportsmen is less severe and generally improves by stopping the activity causing the pain. Surgery is rarely needed [40, 41, 102].

Tip

Calf muscle injuries may be associated or followed by a deep venous thrombosis (DVT). An history of a long flight in the first days of injury may be reported. The diagnosis can be suspected in case of persistent calf pain and increased temperature, tenderness and swelling on palpation. Homan's sign (forced passive dorsiflexion with the knee extended) will be positive. An ultrasound doppler will confirm the diagnosis.

11.5.3 Ankle

Athletes with acute lateral ankle sprains, seen on the sideline, should benefit from rest, icing for 20 min several times a day (e.g., ice packs), compression by a soft bandage and elevation. The objectives of the rehabilitation the following days will be to reduce pain, hemorrhage and swelling and in second stage to improve range of motion, strength and proprioception. Sometimes in lateral ankle sprains, especially in recurrent sprains, the athlete will continue his activity. In this case, taping of the ankle and analgesics can be prescribed. However, in case of a medial ankle sprain or a high ankle sprain, as well as a suspicion of fracture, the medical staff can insist on stopping the activity to avoid aggravation. The ankle will be immobilized with a moon boot or Aircast/taping and crutches will be suggested. An ankle dislocation will require the same management but with an initial attempt to reduce it at the sideline while checking the neurovascular status regularly before and after manual reduction.

In ankle tendinopathies (tibialis posterior and flexor hallucis longus), the management on the sideline will consist of pain relief (e.g., cooling spray or local anesthetics). The risk of tendinous tear should be evaluated and all relevant intrinsic and extrinsic factors should be identified and corrected where possible. Immobilization by Aircast is generally not needed but rather a reduction in training load management. The common treatment is a tailored rehabilitation protocol, based on tendon loading concentric and eccentric exercises.

Sometimes the athlete complains on the sideline of persistent or recurrent ankle pain, several weeks after an acute ankle sprain. This requires further management to exclude an osteochondral lesion or impingement syndrome. On the sideline, the treatment will be only based on pain or symptoms relief and ankle taping.

11.5.4 Foot

Presenting on the sideline, the athlete suffering from plantar fasciitis will be generally advised a load management and avoiding aggravating activities rather than rest. Foot taping and silicone gel heel pads can support the tailored activity. Cryotherapy, stretching of the plantar fascia and calf muscles and self-massage with a frozen golf ball are recommended. Analgesics and NSAIDs can be prescribed to improve tolerance to pain. In the long term, strengthening exercises and risk factors management is advised.

The fad pad contusion requires rest or at least temporary limitation in weightbearing, icing and elevation. Tapping, silicone gel heel pads and appropriate footwear may be useful as well. Analgesics and NSAIDs may be prescribed to decrease the pain. To maintain fitness condition, athletes may opt for non-weightbearing activities such as swimming.

The immediate management of acute and stress fractures as well as uncommon conditions in the foot is similar to what was described above for similar injuries in the leg and ankle.

11.6 Suggested Prevention Measures that Could be Implemented for Early Recognition and Risk Reduction (Attitude, Rules Modification, Referee Instruction)

Prevention of lower limbs injuries should target adjustable risk factors as well as available highest evidence preventive exercises and measures. Current research data does not support any preventative measures for exercise-induced cramps. However, targeted strategies have been suggested including regular static and dynamic stretching, exercises to improve balance, flexibility and posture, physical conditioning, tailored training load, avoidance of drugs causing muscle spasm and maintaining suitable hydration and carbohydrate reserves [98, 103].

In contact sports, it is difficult to avoid abrasions and contusions. However, we can limit them by using protective equipment like safety pads, shin guards, helmets, proper footwear, and others. The athlete will consider the equipment's quality, protection as well as the limitation in mobility and comfort.

Quadriceps muscle strains prevention is based on improving the quadriceps flexibility and core stability, as well as performing eccentric exercise training [1, 104, 105].

To prevent hamstring muscle strains, there is high evidence supporting the practice of eccentric hamstring strengthening exercises including the Nordic hamstring exercise [106–109].

For calf muscle injuries, an initial screening will allow for the implementation of a comprehensive preventative program, based on load management, plyometrics and a selection of strengthening exercises specific to both the specific sport and the specific individual's needs. These exercises should target the loading rates and velocities required by the sport as well as the athlete's weaknesses [71].

To avoid acute fractures, the use of protective equipment (like shin guards) is mandatory, even during training or recreational sessions. For stress fractures, it is important to focus on athletes' education (on optimal training methods and enhancing training load by progressive increments), nutrition, fitness and preventing the female athlete triad [110, 111].

For the medial tibial stress syndrome, a targeted approach to the risk factors is recommended. Recent research suggests the use of shock-absorbing insoles but there is currently no high evidence or consensus across experts on potential preventative equipment [112].

References

1. Mendiguchia J, Alentorn-Geli E, Idoate F, Myer GD. Rectus femoris muscle injuries in football: a clinically relevant review of mechanisms of injury, risk factors and preventive strategies. Br J Sports Med. 2013;47(6):359–66. https://doi.org/10.1136/bjsports-2012-091250.
2. Aronen JG, Garrick JG, Chronister RD, McDevitt ER. Quadriceps contusions: clinical results of immediate immobilization in 120 degrees of knee flexion. Clin J Sport Med. 2006;16(5):383–7. https://doi.org/10.1097/01.jsm.0000244605.34283.94.
3. Lesher JM, Dreyfuss P, Hager N, Kaplan M, Furman M. Hip joint pain referral patterns: a descriptive study. Pain Med. 2008;9(1):22–5. https://doi.org/10.1111/j.1526-4637.2006.00153.x.
4. Boden BP, Osbahr DC, Jimenez C. Low-risk stress fractures. Am J Sports Med. 2001;29(1):100–11. https://doi.org/10.1177/03635465010290010201.
5. Hak DJ, Sanchez A, Trobisch P. Quadriceps tendon injuries. Orthopedics. 2010,33(1):40–6. https://doi.org/10.3928/01477447-20091124-20.
6. Kaufman M, Domroese M. Peripheral nerve injuries of the proximal lower limb in athletes. In: Akuthota V, Herring S, editors. Nerve and vascular injuries in sports medicine. Springer; 2009. p. 161.
7. Seror P, Seror R. Meralgia paresthetica: clinical and electrophysiological diagnosis in 120 cases. Muscle Nerve. 2006;33(5):650–4. https://doi.org/10.1002/mus.20507.
8. Kho KH, Blijham PJ, Zwarts MJ. Meralgia paresthetica after strenuous exercise. Muscle Nerve. 2005;31(6):761–3. https://doi.org/10.1002/mus.20271.
9. Esser S, Thurston M, Nalluri K, Muzaurieta A. "Numb-leg" in a crossfit athlete: a case presentation. PM R. 2017;9(8):834–6. https://doi.org/10.1016/j.pmrj.2017.03.007.
10. Siegel RL, Miller KD, Jemal A. Cancer statistics, 2016. CA Cancer J Clin. 2016;66(1):7–30. https://doi.org/10.3322/caac.21332.
11. Heiderscheit BC, Sherry MA, Silder A, Chumanov ES, Thelen DG. Hamstring strain injuries: recommendations for diagnosis, rehabilitation, and injury prevention. J Orthop Sports Phys Ther. 2010;40(2):67–81. https://doi.org/10.2519/jospt.2010.3047.
12. Yuen EC, Olney RK, So YT. Sciatic neuropathy: clinical and prognostic features in 73 patients. Neurology. 1994;44(9):1669–74. https://doi.org/10.1212/wnl.44.9.1669.
13. Goodacre S, Sutton AJ, Sampson FC. Meta-analysis: the value of clinical assessment in the diagnosis of deep venous thrombosis. Ann Intern Med. 2005;143(2):129–39. https://doi.org/10.7326/0003-4819-143-2-200507190-00012.
14. Maffulli N, Wong J, Almekinders LC. Types and epidemiology of tendinopathy. Clin Sports Med. 2003;22(4):675–92. https://doi.org/10.1016/s0278-5919(03)00004-8.
15. Järvinen M. Epidemiology of tendon injuries in sports. Clin Sports Med. 1992;11(3):493–504.
16. Tarulli AW, Raynor EM. Lumbosacral radiculopathy. Neurol Clin. 2007;25(2):387–405. https://doi.org/10.1016/j.ncl.2007.01.008.
17. Martínez-Navarro I, Montoya-Vieco A, Collado E, Hernando B, Panizo N, Hernando C. Muscle cramping in the marathon: dehydration and electrolyte depletion vs. muscle damage. J Strength Cond Res. 2022;36(6):1629–35. https://doi.org/10.1519/jsc.0000000000003713.
18. Schwellnus MP. Cause of exercise associated muscle cramps (EAMC)—altered neuromuscular control, dehydration or electrolyte depletion? Br J Sports Med. 2009;43(6):401–8. https://doi.org/10.1136/bjsm.2008.050401.
19. Schwellnus MP. Muscle cramping in the marathon: aetiology and risk factors. Sports Med. 2007;37(4–5):364–7. https://doi.org/10.2165/00007256-200737040-00023.
20. Minetto MA, Holobar A, Botter A, Farina D. Origin and development of muscle cramps. Exerc Sport Sci Rev. 2013;41(1):3–10. https://doi.org/10.1097/JES.0b013e3182724817.
21. Acosta I, Bastías P, Matamala JM. [Fasciculations and cramps: physiological bases and clinical approach of a complex phenomenon]. Rev Med Chil. 2021;149(12):1751–64. https://doi.org/10.4067/s0034-98872021001201751.
22. Hutchinson M, Bradshaw C, Hislop M. Leg pain. In: Brukner P, Khan K, editors. Brukner & Khan's clinical sports medicine. McGraw-Hill; 2012.
23. Hotfiel T, Freiwald J, Hoppe MW, Lutter C, Forst R, Grim C, Bloch W, Hüttel M, Heiss R. Advances in delayed-onset muscle soreness (DOMS): part I: pathogenesis and diagnostics. Sportverletz Sportschaden. 2018;32(4):243–50. https://doi.org/10.1055/a-0753-1884.
24. Fields KB, Rigby MD. Muscular calf injuries in runners. Curr Sports Med Rep. 2016;15(5):320–4. https://doi.org/10.1249/jsr.0000000000000292.

25. Green B, Pizzari T. Calf muscle strain injuries in sport: a systematic review of risk factors for injury. Br J Sports Med. 2017;51(16):1189–94. https://doi.org/10.1136/bjsports-2016-097177.
26. Ekstrand J, Hägglund M, Waldén M. Epidemiology of muscle injuries in professional football (soccer). Am J Sports Med. 2011;39(6):1226–32. https://doi.org/10.1177/0363546510395879.
27. Alfredson H, Cook J, Silbernagel K, Karlsson J. Pain in the achilles region. In: Brukner P, Khan K, editors. Brukner & Khan's clinical sports medicine. McGraw-Hill; 2012.
28. Chang WR, Kapasi Z, Daisley S, Leach WJ. Tibial shaft fractures in football players. J Orthop Surg Res. 2007;2:11. https://doi.org/10.1186/1749-799x-2-11.
29. Larsen P, Elsoe R, Hansen SH, Graven-Nielsen T, Laessoe U, Rasmussen S. Incidence and epidemiology of tibial shaft fractures. Injury. 2015;46(4):746–50. https://doi.org/10.1016/j.injury.2014.12.027.
30. Shindle MK, Endo Y, Warren RF, Lane JM, Helfet DL, Schwartz EN, Ellis SJ. Stress fractures about the tibia, foot, and ankle. J Am Acad Orthop Surg. 2012;20(3):167–76. https://doi.org/10.5435/jaaos-20-03-167.
31. Feldman JJ, Bowman EN, Phillips BB, Weinlein JC. Tibial stress fractures in athletes. Orthop Clin North Am. 2016;47(4):733–41. https://doi.org/10.1016/j.ocl.2016.05.015.
32. Winters M. The diagnosis and management of medial tibial stress syndrome: an evidence update. Unfallchirurg. 2020;123(Suppl 1):15–9. https://doi.org/10.1007/s00113-019-0667-z.
33. Järvinen TA, Kannus P, Paavola M, Järvinen TL, Józsa L, Järvinen M. Achilles tendon injuries. Curr Opin Rheumatol. 2001;13(2):150–5. https://doi.org/10.1097/00002281-200103000-00009.
34. Józsa L, Kvist M, Bálint BJ, Reffy A, Järvinen M, Lehto M, Barzo M. The role of recreational sport activity in Achilles tendon rupture. A clinical, pathoanatomical, and sociological study of 292 cases. Am J Sports Med. 1989;17(3):338–43. https://doi.org/10.1177/036354658901700305.
35. Willegger M, Hirtler L, Schwarz GM, Windhager RH, Chiari C. [Peroneal tendon pathologies: from the diagnosis to treatment]. Orthopade. 2021;50(7):589–604. https://doi.org/10.1007/s00132-021-04116-6.
36. Jackson LT, Dunaway LJ, Lundeen GA. Acute tears of the tibialis posterior tendon following ankle sprain. Foot Ankle Int. 2017;38(7):752–9. https://doi.org/10.1177/1071100717701686.
37. Osborn PM, Schmidt AH. Diagnosis and management of acute compartment syndrome. J Am Acad Orthop Surg. 2021;29(5):183–8. https://doi.org/10.5435/jaaos-d-19-00858.
38. Pearse MF, Harry L, Nanchahal J. Acute compartment syndrome of the leg. BMJ. 2002;325(7364):557–8. https://doi.org/10.1136/bmj.325.7364.557.
39. Mauser N, Gissel H, Henderson C, Hao J, Hak D, Mauffrey C. Acute lower-leg compartment syndrome. Orthopedics. 2013;36(8):619–24. https://doi.org/10.3928/01477447-20130724-07.
40. Velasco TO, Leggit JC. Chronic exertional compartment syndrome: a clinical update. Curr Sports Med Rep. 2020;19(9):347–52. https://doi.org/10.1249/jsr.0000000000000747.
41. Vajapey S, Miller TL. Evaluation, diagnosis, and treatment of chronic exertional compartment syndrome: a review of current literature. Phys Sportsmed. 2017;45(4):391–8. https://doi.org/10.1080/00913847.2017.1384289.
42. Verhagen E, Karlsson J. Acute ankle injuries. In: Brukner P, Khan K, editors. Brukner & Khan's clinical sports medicine. McGraw-Hill; 2012.
43. Porter DASL. Baxter's the foot and ankle in sport. Elsevier; 2021.
44. Holzer K, Karlsson J. Ankle pain. In: Brukner P, Khan K, editors. Brukner & Khan's clinical sports medicine. McGraw-Hill; 2012.
45. Arshad Z, Bhatia M. Current concepts in sinus tarsi syndrome: a scoping review. Foot Ankle Surg. 2021;27(6):615–21. https://doi.org/10.1016/j.fas.2020.08.013.
46. Crim J. Medial-sided ankle pain: deltoid ligament and beyond. Magn Reson Imaging Clin N Am. 2017;25(1):63–77. https://doi.org/10.1016/j.mric.2016.08.003.
47. Tourné Y, Molinier F, Andrieu M, Porta J, Barbier G. Diagnosis and treatment of tibiofibular syndesmosis lesions. Orthop Traumatol Surg Res. 2019;105(8s):S275–86. https://doi.org/10.1016/j.otsr.2019.09.014.
48. Bachmann LM, Kolb E, Koller MT, Steurer J, ter Riet G. Accuracy of Ottawa ankle rules to exclude fractures of the ankle and mid-foot: systematic review. BMJ. 2003;326(7386):417. https://doi.org/10.1136/bmj.326.7386.417.
49. Briet JP, Hietbrink F, Smeeing DP, Dijkgraaf MGW, Verleisdonk EJ, Houwert RM. Ankle fracture classification: an innovative system for describing ankle fractures. J Foot Ankle Surg. 2019;58(3):492–6. https://doi.org/10.1053/j.jfas.2018.09.028.
50. Goff JD, Crawford R. Diagnosis and treatment of plantar fasciitis. Am Fam Physician. 2011;84(6):676–82.
51. Carek PJ, Edenfield KM, Michaudet C, Nicolette GW. Foot and ankle conditions: plantar fasciitis. FP Essent. 2018;465:11–7.
52. Trojian T, Tucker AK. Plantar fasciitis. Am Fam Physician. 2019;99(12):744–50.
53. Agosta J, Holzer K. Foot pain. In: Brukner P, Khan K, editors. Brukner & Khan's clinical sports medicine. McGraw-Hill; 2012.
54. Mittlmeier T, Beck M. [Injuries of the midfoot]. Chirurg. 2011;82(2):169–86; quiz 187–8. https://doi.org/10.1007/s00104-009-1866-x.
55. Gorbachova T. Midfoot and forefoot injuries. Top Magn Reson Imaging. 2015;24(4):215–21. https://doi.org/10.1097/rmr.0000000000000058.

56. Flynn TW, Cleland J, Whitman J. Users' guide to the musculoskeletal examination: fundamentals for the evidence-based clinician. Evidence in Motion, Distributed by OPTP; 2008.
57. Tyler P, Saifuddin A. The imaging of myositis ossificans. Semin Musculoskelet Radiol. 2010;14(2):201–16. https://doi.org/10.1055/s-0030-1253161.
58. van Holsbeeck M, Soliman S, Van Kerkhove F, Craig J. Advanced musculoskeletal ultrasound techniques: what are the applications? AJR Am J Roentgenol. 2021;216(2):436–45. https://doi.org/10.2214/ajr.20.22840.
59. Verrall GM, Slavotinek JP, Barnes PG, Fon GT. Diagnostic and prognostic value of clinical findings in 83 athletes with posterior thigh injury: comparison of clinical findings with magnetic resonance imaging documentation of hamstring muscle strain. Am J Sports Med. 2003;31(6):969–73. https://doi.org/10.1177/03635465030310063701.
60. Tenforde AS, Kraus E, Fredericson M. Bone stress injuries in runners. Phys Med Rehabil Clin N Am. 2016;27(1):139–49. https://doi.org/10.1016/j.pmr.2015.08.008.
61. Douis H, Gillett M, James SL. Imaging in the diagnosis, prognostication, and management of lower limb muscle injury. Semin Musculoskelet Radiol. 2011;15(1):27–41. https://doi.org/10.1055/s-0031-1271957.
62. Meek WM, Kucharik MP, Eberlin CT, Naessig SA, Rudisill SS, Martin SD. Calf strain in athletes. JBJS Rev. 2022;10:3. https://doi.org/10.2106/jbjs.Rvw.21.00183.
63. Petraglia F, Ramazzina I, Costantino C. Plantar fasciitis in athletes: diagnostic and treatment strategies. A systematic review. Muscles Ligaments Tendons J. 2017;7(1):107–18. https://doi.org/10.11138/mltj/2017.7.1.107.
64. van Gent RN, Siem D, van Middelkoop M, van Os AG, Bierma-Zeinstra SM, Koes BW. Incidence and determinants of lower extremity running injuries in long distance runners: a systematic review. Br J Sports Med. 2007;41(8):469–80; discussion 480. https://doi.org/10.1136/bjsm.2006.033548.
65. López-Valenciano A, Ruiz-Pérez I, Garcia-Gómez A, Vera-Garcia FJ, De Ste CM, Myer GD, Ayala F. Epidemiology of injuries in professional football: a systematic review and meta-analysis. Br J Sports Med. 2020;54(12):711–8. https://doi.org/10.1136/bjsports-2018-099577.
66. Fong DT, Hong Y, Chan LK, Yung PS, Chan KM. A systematic review on ankle injury and ankle sprain in sports. Sports Med. 2007;37(1):73–94. https://doi.org/10.2165/00007256-200737010-00006.
67. Hägglund M, Waldén M, Ekstrand J. Risk factors for lower extremity muscle injury in professional soccer: the UEFA Injury Study. Am J Sports Med. 2013;41(2):327–35. https://doi.org/10.1177/0363546512470634.
68. Bradley PS, Portas MD. The relationship between preseason range of motion and muscle strain injury in elite soccer players. J Strength Cond Res. 2007;21(4):1155–9. https://doi.org/10.1519/r-20416.1.
69. Orchard JW. Intrinsic and extrinsic risk factors for muscle strains in Australian football. Am J Sports Med. 2001;29(3):300–3. https://doi.org/10.1177/03635465010290030801.
70. Pietsch S, Pizzari T. Risk factors for quadriceps muscle strain injuries in sport: a systematic review. J Orthop Sports Phys Ther. 2022;52(6):389–400. https://doi.org/10.2519/jospt.2022.10870.
71. Green B, McClelland JA, Semciw AI, Schache AG, McCall A, Pizzari T. The assessment, management and prevention of calf muscle strain injuries: a qualitative study of the practices and perspectives of 20 expert sports clinicians. Sports Med Open. 2022;8(1):10. https://doi.org/10.1186/s40798-021-00364-0.
72. Breugem SJ, Hulscher JB, Steller P. Stress fracture of the femoral neck in a young female athlete. Eur J Trauma Emerg Surg. 2009;35(2):192. https://doi.org/10.1007/s00068-008-8034-8.
73. Reinking MF, Austin TM, Richter RR, Krieger MM. Medial tibial stress syndrome in active individuals: a systematic review and meta-analysis of risk factors. Sports Health. 2017;9(3):252–61. https://doi.org/10.1177/1941738116673299.
74. Winkelmann ZK, Anderson D, Games KE, Eberman LE. Risk factors for medial tibial stress syndrome in active individuals: an evidence-based review. J Athl Train. 2016;51(12):1049–52. https://doi.org/10.4085/1062-6050-51.12.13.
75. Newman P, Witchalls J, Waddington G, Adams R. Risk factors associated with medial tibial stress syndrome in runners: a systematic review and meta-analysis. Open Access J Sports Med. 2013;4:229–41. https://doi.org/10.2147/oajsm.S39331.
76. Hubbard TJ, Carpenter EM, Cordova ML. Contributing factors to medial tibial stress syndrome: a prospective investigation. Med Sci Sports Exerc. 2009;41(3):490–6. https://doi.org/10.1249/MSS.0b013e31818b98e6.
77. Kujala UM, Sarna S, Kaprio J. Cumulative incidence of achilles tendon rupture and tendinopathy in male former elite athletes. Clin J Sport Med. 2005;15(3):133–5. https://doi.org/10.1097/01.jsm.0000165347.55638.23.
78. van der Vlist AC, Breda SJ, Oei EHG, Verhaar JAN, de Vos RJ. Clinical risk factors for Achilles tendinopathy: a systematic review. Br J Sports Med. 2019;53(21):1352–61. https://doi.org/10.1136/bjsports-2018-099991.
79. Longo UG, Ronga M, Maffulli N. Achilles tendinopathy. Sports Med Arthrosc Rev. 2018;26(1):16–30. https://doi.org/10.1097/jsa.0000000000000185.
80. Holmes GB, Lin J. Etiologic factors associated with symptomatic achilles tendinopathy. Foot Ankle Int. 2006;27(11):952–9. https://doi.org/10.1177/107110070602701115.

81. Fong DT, Chan YY, Mok KM, Yung PS, Chan KM. Understanding acute ankle ligamentous sprain injury in sports. Sports Med Arthrosc Rehabil Ther Technol. 2009;1:14. https://doi.org/10.1186/1758-2555-1-14.
82. Rano JA, Fallat LM, Savoy-Moore RT. Correlation of heel pain with body mass index and other characteristics of heel pain. J Foot Ankle Surg. 2001;40(6):351–6. https://doi.org/10.1016/s1067-2516(01)80002-8.
83. Riddle DL, Pulisic M, Pidcoe P, Johnson RE. Risk factors for plantar fasciitis: a matched case-control study. J Bone Joint Surg Am. 2003;85(5):872–7. https://doi.org/10.2106/00004623-200305000-00015.
84. Taunton JE, Ryan MB, Clement DB, McKenzie DC, Lloyd-Smith DR, Zumbo BD. A retrospective case-control analysis of 2002 running injuries. Br J Sports Med. 2002;36(2):95–101. https://doi.org/10.1136/bjsm.36.2.95.
85. van Leeuwen KD, Rogers J, Winzenberg T, van Middelkoop M. Higher body mass index is associated with plantar fasciopathy/'plantar fasciitis': systematic review and meta-analysis of various clinical and imaging risk factors. Br J Sports Med. 2016;50(16):972–81. https://doi.org/10.1136/bjsports-2015-094695.
86. Warren BL, Jones CJ. Predicting plantar fasciitis in runners. Med Sci Sports Exerc. 1987;19(1):71–3.
87. Waclawski ER, Beach J, Milne A, Yacyshyn E, Dryden DM. Systematic review: plantar fasciitis and prolonged weight bearing. Occup Med (Lond). 2015;65(2):97–106. https://doi.org/10.1093/occmed/kqu177.
88. Jones MH, Amendola AS. Navicular stress fractures. Clin Sports Med. 2006;25(1):151–8, x–xi. https://doi.org/10.1016/j.csm.2005.08.007.
89. Sanders TG, Williams PM, Vawter KW. Stress fracture of the tarsal navicular. Mil Med. 2004;169(7):viii–xiii.
90. Patel KA, Christopher ZK, Drakos MC, O'Malley MJ. Navicular stress fractures. J Am Acad Orthop Surg. 2021;29(4):148–57. https://doi.org/10.5435/jaaos-d-20-00869.
91. Welck MJ, Hayes T, Pastides P, Khan W, Rudge B. Stress fractures of the foot and ankle. Injury. 2017;48(8):1722–6. https://doi.org/10.1016/j.injury.2015.06.015.
92. Hotfiel T, Carl HD, Jendrissek A, Swoboda B, Barg A, Engelhardt M. [Turf toe injury—extension sprain of the first metatarsophalangeal joint]. Sportverletz Sportschaden. 2014;28(3):139–45. https://doi.org/10.1055/s-0034-1366873.
93. Frimenko RE, Lievers W, Coughlin MJ, Anderson RB, Crandall JR, Kent RW. Etiology and biomechanics of first metatarsophalangeal joint sprains (turf toe) in athletes. Crit Rev Biomed Eng. 2012;40(1):43–61. https://doi.org/10.1615/critrevbiomedeng.v40.i1.30.
94. Osborn CPM, Schmidt AH. Management of acute compartment syndrome. J Am Acad Orthop Surg. 2020;28(3):e108–14. https://doi.org/10.5435/jaaos-d-19-00270.
95. Jackson DW, Feagin JA. Quadriceps contusions in young athletes. Relation of severity of injury to treatment and prognosis. J Bone Joint Surg Am. 1973;55(1):95–105.
96. de Visser HM, Reijman M, Heijboer MP, Bos PK. Risk factors of recurrent hamstring injuries: a systematic review. Br J Sports Med. 2012;46(2):124–30. https://doi.org/10.1136/bjsports-2011-090317.
97. Mason DL, Dickens V, Vail A. Rehabilitation for hamstring injuries. Cochrane Database Syst Rev. 2007;(1):CD004575. https://doi.org/10.1002/14651858.CD004575.pub2.
98. Swash M, Czesnik D, de Carvalho M. Muscular cramp: causes and management. Eur J Neurol. 2019;26(2):214–21. https://doi.org/10.1111/ene.13799.
99. Lewis PB, Ruby D, Bush-Joseph CA. Muscle soreness and delayed-onset muscle soreness. Clin Sports Med. 2012;31(2):255–62. https://doi.org/10.1016/j.csm.2011.09.009.
100. Craig DI. Current developments concerning medial tibial stress syndrome. Phys Sportsmed. 2009;37(4):39–44. https://doi.org/10.3810/psm.2009.12.1740.
101. Winters M, Eskes M, Weir A, Moen MH, Backx FJ, Bakker EW. Treatment of medial tibial stress syndrome: a systematic review. Sports Med. 2013;43(12):1315–33. https://doi.org/10.1007/s40279-013-0087-0.
102. Buerba RA, Fretes NF, Devana SK, Beck JJ. Chronic exertional compartment syndrome: current management strategies. Open Access J Sports Med. 2019;10:71–9. https://doi.org/10.2147/oajsm.S168368.
103. Maughan RJ, Shirreffs SM. Muscle cramping during exercise: causes, solutions, and questions remaining. Sports Med. 2019;49(Suppl 2):115–24. https://doi.org/10.1007/s40279-019-01162-1.
104. LaStayo PC, Woolf JM, Lewek MD, Snyder-Mackler L, Reich T, Lindstedt SL. Eccentric muscle contractions: their contribution to injury, prevention, rehabilitation, and sport. J Orthop Sports Phys Ther. 2003;33(10):557–71. https://doi.org/10.2519/jospt.2003.33.10.557.
105. Brooks JH, Fuller CW, Kemp SP, Reddin DB. Incidence, risk, and prevention of hamstring muscle injuries in professional rugby union. Am J Sports Med. 2006;34(8):1297–306. https://doi.org/10.1177/0363546505286022.
106. Goode AP, Reiman MP, Harris L, DeLisa L, Kauffman A, Beltramo D, Poole C, Ledbetter L, Taylor AB. Eccentric training for prevention of hamstring injuries may depend on intervention compliance: a systematic review and meta-analysis. Br J Sports Med. 2015;49(6):349–56. https://doi.org/10.1136/bjsports-2014-093466.
107. Engebretsen AH, Myklebust G, Holme I, Engebretsen L, Bahr R. Prevention of injuries

among male soccer players: a prospective, randomized intervention study targeting players with previous injuries or reduced function. Am J Sports Med. 2008;36(6):1052–60. https://doi.org/10.1177/0363546508314432.

108. Brukner P. Hamstring injuries: prevention and treatment-an update. Br J Sports Med. 2015;49(19):1241–4. https://doi.org/10.1136/bjsports-2014-094427.
109. Heer ST, Callander JW, Kraeutler MJ, Mei-Dan O, Mulcahey MK. Hamstring injuries: risk factors, treatment, and rehabilitation. J Bone Joint Surg Am. 2019;101(9):843–53. https://doi.org/10.2106/jbjs.18.00261.
110. Nieves JW, Melsop K, Curtis M, Kelsey JL, Bachrach LK, Greendale G, Sowers MF, Sainani KL. Nutritional factors that influence change in bone density and stress fracture risk among young female cross-country runners. PM R. 2010;2(8):740–50; quiz 794. https://doi.org/10.1016/j.pmrj.2010.04.020.
111. Kraus E, Tenforde AS, Nattiv A, Sainani KL, Kussman A, Deakins-Roche M, Singh S, Kim BY, Barrack MT, Fredericson M. Bone stress injuries in male distance runners: higher modified Female Athlete Triad Cumulative Risk Assessment scores predict increased rates of injury. Br J Sports Med. 2019;53(4):237–42. https://doi.org/10.1136/bjsports-2018-099861.
112. Craig DI. Medial tibial stress syndrome: evidence-based prevention. J Athl Train. 2008;43(3):316–8. https://doi.org/10.4085/1062-6050-43.3.316.

Spine Injuries in Sports

12

Guilherme Henrique Ricardo da Costa,
Danilo de Souza Ferronato, Fernando Barbosa Sanchez,
Edelvan Gabana, Vinícius Sabag Machado,
Tarcísio Eloy Pessoa de Barros Filho,
Raphael Martus Marcon,
and Alexandre Fogaça Cristante

12.1 Review of the Clinical Presentation and Differential Diagnosis

Sports practice, from low-performance amateur levels to high-performance professional levels, involves risks of injuries that can be mild, such as muscle pain that can lead to few transient limitations, to severe injuries, with potential risks to the practitioner's life.

In some more popular sports, spinal injuries are less frequent than upper and lower limb injuries. In baseball, only 11.7% of the time, absences from sports at a professional level originate from spinal injuries, while injuries to the upper and lower limbs are responsible for 51.4% and 30.6% of absences [1]. In Soccer, injuries to the thoracic and lumbar spine represent rates between 9% and 14%, while cervical injuries vary from 3% to 7%, reaching 18% due to concussions [2]. They are also less frequent in basketball, despite being responsible for almost the same period of absence from competitions [3]. However, spinal injury rates are quite high in some sports, such as football, ice hockey and gymnastics [4]. Ice hockey has the highest incidence of cervical spine injuries compared to all other sports [5]; meanwhile, the lumbar spine is an uncommon site of injuries in this sport.

We can classify sports injuries to the spine as acute injuries, where there is a specific triggering event or injuries caused by overload and overuse related to repetitive microtrauma and with an insidious evolution [2]. Sports injuries to the spine have a broad spectrum of clinical presentations:

- **Coccydynia**: coccygeal pain, usually related to mechanical overload, instability or local trauma.
- **Contractures and strains**: these are the most frequent injuries. Hyperflexion and hyperextension, as well as torsional movements of the trunk, can lead to excessive loads on the muscular and ligament structures of the spine. Decreased range of motion and local pain are the main symptoms. The diagnosis is usually one of exclusion [2, 6].

G. H. R. da Costa · D. de Souza Ferronato ·
F. B. Sanchez · E. Gabana · V. S. Machado
Spinal Surgery, Institute of Orthopedics and Traumatology, Hospital das Clínicas, University of São Paulo, São Paulo, Brazil

T. E. P. de Barros Filho
Department of Orthopedics and Traumatology, Hospital das Clínicas, University of São Paulo, São Paulo, Brazil

Faculty of Medicine, University of São Paulo, São Paulo, Brazil

R. M. Marcon
Department of Orthopedics and Traumatology, Hospital das Clínicas, University of São Paulo, São Paulo, Brazil

A. F. Cristante (✉)
Faculty of Medicine, University of São Paulo, São Paulo, Brazil

S. Rocha Piedade et al. (eds.), *Sideline Management in Sports*,
https://doi.org/10.1007/978-3-031-33867-0_12

- **Disc herniation and degenerative disc disease**: may present as an axial pain, radiculopathy or myelopathy. Lumbar hernias may present intensified pain complaints in the sitting position when coughing and sneezing. Thoracic hernias have a high rate of associated neurological alterations (60% of cases present neurological deficit), despite being rare and representing 0.25–0.75% of disc hernias [7]. Caused by excessive axial and torsional loads, they are also commonly the result of repetitive trauma. Cervical hernias are prevalent in sports with repetitive head and neck trauma [8]. Frequent trauma can lead to the development of spinal stenosis and, especially if associated with a congenital narrow canal, can lead to neurological changes [9].
- **Stingers/burners**: neuropraxia of a cervical nerve root or brachial plexus, which affects the upper extremities [10]. These are reversible and transient injuries. Two trauma mechanisms have been described: brachial plexus traction and foraminal or spinal canal narrowing [11].
- **Cervical cord neuropraxia**: also known as transient quadriplegia. Caused by hyperextension, hyperflexion or axial load on the cervical spine (Fig. 12.1), characterized by pain, paresthesias and/or motor weakness in more than one extremity, with complete resolution of the condition within 2 days [12].
- **Spondylolysis/spondylolisthesis**: injury to the pars interarticularis is associated with a stress fracture from repetitive trauma in hyperextension and rotational trauma, usually affecting the L5 vertebra [13]. According to pelvic incidence (PI), two mechanisms are described: the "nutcracker" in patients with low PI, and the "shear" in patients with high PI, with this increased risk of slippage [14].
- **Fractures and dislocations**: can present as low-risk injuries, such as spinous apophyses fractures, to catastrophic injuries, usually associated with compression fractures of the subaxial cervical spine related to compression of neurological structures [15]. Several studies have shown tetraplegia as the most common degree of neurological alteration in spinal cord injuries caused by sports trauma [16] (Fact Box 12.1).

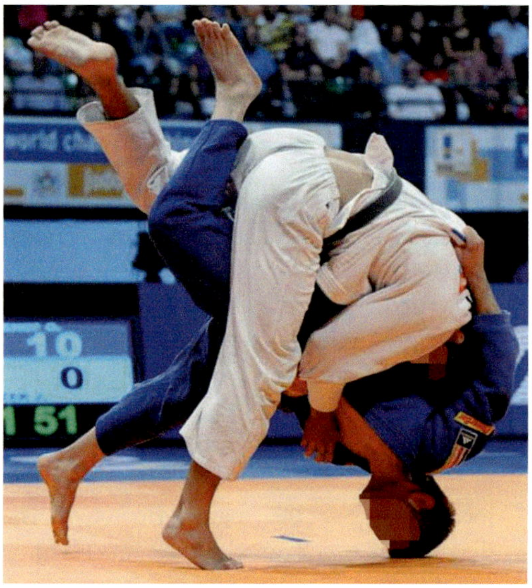

Fig. 12.1 Trauma with axial loading of the cervical spine during a judo match (personal file)

Fact Box 12.1 Sports with the Most Spinal Injuries and Major Injuries

- Ice hockey, football and gymnastics have higher incidences of spinal injuries.
- Main injury: contractures and strains. Decreased range of motion, and local pain are the main symptoms!
- Other injuries that may occur: coccydynia, herniated disc or degenerative disc disease, impingement, cervical spinal neuropraxia, spondylolysis and spondylolisthesis.

12.2 Discussion of Key Physical Examination Pearls and Findings

The assessment of the athlete victim of spinal trauma should initially follow the steps of the ATLS (advanced trauma life support) assessment. The team doctor must be on hand to immediately check for any changes and identify potential problems that need more emergent or urgent care [17].

During sports, the medical team must always be attentive to identify the trauma mechanism that led to the injury (i.e., if there was a fall or a collision with another athlete, for example). Patterns of injury types associated with particular injuries are described, although there is no absolute correlation. The movements and trauma mechanisms associated with spinal injuries are: flexion-compression, vertical or axial compression, flexion-distraction, extension-compression, extension-distraction and lateral flexion [18]. Table 12.1 shows some injuries most commonly related to specific trauma mechanisms. Seeking to standardize the interpretation of different trauma mechanisms and fracture patterns, the AO Spine (*Arbeitsgemeinschaft für Osteosynthesefragen*—Spine) developed classifications for cervical and thoracolumbar fractures. Figure 12.2 demonstrates the AO Spine classification for cervical fractures.

Table 12.1 Mechanisms of trauma and potential injuries (adapted [19])

Region	Trauma mechanism	Characteristic
Cervical	Axial load with hyperflexed neck	Acute disc herniation or spinal cord compression
	Axial load with rotation	Vertebral fractures (most common from C4 to C6)
	Hyperflexion	Atlanto-axial dislocation, odontoid or spinous process fractures
	Hyperflexion with rotation	Facet fracture-dislocation
	Hyperextension	Atlas fracture, hangman's fracture (C2) and posterior arch fractures
	Hypertension with rotation	Fracture of the unciform processes and facet joints
	Isolated axial load	Fractures of vertebral bodies
Thoracolumbar	Axial load	Compression fractures
	Direct posterior trauma	Spinous process avulsion
	Sudden force of flexion, rotation or hyperextension	Spinous process avulsion
	Direct lateral trauma or severe muscle contraction	Transverse process avulsion

Traumatic spinal injuries can often be associated with head trauma (or TBI, traumatic brain injury); thus, loss of consciousness can occur. Therefore, patient assessment is hampered by lack of cooperation. In this scenario, using a cervical collar and transporting to a medical service with a rigid board are fundamental parts of protecting the spine after trauma.

Once other changes are ruled out, the column-specific evaluation begins. The first step is inspection, which seeks to assess the presence of spinal deformities, misalignments with loss of physiological curvatures and skin lesions (such as bulges or blunt wounds). Then, palpation is performed.

Palpate all spinous processes, from the cervical region to the sacro-coccyx, and seek to identify the presence of pain. If positive, it may indicate ligament injury or vertebral fracture. The paravertebral musculature and all the musculature of the back are also palpated, as well as the clavicles, shoulders, scapulae, costal arches and pelvis. Low back pain is the most common cause of acute pain in athletes, being secondary to muscle strain or contracture (spasm) and presenting with pain on local palpation [19].

The pattern of pain provoked has substantial overlap between reference patterns of dermatomes, myotomes and sclerotomes at multiple spine levels and overlapping anatomical structures at the same spinal level, such as intervertebral discs and zygoapophyseal joints [17]. Furthermore, structures with common embryological origin tend to produce a similar pain pattern determined by the nerve that innervates the structure. The location of pain and irradiation are valuable features in identifying the affected spinal level, although it does not indicate which particular structure is the source of the symptom [17].

Afterwards, the spine movement is evaluated. As part of the core, the spine stabilizes the body,

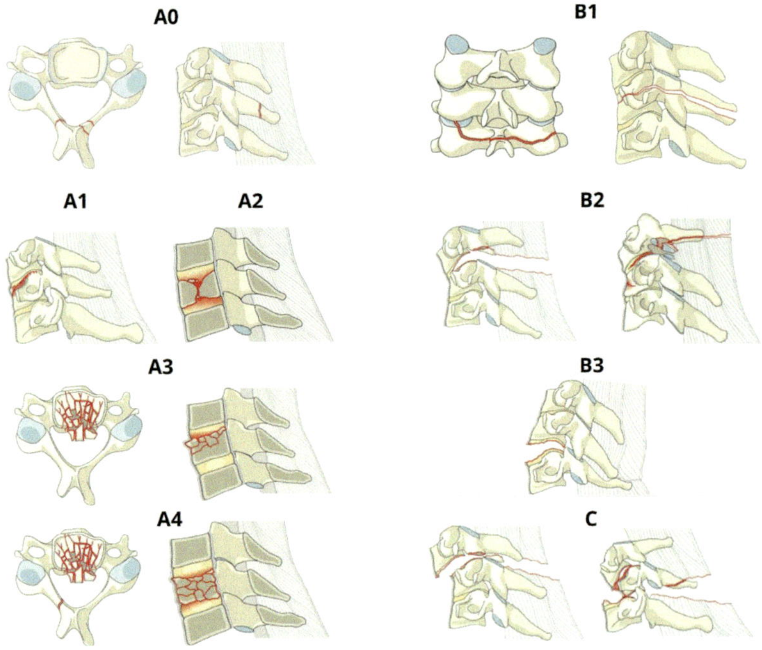

Fig. 12.2 AO Spine classification for cervical fractures. (Adapted with permission from Ref. [20])

Table 12.2 Normal range of motion of spine regions (adapted [21])

Region	Movement	Range of motion
Cervical	Flexo-extension	130°
	Side rotation	80°
	Side tilt	45° to each side
Thoracic	Flexion	45°
	Extension	45°
	Side tilt	45° to each side
Lumbar	Flexion	From 40° to 60°
	Extension	From 20° to 35°
	Side tilt	From 15° to 20°
	Rotation	From 3° to 18°

aids balance, and participates in generating force for the extremities. The range of motion should be evaluated (Table 12.2) and observed for any changes, such as the presence of pain, muscle contracture or movement blockage. How the movement is performed should also be evaluated, whether smoothly and harmoniously or if posture changes are adopted. Movement limitation does not happen specifically due to traumatic changes and may be related to muscle shortening, infection, the presence of tumors or previous degenerative processes, in addition to age.

Finally, the neurological assessment is carried out. At this stage, to guide the assessment, the ASIA (American Spinal Injury Association) score should be used [22], which replaced the Frankel scale and became the gold standard for spinal cord injury assessment [23]. The exam is based on a motor assessment based on myotomes (5 for the upper limbs—from C5 to T1 and 5 for the lower limbs—from L2 to S1), sensory assessment based on dermatomes (28 dermatomes bilaterally) and anorectal examination (voluntary contraction of the external anal sphincter and deep anal sensitivity to pressure). The exam ranks are in Table 12.3.

After this assessment of myothymes and dermatomes, the ASIA classifies spinal cord injuries as complete or incomplete (Table 12.4). In addition, it included a definition in the classification called the neurological level, which is the most caudal functional root level where there is intact sensitivity and motor strength grade 3 or higher.

Another occurrence that may be present in spinal trauma is spinal shock, which is a physiological response to trauma marked by an axonal depolarization immediately after the injury [22]. In the presence of spinal shock, the patient presents with flaccid paralysis and areflexia, notably of the bulbocavernosus reflex. The return of this reflex (which occurs on average after 24–48 h) marks the end of the period of spinal shock. The

Table 12.3 Graduation of scores in the assessment of the ASIA score (adaptation [22])

Evaluation	Score	Maximum score (normal)
Sensitivity	0—Absent 1—Impaired or altered 2—Normal	28 dermatomes × 2 points = 112 112 × 2 (bilateral assessment) = 224
Motor force	0—Absent 1—Visible contraction 2—Movement without gravity 3—Movement against gravity 4—Movement against moderate resistance 5—Normal[a]	10 myotomes × 5 points = 50 50 × 2 (bilateral assessment) = 100
Anorectal	0—Absent 1—Present	1—Normal

[a] Subdivided into completely normal or normal against sufficient resistance in the absence of identifiable inhibitory factors (such as pain or disuse)

Table 12.4 ASIA classification of spinal cord injuries (adapted [22])

Score	Classification	Sensitivity	Motor force
A	Complete	Absent	Absent
B	Incomplete	Present	Absent below the neurological level
C	Incomplete	Present	Present below neurologic level with >50% of muscles with strength grade <3
D	Incomplete	Present	Present below neurologic level with >50% of muscles with strength grade ≥3
E	Normal	Normal	Normal

evaluation to define a complete or incomplete deficit is made after this period, although it is not a definitive criterion of the final status of the neurological picture [24].

It is important to emphasize that the complete evaluation cannot be performed with the patient with altered consciousness (such as in cases of intoxication, TBI or intubation) or in the presence of some other major untreated lesion [22] (Fact Box 12.2).

Fact Box 12.2 Fun Facts About Spine Injuries in Sport

- Football athletes who are subjected to repeated impacts to the skull have an increased risk of developing chronic traumatic encephalopathy (CTE), a neurodegenerative disease associated with repeated traumatic brain injury (in recent studies, CTE alterations were evidenced in 110 of 111 (99%) Former NFL Professional Athletes (National Football League, American Football League) [25].
- Acute disc herniations may present with symptoms of pain associated with radiculopathy (in symptoms of cervicobrachialgia, brachial plexus changes should be ruled out), most often associated with distraction of the C6 root with the contralateral cervical tilt mechanism and downward axial pressure of the ipsilateral shoulder. These changes are usually self-limiting, with a more serious injury being associated with nerve avulsion secondary to vertebral fracture. Also, in more severe cases, spinal cord compression can result in tretaparesis or quadriplegia [19]. In the presence of an acute fissure of the annulus fibrosus, cervical or low back pain with or without irradiation may occur.
- Paralympic athletes with Down syndrome are at increased risk for atlanto-axial dislocation and therefore undergo radiographic screening and are denied participation in the Olympics if the atlanto-odontoid gap is less than 5 mm [19].
- Teardrop fractures are common in rugby and football players and are composed of a fracture of the vertebral body labrum in the frontal plane that protrudes from the body and a sagittal vertebral body fracture. They are considered very unstable fractures and are often associated with stenosis of the canal by

fragments of the fracture or posterior arch [19].

- There is an entity called the spear tackler's spine which is based on radiographic findings: spinal canal narrowing (vertebral canal/vertebral body ratio <0.8), sagittal alignment of the cervical spine or kyphotic and posttraumatic radiographic abnormalities. It is seen in American football athletes and is a contraindication for continued activity [19].
- In some cases, an injury without radiographic signs of abnormality, called SCIWORA (spinal cord injury without radiographic abnormalities) may occur. It is more frequent in children (19–34% of spinal cord injuries) and can have a devastating consequence if there is no rapid diagnosis [19].

12.3 Indications and Benefits of Additional Testing/Imaging (Point of Care or Referral)

All athletes who have suffered spinal trauma should have imaging tests to complement the injury investigation unless the patient is pain-free throughout the range of motion (ROM), is not painful on palpation, is alert and oriented, has injuries from distraction or drunkenness and has no neurologic deficits [26].

The initial evaluation begins with taking radiographs of the entire spine. Anteroposterior (AP) and lateral (P) images of the cervical, thoracic, lumbar and sacrococcyx spine should be performed. X-rays provide helpful information to rule out fractures or dislocations. Lateral flexion and extension radiographs can be taken to investigate images of segment instability (Fig. 12.3).

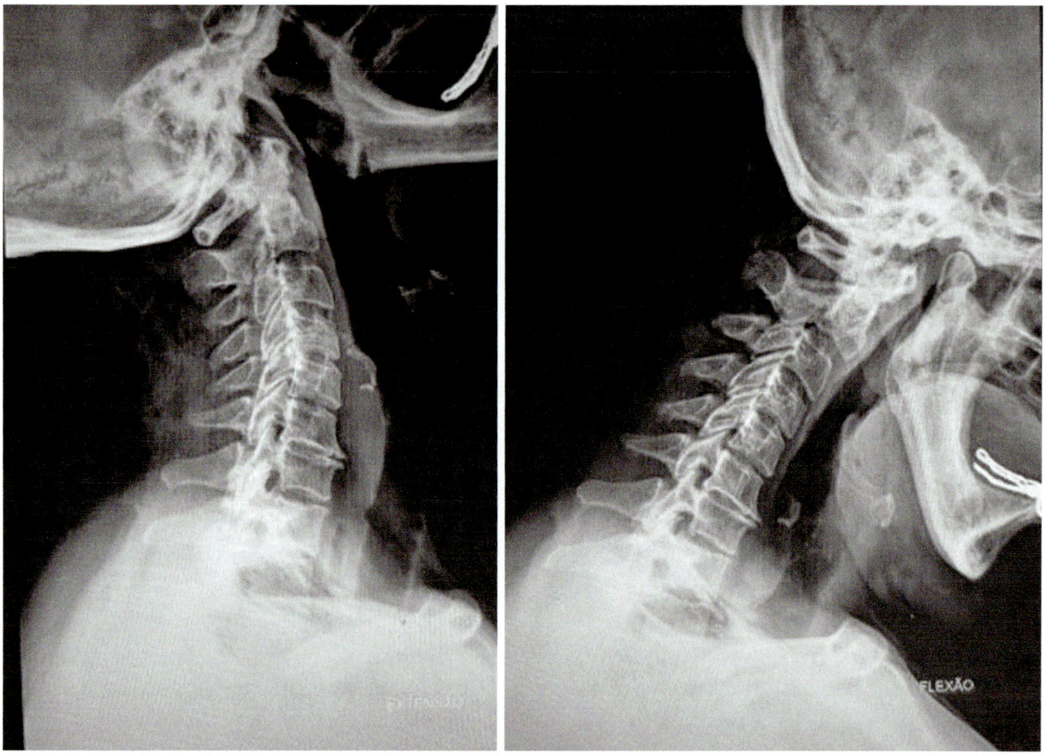

Fig. 12.3 Radiograph in extension and flexion of a former athlete with complaints of refractory neck pain (personal file)

Complementary tests should be requested according to clinical suspicion. Patients with suspected cervicothoracic lesions should undergo computed tomography due to the high rate of lesions not seen on plain radiographs. In addition, the speed and precision in visualizing the cervicothoracic region led CT to replace plain radiographs as a first-line image.

Complementary imaging tests are necessary when neurological or motor dysfunction is present on physical examination. Magnetic resonance imaging (MRI) (Fig. 12.4) allows evaluation of the spinal cord, nerve root compressions, soft tissue injuries and associated ligament injuries.

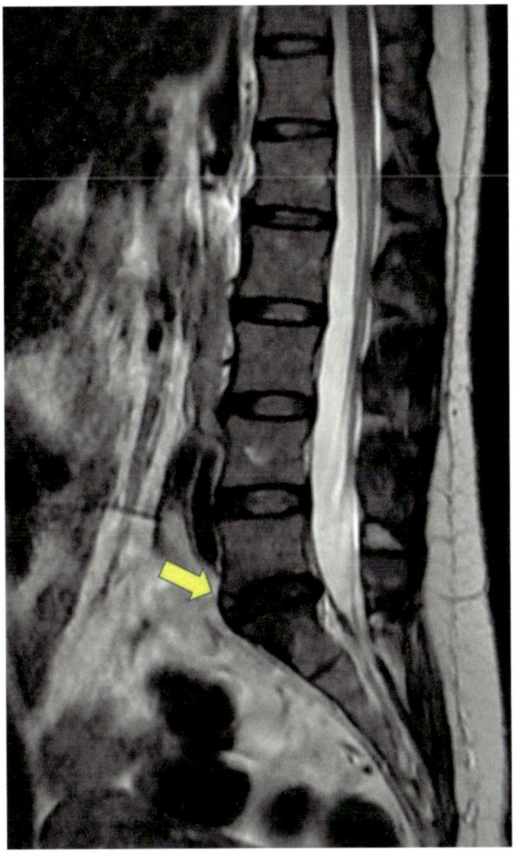

Fig. 12.4 Sagittal magnetic resonance imaging of an athlete victim of a posterior-lateral impact injury in the lumbar region. It is possible to observe a fragment in the lower part of L5's body (personal file)

12.4 Incidence/Prevalence as Well as Predisposing Risk Factors of Each Specific Diagnosis

In general, to compare the prevalence of back pain in different sports, it is essential to consider sport-specific characteristics that may influence prevalence rates. These characteristics are due to differences in training and competition content, body anthropometry and age of peak competitive performance. The most investigated potential risk factors were: load on the spine, age, sex, anthropometry and previous history of back pain [27].

Load on the spine has been investigated in different studies, especially with regard to training volume or experience, loads exerted by different types of training—such as strength training, technique or sport-specific movements [28]. For example, training volume was found to be a risk factor for back pain in speed skaters and rowers but not in Hockey or soccer players. These different results regarding risk factors indicate that sport-specific differences can lead to different loads on the spine [29].

Traumatic spinal injuries and disc abnormalities are more frequent in sports that involve loading the spine during movement (e.g., gymnastics, cricket, weightlifting, rowing) and in sports where the spine is subjected to high-impact loads with sometimes unpredictable landing forces (e.g., horseback riding, volleyball) [30]. There is also some evidence that upright activities such as running may have a protective effect on intervertebral discs or, at an elite level, are less harmful to intervertebral discs than other elite-level sports [31].

Gender and age are often discussed as confounding factors to back pain. Most studies reported higher prevalence for female than male athletes [32]. This is often justified by girls' early maturity or differences in their hormonal changes during puberty compared to boys. Furthermore, the anatomical features of the female body may reinforce the development of back pain, leading to higher prevalence rates in women than in men. In this context, several studies have discussed women's lower muscle mass and bone density, which can destabilize the body and, therefore, insufficient compensation for high loads, menstrual low back pain and pregnancy-related back pain. However, a systematic review did not confirm this hypothesis [33].

Some studies have discussed the high vulnerability of the spine in growing individuals as a risk factor for back pain in young athletes; therefore, the prevalence of back pain in adolescent athletes has been evaluated. However, these studies did not compare their results with an older population [27].

Several anthropometric parameters were examined as risk factors for back pain, including height, weight and body mass index, and results varied between studies. At a high level of competition, anthropometry often differs between different disciplines. For example, basketball players or rowers are usually taller than gymnasts. On the one hand, athletes with typical stature in their discipline (e.g., tall volleyball players) better meet the requirements to become successful (compared to small volleyball players). On the other hand, participation in different sports often leads to adaptation by different stressed body structures. For example, weightlifters' bodies differ significantly from gymnasts. Thus, it is challenging to interpret anthropometric parameters as risk factors in some disciplines. Therefore, we cannot determine whether an anthropometric parameter or sport-specific load is responsible for a back pain problem [27].

Another often-discussed confounding factor for back pain is age. In the general population, the prevalence of back pain in children and adolescents is lower than in adults, but it is increasing [34]. Studies have not found age as a risk factor for back pain [35, 36], while other researchers found [37, 38].

A Player's position is an independent risk factor and likely due to a higher risk of impact; in field soccer specifically, midfielders have higher injury rates, and goalkeepers have a higher risk of low back pain (LBP). Preseason intensity, exercise load as well as past injury history are associated with higher injury rates and more extended restrictions on play [2].

Preseason intensity, exercise load, as well as past injury history are associated with higher injury rates and more extended restrictions on play [2]

Among college and professional baseball players, low back injury rates range from 8.3% to 15% [1, 39]. The prevalence of chronic low back pain ranges from 1% to 40% of baseball players of all experience levels [40, 41].

12.4.1 Muscle Injuries

Cervical strain or sprain describes an injury to the neck's soft tissues, including muscles, tendons and ligaments. Athletes typically experience non-radiating neck pain and decreased range of motion [42].

Thoracic musculoligamentary injuries can occur with both high-energy and high-repetition mechanisms. The repetitive movements involved in rowing were associated with a 22% incidence of back injuries and 9% of rib cage injuries [42].

In field soccer, the spine is a less frequent area of injury, but it can impose severe and debilitating sequelae on athletes. In professional football, 4–6% of lumbar and thoracic injuries have been reported in European leagues [2, 43] and up to 9% in international tournaments [44]. In professional and amateur football, spinal injury rates range from 9% to 14% [2].

12.4.2 Spinal Fractures and Spinal Cord Injury

According to the National Spinal Cord Injury Statistical Center, in 2019, there were approximately 285,000 people with spinal cord injury (SCI) in the United States [45]. Since 2015, car accidents have been the most significant leading cause of injuries (39.3%), followed by falls (31.8%), violence (13.5%) and sports (8%) [45].

In a strictly pediatric population, 5–15 children are expected to experience a traumatic spinal injury experience for every 100,000 sports participants. Football and many other sports have a higher incidence of spinal injuries and can put athletes at risk, including ice hockey, cheerleading and baseball [46].

The majority of spinal cord injuries result in incomplete quadriplegia (47.6%), with complete quadriplegia being the least common (12.3%), with less than 1% of people regaining full neurological function at the time of hospital discharge [45]. A catastrophic cervical spine injury can be defined as a structural distortion of the cervical spine associated with actual or potential damage to the spinal cord [15]. Catastrophic cervical spine injuries include unstable fractures or dislocations, cervical cord neuropraxia (CCN or transient quadriplegia) and intervertebral disc herniations [15].

Additionally, catastrophic spinal cord injury is more likely to result in cervical spine injury than thoracic or low back trauma in sports such as football, ice hockey, free diving, skiing, snowboarding, cheerleading and baseball. A significant axial compressive force placed on the top of the head during neck flexion is a common mechanism of action during sports that can lead to injuries such as quadriplegia [10]. Spinal cord injuries at the thoracic level represent 35.6% of the national spinal cord injury database and evidence suggests that sport-related activities are the second most common cause of total spinal cord injuries in patients >30 years old [47].

In field football, 14 cases of spinal cord injury were found that occurred between 1976 and 2020. The average age at the time of injury was 19 years and 86% of individuals were male. Eight of the 14 subjects had vertebral fracture/dislocation, while two had a concomitant traumatic brain injury. Neurologically, 54% had quadriplegia, 39% had paraplegia, and 8% suffered from hemiplegia and sensory deficit [16].

Spinous process fractures can result from avulsion, hyperflexion or direct blow to the cervical spine [42]. Clay-shoveler fractures, caused by shear forces on the dorsal aspect of the neck, have been documented in sports such as golf, rock climbing, baseball and wrestling [47–49].

Due to the biomechanics of the thoracic spine, injuries sustained in this region, including sports-related injuries, are much less common when compared to those sustained in the cervical and lumbar regions of the spine [50, 51]. The most common injuries to the thoracic spine include musculoligament injuries, herniated discs, fractures and spinal cord injuries [52].

The National Football League reported that herniated thoracic discs account for 2% of all herniated discs. The mechanism of thoracic disc herniation has been linked to blocking, combat and other modes of player-to-player contact [53].

Chest compression fractures, caused by axial loading and flexion, occur in sports such as skiing, rugby and football [51]. Fractures such as burst, translation-rotation and flexion-distraction carry the significant potential to cause spinal cord injury and appear to be most common in the thoracolumbar region of the spine [52].

Stress reactions can occur due to overuse with repetitive mechanical stress that weakens the pars interarticularis and pedicles of the vertebrae. If left untreated, stress reactions can lead to stress fractures and Spondylolysis. There is a consensus that repetitive movements involving lumbar rotation and extension promote Spondylolysis [54–56]. Stress fractures (e.g., pars defects) occur in approximately 3.3% of high school baseball players [57].

Spondylolysis is defined by a fracture or defect of the pars interarticularis and is commonly seen in young athletes due to skeletal immaturity; with 85–95% of cases occurring at L5, followed by 5–15% of cases at L4 and manifesting through repetitive axial loading and hyperextension [50, 58, 59].

In baseball, stress fracture and Spondylolysis are present in 1/3 of athletes with low back pain; the best Diagnosis is made by scintigraphy [6]. As reported by Sakai et al. [2], much higher rates of Spondylolysis (up to 30%) were reported in young athletes and young soccer players in the Japanese pediatric and adolescent population, which was five times the national average [2].

12.4.3 Disc Degeneration and Herniated Discs

Result of compressive forces and rotational forces [6]. Among Japanese baseball players (19.8 ± 0.9 years), 59.7% of the sample had radiographic disc degeneration at one or more levels of the lumbar spine [60]. Most degenerative processes occurred at levels L4/L5 and L5/S1 (57.9% of those with degeneration). The incidence of degeneration in baseball was highest among the sports studied, including swimming, basketball, taekwondo, Soccer and running [60].

The most common herniated cervical disc mechanism seen in National Football League (NFL) athletes is tackle (31%), followed by blocking (25%) [42]. Of NFL athletes, 46% with cervical herniated discs treated without surgery returned to play, while 72% of surgically treated patients returned to play [61]. In addition to a higher rate of return to play than nonsurgical management, these athletes played more games after treatment and had longer careers [61].

According to individual studies, NFL, National Basketball Association (NBA), and Major League Baseball (MLB) athletes have shown lumbar disc herniation and low back strain to be a common injury; with 28% of all spinal injuries in the NFL being herniated discs [42]. Facet pain is typically related to rotation and extension of the spine [6].

Stenosis presents with slowly progressive pain with or without radicular symptoms. Athletes with congenital stenosis may be at increased risk [6].

The literature consensus states that for an athlete to return to play safely, they must not be actively suffering from pain, must have a range of motion and complete return their strength in the absence of neurological deficit [42].

12.5 Sideline Management Guidelines and Suggestions of the Specific Traumatic Injuries and Clinical Issues in Athletes

The successful management of the injured athlete, especially the athlete with a spinal injury, depends on some critical items. Stopping the game immediately to initiate medical care after a suspected spinal injury, similar to the way it is done for suspected brain injury on the field, can help with early recognition and reduction of further damage to the spine/spinal cord.

The organization of the athlete support team must start before the matches. The equipment necessary for handling the injured athlete on the field must be properly organized. A hospital and transport system must be in place if immediate intervention is required.

The first steps in assessing the condition of an injured player, as in all sports, remain the same. The primary goal in early management is to address any life-threatening needs and prevent further injury. It must be done using the Trauma ABCDE approach (ATLS). Checking the patient's airway, breathing, circulation, neurological deficit and exposure is critical regardless of the setting [62]. Pupil examination should also be performed, and notes of size, symmetry and reactivity should be made [63].

In the absence of immediate danger, an athlete with a spinal injury must remain in place until the spine is fully immobilized. During field assessment, all efforts should be based on stabilizing the patient and allowing transport to the hospital. A spinal injury should be assumed to be present until it is ruled out.

The first step in preparing a player for transport is placing him on a rigid board. As a result of trauma from behind, some players are often found in the prone position on the field. It requires a block rolling procedure to place them on the rigid board to avoid unnecessary movements and prevent further damage. The neck is immobilized by placing one hand on each side of the player's head to stabilize the spine.

The main debate is about removing or not safety equipment, with greater emphasis on the helmet. Depending on how tight the helmet is, it may be possible to remove it to complete the neurological assessment or to gain access to the airway. Removing the helmet could increase the angular displacement of the cervical vertebrae and cause a cervical fracture or dislocation [64]. The helmet and shoulder pads should only be removed when the patient is in a controlled environment and the hands of persons trained in such procedures.

A medical specialist should evaluate all athletes with trauma and possible spinal injuries. Correct diagnosis followed by proper treatment is the key to an early return to sport. Spinal injuries, if left untreated, can persist and lead to significant morbidity or loss of participation in future competitions.

The main sport-related spinal injury is muscle strain [10]. Muscle injuries can be carefully treated with nonoperative treatment with physiotherapy, seeking to work the central muscles and painless range of motion associated with symptoms (analgesics, anti-inflammatory drugs, muscle relaxants). Due to the great demand for recovery and athletes, treatment involves more rigorous measures than those used for the general population. Rehabilitation programs are carried out with greater frequency and duration, aiming at the earliest possible clinical success.

Return-to-game decisions can be challenging and high-pressure events. Athletes want to play again, and coaches want their stars back in the game. Returning to the sport generally involves the need for a full, painless range of motion and the absence of neurological deficits. Spine fractures and dislocations prevent a return to play until the spine is stable, the pain has disappeared, and signs of fracture healing are observed.

12.6 Suggested Prevention Measures that Can be Implemented for Early Recognition of Risk Reduction (Attitude, Rule Modification, Referee Instruction)

The prevention of spinal injuries should be a fundamental part of the daily life of athletes. These measures can be divided into general, applicable to different sports, or specific for each sport. The general measures to prevent vertebral injuries, we have:

Muscle strengthening of the CORE and posterior cervical paravertebral musculature. Strengthening and stabilizing the trunk allows greater lumbar and pelvic control, reducing the risk of injury in this region. For specific strengthening of the CORE, the main muscles to be worked are the deep ones of the abdomen: transversus abdominis, internal oblique and multifidus. Strengthening the muscles of the posterior cervical region also contributes decisively to reducing injuries, especially in contact sports. This reduction was observed in several sports, such as baseball, Hockey, basketball and Soccer [2, 6, 13, 65–67].

Some sports federations have invested in research and development of physical preparation techniques that improve performance and prevent injuries. A well-known protocol is FIFA 11+, developed by FIFA (Fédération Internationale de Football Association) after creating the Medical and Research Center (F-MARC) in 1994. This program is divided into three main modules: running and active stretching; strengthening the CORE and legs; cutting and stopping from high speed. When applied to basketball players, the techniques guided in this program also resulted in a reduction in injuries [43, 68].

The development and application of rules for the athlete's safety are essential to avoid spinal injuries, especially in sports with more significant physical contact. Despite the general concepts of protection, the specificities of each modality in its practice lead to the need to develop specific rules. In the case of Hockey, for example, the prohibition of "pushing from behind" (checking from behind) led to a significant reduction in spinal injuries [69].

In the case of Soccer, in addition to the rules already established during the games, care is also oriented when commemorating a goal [16].

In American football, the ban on using the head as a point of support or initial contact in 1976 also significantly reduced the rates of spinal injuries in this sport. Therefore, developing and enforcing rules is critical to ensuring athlete safety.

Rest and recovery time after physical activity. Some studies show that at least one day of muscle rest per week is essential for rehabilitation and injury prevention [70].

For children, attention should be even greater regarding rest time and the number of times they are exposed to physical activities, avoiding excessive wear and the risk of injury. DiFiori et al. [71] proposed a guide to guide children's exposure to basketball; this guide (adapted) is represented in Table 12.5 below:

Prevention measures can also be explicitly adopted for each sport, considering the particularities of movements or positions that are more frequent in each modality. These measures become more important in sports with a higher risk of physical contact between players:

Hockey: mandatory use of a helmet and a face mask that covers the entire face of the player, protecting the largest possible area of contact [69].

American Football: equipment that limits the hyperextension of the neck is indicated for cervical protection. Among the equipment developed explicitly for this purpose, we can mention: Cowboy Collar, Kerr Collar and Bullock Roll, shown in Fig. 12.5 below, adapted from Rowson et al. [72]:

Table 12.5 Guide to guide children's exposure to basketball

Age	Game duration (min)	Number of games per week	Practice duration (min)	Number of workouts per week
7–8	20–28	1	30–60	1
9–11	24–32	1–2	45–75	2
12–14	28–32	2	60–90	2–4
9–12	32–40	2–3	90–120	3–4

Biomechanical analysis has shown that the Kerr Collar has increased protection from impacts to the top and front of the helmet. None of the three above side impacts were superior, except that Kerr Collar reduced the force transmitted to the lower neck [72].

Therefore, considering the importance and potential severity of spinal injuries in sports activities, it is imperative to invest in techniques that increase the prevention and early rehabilitation of these injuries.

Take Home Messages

- Spinal injuries in athletes are frequent; the doctor must be aware of the possibility of their occurrence according to the particularity of the sport in question.
- Evaluation of the patient with a suspected spinal injury must be complete, starting with a detailed physical examination, neurological evaluation and use of complementary imaging methods when necessary.
- Risk factors for injuries, such as gender, age, anthropometric parameters and training volume, may not be so clear.
- A significant axial compressive force placed on the top of the head during neck flexion is a common mechanism of action during sports that can lead to injuries such as quadriplegia. Planning care for athletes with spinal injuries

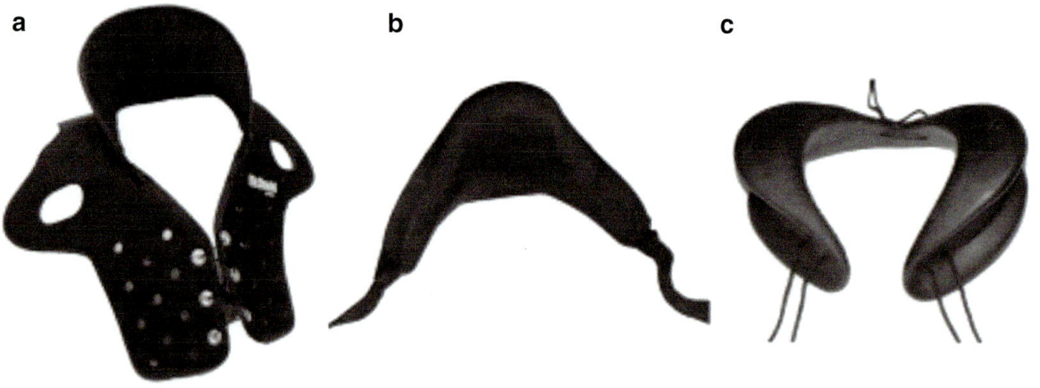

Fig. 12.5 (**a**) Cowboy Collar; (**b**) Bullock Necklace; (**c**) Kerr Collar

must be carried out early, from the preparation of equipment necessary for initial care to a support network with hospitals and rehabilitation clinics.

References

1. Posner M, et al. Epidemiology of major league baseball injuries. Am J Sports Med. 2011;39(8):1675–91.
2. Plais N, et al. Spine injuries in Soccer. Curr Sports Med Rep. 2019;18(10):367–73.
3. Drakos MC, et al. Injury in the National Basketball Association: a 17-year overview. Sports Health. 2010;2(4):284–90.
4. Kim DH, Vaccaro AR, Berta SC. Acute sports-related spinal cord injury: contemporary management principles. Clin Sports Med. 2003;22(3):501–12.
5. Vartiainen M, et al. King–Devick test normative reference values for professional male ice hockey players. Scand J Med Sci Sports. 2015;25(3):e327–30.
6. Camp CL, et al. Epidemiology, treatment, and prevention of lumbar spine injuries in Major League Baseball players. Am J Orthop (Belle Mead NJ). 2016;45:137–43.
7. Court C, et al. Thoracic disc herniation: surgical treatment. Orthop Traumatol Surg Res. 2018;104(1):S31–40.
8. Sortland O, Tysvaer A, Storli OV. Changes in the cervical spine in association football players. Br J Sports Med. 1982;16(2):80–4.
9. Saal JA. Common American football injuries. Sports Med. 1991;12(2):132–47.
10. Boden BP, Jarvis CG. Spinal injuries in sports. Phys Med Rehabil Clin N Am. 2009;20(1):55–68.
11. Zaremski JL, Horodyski M, Herman DC. Recurrent stingers in an adolescent American football player: dilemmas of return to play. A case report and review of the literature. Res Sports Med. 2017;25(3):384–90.
12. Rihn JA, et al. Cervical spine injuries in American football. Sports Med. 2009;39(9):697–708.
13. Yokoe T, et al. Comparison of symptomatic spondylolysis in young Soccer and baseball players. J Orthop Surg Res. 2020;15(1):1–6.
14. Roussouly P, et al. Sagittal alignment of the spine and pelvis in the presence of L5–S1 isthmic lysis and low-grade spondylolisthesis. Spine (Phila Pa 1976). 2006;31(21):2484–90.
15. Banerjee R, Palumbo MA, Fadale PD. Catastrophic cervical spine injuries in the collision sport athlete, part 1: epidemiology, functional anatomy, and diagnosis. Am J Sports Med. 2004;32(4):1077–87.
16. Poudel MK, Sherman AL. Football (Soccer)-related spinal cord injury—reported cases from 1976 to 2020. Spinal Cord Ser Cases. 2020;6(1):1–6.
17. Garfin SR, et al. Rothman-Simeone the spine e-book. Elsevier Health Sciences; 2017.
18. Allen B Jr, et al. A mechanistic classification of closed, indirect fractures and dislocations of the lower cervical spine. Spine (Phila Pa 1976). 1982;7(1):1–27.
19. Barile A, et al. Spinal injury in sport. Eur J Radiol. 2007;62(1):68–78.
20. Vaccaro AR, Koerner JD, Radcliff KE, et al. AOSpine subaxial cervical spine injury classification system. Eur Spine J. 2016;25:2173–84. https://doi.org/10.1007/s00586-015-3831-3.
21. Barros Filho EP, Tarcísio OL, Cristante AF. Exame físico em ortopedia. São Paulo: Sarvier; 2017.
22. Roberts TT, Leonard GR, Cepela DJ. Classifications in brief: American Spinal Injury Association (ASIA) impairment scale. Springer; 2017.
23. van Middendorp JJ, et al. Diagnosis and prognosis of traumatic spinal cord injury. Glob Spine J. 2011;1(1):1–7.
24. Pudles E, Defino HL. A coluna vertebral: conceitos básicos. Artmed Editora; 2014.
25. Simoni CR, et al. Encefalopatia traumática crônica: um impacto do futebol americano. Brazil J Health Rev. 2021;4(3):10818–26.
26. Michaleff ZA, et al. Accuracy of the Canadian C-spine rule and NEXUS to screen for clinically important cervical spine injury in patients following blunt trauma: a systematic review. CMAJ. 2012;184(16):E867–76.
27. Trompeter K, Fett D, Platen P. Prevalence of back pain in sports: a systematic review of the literature. Sports Med. 2017;47(6):1183–207.
28. van Hilst J, et al. Low back pain in young elite field hockey players, football players and speed skaters: prevalence and risk factors. J Back Musculoskelet Rehabil. 2015;28(1):67–73.
29. Eriksson K, et al. Low back pain in elite cross-country skiers: a retrospective epidemiological study. Scand J Med Sci Sports. 1996;6(1):31–5.
30. Belavý DL, et al. Can exercise positively influence the intervertebral disc? Sports Med. 2016;46(4):473–85.
31. Baranto A, et al. Back pain and MRI changes in the thoraco-lumbar spine of top athletes in four different sports: a 15-year follow-up study. Knee Surg Sports Traumatol Arthrosc. 2009;17(9):1125–34.
32. Sato T, et al. Low back pain in childhood and adolescence: assessment of sports activities. Eur Spine J. 2011;20(1):94–9.
33. Noll M, et al. Back pain prevalence and its associated factors in Brazilian athletes from public high schools: a cross-sectional study. PLoS One. 2016;11(3):e0150542.
34. Balague F, Troussier B, Salminen JJ. Non-specific low back pain in children and adolescents: risk factors. Eur Spine J. 1999;8(6):429–38.

35. Maselli F, et al. Low back pain among Italian rowers: a cross-sectional survey. J Back Musculoskelet Rehabil. 2015;28(2):365–76.
36. Ng L, et al. Self-reported prevalence, pain intensity and risk factors of low back pain in adolescent rowers. J Sci Med Sport. 2014;17(3):266–70.
37. Newlands C, Reid D, Parmar P. The prevalence, incidence and severity of low back pain among international-level rowers. Br J Sports Med. 2015;49(14):951–6.
38. Bahr R, et al. Low back pain among endurance athletes with and without specific back loading—a cross-sectional survey of cross-country skiers, rowers, orienteerers, and nonathletic controls. Spine (Phila Pa 1976). 2004;29(4):449–54.
39. Dick R, et al. Descriptive epidemiology of collegiate men's baseball injuries: National Collegiate Athletic Association Injury Surveillance System, 1988–1989 through 2003–2004. J Athl Train. 2007;42(2):183.
40. Bono CM. Low-back pain in athletes. J Bone Joint Surg Am. 2004;86(2):382–96.
41. d'Hemecourt PA, Gerbino PG II, Micheli LJ. Back injuries in the young athlete. Clin Sports Med. 2000;19(4):663–79.
42. Fiani B, et al. Prevalence of sports-related spinal injury stratified by competition level and return to play guidelines. Rev Neurosci. 2021;32(2):169–79.
43. Al Attar WSA, Alshehri MA. A meta-analysis of meta-analyses of the effectiveness of FIFA injury prevention programs in Soccer. Scand J Med Sci Sports. 2019;29(12):1846–55.
44. Kartal A, et al. Soccer causes degenerative changes in the cervical spine. Eur Spine J. 2004;13(1):76–82.
45. NSCISC. Spinal cord injury facts and figures at a glance. 2019 SCI data sheet. Birmingham, AL: University of Alabama at Birmingham; 2020.
46. Puvanesarajah V, et al. Traumatic sports-related cervical spine injuries. Clin Spine Surg. 2017;30(2):50–6.
47. Cantu RC, et al. Return to play after cervical spine injury in sports. Curr Sports Med Rep. 2013;12(1):14–7.
48. Kang D-H, Lee S-H. Multiple spinous process fractures of the thoracic vertebrae (Clay-Shoveler's Fracture) in a beginning Golfer: a case report. Spine (Phila Pa 1976). 2009;34(15):E534–7.
49. Yamaguchi JT, Hsu WK. Intervertebral disc herniation in elite athletes. Int Orthop. 2019;43(4):833–40.
50. Huang P, et al. Return-to-play recommendations after cervical, thoracic, and lumbar spine injuries: a comprehensive review. Sports Health. 2016;8(1):19–25.
51. Albers C, Benneker LM. Sports injuries of the thoracic and lumbar spine. 2019.
52. Menzer H, Gill GK, Paterson A. Thoracic spine sports-related injuries. Curr Sports Med Rep. 2015;14(1):34–40.
53. Gray BL, et al. Disc herniations in the national football league. Spine (Phila Pa 1976). 2013;38(22):1934–8.
54. Laudner K, et al. Thoracolumbar range of motion in baseball pitchers and position players. Int J Sports Phys Ther. 2013;8(6):777.
55. Chosa E, Totoribe K, Tajima N. A biomechanical study of lumbar Spondylolysis based on a three-dimensional finite element method. J Orthop Res. 2004;22(1):158–63.
56. Sairyo K, et al. Three successive stress fractures at the same vertebral level in an adolescent baseball player. Am J Sports Med. 2003;31(4):606–10.
57. Changstrom BG, et al. Epidemiology of stress fracture injuries among US high school athletes, 2005–2006 through 2012–2013. Am J Sports Med. 2015;43(1):26–33.
58. Burnett MG, Sonntag VKH. Return to contact sports after spinal surgery. Neurosurg Focus. 2006;21(4):1–3.
59. Dunn IF, Proctor MR, Day AL. Lumbar spine injuries in athletes. Neurosurg Focus. 2006;21(4):1–5.
60. Hangai M, et al. Lumbar intervertebral disk degeneration in athletes. An J Sports Med. 2009;37(1):149–55.
61. Hsu WK. Outcomes following nonoperative and operative treatment for cervical disc herniations in National Football League athletes. Spine (Phila Pa 1976). 2011;36(10):800–5.
62. Banerjee R, Palumbo MA, Fadale PD. Catastrophic cervical spine injuries in the collision sport athlete, part 2: principles of emergency care. Am J Sports Med. 2004;32(7):1760–4.
63. Daly PJ, Sim FH, Simonet WT. Ice hockey injuries. Sports Med. 1990;10(2):122–31.
64. Prinsen R, Syrotuik DG, Reid DC. Position of the cervical vertebrae during helmet removal and cervical collar application in football and hockey. Clin J Sport Med. 1995;5(3):155–61.
65. Goetzinger S, et al. Spondylolysis in young athletes: an overview emphasizing nonoperative management. J Sports Med (Hindawi Publ Corp). 2020; https://doi.org/10.1155/2020/9235958.
66. Tator CH, et al. Spinal injuries in Canadian ice hockey: documentation of injuries sustained from 1943–1999. Can J Neurol Sci. 2004;31(4):460–6.
67. Arora C, et al. Biomechanics of core musculature on upper extremity performance in basketball players. J Bodyw Mov Ther. 2021;27:127–33.
68. Longo UG, et al. The FIFA 11+ program is effective in preventing injuries in elite male basketball players: a cluster randomized controlled trial. Am J Sports Med. 2012;40(5):996–1005.
69. Benson BW, Meeuwisse WH. Ice hockey injuries. Med Sport Sci. 2005;49:86–119.
70. DiFiori JP, et al. Overuse injuries and burnout in youth sports: a position statement from the American Medical Society for Sports Medicine. Br J Sports Med. 2014;48(4):287–8.
71. DiFiori JP, et al. The NBA and youth basketball: recommendations for promoting a healthy and positive experience. Sports Med. 2018;48(9):2053–65.
72. Rowson S, et al. Biomechanical analysis of football neck collars. Clin J Sport Med. 2008;18(4):316–21.

13 Concussion

Lisa M. Manderino, Jonathan Preszler, and Michael W. Collins

13.1 Introduction

Concussions in athletes are common, though there are numerous factors that complicate its identification during sport participation. Evidence suggests that sport-related concussion is likely to go underreported, due to a combination of lack of knowledge (i.e., of both risks and identifying signs) and reluctance to miss playing time [1, 2]. In the United States, as few as one out of every nine concussions may be reported, though rates of concussion have increased over the past two decades due to increased recognition of the importance of reporting [3, 4]. It is estimated that between 1.1 and 1.9 million pediatric (i.e., in athletes under the age of 18) SRCs occur annually in the US [5], with as many as 1.2 million going unreported [5].When considering all age groups and severities, estimates suggest as many as 3.8 million sports- and recreation-related TBIs occur each year [6]. As many as half of these injuries are never seen in health care settings [6]. While huge strides have been made in recent decades, there remains much room for improvement in our understanding of concussion and our ability to adequately assess this injury on the sideline.

13.2 Overview of Sports-Related Concussion

13.2.1 Diagnostic Criteria

There is no single consensus definition or set of diagnostic criteria for concussion. Numerous research groups have set forth their own clinical definitions and diagnostic guidelines, with some commonalities. Broadly, the effects of concussion are considered to be limited to transient signs and symptoms, without observable structural changes on neuroimaging. Sports-related concussion (SRC), then, refers to concussions that occur in an athletic context. There are unique considerations for the assessment and management of concussion in a sports setting that warrant research and clinical attention. These factors will be discussed herein.

A 2017 systematic review identified 14 manuscripts presenting consensus definitions of concussion from six different organizations [7]. These definitions agree that a concussion presents with impairments of neural functioning as

L. M. Manderino
Concussion & Sports Medicine Institute, Aptiva Health, Louisville, KY, USA
e-mail: lmanderino@aptivahealth.com

J. Preszler
Department of Neuropsychology, Sanford Health, Bismarck, ND, USA
e-mail: Jonathan.Preszler@sanfordhealth.org

M. W. Collins (✉)
Department of Orthopaedic Surgery, UPMC Sports Medicine Concussion Program, University of Pittsburgh Medical Center, Pittsburgh, PA, USA
e-mail: collinsmw@upmc.edu

S. Rocha Piedade et al. (eds.), *Sideline Management in Sports*,
https://doi.org/10.1007/978-3-031-33867-0_13

the result of traumatic, biomechanical forces [8–13]. They also all assert that loss of consciousness may or may not be present at the time of injury. Most of the definitions [8, 11–13] elaborate that impaired neural functioning is identified by the onset of physical symptoms, cognitive and emotional changes, and altered sleep, though two of the definitions [9, 10] do not specify the clinically observable results of this altered neural functioning. Many, but not all, of these definitions note that such impairments are "transient," or "short-lived," though they do not define these terms. Similarly, three of the definitions [8, 9, 12] specify that onset of symptoms must be "rapid," or "immediate," but only one specifies this as meaning "within minutes [11]." Finally, two of the definitions [8, 12] indicate concussion does not present with abnormalities on standard structural neuroimaging techniques (and positive neuroimaging findings would indicate diagnosis of a higher severity TBI).

13.2.2 Pathophysiology

The difficulty in developing a consensus definition for concussion is related to the elusive nature of studying its pathophysiology. Only in the last decade have we begun to understand the neuropathological underpinnings of the clinical presentation. Rather than focal contusion or penetrating injury associated with more severe TBI, the cause of dysfunction in concussion is a nonlinear combination of more diffuse, cellular changes. Initially upon a bump, blow, or jolt to the head, axonal stretching results in ionic flux and depolarization of the neuronal membrane, which causes subsequent depolarization of synapsed neurons, creating a "spreading depression" as downstream neurons are depolarized and unable to fire [14, 15]. In order to restore membrane polarization, glucose metabolism is increased, and intracellular energy stores are quickly depleted [15]. Simultaneous reductions in cerebral blood flow mean that the rate of glucose transport cannot meet the increased energy demands [15]. This paradox is known as "metabolic uncoupling," and is theorized to put an individual at increased vulnerability to second injury during the acute post-injury phase. Animal models have found that impairments in glucose metabolism and associated risk for subsequent concussion can last up to 10 days post-injury [14], though this is suspected to vary between concussive injuries and individuals.

In combination, these metabolic disruptions result in impaired neurotransmission and reduced cellular connectivity in downstream neural systems, producing meaningful functional consequences. For example, both autonomic nervous system dysregulation (including disruptions to the cardiovascular system) [16, 17] and endocrine signaling abnormalities (e.g., within the hypothalamic-pituitary axis) [18, 19] have been observed. In the absence of repetitive injuries to the head during the period of neurometabolic vulnerability, these downstream effects are suspected to be transient and are unlikely to result in cell death or chronic alterations to functioning [14, 20]. Currently, the relationships among clinical signs/symptoms and neurometabolic changes are largely theoretical and remain to be studied empirically.

13.2.3 Epidemiology

As we are yet unable to reliably measure the neurobiological underpinnings of concussive injury in vivo, concussion remains a clinical diagnosis. Study of the epidemiology of SRC is complicated by the multiple definitions and methodology throughout the literature. In athletics, contact sports pose the highest risk for SRC. Boys' American football, rugby, ice hockey, and lacrosse are consistently among the highest risk sports for SRC per athlete exposure, which adjusts for the differing numbers of participants across sports [1, 3, 21]. Figures 13.1 and 13.2 show the high-speed running sports dynamic of American football and rugby: full contact and tackles, respectively.

However, even sports not traditionally considered to be high contact, such as volleyball, gym-

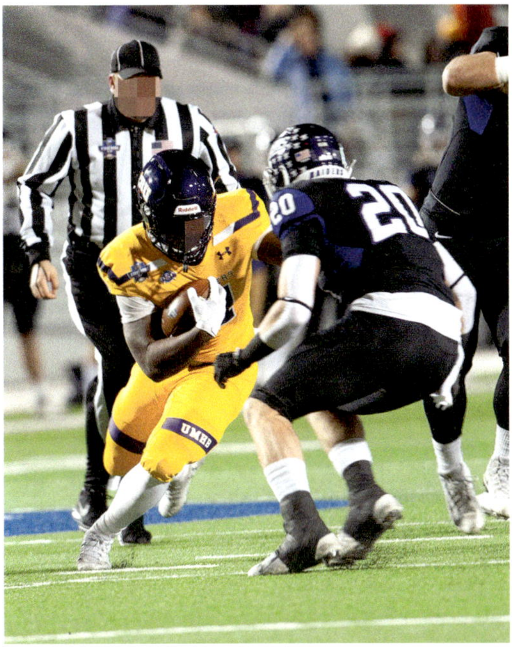

Fig. 13.1 Full contact and tackle in American Football

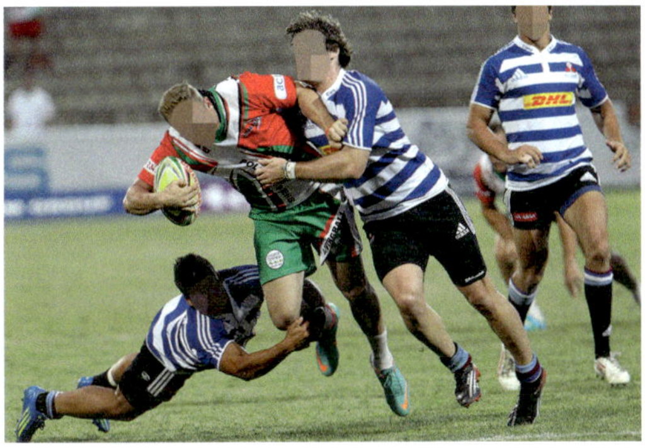

Fig. 13.2 Full contact and tackle in rugby

nastics, and track and field, carry some degree of risk of SRC [1]. Studies also consistently identify greater risk for SRC during game/competition compared to practice participation across sports [1, 21, 22].

Findings regarding age and risk for SRC have been mixed. While some studies find younger athletes may be at greater risk for SRC, other studies find the opposite result [23]. Differences in definition of SRC, research methodology, reporting practices, and medical care-seeking behaviors among youth athletes and their parents are likely accountable for the difficulty in identifying consistent trends in SRC incidence. Data also suggests that female athletes may be at increased risk for sustaining SRC compared to same-sport male counterparts—in one epidemiological study, female high school soccer players experienced 33.0 SRCs per 100,000 athlete exposures (AEs), while male high school soccer players only experienced 19.2 per 100,000 AEs [1]. This trend has been replicated in several other studies of high school and collegiate soccer, as well as basketball [21]. Hypothesized mechanisms for the sex difference include biological differences such as biomechanics, neuroanatomy, and hormone involvement [21, 22]. Others hypothesize that differences in injury rates may be attributable differences in reporting behaviors between men's and women's sports [21, 22]. In combination, these epidemiological findings underscore the risk of SRC to all who engage in sport or recreational activities, as well as the importance of education and access to sideline assessment at all levels of participation.

13.3 Goals of Sideline Assessment

13.3.1 Identification of Suspected SRC

As previously discussed, there has long been concern for underreporting of SRC. Until recently, many athletes and key stakeholders in athletics, such as parents and coaches, were underinformed about SRC. Cultural attitudes towards "toughness," lack of awareness, and reluctance to miss playing time all been cited as reasons that even professional athletes have intentionally hidden SRC symptoms. However, emerging evidence on the pathophysiology of SRC suggests that there is a period of neurologic vulnerability to reinjury after an initial SRC [14, 20]. Given the known risk of athletes underreporting symptoms of SRC, it is important that a thorough and objective sideline assessment be conducted to identify athletes who may be at risk for further injury and poor clinical outcomes. Further, more serious injuries, such as moderate or severe traumatic brain injury, may present similarly to SRC in the acute period (i.e., headache, loss of consciousness).

In this context, the primary goal of sideline assessment is to identify that SRC has occurred. However, as discussed above, the lack of a consensus definition for SRC complicates this pursuit. Generally, assessment focuses on acute symptoms and signs after a traumatic force to the head or body that result in significant jarring of the head and neck. Some acute signs may be observable to on-field healthcare professionals, coaches, or parents. These may include loss of consciousness, confusion (e.g., asking questions repeatedly), disorientation (e.g., unaware of location or identity), clumsiness or balance difficulties, vomiting, and exhibiting a vacant look [12, 24, 25]. Other symptoms may be more subtle, or only noticeable to the athlete. Such physical symptoms include headache, dizziness, nausea, and vision changes (i.e., blurred or double vision). Cognitive symptoms may include feeling mentally slowed down; athletes may express this as feeling "foggy" or "cloudy," or they may feel that they are having difficulty keeping up with gameplay or conversations among teammates. Increased emotionality or emotional lability, and symptoms of fatigue or drowsiness, may also occur. Notably, many of these symptoms are quite abstract. Younger athletes or those with developmental or learning disabilities may have difficulty conceptualizing or verbalizing that they feel "mentally slowed down" or more emotional than usual. Different language or several attempts may be required to assess such symptoms, and in these instances increased weight may be given to collateral report of observable changes from the athlete's typical baseline functioning.

13.3.2 Emergency Referral

It is also important to rule out more serious injuries of the head or cervical spine. A discussion of emergency management assessment and protocol is beyond the scope of this chapter on SRC, though it should be noted that positive findings on such an assessment would take medical priority over a concussion. A qualified medical professional should evaluate the airway, breathing, and circulation of an injured athlete on site [26, 27]. A player should be evaluated for cervical spine injury, including palpation of the cervical spine and assessment of movement and sensation in extremities. Numbness or tingling in the extremities, or midline neck pain or tenderness would be cause for concern for a cervical spine injury [13, 27, 28]. Other signs of a potentially more serious neurological injury are often referred to as "red flag" symptoms. These include loss of consciousness, seizures, worsening mental status, combativeness, and persistent vomiting [27, 28]. While many athletes experience headache acutely after SRC, a headache that is described as severe or as the "worst of the athlete's life," or that continues to worsen after removal from play, would also indicate emergent medical evaluation [27, 28].

13.3.3 Removal from Play

After ruling out more serious injuries, the most important decision point in a sideline assessment for SRC is whether an athlete may be permitted to continue playing. In the short term, continuing to play after sustaining SRC has been linked with adverse outcomes. The direst of these potential outcomes is known as "second impact syndrome," a controversial and poorly studied term referring to catastrophic neurological outcomes (i.e., cerebral edema or subdural hematoma) following a second injury to the head prior to full resolution of an initial SRC. Estimates of the incidence of second impact syndrome vary widely, with the extant literature being plagued by definitional and methodological flaws [29, 30]. Documented cases using strict definitions of second impact syndrome are rare, and appear to be most prevalent in males under 20 years old who play high contact sports (e.g., American football).

Nevertheless, there are well-documented sequelae associated with continued sport participation after SRC aside from second impact syndrome. Most notably, continuing to play after SRC has been linked to higher symptom burden and longer recoveries. Failure to immediately remove an injured athlete from play has been associated with longer days to symptom resolution and return to sport participation, worse neurocognitive test scores post-injury, and greater number and severity ratings of concussion symptoms [31, 32]. One study showed that athletes who were not removed from play immediately were 8.8 times more likely to have protracted recovery [31]. These findings suggest an effective sideline assessment is the best way both keep athletes safe from further injury and improve their recovery trajectories.

13.3.4 Facilitation of Appropriate Treatment Referrals

Significant advancements have been made in the last decade in our understanding of post-acute management of concussion, and many of the long-held recommendations for management have not held up to empirical evaluation [25, 33, 34]. For many years, prescribed cognitive and physical rest (including limited if any participation in academic and athletic activities) were recommended to athletes after SRC. This was presumed to mitigate symptoms and discomfort in the post-acute period, as well as encourage neurobiological resolution of the injury [26]. However, recent evidence suggests that rest does not appear to facilitate recovery, and moreover early return to activities may promote recovery in several ways [25, 33, 34].

Rather, concussion management is leaving a "one size fits all" approach, and research is being done to develop individualized treatment recommendations given an athlete's unique presentation. While it has long been known that SRC presents heterogeneously, only more recently have symptoms been organized into subtypes or profiles [35–37]. Ongoing research seeks to clarify the specific profiles, though existing models include profiles of vestibular, ocular motor, cognitive, migraine, and mood-related symptoms, and some provide for co-occurring modifying factors such as cervical injury and sleep disturbance [35–37]. Early evidence suggests that treatment recommendations can be matched to a specific profile to facilitate recovery. Several important questions remain in the clinical profile literature. Most relevant to the present chapter, it is not yet known at what point post-injury profiles emerge. Sideline assessment will likely continue to play an important role in this evolving body of research; on-field symptoms may ultimately prove helpful in the identification of clinical profiles, and early identification may expedite referrals for appropriate treatment.

In the interim, sideline medical professionals still play an important role in early identification of need for follow-up outpatient evaluation. Athletes who receive earlier referrals to specialty concussion care show more positive recovery trajectories [38, 39]. One study found that athletes who were seen in a specialty concussion clinic within 7 days of injury recovered from their injury an average of 8 days sooner than athletes who presented after 1 week post-injury [39]. Given that sideline assessment does not necessarily result in an emergency department referral for all (or even most) athletes, sideline medical professionals are in the best position to refer for follow-up care.

13.3.5 Relationship to Recovery

Several studies have investigated the relationship between on-field markers and overall severity of SRC, without consistent findings. Research has failed to demonstrate consistent relationships between loss of consciousness and subacute symptom burden, neurocognitive test performances, or time to recovery [40–42]. More recent findings have suggested that on-field dizziness, headache, or post-traumatic amnesia may be more predictive of prolonged recovery [38, 40–42], though these findings again have not been consistently replicated. Pre-injury factors, such as demographics and medical history, individual factors such as reporting style, and treatment variables, such as time to specialty care evaluation, are more consistently found to be related to recovery trajectory in the studies that include them [39, 41, 43]. As such, it appears that the manner in which sideline assessment is best able to facilitate recovery or inform prognosis is through the expeditious identification of injury, swift removal from play, and immediate referral for specialty care.

13.4 Tools for Sideline Assessment

13.4.1 A Note on Psychometrics

For the purposes of the following sections, elements of diagnostic accuracy of a standardized assessment tool warrant a brief introduction. Diagnostic accuracy refers to the ability of an instrument to discriminate between the presence or absence of a condition: in this case SRC. The state of having a SRC is *dichotomous*—an athlete either does or does not have a SRC at any given time. On the other hand, numeric scores on sideline assessments are *continuous*. Diagnostic thresholds or "cutoff scores" are thus developed by researchers to dichotomize these continuous scores. Scores beyond a developed cutoff indicate the presence of SRC, and scores short of the cutoff indicate absence. The effectiveness of such a cutoff is often described in terms of sensitivity and specificity, and these psychometric properties can be directly measured and represented as percentages. Sensitivity reflects the percentage of athletes who are accurately classified by the test as having a SRC (true positives), while specificity reflects the percentage of those who are accurately classified as being healthy (true negatives). It is nearly impossible for any test to possess perfect sensitivity and specificity, and often researchers must make decisions to prioritize one over the other.

As it relates to the sideline assessment of SRC, it has been previously suggested that highly sensitive instruments are preferrable, even at the expense of some degree of specificity. The risks of a false negative (finding that an athlete does not have a SRC, when in fact he does) are considerable: the athlete would not be removed from play, which as discussed earlier increases risk for adverse outcomes. On the other hand, the risks of a false positive (finding that an athlete does have a SRC when in fact, he does not) are relatively smaller: an athlete may miss playing time and unnecessary healthcare resources may be expended to clear the athlete back to play. There are certainly risks in either case, and sideline medical professionals will want to consider carefully the assessments and diagnostic cutoffs they employ with risks of both false positives and false negatives in mind.

13.4.2 Multidimensional Sideline Assessments

13.4.2.1 Sport Concussion Assessment Tool (SCAT)

The Sport Concussion Assessment Tool (SCAT) is one of the longest standing and most researched SRC assessment tools. Initially developed in 1997 as the "Standard Assessment of Concussion," it aimed to standardize the sideline assessment of SRC and incorporate the most useful aspects of various unidimensional assessments. The SCAT has been iteratively modified since its inception, with the latest forms being the Sport Concussion Assessment Tool, 5th Edition (SCAT-5) [28] for athletes aged 13 and older and the Child SCAT-5 version for athletes aged 5–12 years [44]. The current forms are separated into "Immediate/On-Field" and "Office/Off-Field" components. The on-field components of the SCAT-5 include evaluation of red flags, observable signs of concussion, memory assessment, the Glasgow Coma Scale, and a brief cervical spine assessment. The off-field components include a symptom scale, cognitive screen, neurological screen, and balance assessment.

Despite the SCAT being endorsed as the "most well-established and rigorously developed instrument available for sideline assessment" of SRC [24, 26], research has been surprisingly scarce on diagnostic performance of the full SCAT. A study including 166 [45] concussed athletes administered the SCAT-3 one day after injury, but only reported diagnostic values for the components separately. This study found that only the symptom scale component had acceptable diagnostic performance (76% sensitivity, 90% specificity). In perhaps the most compelling study to-date,

Garcia and colleagues studied 941 concussed college athletes who were administered three components of the SCAT (symptom scale, cognitive screen, and balance assessment) within 6 h of injury, finding very high sensitivity (93%) and specificity (96%). Despite these positive results, the models used in this study were complex and included external variables such as sex to augment diagnostic accuracy, rendering it unable to yield any single diagnostic cutoff score for sideline use.

Thus, the SCAT-5 remains without formal guidance for interpretation or data on diagnostic accuracy. Instead, the SCAT's primary utility lies in its broad and comprehensive nature—the inclusion of assessments across many domains, and especially its inclusion of screenings for severe outcomes not necessarily related to SRC (i.e., "red flag" symptoms). However, even with its emphasis on comprehensiveness over diagnostic utility, multidimensional vestibular and oculomotor evaluations remain conspicuously absent from the SCAT, despite research suggesting these domains are commonly disrupted after concussion.

Research on the diagnostic utility of the Child SCAT-5, for use in athletes aged 5–12, is similarly limited. No studies to date have exclusively evaluated its performance in children 12 or younger. Further, test–retest reliability has been found to be poor in a sample of healthy 11–13-year-olds [46]. The only study to report diagnostic utility did so in a sample with an average age of 12, finding that symptoms were the strongest diagnostic predictor with sensitivity of 88% and specificity of 54% [47].

13.4.2.2 ImPACT Quick Test (ImPACT QT)

ImPACT is a well-known and widely used computerized neurocognitive assessment, which assesses several domains of cognitive functioning and concussion symptoms. The traditional ImPACT takes approximately 30 min to complete and requires a quiet testing space with a computer, making it infeasible for use on the sideline. The ImPACT QT is an abbreviated (5–7 min) version administered via a tablet. The QT also includes an optional BESS administration after the neurocognitive elements. While some initial research has examined the normative data of the QT and how it compares to the standard ImPACT [48], no research to-date has evaluated its performance as a diagnostic tool.

13.4.2.3 Vestibular/Ocular Motor Screening (VOMS)

The VOMS is a brief (5 min) screening designed to assess both vestibular and oculomotor dysfunction after concussion. Initially developed as a means of informing appropriate treatment, the VOMS has recently gained attention as a potential diagnostic tool for sideline assessment [49–51]. Diagnostic accuracies have ranged from 0.73 to 0.91 area under the curve (AUC) [49–51]. The only study to date reporting sensitivity and specificity found 77% and 83%, respectively [50]. Studies incorporating a direct comparison have also found that the VOMS outperforms the SCAT3 and the Modified Balance Error Scoring System [50], leading some to suggest its incorporation into the next revision of the SCAT. Further research must establish clear sensitivity and specificity values at ideal cutoffs, determine if the VOMS is confounded by contextual factors, and examine whether VOMS is best as a standalone instrument or included as a component in the SCAT.

13.4.3 Unidimensional Sideline Assessments

In contrast to the lack of published diagnostic findings of the full SCAT and other multidimensional assessment tools, there are more studies evaluating the diagnostic accuracy of unidimensional assessments, many of which comprise the individual components of multidimensional assessments.

13.4.3.1 Post-Concussion Symptom Scale (PCSS)

The PCSS is a self-report symptom inventory including 22 common post-concussion symptoms. Athletes are asked to rate their current symptom severity for each on a Likert scale from 0 (no symptom) to 6 (severe), yielding a total score from 0 to 132. Summarizing the research on the PCSS is difficult, as it has been modified and updated many times, and is typically included as a part of a battery instead of as a standalone instrument. Further, it is researched frequently as an in-office (rather than a sideline) assessment. However, the most recent research has suggested that the PCSS is the best-performing component of the SCAT [45, 52–54], with Harmon reporting up to 91% sensitivity and 97% specificity, though it lacks clear cutoff guidance when used in isolation.

13.4.3.2 Standardized Assessment of Concussion (SAC)

The SAC was developed as a brief cognitive screening tool able to be administered on the sidelines. It includes brief screenings of orientation, attention, immediate memory, and delayed memory. Total scores range from 0 to 30, with lower scores representing poorer performance. Early research on the SAC for use in high school and college athletes was promising, with sensitivity values around 95% and specificity around 76% [55, 56], though more recent studies have been less favorable. Harmon [52] found relatively poor sensitivity and specificity for the SAC (44% and 72%, respectively). Bruce and colleagues [54] also found poor sensitivity (≤62%). Chin [45] found the SAC did not outperform chance in its ability to diagnose concussion.

13.4.3.3 Modified Balance Error Scoring System (mBESS)

The mBESS is a brief balance screening that requires athletes to hold three stances (double leg, single leg, and tandem gait, with eyes closed). In contrast to its predecessor the BESS, which incorporated balancing on a foam surface, the mBESS is conducted only on a firm surface, allowing administration without specialty equipment. Athletes begin each stance with a total score of 10, and deductions are made by the assessor for deviations, yielding a total score between 0 and 30. Harmon [52] looked at three separate cutoffs for the mBESS, and found that each of them sacrificed sensitivity (ranging from 14% to 41%) for higher specificity (ranging from 61 to 97). Similarly, Bruce and colleagues [54] found poor sensitivity for mBESS (≤40%). Further, research has found that mBESS performance can vary depending on a wide number of contextual factors, such as exercise-induced fatigue, location of evaluation (e.g., sideline), equipment worn by the athlete, and non-concussive injuries [57–60].

13.4.3.4 Tandem Gait Task (TGT)

The tandem gait task (TGT) is an optional component of the SCAT that requires heel-to-toe walking with observer assessment of speed and errors/sway. Interestingly, few of the studies mentioned previously that deconstruct the utility of each of the SCAT components include the TGT. However, a number of studies have investigated the TGT in isolation with mixed results. In these studies, sensitivity values of the TGT range from 63% to 88% and specificity from 60% to 72% [61, 62].

13.4.3.5 King-Devick Test (KD Test)

A rapid number naming test relying heavily on the visual system, the King-Devick (KD) assessment can be administered quickly (<5 min), with minimal equipment, by professionals or laypersons [63]. In a very small sample ($N = 22$), Hecimovich [64] found outstanding sensitivity (96%) and specificity (98%) values. Beyond this small sample, research has generally found sensitivity values from 60% to 85% and specificity values from 39% to 90% [65, 66]. Other research has found significant practice effects with re-administration of the KD test [64], potentially undermining its utility.

13.5 Future Directions for Sideline Assessment

13.5.1 Biomarkers

The review of existing assessments above suggests significant room for improvement in sideline assessment tools for SRC. A strong contributing factor to the limited utility of these instruments is the ambiguity in defining concussion, which limits our ability to develop accurate tools for its identification. Until assessments can begin to more directly evaluate the pathophysiology, it is unlikely that sideline diagnostic assessment will make significant progress. Thus, to address this issue, much emerging research focuses on potential biomarkers of concussion in hopes that improving the proximity to the pathophysiology of concussion will improve diagnostic performance.

Biomarkers can be divided into neuroimaging (e.g., CT, MRI, SPECT), neurophysiological (e.g., EEG, eye tracking), and biofluid biomarkers [67]. Neuroimaging and neurophysiological biomarkers are limited in their diagnostic utility of concussion at this time [67], although research is ongoing. The most promising investigations currently come from the biofluid literature. Biofluid biomarkers, broadly speaking, are substances (such as proteins or enzymes) released from the brain when a concussion has occurred that can then be measured in bodily fluids (such as blood or saliva) to indicate the presence of a concussion [67]. Despite promising early research, there are many unresolved obstacles to clinical use of biomarkers. Dozens of potential biomarkers have been identified for traumatic brain injuries of all severities, though the extent to which these would be of use for the identification of concussion specifically is unclear, and measuring biomarkers on the sideline presents a host of logistical challenges. Finally, several studies have found that some proposed biomarkers may not be specific to concussion, as elevated biomarkers have been observed in both uninjured athletes during play [68] and athletes who sustained orthopedic injuries but not concussions [69]. Much research remains to be done before biomarkers can be utilized for sideline assessment of concussion.

13.6 Conclusions

Despite increased attention from the public and scientific community over the past two decades, much remains unknown about SRC. Important cultural changes are occurring and key stakeholders now appreciate the importance of sideline assessment for SRC, given the potential for adverse outcomes should injuries go unidentified. As the importance of and goals for the sideline assessment of SRC become increasingly clear, the available data on even the most well-researched assessment tools lags behind. This places increased importance on the medical training and thoughtful clinical decision making of sideline medical staff to conduct appropriate assessments for this injury, and to rule out more serious co-occurring injuries. Even in the absence of more severe injuries, rapid identification, removal from play, and referral for specialty care is of paramount importance to the trajectory of an athlete's recovery from SRC.

References

1. Gardner AJ, Quarrie KL, Iverson GL. The epidemiology of sport-related concussion: what the rehabilitation clinician needs to know. J Orthop Sports Phys Ther. 2019;49(11):768–78.
2. Cusimano MD, Topolovec-Vranic J, Zhang S, Mullen SJ, Wong M, Ilie G. Factors influencing the underreporting of concussion in sports. Clin J Sport Med. 2017;27(4):375–80.
3. Pierpoint LA, Collins C. Epidemiology of sport-related concussion. Clin Sports Med. 2021;40(1):1–18.
4. Centers for Disease Control and Prevention. National Concussion Surveillance System. 2021.
5. Bryan MA, Rowhani-Rahbar A, Comstock RD, Rivara F. Sports- and recreation-related concussions in US youth. Pediatrics. 2016;138(1):e20154635.
6. Langlois JA, Rutland-Brown W, Wald MM. The epidemiology and impact of traumatic brain injury. J Head Trauma Rehabil. 2006;21(5):375.
7. McCrory P, Feddermann-Demont N, Dvořák J, Cassidy JD, McIntosh A, Vos PE, et al. What is the definition of sports-related concussion: a systematic review. Br J Sports Med. 2017;51(11):877–87.
8. Herring SA, Bergfeld JA, Boland A, Boyajian-O'Neill LA, Cantu RC, Hershman E, et al. Concussion (mild traumatic brain injury) and the team physician. Med Sci Sports Exerc. 2006;38(2):395–9.
9. Gurdjian ES, Volis HC. Congress of Neurological Surgeons Committee on head injury nomenclature: glossary of head injury. Clin Neurosurg. 1966;12:386–94.
10. Broglio SP, Cantu RC, Gioia GA, Guskiewicz KM, Kutcher J, Palm M, et al. National athletic trainers' association position statement: management of sport concussion. J Athl Train. 2014;49(2):245–65.

11. Giza CC, Kutcher JS, Ashwal S, Barth J, Getchius TSD, Gioia GA, et al. Summary of evidence-based guideline update: evaluation and management of concussion in sports: report of the guideline development Subcommittee of the American Academy of Neurology. Neurology. 2013;80(24):2250–7.
12. McCrory P, Meeuwisse WH, Aubry M, Cantu RC, Dvořák J, Echemendia RJ, et al. Consensus statement on concussion in sport—the 4th international conference on concussion in sport held in Zurich, November 2012. PM R. 2013;5(4):255–79.
13. Harmon KG, Drezner JA, Gammons M, Guskiewicz KM, Halstead M, Herring SA, et al. American Medical Society for Sports Medicine position statement: concussion in sport. Br J Sports Med. 2013;47(1):15–26.
14. Giza CC, Hovda DA. The new neurometabolic cascade of concussion. Neurosurgery. 2014;75(Suppl 4):S24–33.
15. Seifert T, Shipman V. The pathophysiology of sports concussion. Curr Pain Headache Rep. 2015;19(8):36.
16. Hilz MJ, DeFina PA, Anders S, Koehn J, Lang CJ, Pauli E, et al. Frequency analysis unveils cardiac autonomic dysfunction after mild traumatic brain injury. J Neurotrauma. 2011;28(9):1727–38.
17. Leddy JJ, Kozlowski K, Fung M, Pendergast DR, Willer B. Regulatory and autoregulatory physiological dysfunction as a primary characteristic of post concussion syndrome: implications for treatment. NeuroRehabilitation. 2007;22(3):199–205.
18. Dedovic K, D'Aguiar C, Pruessner JC. What stress does to your brain: a review of neuroimaging studies. Can J Psychiatry. 2009;54(1):6–15.
19. Purkayastha S, Stokes M, Bell KR. Autonomic nervous system dysfunction in mild traumatic brain injury: a review of related pathophysiology and symptoms. Brain Inj. 2019;33(9):1129–36.
20. Howell DR, Southard J. The molecular pathophysiology of concussion. Clin Sports Med. 2021;40(1):39–51.
21. Clay MB, Glover KL, Lowe DT. Epidemiology of concussion in sport: a literature review. J Chiropr Med. 2013;12(4):230–51.
22. Covassin T, Moran R, Elbin RJ. Sex differences in reported concussion injury rates and time loss from participation: an update of the National Collegiate Athletic Association Injury Surveillance Program from 2004–2005 through 2008–2009. J Athl Train. 2016;51(3):189–94.
23. Tsushima WT, Siu AM, Ahn HJ, Chang BL, Murata NM. Incidence and risk of concussions in youth athletes: comparisons of age, sex, concussion history, sport, and football position. Arch Clin Neuropsychol. 2019;34(1):60–9.
24. Yue JK, Phelps RRL, Chandra A, Winkler EA, Manley GT, Berger MS. Sideline concussion assessment. Neurosurgery. 2020;87(3):466–75.
25. Harmon KG, Clugston JR, Dec K, Hainline B, Herring S, Kane SF, et al. American Medical Society for Sports Medicine position statement on concussion in sport. Br J Sports Med. 2019;53(4):213–25.
26. McCrory P, Meeuwisse W, Dvorak J, Aubry M, Bailes J, Broglio S, et al. Consensus statement on concussion in sport—the 5th international conference on concussion in sport held in Berlin, October 2016. Br J Sports Med. 2017;51:838.
27. Nicholson CA, Weber KM, Pieroth EM. Sideline assessment of concussion. Oper Tech Sports Med. 2022;30(1):150893.
28. Sport concussion assessment tool—5th edition. Br J Sports Med. 2017;51:851–8.
29. Engelhardt J, Brauge D, Loiseau H. Second impact syndrome. Myth or reality? Neurochirurgie. 2021;67(3):265–75.
30. Stovitz SD, Weseman JD, Hooks MC, Schmidt RJ, Koffel JB, Patricios JS. What definition is used to describe second impact syndrome in sports? A systematic and critical review. Curr Sports Med Rep. 2017;16(1):50–5.
31. Elbin RJ, Sufrinko A, Schatz P, French J, Henry L, Burkhart S, et al. Removal from play after concussion and recovery time. Pediatrics. 2016;138(3):e20160910.
32. Asken BM, Bauer RM, Guskiewicz KM, McCrea MA, Schmidt JD, Giza CC, et al. Immediate removal from activity after sport-related concussion is associated with shorter clinical recovery and less severe symptoms in collegiate student-athletes. Am J Sports Med. 2018;46(6):1465–74.
33. Chan C, Iverson GL, Purtzki J, Wong K, Kwan V, Gagnon I, et al. Safety of active rehabilitation for persistent symptoms after pediatric sport-related concussion: a randomized controlled trial. Arch Phys Med Rehabil. 2018;99(2):242–9.
34. Schneider KJ, Leddy JJ, Guskiewicz KM, Seifert T, McCrea M, Silverberg ND, et al. Rest and treatment/rehabilitation following sport-related concussion: a systematic review. Br J Sports Med. 2017;51(12):930–4.
35. Lumba-Brown A, Teramoto M, Bloom OJ, Brody D, Chesnutt J, Clugston JR, et al. Concussion guidelines step 2: evidence for subtype classification. Neurosurgery. 2020;86(1):2–13.
36. Langdon S, Königs M, Adang EAMC, Goedhart E, Oosterlaan J. Subtypes of sport-related concussion: a systematic review and meta-cluster analysis. Sports Med. 2020;50(10):1829–42.
37. Collins MW, Kontos AP, Reynolds E, Murawski CD, Fu FH. A comprehensive, targeted approach to the clinical care of athletes following sport-related concussion. Knee Surg Sports Traumatol Arthrosc. 2014;22(2):235–46.
38. Bock S, Grim R, Barron TF, Wagenheim A, Hu YE, Hendell M, et al. Factors associated with delayed recovery in athletes with concussion treated at a pediatric neurology concussion clinic. Childs Nerv Syst. 2015;31(11):2111–6.

39. Eagle SR, Puligilla A, Fazio-Sumrok V, Kegel N, Collins MW, Kontos AP. Association of time to initial clinic visit with prolonged recovery in pediatric patients with concussion. J Neurosurg Pediatr. 2020;26(2):165–70.
40. Collins MW, Iverson GL, Lovell MR, McKeag DB, Norwig J, Maroon J. On-field predictors of neuropsychological and symptom deficit following sports-related concussion. Clin J Sport Med. 2003;13:222–9.
41. Meehan WP, O'Brien MJ, Geminiani E, Mannix R. Initial symptom burden predicts duration of symptoms after concussion. J Sci Med Sport. 2016;19(9):722–5.
42. Teel EF, Marshall SW, Shankar V, McCrea M, Guskiewicz KM. Predicting recovery patterns after sport-related concussion. J Athl Train. 2017;52(3):288–98.
43. Kontos AP, Elbin RJ, Sufrinko A, Marchetti G, Holland CL, Collins MW. Recovery following sport-related concussion: integrating pre- and postinjury factors into multidisciplinary care. J Head Trauma Rehabil. 2019;34(6):394–401.
44. Sport concussion assessment tool for childrens ages 5 to 12 years. Br J Sports Med. 2017;51:862–9.
45. Chin EY, Nelson LD, Barr WB, McCrory P, McCrea MA. Reliability and validity of the sport concussion assessment tool-3 (SCAT3) in high school and collegiate athletes. Am J Sports Med. 2016;44(9):2276–85.
46. Kelshaw PM, Cook NE, Terry DP, Cortes N, Iverson GL, Caswell SV. Interpreting change on the Child Sport Concussion Assessment Tool 5th edition. J Sci Med Sport. 2022;25(6):492–8.
47. Erdman NK, Kelshaw PM, Hacherl SL, Caswell SV. Symptoms are the most effective child SCAT5 component for recognizing concussion on the day of injury. 2021.
48. Elbin RJ, D'Amico NR, McCarthy M, Womble MN, O'Connor S, Schatz P. How do ImPACT quick test scores compare with ImPACT online scores in non-concussed adolescent athletes? Arch Clin Neuropsychol. 2020;35(3):326–31.
49. Elbin RJ, Eagle SR, Marchetti GF, Anderson M, Schatz P, Womble MN, et al. Using change scores on the vestibular ocular motor screening (VOMS) tool to identify concussion in adolescents. Appl Neuropsychol Child. 2021;11:1–7.
50. Ferris LM, Kontos AP, Eagle SR, Elbin RJ, Collins MW, Mucha A, et al. Utility of VOMS, SCAT3, and ImPACT baseline evaluations for acute concussion identification in collegiate athletes: findings from the NCAA-DoD Concussion Assessment, Research and Education (CARE) Consortium. Am J Sports Med. 2022;50(4):1106–19.
51. Kontos AP, Monti K, Eagle SR, Thomasma E, Holland CL, Thomas D, et al. Test–retest reliability of the Vestibular Ocular Motor Screening (VOMS) tool and modified Balance Error Scoring System (mBESS) in US military personnel. J Sci Med Sport. 2021;24(3):264–8.
52. Harmon KG, Whelan BM, Aukerman DF, Bohr AD, Nerrie JM, Elkinton HA, et al. Diagnostic accuracy and reliability of sideline concussion evaluation: a prospective, case-controlled study in college athletes comparing newer tools and established tests. Br J Sports Med. 2022;56(3):144–50.
53. Garcia GGP, Broglio SP, Lavieri MS, McCrea M, McAllister T. Quantifying the value of multidimensional assessment models for acute concussion: an analysis of data from the NCAA-DoD Care Consortium. Sports Med. 2018;48(7):1739–49.
54. Bruce JM, Thelen J, Meeuwisse W, Hutchison MG, Rizos J, Comper P, et al. Use of the Sport Concussion Assessment Tool 5 (SCAT5) in professional hockey, part 2: which components differentiate concussed and non-concussed players? Br J Sports Med. 2021;55(10):557–65.
55. Barr WB, McCrea M. Sensitivity and specificity of standardized neurocognitive testing immediately following sports concussion. J Int Neuropsychol Soc. 2001;7(6):693–702.
56. McCrea M. Standardized mental status testing on the sideline after sport-related concussion. J Athl Train. 2001;36(3):274–9.
57. Rahn C, Munkasy BA, Barry Joyner A, Buckley TA. Sideline performance of the balance error scoring system during a live sporting event. Clin J Sport Med. 2015;25(3):248–53.
58. Docherty CL, Valovich McLeod TC, Shultz SJ. Postural control deficits in participants with functional ankle instability as measured by the balance error scoring system. Clin J Sports Med. 2006;16:203–8.
59. Wilkins JC, Valovich McLeod TC, Perrin DH, Gansneder BM. Performance on the balance error scoring system decreases after fatigue. J Athl Train. 2004;39(2):156–61.
60. Azad AM, al Juma S, Bhatti JA, Delaney JS. Modified Balance Error Scoring System (M-BESS) test scores in athletes wearing protective equipment and cleats. BMJ Open Sport Exerc Med. 2016;2(1):e000117.
61. Oldham JR, Difabio MS, Kaminski TW, Dewolf RM, Howell DR, Buckley TA. Efficacy of tandem gait to identify impaired postural control after concussion. Med Sci Sports Exerc. 2018;50(6):1162–8.
62. van Deventer KA, Seehusen CN, Walker GA, Wilson JC, Howell DR. The diagnostic and prognostic utility of the dual-task tandem gait test for pediatric concussion. J Sport Health Sci. 2021;10(2):131–7.
63. Leong DF, Balcer LJ, Galetta SL, Liu Z, Master CL. The King-Devick test as a concussion screening tool administered by sports parents. J Sports Med Phys Fitness. 2014;54(1):70–7.

64. Hecimovich M, King D, Dempsey AR, Murphy M. The King–Devick test is a valid and reliable tool for assessing sport-related concussion in Australian football: a prospective cohort study. J Sci Med Sport. 2018;21(10):1004–7.
65. Fuller GW, Cross MJ, Stokes KA, Kemp SPT. King-Devick concussion test performs poorly as a screening tool in elite rugby union players: a prospective cohort study of two screening tests versus a clinical reference standard. Br J Sports Med. 2019;53(24):1526–32.
66. Galetta KM, Liu M, Leong DF, Ventura RE, Galetta SL, Balcer LJ. The King-Devick test of rapid number naming for concussion detection: meta-analysis and systematic review of the literature. Concussion. 2016;1(2):CNC8.
67. Wilde EA, Wanner IB, Kenney K, Gill J, Stone JR, Disner S, et al. A framework to advance biomarker development in the diagnosis, outcome prediction, and treatment of traumatic brain injury. J Neurotrauma. 2022;39(7–8):436–57.
68. Otto M, Holthusen S, Bahn E, Söhnchen N, Wiltfang J, Geese R, et al. Boxing and running lead to a rise in serum levels of S-100B protein. Int J Sports Med. 2000;21(8):551–5.
69. Anderson RE, Hansson LO, Nilsson O, Dijlai-Merzoug R, Settergren G. High serum S100B levels for trauma patients without head injuries. Neurosurgery. 2001;48(6):1255–60.

Injuries to the Face

Facial

14

Sanmisola George and Mark R. Hutchinson

14.1 Introduction

Injures to the head and face can be common in contact sports and need to be assessed properly in order to expedite treatment and prevent severe complications. Although concussion is the most common head trauma in sports, there are many other face and head injuries that can occur. The focus of this chapter will be to discuss the less common face and head injuries and their management (Fig. 14.1).

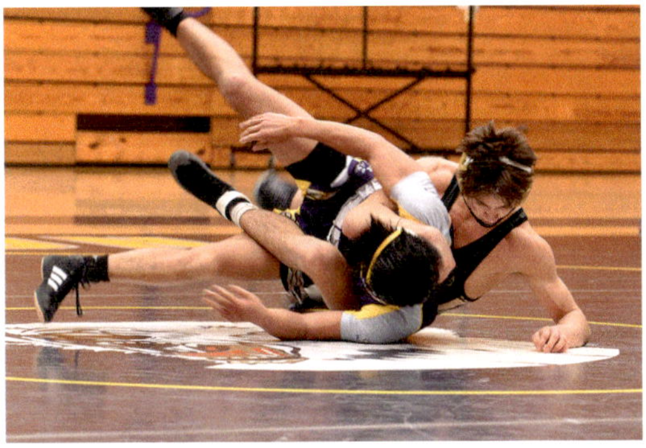

Fig. 14.1 Depiction of wrestling athletes during a match

14.2 Lacerations of the Face

Incidence/Prevalence as Well as Predisposing Risk Factor

Of all facial injuries, 29% occur during sports. Athletics like football, baseball, and hockey account for a high percentage of facial injuries among young adults. The face, however, has excellent blood flow, therefore wound healing is accelerated and infections are uncommon.

14.2.1 Eye Lid Lacerations

Eye lid lacerations are common with blunt or penetrating trauma, therefore globe rupture and foreign bodies must be excluded prior to management of laceration. If laceration is superficial, involving <25% of the eye lid, then the laceration can heal with secondary intention and use of topical antibiotics. However, if laceration is >25%, primary closure is recommended (see sideline management for closure methods). Referrals to ophthalmology should be made for laceration of the lid margin, presence of orbital fat, laceration of the medial canthus, ptosis, or laceration of the lacrimal duct. Primary closure of lesion must be initiated within 36 h.

S. George (✉)
Advocate Lutheran Sports Medicine, Park Ridge, IL, USA

M. R. Hutchinson
Orthopaedics and Sports Medicine, University of Illinois at Chicago, Chicago, IL, USA

S. Rocha Piedade et al. (eds.), *Sideline Management in Sports*, https://doi.org/10.1007/978-3-031-33867-0_14

14.2.2 Laceration of the Ears

Ear lacerations can result from isolated trauma, therefore serious head or middle ear injury must be excluded prior to addressing an ear laceration. Primary closure of uncomplicated ear laceration is appropriate. However, patients with auricular avulsion, split ear lobe (usually from earrings), or laceration extending into the external canal should be referred to ENT.

14.2.3 Laceration of the Lips

Most buccal mucosa lacerations heal rapidly without repair and do not warrant primary closure. If intraoral lacerations are >2 cm, it should be approximated in order to reduce incidence of retaining food particles or other foreign debris. Lip lacerations may be associated with injuries to surrounding structures, therefore be sure to assess for dental fractures, gingival bleeding, trauma to salivary glands, and mandibular or maxillary fractures prior to addressing laceration.

Indications and Benefits of Additional Testing/Imaging (Point of Care or Referral)
Athletes with clinical findings that suggest the presence of a foreign body or bony injury warrant appropriate imaging and appropriate specialist evaluation.

Signs and symptoms that warrant imaging or referral include but are not limited to:

- Amber or clear middle ear effusion
- Otorrhea (clear or bloody ear canal drainage)
- Hearing defect
- Nystagmus
- Ataxia
- Confusion
- Retro-auricular hematoma, battle sign (typically appears 6–48 h after injury)
- Cranial nerve dysfunction
- Vision loss or change
- Ptosis
- Malocclusion or abnormal bite
- Palpable step-off

Sideline Management Guidelines (Suggestions and Clinical Issues in Athletes)
Direct pressure can be applied to bleeding laceration; however, ensure there is no underlying fracture.

In general, facial lacerations without risk factors for infection can be closed within 24–48 h if appropriate.

Appropriate irrigation and debridement of wound are required prior to closure.

Prophylactic topical or oral antibiotics can be considered for infection.

Tetanus prophylaxis should be provided for all wounds if indicated.

Methods of wound closure to consider:

A. Simple interrupted suture placement provides good cosmetic skin closure.
B. Tissue adhesives are effective in the closure of straight, low tensile facial lacerations without dermal or subcutaneous involvement.
C. Adhesive tapes are cost effective, time saving, and significantly less painful than sutures. There are no significant differences between results of adhesive tapes versus tissue adhesives.

Prevention Measures that Could be Implemented for Early Recognition of Risk Reduction (Attitude, Rules Modification, Referee Instruction)
Lacerations to the eyes and buccal mucosa can be prevented with eye protection and mouth guards when applicable.

Take Home Messages

- Sports like football, baseball, and hockey account for a high percentage of facial injuries among young adults.
- Athletes with clinical findings that suggest the presence of a foreign body or bony injury warrant appropriate imaging and specialty evaluation.
- In general, facial lacerations without risk factors for infection can be closed within 24–48 h; if appropriate, cleansing is performed [1].

14.3 Ocular Injuries

Incidence/Prevalence as Well as Predisposing Risk Factor

Athletes with contacts, myopia or hyperopia, or h/o eye surgery or eye disease have an increased risk of ocular injury. Annual rate for all cause ocular injuries presenting to the ED was 37.6 per 10,000 and sports are responsible for 1/3 of ocular injuries that lead to blindness. High-risk sports include Boxing, MMA, wrestling, baseball/softball, basketball, lacrosse, racquetball, and hockey. A 2018 study in the Journal of Pediatrics found that basketball caused almost 16% of eye injuries in kids between 1990 and 2012.

Review of Clinical Presentation

Eye injury commonly presents with symptoms that include decreased visual acuity, diplopia, flashers, floaters, photophobia, and halos around lights.

Differential Diagnosis for Eye Injuries

Conjunctival laceration—Full thickness break of the conjunctiva

Partial thickness scleral laceration—Incomplete scleral break not to the level of the choroid

Partial thickness corneal laceration—Incomplete corneal break without loss of aqueous humor

Conjunctival abrasion—Injury to the epithelium of the conjunctiva

Corneal abrasion—Injury to the epithelium of the cornea

Corneal Foreign Body

Hyphema—Blood in the anterior chamber of the eye

Traumatic iritis—Inflammation in the anterior chamber resulting from trauma

Traumatic mydriasis—Chronic pupil dilation usually from iris sphincter damage

Lens dislocation—Native or artificial lens implant displacement from its original location

Vitreous hemorrhage—Bleeding into the vitreous cavity

Commotio retinae—Retinal whitening due to trauma-associated retinal edema

Retinal detachment—Separation of the retina from the underlying choroid and sclera

Global Eye Rupture (Fig. 14.2)

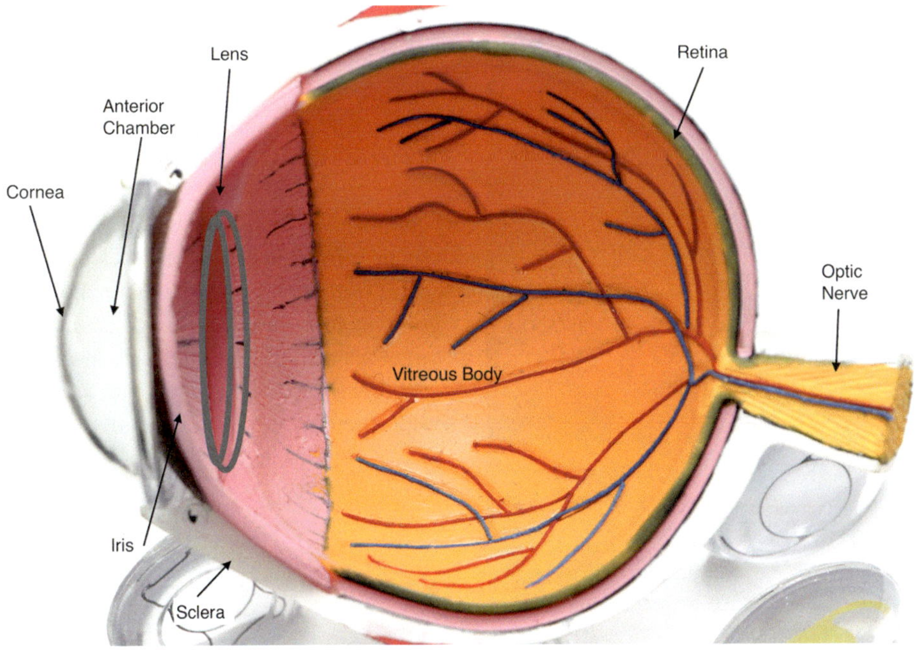

Fig. 14.2 Anatomical cross-section of the eye. (Singh, Harpreet. "Red and White Round Plastic Toy Photo—Free Lens Image on Unsplash." *Beautiful Free Images & Pictures | Unsplash*, 12 Mar. 2021, https://unsplash.com/photos/ioYYWWX2fjk)

Key Physical Examination Pearls and Findings

- Visual acuity test is the single most important test as it can be compared to the athletes' baseline.
- Visual fields defect and extraocular motion abnormality may indicate entrapment secondary to fracture or nerve injury.
- Anisocoria diagnosed via swinging light test may indicate ocular nerve injury.
- Although fundoycopic exam may be difficult to do on the sideline, it can be a helpful tool for acute visual loss and aides in assessing optic disc, vessels, and retina looking for retinal edema or detachment, hemorrhage.
- Tonometry assesses for eye pressure that may be elevated in hemorrhage or internal orbital edema.
- Fluorescein stain with woods lamp to assess for corneal abrasion (Fig. 14.3).

14.3.1 Corneal Abrasions

Corneal abrasions result from cutting or scratching of the anterior surface of the ocular epithelium. This may present with acute pain, photophobia, redness, tearing, and decreased visual acuity that worsen with light exposure and blinking. Risk factors include use of contact lens or previous history of corneal abrasion.

If concerned for corneal abrasion at sideline, take the following steps:

- Evaluate for foreign body. If foreign body is identified, it can be easily removed with carful use of Q-tip. Doing so may prevent further damage
- Conduct fluorescein stain exam under blue light in order to diagnose corneal abrasion. Abrasion will illuminate using black light exposing abrasion or foreign body
- If abrasion is identified, treat with topical antibiotics (erythromycin ointment or fluoroquinolones)
  - Topical NSAIDs may help with pain control
- Eye patch is not indicated or useful; however, it is recommended for athlete to avoid rubbing
- Avoid contacts use until abrasion has healed
- Consult ophthalmology for large lesions, unchanged, or worsening symptoms after 24 h
- Anesthetic is often needed to complete a full exam; however, global eye rupture must be excluded prior to use

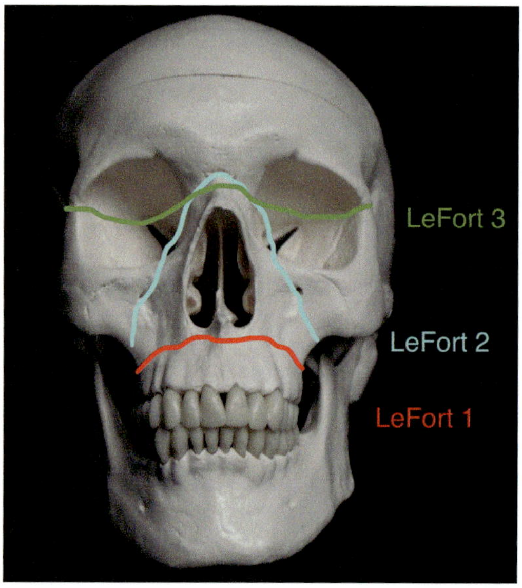

Fig. 14.3 Frontal view of the human skull depicting the anatomical locations of the three different types of LeFort fractures

14.3.2 Conjunctival Hemorrhage

A conjunctival hemorrhage is a common finding that occurs from trauma or spontaneously. Athletes are usually asymptomatic; however, it is important to ensure that visual acuity is intact. Symptoms resolve spontaneously in 2–3 weeks.

Note, hemorrhage that surrounds entire sclera (hemorrhagic chemosis) may indicate globe rupture which will need urgent referral to ophthalmology.

14.3.3 Retinal Detachment

Retinal detachment produces immediate loss of visual. It can be caused by retinal instability, trauma, increase in intraocular pressure, decreased oxygen saturation, or elevated venous pressure from valsalva maneuvers (seen in mountain climbing and weightlifting).

Involvement with macula results in decreased visual acuity or distortion of visual perception. Athletes will usually describe vision as containing floaters, haze, smoke, shadows, flashing lights, or cobwebs. Waving, black curtain encroaching on central vision, has also been described.

If concern for retinal detachment is on sideline, take the following steps:

- Assess visual field and acuity.
- Conduct additional exams including:
  - Funduscopic examination which can reveal hemorrhages. It is necessary to dilate the pupil widely to visualize a retinal detachment during its early stages because detachments begin in the far periphery.
  - Point of care ultrasound can be diagnostic.
- Emergent referral to ophthalmology is needed.
  - Symptomatic athletes need surgical intervention.
  - In asymptomatic athletes, surgery may not be indicated. Close observation for 1–2 weeks may be recommended.

14.3.4 Hyphema

Hyphema is classified as a hemorrhage into the anterior chamber of the eye. It can be caused by a tear in peripheral iris vessels. Projectiles that strike the exposed portion of the eye are a common cause of hyphema. Common symptoms are reduced visual acuity, discomfort, tearing, and photophobia. Penlight exam can identify macroscopic hyphema in acute settings; however, small amounts of fluid can often be overlooked and recurrent hyphema can lead to permanent vision loss. After sustaining projectile trauma, the athlete must be examined via slit lamp examination to identify microscopic hyphema.

If concern for hyphema after projectile trauma on sideline, take the following steps:

- Assess visual acuity
- Shielding of the eye with rigid eye shield should be placed for protection, can be used for 2 weeks
- Refer to ophthalmology for slit lamp examination and treatment
  - Topical atropine sulfate twice daily for 2 weeks and topical corticosteroids may be recommended
- Avoid salicylates and NSAID as this may contribute to increased bleeding

Note that recurrent bleeding is most common during first 5 days after injury; therefore, close observation is needed. It is also associated with vitreous hemorrhage, retinal hemorrhage, and can contribute to glaucoma. Close observation is needed.

Sideline Management Guidelines (Suggestions and Clinical Issues in Athletes)
Sideline management of eye injury is dependent on mechanism and presentation. Generally, sideline eye exam should avoid physical manipulation of the affected eye. Do not manipulate or forcibly open an eye if mechanism and exam cannot rule out a ruptured globe. If an open globe is present on gross eye inspection, eye irrigation and solutions should be avoided so as not to further contaminate the wound. Place protective eye shield over the and refer emergently to opthalmology.

Prevention Measures that Could be Implemented for Early Recognition of Risk Reduction (Attitude, Rules Modification, Referee Instruction)
All athletes should wear sports eye protection that meets requirements set by appropriate organizations. Athletes who wear contacts or glasses should also wear appropriate protective eyewear. Protective sports glasses with shatterproof plastic, called polycarbonate lenses, should be worn for sports such as basketball, racquet sports, soccer, and field hockey. Choose eye protectors that have been tested to meet the American Society of Testing and Materials (ASTM) standards.

Take Home Messages

- High-risk sports include Boxing, MMA, wrestling, baseball/softball, basketball, lacrosse, racquetball, and hockey.
- Sideline management of eye injury is dependent on mechanism and presentation.
- Never manipulate or forcibly open an eye if mechanism and exam cannot rule out a ruptured globe.
- Do not use topical anesthetic if ruptured globed cannot be ruled out. Anesthetic can further damage the retina.
- All athletes should wear sports eye protection that meets requirements set by appropriate organizations [2–6].

14.4 Fractures of the Face

The facial structure is undoubtedly important for appearance, but is also integral for the function of the face. It is important for proper mastication, speech, airway, expression, and other functions; therefore the initial treatment of any facial injuries should focus on maintaining function and then secondary cosmetics. Maxillofacial injuries account for an estimated 11% of National Collegiate Athletic Association (NCAA) sport-related injuries and occur at a rate of 0.2–1.5 injuries per 1000 athletic events/exposures [7].

Incidence/Prevalence as Well as Predisposing Risk Factor

A study showed that the highest frequency of sports-related facial bone fractures was in the age group 11–20 years. The most common causes of the injury were soccer (38.1%), baseball (16.1%), basketball (12.7%), martial arts (6.4%), and skiing or snowboarding (11%). Fractures of the nasal bone were the most common in all sports. Mandible fractures were common in soccer and martial arts. Orbital bone fractures were common in baseball, basketball, and ice sports. Fractures of the zygoma were frequently seen in soccer and martial arts [8].

Key Physical Examination Pearls and Findings

Overall, initial examination for suspected facial trauma will indicate area of suspected injury and is as follows:

- Inability to breath out both sides of the nose is consistent with nasal fracture (see Sect. 14.5 for more details)
- Trismus or difficulty speaking suggests a mandibular fracture
- Diplopia or visual changes are common in patients with orbital fractures
- Distorted hearing may indicate tympanic membrane injury
- Facial paresthesias can occur from a number of facial fractures
- Malocclusion suggests a mandibular fracture. Occlusion can be evaluated by asking the patient if his or her bite has changed since the injury (Sect. 14.7)
- Painful or loose teeth should prompt the examiner to evaluate for a mandibular alveolar injury
- Bleeding from your mouth, nose, or ears [9]?

14.4.1 Mandibular Fractures

Mandibular fracture usually occurs with direct trauma to the mandible from projectile object or fall. Athletes may complain of skin laceration associated with loose jaw, crepitus, or inability to flush teeth together. On examination, you may be able to elicit pain with palpation or appreciated loose teeth and/or numbness due to injury to the mandibular nerve.

Once a potential mandibular fracture has been identified on the sideline, take the following steps:

- Protect airway, allow the athlete to sit in a position most comfortable to them.
- If needed, place the athlete in a forward sitting position to allow blood to drain out if applicable
- Immobilize with As long as there is no nasal drainage and the patient can breath, immobilize with an ace wrap
- Transport for further imaging:
  - Athletes will need imaging to confirm, via panorex X-ray or CT scan [10]
- All athletes with mandibular fractures warrant evaluation and treatment by an oral and maxillofacial surgeon

Unilateral/Bilateral Malocclusion or condylar fracture—treated with 7–10 days of immobilization by intermaxillary fixation or maxilla-mandibular fixation followed by guiding elastics and movement exercises [9].

Return to noncontact sports in 4 weeks; contact sports in 2–3 months.

14.4.2 Maxillary "LeFort" Fractures

LeFort fractures are those of the midface that involves the maxillary segment. There are three types (Fig. 14.4)

- LeFort I "transverse" injuries involve a transverse fracture through the maxilla above the roots of the teeth. The injury may be unilateral or bilateral. Athletes may complain of malocclusion. The clinician may detect motion in the maxilla when the upper teeth are grasped while the forehead is held stationary.
- LeFort II "pyramidal" injuries are typically bilateral and involve fractures that extend superiorly in the midface to include the nasal bridge, maxilla, lacrimal bones, orbital floor, and rim. When examined, the nasal complex moves as a unit with the maxilla when the teeth are grasped while the forehead is held stationary.

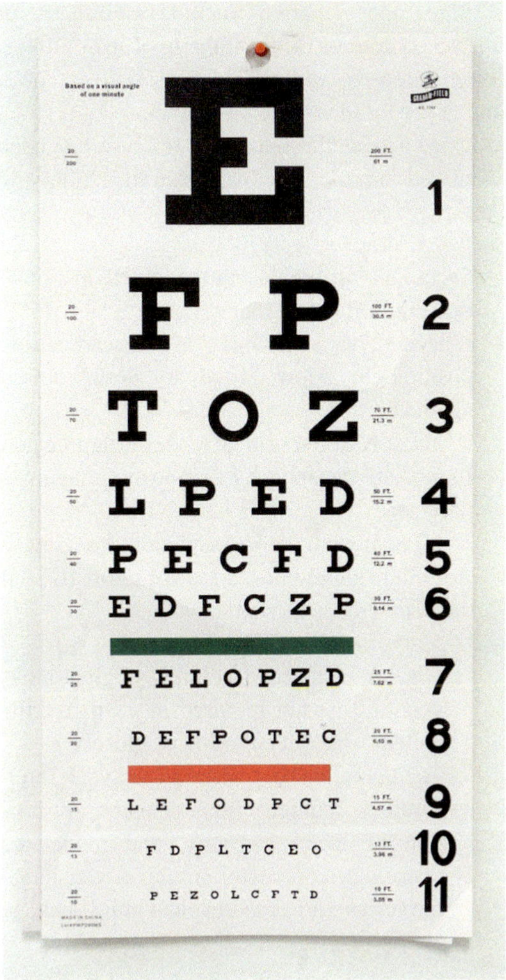

Fig. 14.4 Image of a Snellen Eye chart which is used for the assessment of visual acuity

- LeFort III "craniofacial" injuries are rare and involve fractures that result in discontinuity between the skull and the face. The fractures begin at the bridge of the nose and extend posteriorly along the medial wall of the orbit and the floor of the orbit, and then through the lateral orbital wall and the zygomatic arch. Intranasally, they extend through all the lesser bones to the base of the sphenoid and are frequently associated with a cerebrospinal fluid (CSF) leak [11, 12–15].

Signs and symptoms include asymmetry or altered contour of face, flattening of the midface, loose dentition, and altered sensation of cheek and upper lip (due to nerve injury).

Once a potential maxillary fracture has been identified on the sideline, take the following steps:

- Secure airway by placing the athlete in a position comfortable to that athlete
- If needed, place the athlete in a forward sitting position to allow blood to drain out if applicable

  Note: Nasotracheal airway contraindicated
- Immediate transport for diagnostic imaging is need

  CT scan with coronal and axial imaging
- Antibiotic should be started if LeFort III or if there are any open/visible wounds
- Urgent referral to ENT is required
  - For non-displaced fractures, surgical interventions are not required in a trustworthy patient who can be followed closely
  - For complicated fractures, surgical interventions required (malocclusion, disruption of facial harmony, and associated neurologic complication such as visual disturbances and cerebrospinal fluid leakage [16])

Return to play is dependent on the severity of injury. Evidence-based research to establish return to play guidelines is limited. Recovery periods of up to 6 weeks have been reported in literature [16].

14.4.3 Orbital Fracture

It is important to be able to identify orbital fractures as there are several complications associated that can ultimately lead to blindness. They are often associated with nosebleed and nasal fractures. Common signs and symptoms of orbital fracture include bony tenderness, reduced visual acuity, swelling, periocular ecchymosis, diplopia, and decreased sensation in the distribution of the infraorbital or supraorbital nerves. During palpation of the face, deformity, tenderness, crepitus, and/or step-off on palpation may be noted. Enophthalmos is a posterior displacement of the eye which may have the appearance of relative ptosis.

If orbital fracture is suspected, take the following steps:

- Place the athlete in a comfortable position, keep the head of the bed elevated in order to reduce periorbital swelling
- Rule out ruptured globe, do not forcefully open or manipulate the eyes; this may cause additional damage and potential rupture
- In addition to standard eye exam, it is important to assess extraocular movements; reduced ocular motion indicated ocular muscle entrapment and likely fracture
- Assess ocular pressure with tonometry, if intraocular pressure is increased, emergent referral to ophthalmology is needed
- Transport patient to ED for urgent imaging and ophthalmology consultation. Can use ice during transport in order to reduce periorbital swelling
  - Standard imaging is CT [10]

Complications of orbital fracture:

1. Orbital fractures can cause a hematoma within the orbit, behind the globe potentially causing acute exophthalmos leading to neurapraxia of the retinal nerve and compression of the retinal artery. In all orbital fractures, emergency evaluation is required to prevent blindness.
2. Orbital floor fracture "blowout fractures" most commonly occur when a small, round object (e.g., a baseball) strikes the eye. This may lead to entrapment of the inferior rectus muscle and/or orbital fat. Subsequent loss of muscle function leads to restricted vertical gaze and diplopia. Additional symptoms suggestive of injury are diplopia, especially with upward gaze, and ipsilateral nosebleed. Prolonged tissue entrapment and inflammation can result in fibrosis and contracture which can lead to permanent functional disabilities.

Return to Play

6–8 weeks after injury, protective gear recommended [10].

Prevention Measures that Could be Implemented for Early Recognition of Risk Reduction (Attitude, Rules Modification, Referee Instruction)

There is evidence that eye protection, mouth guards, helmets, and face guards are effective in reducing the risk of facial injury. However, these safety practices are not adopted universally by all athletes or by all sports [17].

Take Home Messages

- Facial fractures are most common in soccer (38.1%), baseball (16.1%), basketball (12.7%), martial arts (6.4%), and skiing or snowboarding (11%)
- First step in assess a facial fracture is to protect the airway
- All athletes with mandibular fractures warrant evaluation and treatment by an oral and maxillofacial surgeon
- LeFort fracture is associated with asymmetry or altered contour of face or flattening of the midface
- Orbital fracture can be associated with nosebleed and nasal fractures
- Do not forcefully open or manipulate the eyes; this may cause additional damage and potential rupture
- Eye protection, mouth guards, helmets, and face guards are effective in reducing the risk of facial injury

14.5 Nasal Injuries

Incidence/Prevalence as Well as Predisposing Risk Factor

Almost 40% of all facial fractures involve the nasal bones [18]. Nasal injuries are among the most common sports injuries and most common in contact sports. Studies have shown that majority of nasal injuries occurred in females and in basketball. Sixty-four percent of nasal injuries are fractures [19].

Differential Diagnosis

Facial laceration
Facial fracture
Contusion

Key Physical Examination Pearls and Findings

In nasal trauma, exam findings may include edema and ecchymosis at the nose and periorbital structures. Palpation of the nasal structures should be done to elicit any crepitus, indentation, or irregularity of the nasal bone. Uncommon findings such as a cerebrospinal fluid (CSF) leak posing as clear rhinorrhea, subcutaneous emphysema, mental status changes, new malocclusion, or limited extraocular movement should prompt immediate subspecialty referral. External and internal examination may be difficult following nasal injury because of ecchymoses, edema, epistaxis, and dried blood. However, be sure to assess for septal hematoma via direct visualization into the nares.

Indications and Benefits of Additional Testing/Imaging (Point of Care or Referral)

Imaging is rarely needed for nasal injury due to poor sensitivity and specificity with plain radiograph. Diagnosis can be made with physical exam. Plain radiography does not identify cartilaginous disruptions and physicians may misinterpret normal suture lines as non-displaced fractures.

Imaging is, however, indicated with complicated fractures including finding constant with cranial or cranial fracture or ophthologic injury. Examples of concerning findings include CSF rhinorrhea, extraocular movement abnormalities, or malocclusion. If identified, CT is indicated to assess for facial and mandibular fracture [20].

14.5.1 Epistaxis

Epistaxis usually occurs spontaneously at Kiesselbach's plexus on nasal septum in area of thin nasal mucosa overlying blood vessels. Trauma is second most common cause of epistaxis. Note that epistaxis can occur without nasal fracture. Posterior bleeding is less common and can be difficult to control [10].

If epistaxis is observed, the following steps can be taken:

- Secure airway
- Position the athlete in seated position bent forward at the waist. This will minimize bleeding to the oral cavity avoiding aspiration and ingestion of blood
- If direct facial trauma is observed, assess for nasal and other facial fractures
- Pinch the nostrils against the nasal septum, below the bony portion of the nose
- If hemostasis is not achieved within 10 min of direct pressure, consider topical vasoconstriction medications
  - Oxymetazoline (Afrin spray) followed by 10 more minute of compression [21]
- Anterior nasal bleeding that does not stop with these maneuvers can be treated with nasal packing
- Nosebleeds that do not stop with above treatment need urgent visit to the ED for evaluation by an otolaryngologist

Note, vaseline applied nightly to the nasal septum can prevent drying and cracking of the nasal mucosa, which may help prevent recurrent epistaxis.

14.5.2 Nasal Fracture and Septal Hematoma

Epistaxis, nasal asymmetry, crepitus on palpation, swelling, and nasal airway obstruction are signs and symptoms of nasal fracture. Nasal fractures can often be associated with adjacent fractures such as orbital and mid face fractures; therefore, it is very important to assess for additional fractures. Nasal fractures are also highly associated with septal hematoma which if present can result in necrosis of the septum. If a septal hematoma is identified, it must be drained immediately to avoid complications.

Pain, tenderness, and swelling to the nasal bridge are diagnostic. X-rays may show fracture, but are not necessary and required.

Once nasal fracture is identified, the following steps can be taken:

- Secure airway
- Place athlete in comfortable position with head elevated to decrease swelling
- Place ice over nasal bridge/nose. Prior to reduction and after initial injury, it is recommended that the athlete rest, apply ice, and maintain head elevation
- ED evaluation will be needed
  - Evacuation and treatment of septal hematoma within 24–48 h
  - Otolaryngologists prefer to wait for 3–7 days to allow swelling to resolve
  - Follow-up evaluation and management of nasal fracture reduction can be safely scheduled after the swelling resolve, between 5 and 7 days
- Nasal splint is recommended for protection.

Athletes can return to contact/collision sports with a face mask in approximately 4 weeks.

Perforated septal injuries may be identified during patient evaluation. They should be referred to an otolaryngologist for outpatient management within 3–5 days [20].

Prevention Measures that Could be Implemented for Early Recognition of Risk Reduction (Attitude, Rules Modification, Referee Instruction)

There is evidence that eye protection, mouth guards, helmets, and face guards are effective in reducing the risk of facial injury. However, these safety practices are not adopted universally by all athletes or by all sports [17].

Take Home Messages

- Almost 40% of all facial fractures involve the nasal bones
- First step to assess a facial fracture is to protect the airway
- Epistaxis and Nasal Fractures can be diagnosed clinically
- Imaging is rarely needed for nasal injury due to poor sensitivity and specificity with plain radiograph
- Complicated fractures need imaging and further evaluation by appropriate specialist
- Always evaluate for septal hematoma, if identified it must be drained immediately to avoid necrosis of the septum
- Eye protection, mouth guards, helmets, and face guards are effective in reducing the risk of facial injury

14.6 Ear Injuries

Many different types of accidents can damage your ear canal, eardrum, cartilage, and skin around your ear. The ear canal is a passageway of bone, skin, and cartilage that leads from the exterior ear to the middle ear, where your eardrum sits [22].

14.6.1 Auricular Hematoma and Cauliflower Ear

Auricular hematoma describes a collection of blood within the cartilaginous outer ear. Cauliflower ear is the permanent deformity caused by fibrocartilage overgrowth if an auricular hematoma is not fully drained or is untreated [23]. Auricular hematoma is caused by shear forces on ear. This can most commonly be seen in wrestlers, boxers, or mixed martial arts; clinical diagnosis of swelling or fluctuant area in cartilaginous area of ear.

Once an auricular hematoma is identified, the following steps can be taken:

- Cleanse the ear with antiseptic
- Provide local anesthesia
- Identify and aspirate the most fluctuant part of the hematoma with an 18 gauge needle while milking the hematoma to ensure complete drainage
- After needle aspiration, apply pressure for 5–10 min
- Place sterile gauze with the center cut out to provide padding behind the ear
- Mold sterile petrolatum-impregnated gauze or saline-soaked cotton balls within the contours of the auricle. If the skin was incised, this portion of the dressing needs to re-approximate the skin at the incision site
  - Hematoma will reoccur if not bolstered; therefore bolster should be in place for 7 days
- Place sterile gauze over the entire ear
- Wrap the ear and head with sterile rolled gauze to hold in place [23]
- Consider use of prophylactic antibiotics with Staphylococcus coverage

Return to Play
No restrictions.

Prevention
Proper headgear use.

14.6.2 Otitis Externa "Swimmer's Ear"

Otitis externa is infection of the ear canal commonly seen in water sport athletes. The most common causative organisms are Pseudomonas aeruginosa or *Staphylococcus aureus*. Athletes may present with pain and discomfort with motion of pinna and drainage from the ear canal. On inspection, visualization of a swollen erythematous external auditory canal or pinna with or without associated purulent discharge is diagnostic. Attempts to visualize TM may not be possible due to swelling; however, with suspected or confirmed TM rupture, it is important to avoid aminoglycosides or alcohol as it may reach the middle ear resulting in ototoxicity.

Topical antibiotics and topical corticosteroid are highly effective treatments. There are multiple solution combinations that can be used; therefore, it is important to consider coverage of specific pathogens, most commonly Pseudomonas aeruginosa or *Staphylococcus aureus*. Recommended topical antibiotic for water sport athletes is a fluoroquinolone (Ofloxacin and ciprofloxacin) which provides coverage against both pathogens. Antibiotics can be combined with glucocorticoids (hydrocortisone, dexamethasone, or prednisone). Glucocorticoids reduce symptoms caused by inflammation. Treatment duration is for 5–7 days. Cortisporin (e.g., hydrocortisone polymyxin neomycin) is commonly used for treatment of otitis externa in the outpatient setting; however, it should be used with caution. Attempts to visualize TM may not be possible due to swelling; however, with suspected or confirmed TM rupture, it is important to avoid aminoglycosides or alcohol as it may reach the middle ear resulting in ototoxicity. For severe infections, oral antibiotic can be considered.

Return to Play

- After resolution of symptoms.
- The athlete must be fever-free before returning to sports or recreation.
- Those involved in water sports should not return to activity until the ear drum is moving normally and shows no signs of tearing or perforation [24].

Prevention

Dry ears after swimming or after water exposure. A hair dryer to ear can help reduce moisture.

14.6.3 Otitis Media

Otitis media is an infection of the middle ear. It is important to understand that symptoms of ear infection can appear differently for children and adults. Child athletes may present with ear pain, tugging in the ear, difficulty sleeping, irritable, difficulty hearing, dizziness, drainage of fluids from ears, headache, and loss of appetite. Adult athletes may have ear pain, fullness in ear, drainage of fluids from ears, diminished hearing, and dizziness. Middle ear infection is clinically diagnosed using an otoscope to look into the ear where a bulging tympanic membrane, erythema of tympanic membrane, or reduced mobility of the tympanic membrane can be observed.

Risk factors for ear infections are:

- Younger age
- Seasonal or environmental allergies
- Exposure to cigarette smoke
- Gastroesophageal reflux
- Immunodeficiency
- Recent illness such as upper respiratory infection or sinus infection
- Swimming
- Cerumen impaction

Treatment

Acetaminophen or ibuprofen can be used to relieve pain and reduce fever if present. Oral antibiotics is recommenced to treat infection. Amoxicillin 875 mg with clavulanate 125 mg orally twice daily for 7–10 days is standard treatment. If athlete is allergic to penicillin, then cephalosporins can be used as alternative antibiotic.

Injury Prevention

- Regular hand washing to prevent viral infections.
- Avoid second hand smoke exposure.
- Dry ears after swimming. A hair dryer to ear can help reduce moisture.

Return to Play

- The decision to resume activity varies depending on any coexisting illness or associated complications.
- The athlete must be fever-free before returning to sports or recreation.
- Those involved in water sports should not return to activity until the ear drum is moving normally and shows no signs of tearing or perforation [24].

14.6.4 Tympanic Membrane Perforation/Rupture

Tympanic membrane perforation mechanism of injury can be caused by infection, trauma, or rapid changes in pressure, leading to sudden otalgia, otorrhea, tinnitus, and vertigo. Activities such as skydiving or scuba diving with pressure changes barotrauma can cause injury. A direct blow to the ear by a large ball or in boxing may also cause damage [25]. Athletes can present with hearing loss, serous or bloody drainage from ear, hole visible in tympanic membrane, and/or vertigo. Diagnosis is made with direct visualization of rupture with pneumatic otoscope [25].

Treatment

Most TM perforation or rupture (85–90%) will heal without treatment, resolve spontaneously, and without complications. In TM rupture, it is important to avoid topical aminoglycosides or alcohol as it may reach the middle ear resulting in ototoxicity. If no healing occurs within 2–3 weeks, refer to otolaryngologist. Complications, if not treated, can lead to prolonged hearing loss, chronic otitis media, cholesteatoma, and mastoiditis [25]. If there is persistent hearing loss or suspicion for ossicular disruption, the athlete needs immediate referral to otolaryngologist.

Return to Play

The ear should be kept dry until TM has completely healed, otherwise wet/moist ear increases risk for infection [25].

14.6.5 Diver's Ear/Barotrauma

SUBA diving is a popular attraction for many people. According to the Divers Alert Network, there is an average fatality rate of 1.8 per 100,000 divers per year. Although mortality rates are low, diving-related injuries and illnesses may occur, including barotrauma, arterial gas embolism, decompression sickness, nitrogen narcosis, and pulmonary edema.

The middle and outer ear is separated by the TM and the eustachian tube helps to establish an equilibrium between the pressures across the membrane. Diving can cause a disequilibrium between the outer and inner ear causing barotrauma/tympanic membrane rupture, potentially affecting or causing damage to the inner ear as well. Symptoms include ear pain, ear pressure, vertigo, nausea, or disorientation.

Treatment of middle ear barotrauma consists of topical and systemic decongestants, analgesics, and antihistamines. Antibiotics should be used if purulent otorrhea is observed. Most tympanic membrane ruptures heal spontaneously if normal eustachian tube function is restored and infection is controlled [26]. Avoid air travel a least 12 h after one diving experience and at least 48 h after more than one diving experience to avoid fatal complications.

Indications and Benefits of Additional Testing/Imaging (Point of Care or Referral)

Imaging is neither recommended or needed for ear trauma unless complicating factors are parent such as concern for facial fracture or if cerebral spinal fluid is suspected/present. Many ear injuries can be diagnosed clinically.

Prevention Measures that Could be Implemented for Early Recognition of Risk Reduction (Attitude, Rules Modification, Referee Instruction)

- Avoiding loud noises, wearing noise cancelling ear protection, or lowering the volume on earbuds and headphones.
- Getting special earplugs, chewing gum, or yawning to reduce pressure when flying on an airplane.
- Using a helmet for sports involving bike riding, skateboard, or motorcycle.
- Wearing protective headgear during contact sports such as boxing, rugby, and wrestling.
- Dry ears after water activity.
- Avoiding putting anything into the ears [22].

Take Home Messages
- Ear injuries can occur in sports associated with direct combat and in water sports.
- It is important to rule out infection in athletes presenting with ear pain or hearing loss.
- Imaging is not needed to diagnosis ear injury unless there is evidence of fracture or CSF is present.
- Ear injury is preventable in athletes by wearing proper head gear and drying ears after water activity.
- For persistent hearing loss greater than 4 weeks or persistent vertigo >1 week, refer patient to otolaryngologist as this can indicate inner ear damage.

14.7 Dental Injuries

Incidence/Prevalence as Well as Predisposing Risk Factor

The most commonly injured teeth are the maxillary central incisors, followed by the maxillary lateral incisors and the mandibular incisors. Falls are the most frequent cause of dental trauma among preschool and school-age children. Sports-related dental injuries are more common etiologies in adolescents [27].

Review of Clinical Presentation and Physical Exam

High force injuries to the teeth are associated with the potential for head, neck, and facial bone trauma; therefore, assess for additional injuries if tooth injury is suspected.

- Common signs and symptoms of tooth injury include the following:
- Spontaneous pain or sensitivity to hot/cold to any teeth after injury which would indicate dentin or pulp exposure.
- Bleeding from fracture site which would indicate pulp involvement.
- Teeth that are tender to touch or painful when eating which would indicate periodontal ligament damage.
- Occlusion or change in the athlete's bite which may indicate displaced teeth or jaw dislocation [27].

14.7.1 Tooth Crown Fractures

The crown of the tooth refers to the most visible portion of the tooth usually covered by enamel (Fig. 14.5).

If a crown fracture is suspected, take the following steps:

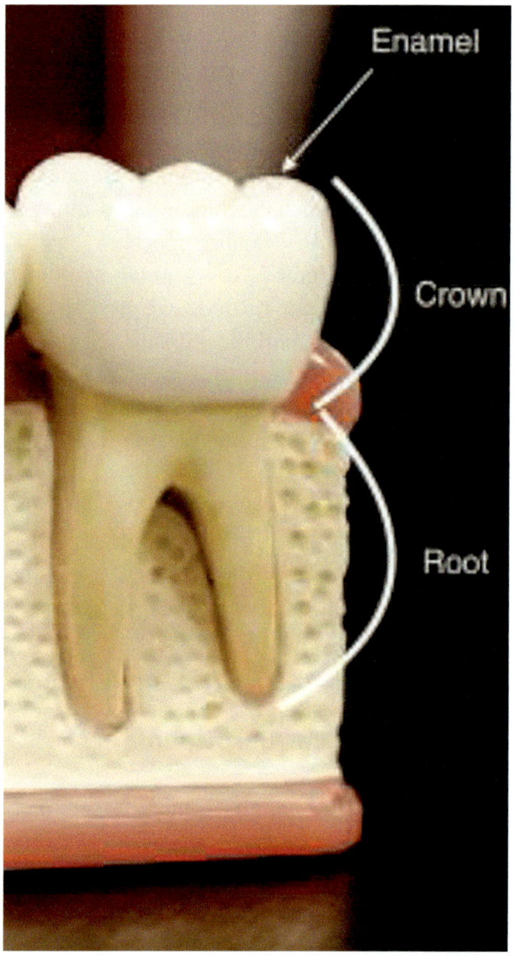

Fig. 14.5 Model of a molar tooth illustrating various sections of the tooth anatomy

- Examine teeth for fractures and laxity.
- Transport fractured teeth in culture medium (hanks balanced salt solution), cold milk, or physiological sterile saline [10].
- Radiographs should assess extent of fracture (crown, enamel, or root fractures).
- Refer to dentist
  - Crown fractures that involve only the enamel do not require specific treatment unless there is a sharp or rough edge; however, cosmetic treatment may be desired.
  - Fractures with exposed dentin, referral to a dentist within a few days is warranted in order to prevent infection.
  - Complicated fractures which are fractures that include pulp exposure or extend into the root require immediate dental referral in order to avoid pulp necrosis.
  - Prophylactic antibiotics is needed for fractures involving the dentin or pulp (Fig. 14.6).

14.7.2 Tooth Avulsion

A tooth avulsion refers to when a tooth is partially or completely dislodged from its socket.

If a tooth avulsion is suspected, take the following steps:

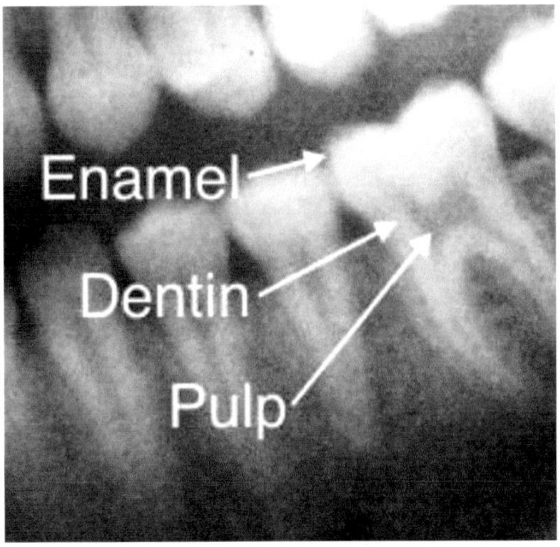

Fig. 14.6 X-Ray image of a portion of the mandible which displays the tooth anatomy. In this image, the delineation between the three areas of the tooth can be observed

- If it is not certain whether the tooth is primary or permanent, the tooth should be gently replanted and the patient referred emergently to a dentist [27].
  - Avulsed or displaced permanent teeth should be reimplanted immediately if possible. Tooth survival diminishes quickly with the amount of time out of the socket with small chance of survival after 1 h out of the socket [10].
  - Avulsed primary teeth should not be replanted because of the potential for injury to the developing tooth bud [27]
- If permanent tooth is sublimed do not try to straighten, refer to dentist. Place gauze pad in mouth and have the athlete gently bit down to hold tooth in place until they are seen urgently by a dentist
- If permanent tooth is completely avulsed, handle tooth by the crown
  - Do not rinse with saline or tap water
  - Do not rub or sterilize root
  - If immediate reimplantation is not possible, the tooth should be stored in culture medium (hanks balanced salt solution), cold milk, or physiological sterile saline [10]
- Emergently evaluated by a dentist [27]
- Radiographs may be obtained
- Prophylactic antibiotics is needed

14.7.3 TMJ Dislocations

Dislocation of the TMJ is usually an anterior dislocation. Dislocations can be caused by trauma or any action involving opening the mouth including yawning, laughing, or singing. Spontaneous reduction is rare due to muscles of mastication spasm. Patients with TMJ dislocation will present with inability to close the mouth in bilateral or with the jaw rotated laterally with a unilateral dislocation. Abnormal speech and drooling may also be present.

If the dislocation is suspected due to trauma, take the following steps:

- Obtain plain X-ray to rule out fractures

– Should be obtained before reduction is attempted to determine the presence of a fracture
– Refer to oral surgeon

Trauma to the temporomandibular joint (TMJ) may result in soft tissue injury, fracture, or dislocation. Injuries to the meniscus or collateral ligaments can cause malposition of the jaw, resulting in clicking or popping or the inability to open the mouth fully. Patients without a fracture or dislocation but with pain can be treated by limiting their diet to soft foods and avoiding yawning or straining to open their mouths wide. Follow-up with an oral surgeon is recommended within 2 weeks.

Indications and Benefits of Additional Testing/Imaging (Point of Care or Referral)

Indications for referral to dentist included:

– Avulsed permanent tooth
– Extrusion >3 mm or interfering with bite
– Displaced teeth that interfere with bite
– Fractured teeth with exposed pulp
– Fractured permanent teeth
– Suspected root fracture
– Intrusion of the tooth

Note, for athletes under 13 years of age, a pediatric dentist is preferred.

Prevention Measures that Could be Implemented for Early Recognition of Risk Reduction (Attitude, Rules Modification, Referee Instruction)

Mouth guards can prevent dental injury [10]. Athletes who do not wear mouth guard are two times more likely to have injury. American dental Association estimated that mouth guards prevent approximately 200,000 injuries per year in high school and collegiate football players. NCAA require mouth guards for football, hockey, and lacrosse. In addition, most high schools require mouth guards for wrestlers with braces.

Take Home Messages

- Tooth injury has a high association with head, neck, and facial injury and fractures, be sure to assess.
- Only handle tooth fracture or avulsion by the crown.
- Do not rinse tooth with saline or tap water and do not rub or sterilize root.
- Immediately reimplant permanent avulsed teeth as soon as possible.
- Transfer or storage of tooth should be done within culture medium (hanks balanced salt solution), cold milk, or physiological sterile saline.
- TMJ dislocation will need urgent referral to oral surgeon.

References

1. UpToDate. n.d. Retrieved 12 Nov 2022, from https://www.uptodate.com/contents/assessment-and-management-of-facial-lacerations?search=lacerations+of+the+face&source=search_result&selectedTitle=1~150&usage_type=default&display_rank=1#H22537793.
2. American Academy of Ophthalmology: protecting sight. Empowering lives—American Academy of Ophthalmology. n.d. Retrieved 12 Nov 2022, from https://www.aao.org/.
3. UpToDate. n.d. Retrieved 12 Nov 2022, from https://www.uptodate.com/contents/open-globe-injuries-emergency-evaluation-and-initial-management?search=Sports+related+eye+injuries+&source=search_result&selectedTitle=3~150&usage_type=default&display_rank=3.
4. Medeiros S. Basketball is the leading cause of eye injuries. American Academy of Ophthalmology; 2022. Retrieved 12 Nov 2022, from https://www.aao.org/eye-health/tips-prevention/madness-basketball-is-leading-cause-of-eye-injurie
5. UpToDate. n.d. Retrieved 12 Nov 2022, from https://www.uptodate.com/contents/overview-of-eye-injuries-in-the-emergency-department?search=Sports+related+eye+injuries+&source=search_result&selectedTitle=1~150&usage_type=default&display_rank=1#H1582332316.
6. Publications.aap.org. n.d. Retrieved 12 Nov 2022, from https://publications.aap.org/view-large/6602957.

7. Mertz KC, Bolia IK, English MG, Cho AW, Trasolini N, Hasan LK, Haratian A, Diaz P, Romano R, Gamradt SC, Weber AE. Epidemiology and outcomes of maxillofacial injuries in NCAA Division I athletes participating in 13 sports. Orthop J Sports Med. 2022. Retrieved 12 Nov 2022, from https://www.ncbi.nlm.nih.gov/pmc/articles/PMC8949702/.
8. Hwang K, You SH, Lee HS. Outcome analysis of sports-related multiple facial fractures. J Craniofac Surg. 2009. Retrieved 12 Nov 2022, from https://pubmed.ncbi.nlm.nih.gov/19352203/.
9. UpToDate. n.d. Retrieved 12 Nov 2022, from https://www.uptodate.com/contents/initial-evaluation-and-management-of-facial-trauma-in-adults/abstract/10-16.
10. Madden CC, Putukian M, McCarty EC, Young CC, Netter FH, Machado CAG, Craig JA, Marzejon KW, DaVanzo TS, Perkins JA. Netter's sports medicine. Elsevier; 2023.
11. UpToDate. n.d. Retrieved 12 Nov 2022, from https://www.uptodate.com/contents/mandibular-jaw-fractures-in-children?search=mandibular+fracture&source=search_result&selectedTitle=2~41&usage_type=default&display_rank=2.
12. Kim, H. S., Kim, S. E., & Lee, H. T. (2017). Management of Le Fort I fracture. Arch Craniofacial Surg. Retrieved 12 Nov 2022, from https://www.ncbi.nlm.nih.gov/pmc/articles/PMC5556744/.
13. Perkins SW, Dayan SH, Sklarew EC, Hamilton M, Bussell GS. The incidence of sports-related facial trauma in children. Ear Nose Throat J. 2000. Retrieved 12 Nov 2022, from https://pubmed.ncbi.nlm.nih.gov/10969474/.
14. UpToDate. n.d. Retrieved 12 Nov 2022, from https://www.uptodate.com/contents/orbital-fractures?search=factures+of+the+face+&topicRef=343&source=see_link#H13.
15. Fellowship SM. Ear problems and injuries in athletes. Curr Sports Med Rep. 2014. Retrieved 12 Nov 2022, from https://journals.lww.com/acsm-csmr/fulltext/2014/01000/ear_problems_and_injuries_in_athletes.8.aspx.
16. Henry Ford Health Scholarly Commons. Site. n.d. Retrieved 12 Nov 2022, from https://scholarlycommons.henryford.com/.
17. Black AM, Patton DA, Eliason PH, Emery CA. Prevention of sport-related facial injuries. Clin Sports Med. 2017. Retrieved 12 Nov 2022, from https://pubmed.ncbi.nlm.nih.gov/28314416/.
18. Hoffmann JF. An algorithm for the initial management of nasal trauma. Facial Plast Surg. 2015. Retrieved 12 Nov 2022, from https://www.thieme-connect.de/products/ejournals/html/10.1055/s-0035-1555618.
19. Cannon CR, Cannon R, Young K, Replogle W, Stringer S, Gasson E. Characteristics of nasal injuries incurred during sports activities: analysis of 91 patients. Ear Nose Throat J. 2011. Retrieved 12 Nov 2022, from https://pubmed.ncbi.nlm.nih.gov/21853433/.
20. Kucik CJ, Clenney T, Phelan J. Management of acute nasal fractures. Am Fam Physician. 2004. Retrieved 12 Nov 2022, from https://www.aafp.org/pubs/afp/issues/2004/1001/p1315.html.
21. UpToDate. n.d. Retrieved 12 Nov 2022, from https://www.uptodate.com/contents/management-of-epistaxis-in-children?search=Epistaxis+sports&source=search_result&selectedTitle=2~150&usage_type=default&display_rank=2#H2.
22. Ear injuries and trauma. Cleveland Clinic. n.d. Retrieved 12 Nov 2022, from https://my.clevelandclinic.org/health/diseases/17574-ear-injuries-and-trauma.
23. UpToDate. n.d. Retrieved 12 Nov 2022, from https://www.uptodate.com/contents/assessment-and-management-of-auricular-hematoma-and-cauliflower-ear?search=ear+injury+&source=search_result&selectedTitle=2~150&usage_type=default&display_rank=2#H3540956.
24. Ear infections (otitis media). Sports Medicine Today. n.d. Retrieved 12 Nov 2022, from https://www.sportsmedtoday.com/ear-infections-otitis-media-va-213.htm.
25. Tympanic membrane perforations. StatPearls. n.d. Retrieved 12 Nov 2022, from https://www.ncbi.nlm.nih.gov/books/NBK557887/.
26. UpToDate. n.d. Retrieved 12 Nov 2022, from https://www.uptodate.com/contents/complications-of-scuba-diving?search=Divers+ear&source=search_result&selectedTitle=1~150&usage_type=default&display_rank=1#H7.
27. UpToDate. n.d. Retrieved 12 Nov 2022, from https://www.uptodate.com/contents/evaluation-and-management-of-dental-injuries-in-children?search=Dental+and+Orofacial+Injuries+in+sport&source=search_result&selectedTitle=5~150&usage_type=default&display_rank=5.

Further Reading

Unsplash. Beautiful free images & pictures. Unsplash. n.d. Retrieved November 25, 2022, from https://unsplash.com/.

Airway Management

15

Michael Edgar, Luke Zabawa, Sam Jiang,
Salma Mumuni, and Mark R. Hutchinson

15.1 Overview

Alongside cardiopulmonary arrest, airway management necessitates immediate attention regarding sideline care [1–4]. In situations where little evidence of injury may be available, the true severity of injury may not be apparent [1, 3, 4]. In these situations, it becomes necessary to use professional judgment, as maximal damage may not manifest for up to 48 h [1, 3, 4]. Airway emergencies can occur due to a variety of reasons, which may initially present with sudden collapse. This could be due to issues such as heat exhaustion, stroke, cardiac dysrhythmia, seizure, anaphylaxis, status asthmaticus, and convulsion [1, 5, 6]. Other injuries may fall into direct or indirect airway trauma, for example, throat and facial injuries compared to pneumothorax and flail chest [1, 7]. Although one may not typically view some of these as standard airway issues, presentation can involve the loss of tongue muscle tone, which leads it to fall back and obstruct the airway [1, 3, 4]. Moreover, conditions such as these can present with blood and emesis in the airway further complicating the presentation [1, 8].

M. Edgar · L. Zabawa · S. Jiang · S. Mumuni
University of Illinois, Chicago, IL, USA
e-mail: medgar3@uic.edu; zabawa2@uic.edu; sjiang@uic.edu

M. R. Hutchinson (✉)
Sports Medicine, University of Illinois,
Chicago, IL, USA

The appropriate management of emergent airway conditions begins with a proper history and physical exam [1, 9, 10]. A history may be brief given the time-sensitive nature of the condition [1, 9, 10]. Simply having the ability to speak demonstrates a patent airway and may allow for one to discover precipitating events and relevant medical history [1, 9, 10]. In regard to the physical exam, the Advanced Trauma Life Support (ATLS) can allow one to secure a patent area amidst potential injury [1, 9, 10]. This typically starts with the 'ABC' approach by assessing airway, breathing, and circulation [1, 9, 10]. Observations can involve changes in skin color, such as cyanosis, distress, stridor (high-pitched noisy breathing from potential obstruction), and the ability to phonate [1, 9, 10]. Other observations may include signs of tracheal deviation, chest wall motion, breath sounds, accessory respiratory muscle use, and jaw malocclusion [1, 9, 10]. Although this is not a laundry list of observations, each offers insight into the underlying cause of the issue. For example, tracheal deviation and decreased breath sounds may be evident with a tension pneumothorax, whereas jaw malocclusion may indicate a mandibular fracture.

When examining various issues and injuries when performing sideline management, appropriate equipment is necessary. In regard to airway management, necessary equipment typically revolves around cardiopulmonary care [3, 11–14]. This can involve airway equipment, such as

S. Rocha Piedade et al. (eds.), *Sideline Management in Sports*,
https://doi.org/10.1007/978-3-031-33867-0_15

a cricothyrotomy kit, large bore angiocatheter for tension pneumothorax, mouth-to-mouth masks, and short-acting beta-2 agonists [3, 11–14]. It may also involve ACLS drugs and equipment, an automated external defibrillator (AED), blood pressure cuff, prepackaged epinephrine, IV fluids, and a stethoscope [3, 11–14]. Given the immediate emergency of both cardiovascular and pulmonary issues, equipment should be stored together and checked regularly [3, 11–14].

For sideline management of airway problems, the 'ABC' approach is the first step in proper management. This may mean inspection of the mouth and throat to observe for foreign body obstruction, which may be removed manually or with forceps [15–18]. Breathing management may also be managed by lying someone in the recovery position, if one has spontaneous and effective breathing, in order to aid in fluid and foreign material drainage [15–18]. All these maneuvers should be performed while maintaining stabilization of the cervical spine if spinal trauma is suspected. This is performed by keeping the head in a neutral position with one's hands and arms being utilized to stabilize the individual's head, neck, and shoulders [15–18]. Concurrently, someone should have called emergency medical services (EMS) to further handle the issue in an appropriate facility. Despite this, there have been recent controversy over the use of spine immobilization devices such as spine boards and cervical collars when concurrent vascular and airway compromise is present [19, 20]. Several studies have found an increased risk of death with their use given the potential for delayed emergent care or hiding additional severe injuries [19, 20].

If there is airway compromise, there are two simple primary maneuvers. These are the head tilt and chin lift maneuver, and the jaw thrust maneuver (Figs. 15.1, 15.2, 15.3 and 15.4) [15–18]. The latter is the procedure of choice when there is suspected concomitant spinal trauma [15–18]. If the airway is open and ventilation is adequate after performing one of these maneuvers, simply focus on airway maintenance and monitoring their condition. If the airway is open with inadequate ventilation, rescue breathing can

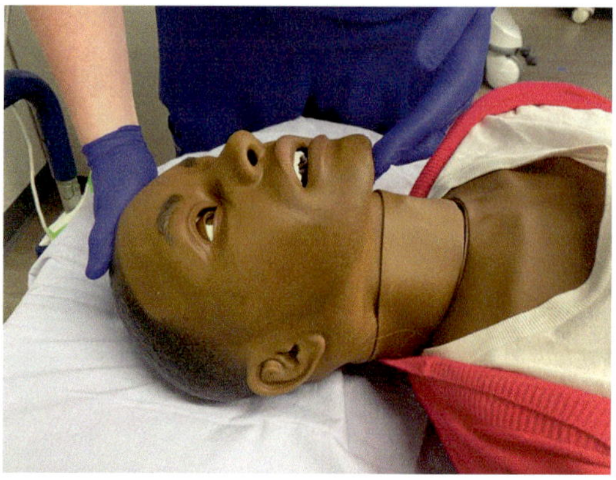

Fig. 15.1 Head tilt adult

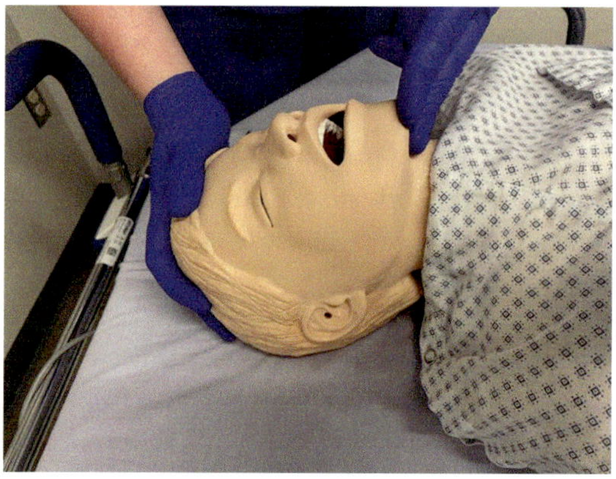

Fig. 15.2 Head tilt child

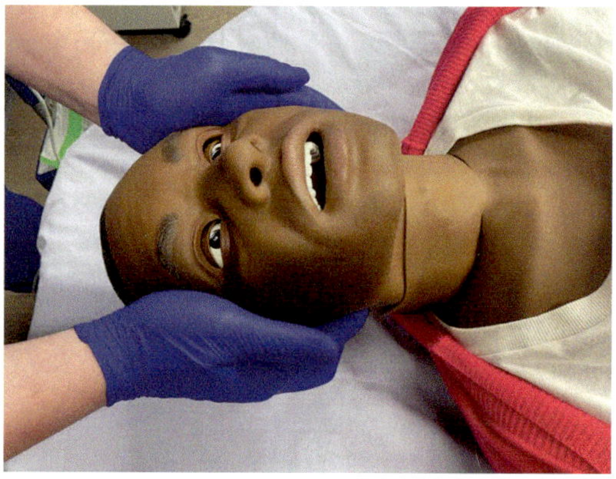

Fig. 15.3 Jaw thrust adult

be performed, with progression to bag ventilation using a mask (Figs. 15.5 and 15.6) [8, 21–23]. Bag mask ventilation should use 100% supplemental oxygen whenever possible [8, 21–23].

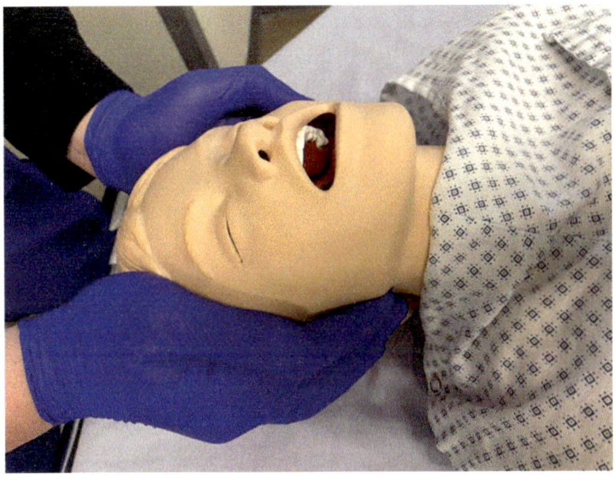

Fig. 15.4 Jaw thrust child

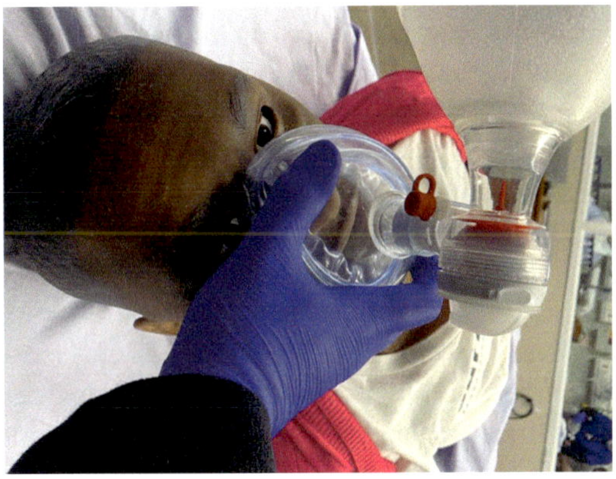

Fig. 15.5 Masking adult

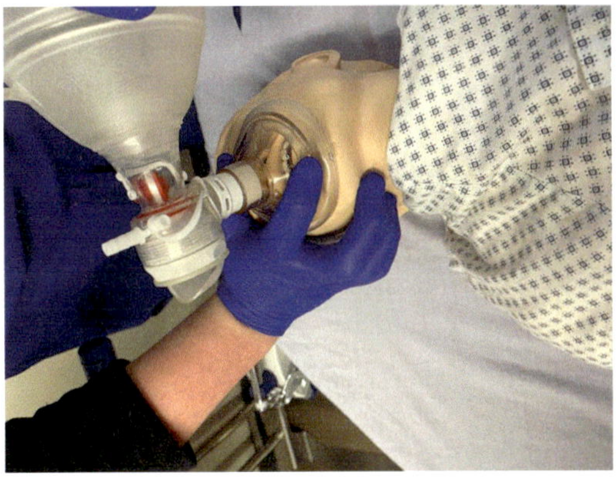

Fig. 15.6 Masking child

Ideally, this should be used alongside an oropharyngeal or nasopharyngeal airway to improve ventilation and prevent the tongue from obstructing the airway, which becomes key in unconscious individuals. Recent literature has also demonstrated additional ease with placement of a nasopharyngeal tube when used alongside a guidewire compared to the conventional neck flexing technique when dealing with unconscious patients [24]. It has also been shown to cause less trauma and complications, both pertinent in an athletic setting when additional bodily trauma may be present [24].

If ventilation is still inadequate, several options exist, including a laryngeal mask, combitube, intubation, or a surgical airway by needle cricothyrotomy or standard cricothyrotomy [3, 21, 25]. A laryngeal mask is an inflatable mask that is passed blindly into the respiratory tract and then the cuff of the mask is inflated [3, 21, 25]. It typically is useful in patients with facial hair as a secure facial seal is not possible with a bag valve mask, although risk of aspiration is possible [3, 21, 25]. An endotracheal tube involves orotracheal intubation which requires a laryngoscope for proper placement [3, 21, 25]. A combitube is described as an esophageal tracheal double lumen airway and used when a patient cannot be endotracheally intubated from direct laryngoscopy [3, 21, 25]. It is typically blindly passed into the oropharynx with a chin-lift maneuver [3, 21, 25].

Finally, a surgical airway may be performed when intubation is not possible, which is typical with hemorrhage, laryngeal edema, or fracture obstruction [21, 26, 27]. The two primary options of percutaneous needle cricothyrotomy and standard cricothyrotomy are typically used in emergent settings, although optimal use depends on the age of the patient [21, 26, 27]. Percutaneous needle cricothyrotomy involves the use of a large bore, catheter-over-needle device through the cricothyroid membrane and is preferred in patients less than 12 years old [21, 26, 27]. A standard surgical cricothyrotomy is preferred in individuals over 12 years of age as it allows for a cricothyroid membrane (CTM) tube large enough for ventilation [21, 26, 27]. Equipment needed for a standard cricothyrotomy involves a #10-blade scalpel, hemostats, a tracheal hook, and endotracheal tube (ETT) or tracheostomy tube [21, 26, 27]. Additionally, a tracheostomy is possible but highly advised against, given the dangers of the procedure when performed within an emergency setting [21, 26, 27].

Finally, in sporting environments with helmet use, unless there are signs of airway compromise, do not remove the helmet prior to the hospital given the risk of spinal trauma. This is in contrast to face masks that should be removed for appropriate assessment by cutting or unscrewing the loops that attach the mask to the helmet [28, 29].

Key Points

- A variety of conditions can compromise the airway both directly and indirectly.
- A prompt history and 'ABC' approach to airway management is key given time sensitivity.
- Simple primary maneuvers include the head tilt and chin lift or the jaw thrust maneuver.
- Surgical airways can be performed with a percutaneous needle cricothyrotomy or standard cricothyrotomy.
- Do not remove the helmet prior to hospital admission given the risk of spinal trauma.

15.2 Throat Injuries

In regard to airway injuries, several forms of traumatic injury are typical [1, 30]. These can involve facial fractures, throat injuries, which can involve larynx fractures, and laryngotracheal junction disruption and soft tissue injury in the respective locations [1, 30–32]. Laryngeal trauma accounts for approximately 1% of blunt and 7% of penetrating trauma, with only 10% being due to athletic injury [1, 30–32]. Despite this, mortality rates for laryngeal trauma can approach 40%, highlighting the severity of the injury [30–32]. Although rare, they are relatively more predominant in sports such as football, hockey, lacrosse, and full contact martial arts [1]. Specific to the United States, football and soccer account for the highest rates of head and neck injury, due to aerial challenges for the ball [30–32]. In general, children sustain fewer laryngeal injuries than adults which is believed to be due to their more elastic skeleton and higher proportion of subcutaneous fat [30–32]. Males also generally sustain a higher proportion of face and neck injuries, accounting for 60–88% of trauma in this region [30–32]. Despite the lower occurrence in females, the highest rate of laryngotracheal injuries are experienced by cheerleaders in this athletic population [30–32].

Throat injuries are typically blunt trauma, and those that go through the platysma, or cross the midline of the neck typically are associated with a higher degree of injury [15, 31, 32]. This typically involves injury to the anterolateral neck region as four major groups of structures are present [15, 31, 32]. These involve the larynx and trachea, tracheobronchial transection, vascular structures, and esophagus and gastrointestinal tract [15, 31, 32]. For penetrating injuries in this region, always inspect for foreign bodies and remove anything that is deeply embedded [15, 31, 32].

Blunt injuries can appear less severe but can be just as fatal and may appear with hoarseness or a weak voice, difficulty breathing due to laryngospasm, or difficulty swallowing due to leak from a gas-containing structure [1, 30–32]. Blunt throat injuries can include laryngeal contusions, laryngeal fracture which may present with a palpable step defect of the thyroid cartilage [1, 30–32]. Additionally, laryngotracheal injuries involving thyroid cartilage fracture can lead to submucosal hemorrhage and rapid edema [1, 30–32]. The individual may also present with dyspnea, hemoptysis, dysphonia, anterior neck tenderness, subcutaneous emphysema, and loss of the normal laryngeal architecture [1, 30–32]. Despite appropriate measures, tracheobronchial injuries typically have a high rate of mortality and a high risk of failure with endotracheal suction.

Given the nature of neck injuries, it becomes pertinent to also recognize other issues which may occur in the vicinity of the airway [1, 30–32]. Vascular injuries such as a carotid artery dissection or aneurysm are typically described as sudden onset throbbing or sharp neck pain and occur at two distinct times, immediately at the time of injury or several hours to days later [1,

30–32]. Due to the rapid lateral flexion, hyperextension and hyperflexion of the neck with some contact sports, such as football and wrestling, an appropriate understanding of the mechanism of injury is necessary to diagnose this as a potential sequelae [1, 30–32]. Finally, aerodigestive issues can be confused with respiratory and airway injuries as they often occur in conjunction with pharyngeal or laryngeal injuries. Injury involves rupture of the esophagus with release of gas into the mediastinum, presenting with emphysema, dysphonia, and dysphagia [1, 30–32]. These injuries typically are not as acute as true tracheobronchial injuries, but can present after hours to days with sequelae such as sepsis [1, 30–32].

Following appropriate assessment and management of neck injuries, several additional imaging modalities may be beneficial. Plain radiographs can offer a means to detect hyoid bone elevation, suggesting cricotracheal separation [1, 33]. Computed tomography (CT) can be used for the initial workup of a suspected laryngeal trauma when no obvious fracture or lacerations are identified during the sideline examination [1, 33]. Finally, fibroscopic endoscopy can help determine the extent of the laryngeal damage or presence of additional mucosal injuries [1, 33].

To appropriately prevent laryngotracheal injury, several steps can be taken [1, 31, 32]. Equipment must be well-maintained, especially for contact sports [1, 31, 32]. Athletic regulators must also adequately enforce existing rules of contact, such as spearing with the head in football [1, 31, 32]. In conjunction, football players and coaches need to be cognizant and adhere to proper blocking and tackling techniques to decrease the likelihood of head and neck injuries [1, 31, 32]. This can be enforced by having athletes utilize proper conditioning, warm-up, and technique play [1, 31, 32]. Finally, appropriate use of equipment, such as helmets, face masks, neck guards, and other protective equipment, can help prevent injuries to the neck [1, 31, 32].

Key Points

- Laryngeal injuries are rare but mortality rates can approach 40%.
- Laryngeal injuries are typically from blunt trauma and may appear less severe despite being just as fatal.
- Prompt CT scan can allow for appropriate initial workup of a suspected laryngeal trauma.

15.3 Facial Injuries

Facial injuries offer another potential for airway compromise. Typically, these injuries occur to the lower third of the face and can present with cyanosis, breathing difficulty, or altered breathing patterns. Sporting activities account for between 3% and 29% of facial injuries and 10% and 42% of facial fractures [30, 34, 35]. These injuries are more common in contact sports and younger male athletes, demonstrating similar prevalence to throat injuries [30, 34, 35].

A first step in sideline examination involves inspection of open or crossbite deformities of the jaw to detect mandibular fractures. There may also be displaced teeth, pain with jaw motion, subjective sensation of an altered bit, or palpable 'step defect' in the dental arch [30, 34, 35]. The individual may also present with numbness to the lip or chin due to inferior alveolar nerve branch damage [30, 34, 35]. Indirect signs of injury can be seen with inspection of the ears and nose due to cerebrospinal fluid leakage. Bruising around the ear and eyes also indicate potential fracture, known as Battle's sign and raccoon eyes, respectively [30, 34, 35]. An otoscope may also reveal blood in the canal or behind an intact eardrum (hemotympanum) [30, 34, 35]. These signs detected by inspection of the ear can be indicative of a fracture of the base of the cranium, known as a basilar fracture [30, 34, 35]. Despite the injuries occurring on the face, patients can present with neck tenderness or pain on movement, due to consequent airway swelling and compromise.

Mandibular fractures can be panfacial fractures with gross displacement, mobility, and swelling due to profuse bleeding from the comminuted mandibular fracture [36, 37]. These injuries most often occur after falls or high-energy blows to the chin and are most common at the body of the mandible (35%), angle (25%), condyle (15%), symphysis (10%), and ramus (5%) [36, 37]. High risk of airway compromise occurs with bilateral anterior mandibular fractures as they can lead to loss of anterior support of the tongue, causing it to fall back and obstruct the airway, which in conjunction with soft tissue swelling leads to an emergent issue.

Although not as common, injury to the upper and middle third of the face can also present with airway obstruction. Typically, these are Le Fort (LF) II and III fractures which are classified by the line of the fracture along the face [36, 37]. LFII fractures typically present with bilateral subconjunctival hematomas and diplopia, periorbital bruising, a symmetric and palpable step deformity of the orbital rims, zygomatic arches, nose, and maxilla with infraorbital nerve damage [36, 37]. LFIII fractures typically present similarly, but are considered more severe with some individuals being unconscious upon inspection [36, 37].

Although sideline assessment and care of these conditions are necessary first steps, hospital admission is required for appropriate management, as greater than 50% of mandibular fractures require surgical repair [30, 34, 35]. As such, plain radiographs can allow for general assessment of the facial fracture locations, while a CT can allow for more specific detail to be noted for bony abnormalities [30, 34, 35]. Appropriate prevention of facial injuries follows similar principles to throat injuries given the traumatic nature of the condition. Additional emphasis should be placed on equipment that protects the face, such as helmets, visors, and safety glasses [34–36].

Key Points

- Facial injuries typically occur in the lower third of the face.
- Inspect jaw malocclusion and intraorally for additional trauma.
- Understand that bilateral mandibular fracture has a high rate of concurrent airway compromise.
- Facial fractures can be categorized using the Le Fort classification system.

15.4 Indirect Injuries

A variety of other injuries may also indirectly lead to airway and respiratory issues. For example, pneumothorax, cervical spine injury, chest trauma that may lead to airway swelling, and spinal shock can present with decreased respiratory drive [15, 38]. For traumatic injury or spontaneous breathing issues, pneumothorax should be suspected in tall, thin, young males who present with signs of breathlessness, chest pain, dry cough, increased heart rate and breathing rate, and diminished breath sounds and chest hyperresonance on physical exam [39, 40]. Although rare, 2% of adult pneumothorax are associated with sport [39, 40]. Pneumothorax can also occur secondary to traumatic injuries such as rib fracture, in which bone fragments can pierce the pleural lining [38]. As such, it is important to be aware of potential secondary injury in the area.

A more severe form of pneumothorax known as tension pneumothorax revolves around increased air collection in the pleural space of the chest cavity which leads to increased pressure. This in turn causes mediastinal shift and compression of trachea and cardiovascular vessels which can lead to issues such as obstructive shock [39, 40]. As such, this condition needs to be treated as a medical emergency, especially if signs such as jugular venous distension and tracheal deviation are noted [39, 40]. A condition which may appear as pneumothorax at first observation is pneumomediastinum, in which air collects in the mediastinal area after a traumatic injury in sport [39, 40]. Typically, some unique findings include dysphagia, dysphonia, voice hoarseness, and subcutaneous emphysema, in which crackles of air can be felt beneath the skin [39, 40]. Given its rare occurrence, no epidemiological data exist for its prevalence within various sports [39].

Given that pneumothorax may occur secondary to rib fracture, it is paramount to understand potential respiratory sequelae directly related to the traumatic injury [41, 42]. Severe compressive injury to the chest wall can lead to multiple sequential rib fractures, which may cause a condition known as flail chest [41, 42]. Flail chest is described as four or more consecutive rib fractures in at least two places [41, 42]. The issue that arises from this is paradoxical breathing, in which the affected portion of the chest wall collapses during inspiration and expands during expiration [41, 42]. Rib fractures and flail chest tend to occur after force is directed to the chest wall anteriorly at a 60° rotation from the sternum, which may occur in high-impact contact sports [41, 42]. If forces are strong enough, they may also disrupt the sternochondral junction, which is the point where the rib attaches to the sternum, causing increased breathing problems [41, 42]. In regard to sport, high-impact chest trauma typically results from direct impact and rapid deceleration to the chest wall [43]. This can be from impact with another competitor, contact with fixed sporting equipment such as a goalpost, or sport projectile such as a baseball [43]. Athletes that experience serious chest wall injuries typically lack sufficient external protection [43]. Despite its rare occurrence in sport, general epidemiology demonstrates that flail chest occurs in up to 10% of chest wall trauma and has a mortality rate ranging between 10% and 15% highlighting its severity [41, 42].

During physical examination, paradoxical chest movement with normal respiration can be noted. In addition, the individual may describe severe chest wall pain and show signs of respiratory insufficiency such as increased breathing rate [41, 42]. This can be in conjunction to decreased breath sounds that may indicate a pneumothorax, pulmonary contusion, or hemothorax, as previously described [41, 42]. Initial sideline management of flail chest, pneumothorax, and hemothorax is focused primarily on maintaining appropriate ventilation given the impaired breathing mechanics and lung compliance [41, 42]. Pain management is also recommended for conditions such as flail chest, in which nonsteroidal anti-inflammatory drugs (NSAIDs) may be prescribed for use [41, 42]. Upon hospital arrival, emergent imaging typically involves chest radiographs which demonstrate the rib fractures along the lateral and posterior aspects of the rib [41, 42]. In addition, a chest and abdominal CT are typically performed to investigate other potential sequelae of the injury, such as aortic dissection, pneumothorax, and hemothorax. To better protect athletes and prevent injuries to this region, improved education on protective equipment to the thorax should be considered, especially in sports with high-speed collisions or projectiles.

Key Points

- Indirect trauma such as pneumothorax and severe rib fractures can present additional challenges for airway patency.
- Remember to inspect other body regions and not simply the face and throat in isolation.

15.5 Allergies and Autoimmune Airway Compromise

Moreover, asthma and other respiratory emergencies should be suspected if there was no trauma present. Acute asthma (status asthmaticus) affects 3–50% athletes and typically presents with laryngeal edema, bronchospasm, stridor, wheezing, cyanosis, and potentially shock [15, 44]. Timely use of an inhaled ß-2 sympathomimetics should be used until there is improvement [15, 44, 45]. A milder form of this may also present as exercise-induced bronchospasm which presents in 30–70% of athletes or acute respiratory difficulty due to air pollution [40].

Although similar, anaphylaxis may also present similarly, although the etiology usually involves contact with an allergen. Anaphylaxis typically occurs in females with a 2:1 ratio, with a mean age of 37.5 years. It is more pronounced in submaximal sporting activities such as jogging, running, dancing, tennis, cycling, swimming, and skiing [45, 46]. In children, 5–15% of anaphylactic episodes due to a food allergen can be exacerbated by exercise or can be triggered by the combination of both but by neither in isolation [44–47]. Anaphylaxis typically presents with airway, lip, tongue, and pharyngeal and epiglottic swelling [15, 44]. They may also experience cardiovascular compromise due to peripheral vasodilation, which presents with redness and warmth when touched [15, 44]. Other signs of laryngeal edema, bronchospasm, stridor, hoarseness, wheezing, cyanosis, and shock will present similarly to asthma [15, 44]. In order to adequately treat anaphylaxis, there should be urgent administration of 0.5 mg of adrenaline by intramuscular injection [15, 44].

Key Points

- Clinicians should be up-to-date on the medical history of athletes on the field.
- Airway compromise can be nontraumatic in a sports setting.

15.6 Miscellaneous Respiratory Issues

There are a myriad of conditions which can lead to airway compromise issues that are not typically considered related to sideline care. That being said, an astute clinician should always keep a large differential given the difference in management needed for appropriate care of unique conditions. Issues such as pulmonary embolism should be suspected when there is a history of travel, bed rest, or recent surgery, in conjunction with signs of dyspnea, or pleuritic chest pain without any trauma. In such situations, the patients should be laid supine and given oxygen by facemask [48, 49]. Although rates of pulmonary embolism in sport are limited, data suggest a rare incidence of 1.27–2.06 cases per 1000 players per year in the National Basketball Association (NBA) [48, 49]. It has also been found that men (66.7%) are predominantly affected in basketball with a mean age for men being 28.8 years old and 20.4 years old in women [48, 49]. Typically, treatment for massive, life-threatening embolism is treated with intra-arterial thrombolytics which destroy the blood clot, or more invasive interventions such as a thrombectomy, to directly remove the thrombus [49, 50].

Convulsions offer another important condition to consider when managing airway compromise in sport [15, 51]. Sport-related convulsions are considered more common in full contact sports such as hockey, mixed martial arts, boxing, rugby, Australian football, wrestling, and soccer [15, 51]. It typically affects younger adults around 23–24 years old and mainly presents with posturing, which involves tonic contraction of the limbs [15, 51]. Less common presentations involve focal motor, generalized tonic clonic and myoclonic seizures. After concussive convulsion, the mean time until return to play is approximately 15 days [51].

Convulsions can appear very dramatic in the moment, but keeping a level head when approaching an individual experiencing one is key to management [51]. For sideline management, superficial suction of secretions or blood should be done to avoid aspiration and to maintain a clear airway [51]. Additionally, antiepileptic medications can be used, although bite sticks are no longer recommended for individuals currently having a convulsion [51]. Additional testing and imaging typically involve electroencephalography (EEG) and brain imaging which typically involves CT or MRI [51]. Despite resolution of the condition, long-term sequelae of post-concussive convulsions can present in up to 7% of patients. This can involve conditions such as post-traumatic encephalopathy and recurrent seizures are common sequelae [51]. Given long-term sequelae, an appropriate record of athletes who have experienced convulsions in the past is appropriate for prevention and prompt management if they occur again.

Key Points

- Be aware of other conditions which may present with airway compromise such as pulmonary embolism and convulsions.

15.7 Conclusion

Overall, there are a variety of injuries that both directly and indirectly compromise the airway or breathing ability of athletes. Prompt diagnosis and treatment is necessary to avoid devastating consequences. Being aware of the various injuries more common to specific sports or athletic populations can help the astute clinician when guiding sideline management. Currently, the IOC and NCAA both have the most extensive manuals dedicated to airway injuries. They may offer a consolidated resource for airway injury diagnosis, treatment protocols, and preventative strategies that sporting institutions can use to prevent their occurrence. Additional research should aim to better organize the various injuries which may compromise the airway and guidelines should be developed and appropriately applied to better prevent their occurrence within sport.

References

1. Paluska SA, Lansford CD. Laryngeal trauma in sport. Curr Sports Med Rep. 2008;7(1):16–21.
2. Jaworski CA. Advances in emergent airway management. Curr Sports Med Rep. 2002;1(3):133–40.
3. Waterbrook AL, Davenport M. Initial evaluation, resuscitation, and acute management. In: Sports-related fractures, dislocations and trauma. Cham: Springer; 2020. p. 3–9.
4. Conway D, Urquhart CS. Airway trauma. Anaesth Intensive Care Med. 2017;18(4):199–201.
5. Adams WM. Exertional heat stroke within secondary school athletics. Curr Sports Med Rep. 2019;18(4):149–53.
6. Carter JM, McGrew C. Seizure disorders and exercise/sports participation. Curr Sports Med Rep. 2021;20(1):26–30.
7. Dobitsch AA, Oleck NC, Liu FC, Halsey JN, Hoppe IC, Lee ES, Granick MS. Sports-related pediatric facial trauma: analysis of facial fracture pattern and concomitant injuries. Surg J. 2019;5(04):e146–9.
8. Madkhali EE, Albati SA, Ahmad HF, Alzhrani SM, Nassir AY, Albalawi BM, Heji AS, Alhashim AG, Alarfaj AA, Alsaffar AH, Alharbi MG. Emergency airway management in neck trauma. Egypt J Hosp Med. 2018;70(3):409–13.
9. Ahmad I, Onwochei DN, Muldoon S, Keane O, El-Boghdadly K. Airway management research: a systematic review. Anaesthesia. 2019;74(2):225–36.
10. Kovacs G, Sowers N. Airway management in trauma. Emerg Med Clin. 2018;36(1):61–84.
11. Olympia RP, Brady J. Emergency preparedness in high school–based athletics: a review of the literature and recommendations for sport health professionals. Phys Sportsmed. 2013;41(2):15–25.
12. Micheo W. Sports coverage: the handbook for the sports medicine clinician. Springer Publishing Company; 2020.
13. Stuart MJ. Facial injuries in sports, an issue of clinics in sports medicine. Elsevier Health Sciences; 2017.
14. Callender SS. Being a team physician. Curr Sports Med Rep. 2018;17(2):39–40.
15. McDonagh DO, Zideman DA. The IOC manual of emergency sports medicine. John Wiley & Sons; 2015.
16. Colbenson K. An algorithmic approach to triaging facial trauma on the sidelines. Clin Sports Med. 2017;36(2):279–85.
17. Ray R, Luchies C, Bazuin D, Farrell RN. Airway preparation techniques for the cervical spine-injured football player. J Athl Train. 1995;30(3):217.
18. Van de Vliet P, Wilkinson M. Emergency medical care in paralympic sports. In: The IOC manual of emergency sports medicine. Wiley Blackwell; 2015. p. 212–9.
19. Vanderlan WB, Tew BE, McSwain NE Jr. Increased risk of death with cervical spine immobilisation in penetrating cervical trauma. Injury. 2009;40(8):880–3.
20. Walters BC, Hadley MN, Hurlbert RJ, Aarabi B, Dhall SS, Gelb DE, Harrigan MR, Rozelle CJ, Ryken TC, Theodore N. Guidelines for the management of acute cervical spine and spinal cord injuries: 2013 update. Neurosurgery. 2013;60(CN_Suppl_1):82–91.
21. Norris RL, Peterson J. Airway management for the sports physician: part 1: basic techniques. Phys Sportsmed. 2001;29(10):23–9.
22. Way DP, Panchal AR, Finnegan GI, Terndrup TE. Airway management proficiency checklist for assessing paramedic performance. Prehosp Emerg Care. 2017;21(3):354–61.
23. Mendis D, Anderson JA. Blunt laryngeal trauma secondary to sporting injuries. J Laryngol Otol. 2017;131(8):728–35.
24. Baratlou A, Mokhlesian M, Khajavi M, Behseresht A. Nasopharyngeal tube placement in emergency intubated patients with decreased consciousness with a new guidewire: a prospective randomized controlled trial. Tehran Univ Med J. 2021;78(10):678–83.
25. Asimakopoulos P, Montague ML. Acute airway conditions. In: ENT head & neck emergencies. CRC Press; 2018. p. 215–24.
26. Zasso FB, You-Ten KE, Ryu M, Losyeva K, Tanwani J, Siddiqui N. Complications of cricothyroidotomy versus tracheostomy in emergency surgical airway management: a systematic review. BMC Anesthesiol. 2020;20(1):216.
27. Eng J, Sivam S. General overview of the facial trauma evaluation. Facial Plast Surg Clin. 2022;30(1):1–9.
28. Hersch RF. Cervical spine motion and collegiate athletic trainer confidence during helmet removal: a multi methods study.
29. Waninger KN. Management of the helmeted athlete with suspected cervical spine injury. Am J Sports Med. 2004;32(5):1331–50.

30. Viozzi CF. Maxillofacial and mandibular fractures in sports. Clin Sports Med. 2017;36(2):355–68.
31. Iarocci AL, Winters RD. Laryngeal trauma: a review of current diagnostic and management strategies. Curr Opin Otolaryngol Head Neck Surg. 2022;30(4):276–80.
32. Lane AD. Soft tissue neck injury. In: Sports-related fractures, dislocations and trauma. Cham: Springer; 2020. p. 803–10.
33. Henry M, Hern HG. Traumatic injuries of the ear, nose and throat. Emerg Med Clin. 2019;37(1):131–6.
34. Hwang K. Field management of facial injuries in sports. J Craniofac Surg. 2020;31(2):e179–82.
35. Chukwulebe S, Hogrefe C. The diagnosis and management of facial bone fractures. Emerg Med Clin. 2019;37(1):137–51.
36. Reehal P. Facial injury in sport. Curr Sports Med Rep. 2010;9(1):27–34.
37. Gómez Roselló E, Quiles Granado AM, Artajona Garcia M, Juanpere Martí S, Laguillo Sala G, Beltrán Mármol B, Pedraza GS. Facial fractures: classification and highlights for a useful report. Insights Imaging. 2020;11(1):1–5.
38. Alent J, Narducci DM, Moran B, Coris E. Sternal injuries in sport: a review of the literature. Sports Med. 2018;48(12):2715–24.
39. Curtin SM, Tucker AM, Gens DR. Pneumothorax in sports: issues in recognition and follow-up care. Phys Sportsmed. 2000;28(8):23–32.
40. Gonzalez A, Mares AV, Espinoza DR. Common pulmonary conditions in sport. Clin Sports Med. 2019;38(4):563–75.
41. Pettiford BL, Luketich JD, Landreneau RJ. The management of flail chest. Thorac Surg Clin. 2007;17(1):25–33.
42. Baiu I, Spain D. Rib fractures. JAMA. 2019;321(18):1836.
43. Thomas RD, De Luigi AJ. Chest trauma in athletes. Curr Sports Med Rep. 2018;17(8):251–3.
44. Christensen MJ, Eller E, Kjaer HF, Broesby-Olsen S, Mortz CG, Bindslev-Jensen C. Exercise-induced anaphylaxis: causes, consequences, and management recommendations. Expert Rev Clin Immunol. 2019;15(3):265–73.
45. Chenuel B. Induced asthma and sport. Rev Prat. 2020;70(9):997–1004.
46. Bonini M, Palange P. Anaphylaxis and sport. Curr Opin Allergy Clin Immunol. 2014;14(4):323–7.
47. Toit GD. Food-dependent exercise-induced anaphylaxis in childhood. Pediatr Allergy Immunol. 2007;18(5):455–63.
48. Casals M, Martínez JA, Caylà JA, Martín V. Do basketball players have a high risk of pulmonary embolism? A scoping review. Med Sci Sports Exerc. 2016;48(3):466–71.
49. Bishop M, Astolfi M, Padegimas E, DeLuca P, Hammoud S. Venous thromboembolism within professional American sport leagues. Orthop J Sports Med. 2017;5(12):2325967117745530.
50. Lapner ST, Kearon C. Diagnosis and management of pulmonary embolism. BMJ. 2013;346:f757.
51. Kuhl NO, Yengo-Kahn AM, Burnette H, Solomon GS, Zuckerman SL. Sport-related concussive convulsions: a systematic review. Phys Sportsmed. 2018;46(1):1–7.

16 Thorax, Abdomen, and Genital

Sérgio Rocha Piedade, Rogério Fortunato de Barros, Ricardo Kalaf, and Daniel Miranda Ferreira

16.1 Introduction

Sports trauma is not restricted to the musculoskeletal system; it could also result in injuries to the thorax, abdomen, and genitals and affect their internal organs [1].

Each of these areas has its particular anatomy, bone framework, and sheltered internal organs. In sports, the primary mechanisms for thorax injury are direct trauma and sudden deceleration and high or low-energy trauma to the abdomen, such as a direct blow, deceleration, or penetration [2].

S. R. Piedade (✉)
Exercise and Sports Medicine, Department of Orthopedics, Rheumatology and Traumatology, University of Campinas—UNICAMP, Campinas, SP, Brazil
e-mail: piedade@unicamp.br

R. F. de Barros
São Leopoldo Mandic Faculty of Medicine, Campinas, SP, Brazil

R. Kalaf
Thoracic Surgery Division, State University of Campinas—UNICAMP, Campinas, SP, Brazil

D. M. Ferreira
Exercise and Sports Medicine, Department of Radiology, University of Campinas—UNICAMP, Campinas, SP, Brazil

Radiology at São Leopoldo Mandic Faculty of Medicine, Campinas, SP, Brazil

The thorax presents a ribcage with the heart, lungs, oesophagus, trachea, and other organs and structures [3]. Despite the protection of these internal organs provided by this bone structure, it is limited to the chest wall integrity, Fig. 16.1. When high-energy trauma damages this cage causing a bone fracture, the dislocation of fragments may injure these internal organs.

Moreover, in the female athlete, the trauma on the thorax may cause a breast contusion and hematoma, clinically manifested by pain, discomfort, and sensibility [4, 5].

The abdomen is between the thorax and the pelvis, and its cavity shelters most digestive organs, such as the intestine, stomach, liver, gallbladder, and pancreas (Fig. 16.2) [6]. Although most injuries result from muscle strains and contusions, anatomically, the abdomen does not have a bone framework surrounding its internal organs, making it more vulnerable to direct trauma [7, 8]. Despite its minor anatomical protection and vulnerability to sports trauma, most sports modalities do not require the regular use of abdominal protective equipment.

In sports, genital injuries are less frequently reported than others [9]. However, they could occur in traumas involving athlete collisions, kicks, and falls, particularly in contact sports, and sometimes problems related to the sports equipment. While in females, the genitals are anatomically internal and externally located, in males, the

S. Rocha Piedade et al. (eds.), *Sideline Management in Sports*,
https://doi.org/10.1007/978-3-031-33867-0_16

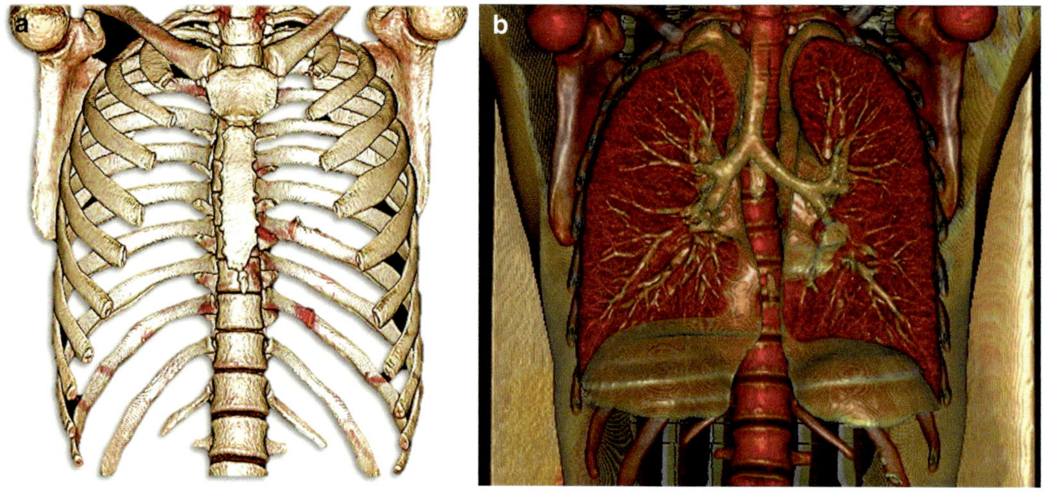

Fig. 16.1 Full-field view computed tomography of the thorax in a 3D volume rendered image using a high opacity threshold for bone (**a**) and a low opacity for internal soft tissues (**b**)

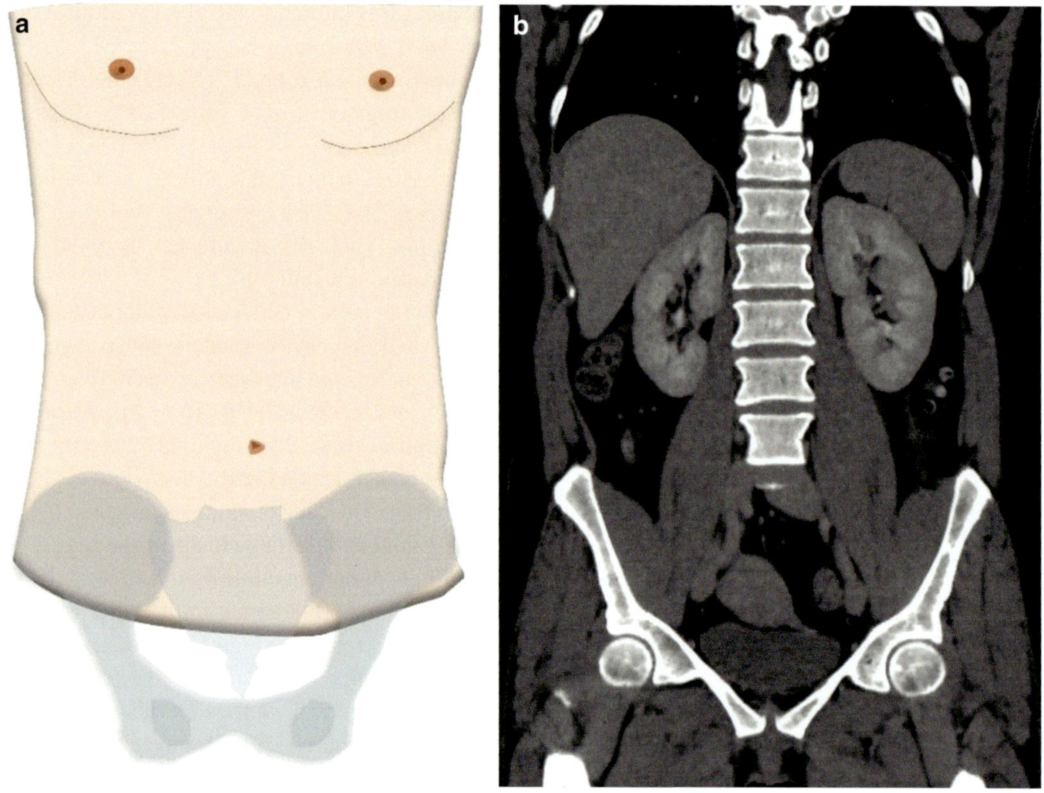

Fig. 16.2 (**a**) Drawing showing the relationship between the abdomen and the pelvis bone. (**b**) Coronal CT scan image of normal abdominal in soft tissue window for visualization of internal parenchymal organs

genital is more exposed to trauma and injuries due to their external location [10].

This chapter approaches the initial physical assessment, the most common sports injuries on the thorax, abdomen, and genital, discussing the initial assessment and proper investigation of athletes' clinical complaints and findings, followed by a well-practised intervention protocol that will play an essential role in optimizing the outcome of each case.

16.2 Initial Physical Assessment

The sports physician guides the initial physical assessment by carefully inspecting the athlete's reported complaints of local pain and discomfort and performing clinical manoeuvres to search for specific injuries related to the trauma mechanism [11–13].

In sports trauma, most of the injuries in the thorax, abdomen, and genital areas are restricted to skin abrasions, swelling, muscle strains, and contusions and, therefore, do not prevent the athlete from returning to the field of play [14].

However, the thorax and abdominal injuries caused by the considerable kinetic energy of trauma can cause life-threatening conditions [15–17]. Therefore, in these cases, the physician must pay close attention when assessing an athlete with suspicion of intra-thoracic or abdominal injury to identify any clinical signs of hemodynamic instability such as an abnormal heartbeat, shortness of breath, pulmonary congestion, or cold extremities—suggesting internal bleeding or shock [14, 17–19].

16.3 Thoracic Injuries in Sports

The skin, muscle, and ribcage are the structures of the first protection line of the thorax against external trauma [3]. Consequently, skin abrasions, contusions, and fractures are the primary clinical events reported in sports practice, and the level of trauma energy determines the injury's complexity [13].

Blunt trauma to the thoracic wall is the primary mechanism of chest injuries in sports [18]. They may result in contusions or fractures in the clavicle, ribs, sternoclavicular joint, and sternal manubrium. In general, they are a single injury and could be diagnosed quickly by the physician by assessing the site of pain, ecchymosis, or bone crepitation [20]. Although most of these injuries do not risk an athlete's life, the physician should be aware of high-energy traumas or perforating ones, such as hemothorax, pneumothorax, or even pulmonary contusion [2, 14, 21]. Therefore, the physician should be mindful of any sign of athlete's dyspnea, hypoxia, tachypnea, blood-tinged sputum, and chest pain. Remember: look, feel, listen, percuss!

An example is the paradoxical chest movement ("fail chest") that results from various rib fractures in two or more chest locations that harm the pulmonary function, worsening the ventilation and gas exchange [22] (Fig. 16.3).

The initial assessment of sports thorax trauma starts by checking whether the athlete's breathing pattern is regular or has any abnormality such as difficulty or even pain; the athlete is holding his chest wall; a thorax asymmetry when breath-

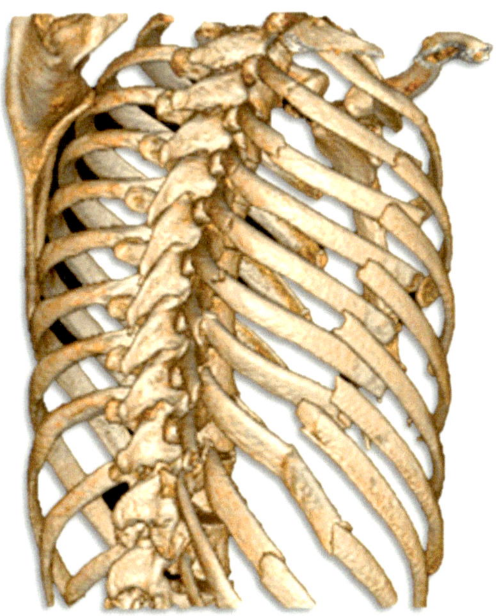

Fig. 16.3 Full-field view computed tomography of the thorax in a 3D volume rendered image using a high opacity threshold for bone, demonstrating fractures of multiple ribs

ing—**red flags** [11, 23]. The evaluation follows by palpating areas of tenderness in the ribs, intercostal spaces, sternum, and costochondral joints and performing anterior-posterior pressure on the chest wall to check the presence of rib fractures [23]. Some thoracic trauma injuries and their main clinical and radiological findings are presented in Table 16.1.

Table 16.1 Thoracic trauma injuries' main clinical and radiological findings

	Diagnosis	
Thoracic trauma	Main clinical findings	Radiology
Pulmonary contusion and respiratory distress	Hypoxemia, hypercarbia, and an increase in laboured breathing	Consolidation patterns ("traumatic pneumonia") typically appear within 4–6 h after injury, but only 47% of lesions are detected at the time of admission, whereas 92% are seen 24 h after injury. In **CT scan—**focal, non-segmental areas of parenchymal opacification (typically crescentic), peripheral, posteriorly, and in lower lobes.
Pneumothorax	Dyspnea and chest pain. In tension pneumothorax, patients are distressed with rapid, laboured respirations, cyanosis, profuse diaphoresis, and tachycardia.	A thin discrete radiopaque line parallel to the chest wall, absent peripheral vessel markings. Subtle findings of pneumothorax may be non-identified at radiography. However, a **CT scan** should be performed if tension pneumothorax is clinically suspected.
Hemothorax	Broad and overlapping pneumothorax; respiratory distress, tachypnea, decreased or absent breath sounds, dullness to percussion, chest wall asymmetry, tracheal deviation, hypoxia, narrow pulse pressure, and hypotension	Costophrenic angle blunting, hemidiaphragm obscuration, homogeneous hemithorax opacity, fluid within the interlobar fissures, or an apical cap. **Thoracic FAST** has a sensitivity equivalent to or greater than that of radiography. **CT scan** has the highest sensitivity for hemothorax and can also provide clues about a time frame. An extrapleural hematoma can mimic a hemothorax and is present in approximately 7% of cases of traumatic thoracic injury
Commotio cordis	Presumptively made based upon the clinical scenario available electrocardiographic (ECG) data demonstrating ventricular fibrillation and the absence of structural heart disease or myocardial trauma on imaging studies.	Absence of structural heart damage on imaging studies (echocardiogram, computed tomography of the chest)
Traumatic diaphragmatic hernia	In some cases, there may be no initial symptoms or signs suggesting a diaphragm injury. With time, the diaphragmatic defect increases, and abdominal organs are likely to be herniated, mainly on the left-sided diminished breath sounds. In case of a herniated stomach, air injected into the nasogastric tube may be heard in the chest upon auscultation, although this finding is nonspecific.	**CXR**: Diaphragmatic can be as obvious as visualization of the stomach or other abdominal organs in the chest. **US exam**: Discontinuity of the diaphragm, herniation of the liver or bowel loops through a diaphragmatic defect, floating diaphragm, or non-visualization of the diaphragm. **CT scan** detects diaphragm injury and helps assess the posterior lumbar elements of the diaphragm (crura and arcuate ligaments) **MRI** does not play a significant role in the initial evaluation of the injured patient.

Table 16.1 (continued)

	Diagnosis	
Thoracic trauma	Main clinical findings	Radiology
Cardiac tamponade	Beck's triad, namely low arterial blood pressure, dilated neck veins and muffled heart sounds, chest pain Syncope or presyncope Dyspnea and tachypnea Tachycardia Peripheral edema Pulsus paradoxal Narrow pulse pressure	**CXR**: Enlarged cardiac silhouette with clear lung fields. In general, however, the findings on a chest radiograph are neither sensitive nor specific for diagnosing cardiac tamponade. Although cardiac tamponade is a clinical diagnosis, two-dimensional and Doppler echocardiography play a major role in identifying pericardial effusion and assessing hemodynamic significance. If echocardiography is available, other imaging techniques, such as CT scan and MR, are not usually necessary for pericardial effusion evaluation.

Abbreviations: *CT scan* computed tomography, *Thoracic FAST* thoracic focused assessment with sonography for trauma, *CXR* chest X-ray, *US exam* ultrasonography, *MRI* magnetic resonance imaging [24, 25]

16.3.1 Key Points in Assessing Sports Thorax Injuries on the Sideline

If the athlete is dyspneic, offer oxygen support.

In the case of pneumothorax and hemothorax, the focus of acute treatment is the hemodynamic stabilization of the athlete. Therefore, ABSc life support begins with airway management and simultaneously the diagnosis determination before hospital transfer.

If a **tension pneumothorax is clinically suspected** (distressed with rapid, laboured respirations, cyanosis, profuse diaphoresis, and tachycardia), a needle decompression should be performed by inserting a 14 or 18-gauge needle into the second intercostal space in the midclavicular line just above the third rib [26, 27].

In case of "fail chest" (unstable thorax due to multiple rib fractures), perform a manual stabilization or apply a bulky dressing to fail segment to transfer to a hospital facility [28].

16.3.2 Abdominal Injuries in Sports

Sports-related abdominal trauma often results from falls and blunt trauma mechanisms- involving minor injuries such as muscle strains and contusions, quickly diagnosed and managed conservatively. Nevertheless, in high-energy sports trauma, deceleration or penetrating trauma mechanisms on the abdomen may become a real challenge to evaluate the athlete on the sideline sports scene [13, 29].

Regarding high-energy trauma, children and young athletes are more vulnerable to severe abdominal injury because their abdominal wall is thinner, and their ribs are less robust than adults' ones [30]. Moreover, symptoms of abdominal injuries following blunt trauma may not be obvious, and clinical signs or symptoms may appear hours or days later, explaining some misdiagnoses. Besides that, the sports physician should remember that spleen, liver, and kidney injuries are closely related to high-energy abdominal trauma [31]. Eventually, the small bowel, pancreas, or bladder may rupture intra or retroperitoneally and delay the diagnosis [32, 33].

16.4 Abdominal Physical Assessment

The abdomen's sports trauma assessment begins with a careful clinical inspection, searching for abrasions, bruising, lacerations, penetration and/or punctures, tenderness, swelling, deformities, and asymmetry [29, 34]. Moreover, with close attention to local ecchymosis that, when present in the periumbilical area (Cullen's sign) and the flanks (Grey-Turner's sign), could suggest a retroperitoneal haemorrhage [35]. Patterned bruising of abdominal wall in blunt trauma is called London sign. It indicates that the impacting force is sharp and severe enough to cause visceral injury, such as an intestine perforation [36]. Moreover, it is mandatory to assess the stability of the pelvic ring, particularly in cases of suspicious pelvic or lower limb fractures. Therefore, a gentle manual maneuver pushing the pelvis and the iliac crest inward and outward allows for identifying any instability or bone crepitus of the pelvis ring.

Another point to assess is the abdominal shape and the presence of abdominal distension because asymmetrical distension could be high-suspicious internal bleeding. The abdomen auscultation will be more adequately performed out of the field of play, with close attention to bowel sounds, because its absence may signal free peritoneal blood. The physical examination is followed by abdomen percussion and palpation, checking areas of tenderness, guarding, pain elicited by activity, fulness, crepitation, and peritonism. The sports physician should be aware of clinical signs of hemodynamic instability, clinically manifested by a progressive increase of abdominal discomfort and pain in the left shoulder or proximal arm (Kehr's sign—splenic injury), focal pain, tenderness, a palpable or visible tender mass, nausea, vomiting guarding, and abdomen rigidity [36–39]. Table 16.2 summarizes the decision-making in abdominal trauma in athletes based on the clinical findings.

Table 16.2 Clinical findings and decision-making in abdominal trauma in athletes

Athlete's abdominal trauma	
Clinical findings and complaints	Decision-making
Transient complaints, normal abdomen status, hemodynamically stable, and no additional injury	May return to the field of play
Equivocal findings Normal hemodynamic status	**The athlete should be removed from the game** Further investigation in the trauma care center
Evident abdominal injury	**Immediately transferred** **To a hospital or trauma center**

16.4.1 Genital Injury

Genital injuries in athletes are less commonly reported than musculoskeletal ones, and in more than 80% of cases, blunt trauma is the primary mechanism of injury. Although genital penetrating trauma is less reported, these injuries may require tissue debridement according to the tissue damage [40].

In clinical practice, the trauma energy will result in more or less significant injury. It may be commonly manifested by local pain, tenderness to palpation, swelling, and sometimes ecchymosis. The localization of the swelling helps guide the physical assessment. When located distally to the neck of the scrotum, it may implicate testicular injury, epididymal injury, or hydrocele, whereas the presence of swelling above this location may be related to incarcerated hernia or spermatic cord injury [41].

16.4.2 Scrotal Trauma

A scrotal trauma may result in a hematoma, hydrocele, hematocele, testicular fracture, rupture, or torsion, and pain and swelling will occur quickly. A hemiscrotal hematocele may present as a large tender mass associated with loss of the scrotum rugae. Moreover, hematocele may be related to testicular rupture, and in these cases, the ultrasound exam will show an echogenic discontinuity of tunica albuginea. The early diagnosis of testicular rupture is critical because emergent surgery results in testis salvage in more than 80% of cases [42].

The physical findings of testicular torsion and scrotal trauma may be similar. At the same time, a painful scrotum may result from testicular torsion, epididymitis, or contusion of the scrotum wall and scrotal hematocele with or no testis rupture.

The outcomes are strictly related to the early diagnosis, and testicular exploration should promptly indicate in case of testicular torsion because a gradual testicular death takes place after 6 h, and survival reduces drastically after 24 h [43–45].

16.4.3 Labial and Penile Trauma

The trauma of the vaginal labial may curse with severe hematomas, and an adequate clinical evaluation will require local anaesthesia on the vagina and/or urethra. Large hematoma may cause urinary retention; sometimes, catheter drainage will be necessary.

When the hematoma is extensive, there is a risk for urinary retention, and sometimes urethral catheter drainage is indicated. Antibiotics prescription will be guided by assessing the local tissue conditions and considering trauma energy characteristics.

Penis injury is uncommon in sports, and an operation is rarely needed. It may occur after zipper injuries that are easily managed by opening the zipper on both sides, which solves this type of problem. However, in case of severe penis injuries, an individualized surgical approach is needed, and microvascular repair and skin grafting may be required [46] Regarding genital neuropathies, cycling has been associated with them and erectile dysfunction in males. Women riders also have decreased genital sensation due to repetitive low-energy trauma [47, 48].

Take Home Messages

- The level of kinetic energy involved in the trauma mechanism will help identify the red flags and minimize the risks to the athlete's health.
- Thorax trauma starts by checking whether the athlete's breathing pattern is regular or has any abnormality.
- The presence of ecchymosis in the periumbilical or flank of the abdomen could indirectly signal a retroperitoneal haemorrhage.
- The physical findings of testicular torsion and scrotal trauma may be similar.
- In case of testicular torsion, the outcomes are strictly related to the early diagnosis and prompt testicular exploration.
- In vaginal labial trauma, large hematoma may cause urinary retention, and sometimes, catheter drainage will be necessary.
- In case of severe penis injuries, an individualized surgical approach is needed.

References

1. Kudzinskas A, Callahan AL. Anatomy, thorax. Treasure Island, FL: StatPearls Publishing; 2022.
2. Phillips NR, Kunz DE. Chest trauma in athletic medicine. Curr Sports Med Rep. 2018;17:90–6. https://doi.org/10.1249/JSR.0000000000000464.
3. Tang A, Bordoni B. Anatomy, thorax, muscles. Treasure Island, FL: StatPearls Publishing; 2022.
4. Obourn PJ, Benoit J, Brady G, Campbell E, Rizzone K. Sports medicine-related breast and chest conditions-update of current literature. Curr Sports Med Rep. 2021;20:140–9. https://doi.org/10.1249/JSR.0000000000000824.
5. Krajcová A, Hurt K, Kufa R, Molitor M. Breast implant rupture: a sports trauma report. Ces Gynekol. 2020;85:116–9.
6. Marsland MJ, Tomic D, Brian PL, Lazarus MD. Abdominal anatomy tutorial using a medical imaging platform. MedEdPORTAL J Teach Learn Resour. 2018;14:10748. https://doi.org/10.15766/mep_2374-8265.10748.
7. Sido B, Grenacher L, Friess H, Büchler MW. [Abdominal trauma]. Orthopade. 2005;34:880–8. https://doi.org/10.1007/s00132-005-0846-1.
8. Feliciano DV. Abdominal trauma revisited. Am Surg. 2017;83:1193–202.
9. Bagga HS, Fisher PB, Tasian GE, Blaschko SD, McCulloch CE, McAninch JW, et al. Sports-related genitourinary injuries presenting to United States emergency departments. Urology. 2015;85:239–44. https://doi.org/10.1016/j.urology.2014.07.075.
10. Bieniek JM, Sumfest JM. Sports-related testicular injuries and the use of protective equipment among young male athletes. Urology. 2014;84:1485–9. https://doi.org/10.1016/j.urology.2014.09.007.
11. Smith D. Chest injuries, what the sports physical therapist should know. Int J Sports Phys Ther. 2011;6:357–60.

12. Intravia JM, DeBerardino TM. Evaluation of blunt abdominal trauma. Clin Sports Med. 2013;32:211–8. https://doi.org/10.1016/j.csm.2012.12.001.
13. Chen AW, Archbold CS, Hutchinson M, Domb BG. Sideline management of nonmusculoskeletal injuries by the orthopaedic team physician. J Am Acad Orthop Surg. 2019;27:e146–55. https://doi.org/10.5435/JAAOS-D-17-00237.
14. Gregory PL, Biswas AC, Batt ME. Musculoskeletal problems of the chest wall in athletes. Sports Med. 2002;32:235–50. https://doi.org/10.2165/00007256-200232040-00003.
15. Yamamoto L, Schroeder C, Morley D, Beliveau C. Thoracic trauma: the deadly dozen. Crit Care Nurs Q. 2005;28:22–40. https://doi.org/10.1097/00002727-200501000-00004.
16. Maron BJ, Link MS. Don't forget commotio cordis. Am J Cardiol. 2021;156:134–5. https://doi.org/10.1016/j.amjcard.2021.05.053.
17. Adam J, De Luigi AJ. Blunt abdominal trauma in sports. Curr Sports Med Rep. 2018;17:317–9. https://doi.org/10.1249/JSR.0000000000000519.
18. Varada SL, Popkin CA, Hecht EM, Ahmad CS, Levine WN, Brown M, et al. Athletic injuries of the thoracic cage. Radiographics. 2021;41:E20–39. https://doi.org/10.1148/rg.2021200105.
19. Gosteli G, Yersin B, Mabire C, Pasquier M, Albrecht R, Carron P-N. Retrospective analysis of 616 air-rescue trauma cases related to the practice of extreme sports. Injury. 2016;47:1414–20. https://doi.org/10.1016/j.injury.2016.03.025.
20. Thomas RD, De Luigi AJ. Chest trauma in athletes. Curr Sports Med Rep. 2018;17:251–3. https://doi.org/10.1249/JSR.0000000000000503.
21. Sano A, Yotsumoto T. Chest injuries related to surfing. Asian Cardiovasc Thorac Ann. 2015;23:839–41. https://doi.org/10.1177/0218492315591103.
22. de Campos JRM, White TW. Chest wall stabilization in trauma patients: why, when, and how? J Thorac Dis. 2018;10:S951–62. https://doi.org/10.21037/jtd.2018.04.69.
23. Pettiford BL, Luketich JD, Landreneau RJ. The management of flail chest. Thorac Surg Clin. 2007;17:25–33. https://doi.org/10.1016/j.thorsurg.2007.02.005.
24. Rashid MA, Wikström T, Ortenwall P. Nomenclature, classification, and signficance of traumatic extrapleural hematoma. J Trauma. 2000;49:286–90. https://doi.org/10.1097/00005373-200008000-00016.
25. Maron BJ, Gohman TE, Kyle SB, Estes NAM 3rd, Link MS. Clinical profile and spectrum of commotio cordis. JAMA. 2002;287:1142–6. https://doi.org/10.1001/jama.287.9.1142.
26. Jalota Sahota R, Sayad E. Tension pneumothorax. Treasure Island, FL: StatPearls Publishing; 2022.
27. Azizi N, Ter Avest E, Hoek AE, Admiraal-van de Pas Y, Buizert PJ, Peijs DR, et al. Optimal anatomical location for needle chest decompression for tension pneumothorax: a multicenter prospective cohort study. Injury. 2020; https://doi.org/10.1016/j.injury.2020.10.068.
28. Dehghan N, Nauth A, Schemitsch E, Vicente M, Jenkinson R, Kreder H, et al. Operative vs nonoperative treatment of acute unstable chest wall injuries: a randomized clinical trial. JAMA Surg. 2022;157:983–90. https://doi.org/10.1001/jamasurg.2022.4299.
29. Barrett C, Smith D. Recognition and management of abdominal injuries at athletic events. Int J Sports Phys Ther. 2012;7:448–51.
30. Sanchez JI, Paidas CN. Childhood trauma. Now and in the new millennium. Surg Clin North Am. 1999;79:1503–35. https://doi.org/10.1016/s0039-6109(05)70090-6.
31. Diamond DL. Sports-related abdominal trauma. Clin Sports Med. 1989;8:91–9.
32. Gad MA, Saber A, Farrag S, Shams ME, Ellabban GM. Incidence, patterns, and factors predicting mortality of abdominal injuries in trauma patients. N Am J Med Sci. 2012;4:129–34. https://doi.org/10.4103/1947-2714.93889.
33. Ribas-Filho JM, Malafaia O, Fouani MM, da Justen MS, Pedri LE, da Silva LMA, et al. Trauma abdominal: estudo das lesões mais frequentes do sistema digestório e suas causas. ABCD Arq Bras Cir Dig (São Paulo). 2008;21:170–4. https://doi.org/10.1590/S0102-67202008000400004.
34. Haycock CE, How I. Manage abdominal injuries. Phys Sportsmed. 1986;14:86–99. https://doi.org/10.1080/00913847.1986.11709102.
35. Guldner GT, Magee EM. Grey-Turner sign. StatPearls; 2022.
36. Raveenthiran V. The London sign (patterned bruising of blunt abdominal trauma). J Pediatr Surg. 2018;53:1252–3. https://doi.org/10.1016/j.jpedsurg.2018.03.013.
37. Harmsen AMK, Giannakopoulos GF, Moerbeek PR, Jansma EP, Bonjer HJ, Bloemers FW. The influence of prehospital time on trauma patients outcome: a systematic review. Injury. 2015;46:602–9. https://doi.org/10.1016/j.injury.2015.01.008.
38. Kotwal RS, Howard JT, Orman JA, Tarpey BW, Bailey JA, Champion HR, et al. The effect of a golden hour policy on the morbidity and mortality of combat casualties. JAMA Surg. 2016;151:15–24. https://doi.org/10.1001/jamasurg.2015.3104.
39. Farhat GA, Abdu RA, Vanek VW. Delayed splenic rupture: real or imaginary? Am Surg. 1992;58:340–5.
40. Sacco E, Marangi F, Pinto F, D'Addessi A, Racioppi M, Gulino G, et al. [Sports and genitourinary traumas]. Urologia. 2010;77:112–25.
41. Randhawa H, Blankstein U, Davies T. Scrotal trauma: a case report and review of the literature. Can Urol Assoc J. 2019;13:S67–71. https://doi.org/10.5489/cuaj.5981.
42. Deurdulian C, Mittelstaedt CA, Chong WK, Fielding JR. US of acute scrotal trauma: optimal technique, imaging findings, and management. Radiographics. 2007;27:357–69. https://doi.org/10.1148/rg.272065117.
43. Sandella B, Hartmann B, Berkson D, Hong E. Testicular conditions in athletes: torsion, tumors,

and epididymitis. Curr Sports Med Rep. 2012;11:92–5. https://doi.org/10.1249/JSR.0b013e31824c8886.
44. Seng YJ, Moissinac K. Trauma induced testicular torsion: a reminder for the unwary. J Accid Emerg Med. 2000;17:381–2. https://doi.org/10.1136/emj.17.5.381.
45. Mellick LB, Sinex JE, Gibson RW, Mears K. A systematic review of testicle survival time after a torsion event. Pediatr Emerg Care. 2019;35:821–5. https://doi.org/10.1097/PEC.0000000000001287.
46. Hunter SR, Lishnak TS, Powers AM, Lisle DK. Male genital trauma in sports. Clin Sports Med. 2013;32:247–54. https://doi.org/10.1016/j.csm.2012.12.012.
47. Partin SN, Connell KA, Schrader S, LaCombe J, Lowe B, Sweeney A, et al. The bar sinister: does handlebar level damage the pelvic floor in female cyclists? J Sex Med. 2012;9:1367–73. https://doi.org/10.1111/j.1743-6109.2012.02680.x.
48. Dettori JR, Koepsell TD, Cummings P, Corman JM. Erectile dysfunction after a long-distance cycling event: associations with bicycle characteristics. J Urol. 2004;172:637–41. https://doi.org/10.1097/01.ju.0000130749.37731.9f.

Part III

Evaluation and Management Athlete's Health and Illness

17 Importance of PPE, Athlete Medical History, Family History, Identifying Predisposing Factors and Potential Red Flags

Sérgio Rocha Piedade
and Daniel Miranda Ferreira

17.1 Introduction

Sports practice drives us to challenges and achievements, pushing us to invest in health; however, this physical activity is not free from injuries. Each sports modality has a particular level of intensity (judo, soccer, American football, tennis, swimming), physical demands (running, triathlon), practice environment (indoor or outdoor), material (racquet, gloves, ball, skate, sports clothes, and shoes), and even specific sports-related injuries that define the DNA of sports modality [1–4].

Over time, measures of adjustments in the rules of the sport, improvement and implementation of protective measures (mouth guards, helmets, gloves), and rest intervals during the games have contributed to reducing the occurrence and minimizing **sports** injuries **during training and competition**.

S. R. Piedade (✉)
Exercise and Sports Medicine, Department of Orthopedics, Rheumatology, and Traumatology, University of Campinas—UNICAMP, Campinas, SP, Brazil
e-mail: piedade@unicamp.br

D. M. Ferreira
Exercise and Sports Medicine, Department of Radiology, University of Campinas—UNICAMP, Campinas, SP, Brazil

Radiology at São Leopoldo Mandic, Faculty of Medicine, Campinas, SP, Brazil

However, the sports physician should keep in mind that sports injuries are not restricted to trauma events, and nontraumatic injuries are also part of an athlete's life. Aging, being overweight, previous injuries, handicaps, and chronic diseases such as diabetes, hypertension, and heart disease may negatively impact an athlete's health. Therefore, any measure to assess and monitor the athlete's health is welcome and necessary, mainly for professional athletes who constantly push their body limits through high physical demands and substantial psychological distress.

This fact reinforces the importance of athletes' pre-participation and periodic clinical assessment. On the other hand, recreational and regular sports practitioners should not be excluded from this evaluation, and a pre-participation assessment should be performed before starting regular sports practice.

The pre-participation evaluation is the cornerstone of sports injury prevention. It is crucial in assessing athletes' global health, screening, and recognizing clinical comorbidities, handicaps, or underlying conditions that may be life-treating or impose relative or formal contraindication to sports practice. PPE has become an essential tool for monitoring athletes' health during their sports lifetime, defining medical recommendations and strategies to reduce the risk of exposing an athlete to an adverse clinical condition [5–9].

Athletes should be conscious that PPE does not preclude them from sports practice. Still, it

S. Rocha Piedade et al. (eds.), *Sideline Management in Sports*,
https://doi.org/10.1007/978-3-031-33867-0_17

allows the physician to diagnose a clinical condition, comorbidity, or even an underlying disease to assess and treat it adequately [10–13].

The chapter approaches the PPE in athletes and calls attention to points of athletes' and family medical history, oral and physical assessment, and the importance of screening predisposing diseases and potential red flags.

17.2 Pre-participation Evaluation

The pre-participation assessment starts with recording information about the athlete's medical and injury history and family medical history to screen possible **cardiovascular underlying disease related to sudden cardiac arrest**. Moreover, it helps to tailor the PPE for each specific athlete's population regardless of age, gender, sports modality, clinical comorbidities, previous injuries, and level of sports practice (professional or recreational).

17.3 When Should PPE Be Performed?

In clinical practice, a period of 6–8 weeks before starting sports practice or a new program involving higher physical demands is an adequate time for injury rehabilitation, screening, and managing medical disorders that could affect an athlete's performance and predispose them to injuries, even adverse health conditions.

Broadly speaking, decision-making involves identifying formal risks to the athlete's health, considering that the athlete will be safe:

- Under medical treatment
- Participating in other sports
- Cleared for some specific physical activities or sports
- Because this problem does not expose them to the risk of injury or loss of life

17.4 The Three-Key Points of Anamnesis

The anamnesis is structured into three-key points to screen an underlying disease and record the athlete's medical history, previous and new injuries and complaints related to sports practice, and also family health history [14–17]. These reported data will guide the sports physician to perform the physical evaluation. Anamnesis should be carried out in a pleasant and friendly environment, making the athlete more confident and comfortable to informally reply the questions about their motivation to practice sports, sport/quality of life, and health concerns. The athlete's answer should be graded from 0 to 10:

- How motivated are you to play sports?
- Do you feel in good shape to **practice sports**?
- Have you been sleeping well?
- Do you have any **concerns** with healthy eating?
- Do you have any **complaints** when playing sports?

Table 17.1 summarizes potential disease and potential red flags to be screening in athlete's anamnesis.

17.4.1 The Athletes' Health History

Recorded data of an athlete's health history aim to identify the complaints and disorders related to their physical activity and psychological distress in sports practice and to investigate how these conditions occur or could be relieved. Damasceno et al. pointed out that assessing the athlete's nutritional deficiencies through oral health evaluation is crucial. Moreover, it is essential to identify previous and new injuries and complaints related to chest pain, fatigue, and breathing difficulties when performing high-intensity physical activity. Table 17.1 highlights relevant points to be explored in athletes' health history [18].

Table 17.1 Screening predisposing diseases and potential reds flags

Neurological	
	Mental confusion or memory loss after head trauma, suspicious of sports-related concussion
Psychological distress or disorders	
	Anxiety, depression, OCD, eating disorders, anorexia, REDS
Skin	
	Dermatitis, allergies (triggered by food, insects, medicines), infections (bacteria, virus), acne (wrestlers), surgical scars
Oral (7-Oral Health Assessment)	
	Tooth pain, gingivitis, tooth loss, simplex herpes
Gastrointestinal disorders	
	Gastrite, hepatitis, abdomen tenderness, or masses
Cardiovascular	
	Shortness of breath and fatigue with exertion, exertional chest pain, irregular heartbeat, syncope
Respiratory	
	Exercise-induced bronchospasm, chronic respiratory problems (asthma, bk) or acute (infections, pneumonia)
Urinary	
	Infections, calculus, nephritis, kidney agenesis
Endocrinological	
	Diabetes, hyperparathyroidism, hypercholesterolemia
Special clinical signs in females	
	Menstrual dysfunction, amenorrhea or oligomenorrhea, osteoporosis (young female)
Musculoskeletal	
	Muscle injury, sprain, ligament injury, prior fracture, hernia, rheumatologic diseases, myopathy, arthrosis
Regular medication use (chronic diseases)	
	Antidepressive, steroids, anti-inflammatory drugs, beta blocker, diuretic, etc.
Hospitalization/previous surgeries/injuries under treatment	
	Fracture, ligament reconstruction, arthrodesis, heart revascularization, transfusion
Vaccination history	
	Hepatitis A; hepatitis B; ACWY meningitis and meningitis B; triple virus (MMR), etc.

17.4.2 Family Medical History

Members from the same family have more than genetics; they also share the same environment, lifestyle, nutrition and, therefore, genes and social habits that build their body development and guide health. These reports may help consider and identify possible underlying diseases, such as cardiovascular (hypertension, myocardiopathy), asthma and exercise-induced bronchospasm, diabetes, hematological, gastrointestinal, neurological, eating, or even a psychiatric one that could be involved in the athlete's complaints.

17.4.3 Physical Assessment

The physical assessment is optimized by the information obtained in the anamnesis: athlete's complaints, medical history, and family medical reports.

17.4.4 Oral Health Assessment

In this context, as pointed out by Damasceno et al. [19], oral health plays a crucial role in an athlete's health because it can assess an athlete's oral hygiene and identify indirect signs of an underlying disease and dietary deficiency. Damasceno et al. [19] propose a systematic assessment of seven-oral health points to address the athletes' oral hygiene and maintenance (periodical exams) and identify clues of systemic diseases that may impact the athletes' performance. The 7-oral health assessment covers the entire oral cavity topography (Fig. 17.1a): extraoral region (1), lips (2), teeth (3), gingiva (4), tongue and oropharynx (5), other mucosae (6), and saliva (7). Table 17.2 presents the 7-oral health assessment and addressed points [19].

The sports physician should be aware of the status and color of the lips, mucosas, teeth conditions (normal structural integrity (a), dental plaque (biofilm stagnation) and/or the presence of calculus (tartar) (b), dental loss (c), and also tooth wear (indirect signs of anxiety, depression, or stress that could commonly be associated with bruxism) (d), and also athlete's oral hygiene.

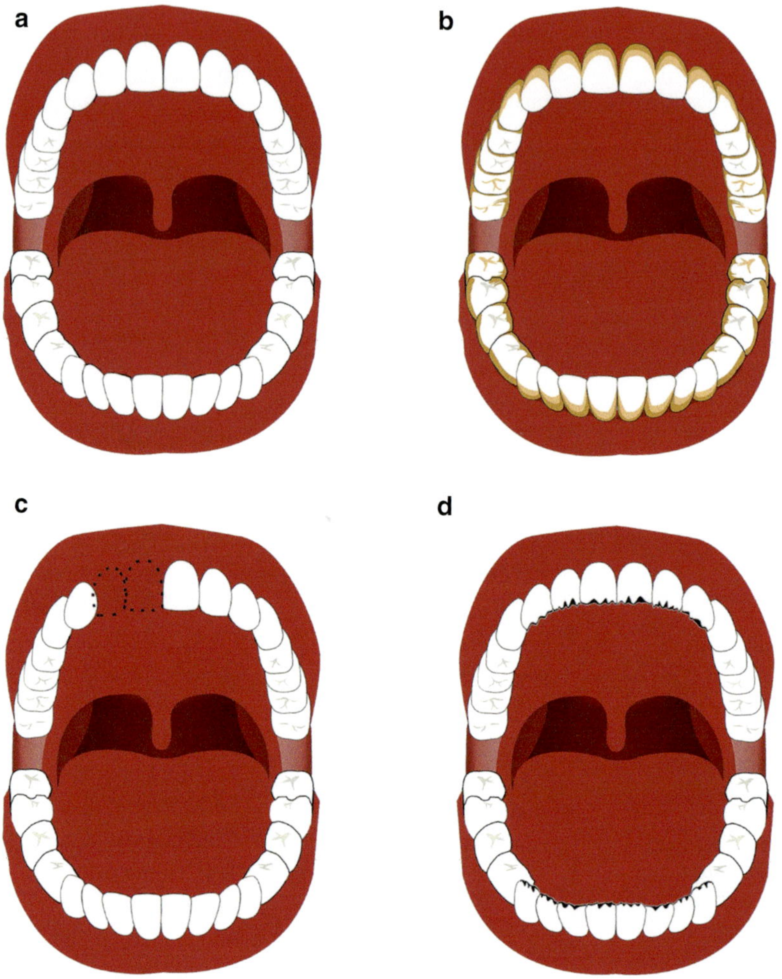

Fig. 17.1 Oral cavity assessment showing four different conditions: (**a**) a healthy month, (**b**) dental tartar, (**c**) dental loss, and (**d**) bruxism. (Source: Ana Karina Piedade)

17.4.5 Musculoskeletal Physical Assessment

With the athlete standing, wearing underwear and no shirt, the physician inspects a general view of the body. The skin is screened for lesions and scars. The **dynamic physical evaluation starts with** the sports physician seeking to identify any changes in gait, such as limping. Then, the spine motion is assessed (Fig. 17.2). It is followed by the upper limbs and **finishes** with the lower limbs (Fig. 17.3).

Muscle balance, strength asymmetry, and joint range of motion between limbs are systematically evaluated to screen and identify muscle weakness, stretching deficit, uni or bilateral joint motion restriction, limb discrepancy or malalignment, and collagen disease (such as Marfan disease) that will expose the athlete to injuries (Fig. 17.3).

Table 17.2 Seven-oral health assessment and addressed points

Seven-oral health assessment	Addressed points
Extraoral region	Salivary glands Lymph nodes Temporomandibular joint **Oral breathing pattern**
Lips	**Painful fissures** (**cheilitis** → unilateral or bilateral chronic lesion with painful fissures in labial commissure and can be associated with atrophy, ulceration, candidiasis, and bacterial infection) **Labial edema** (immunological disorder) **Ulcers** (**painless** → chronic trauma, syphilitic cancer, oral squamous cell carcinoma) **Aphthous ulcer** **Vesicles** (simplex herpes)
Teeth	Integrity, biofilm stagnation (bacterial plaque), presence of calculus (tartar), and dental losses
Gingiva	Chronic gingivitis is painless with a red-swollen appearance and presents gingival bleeding during dental brushing
Tongue and oropharynx	The presence of pus in the tonsils and oropharynx associated with palpable painful cervical lymph nodes indicates bacterial pharyngotonsillitis
Other mucosae	Alveolar and jugal mucosae and hard palate
Saliva	*Identify clinical and adverse conditions* **Cortisol and testosterone** (physiological indexes of sports performance) **Alpha-amylase** (a biomarker of physical stress) **Reduction of IgA-s** (↑↑ susceptibility to infection)

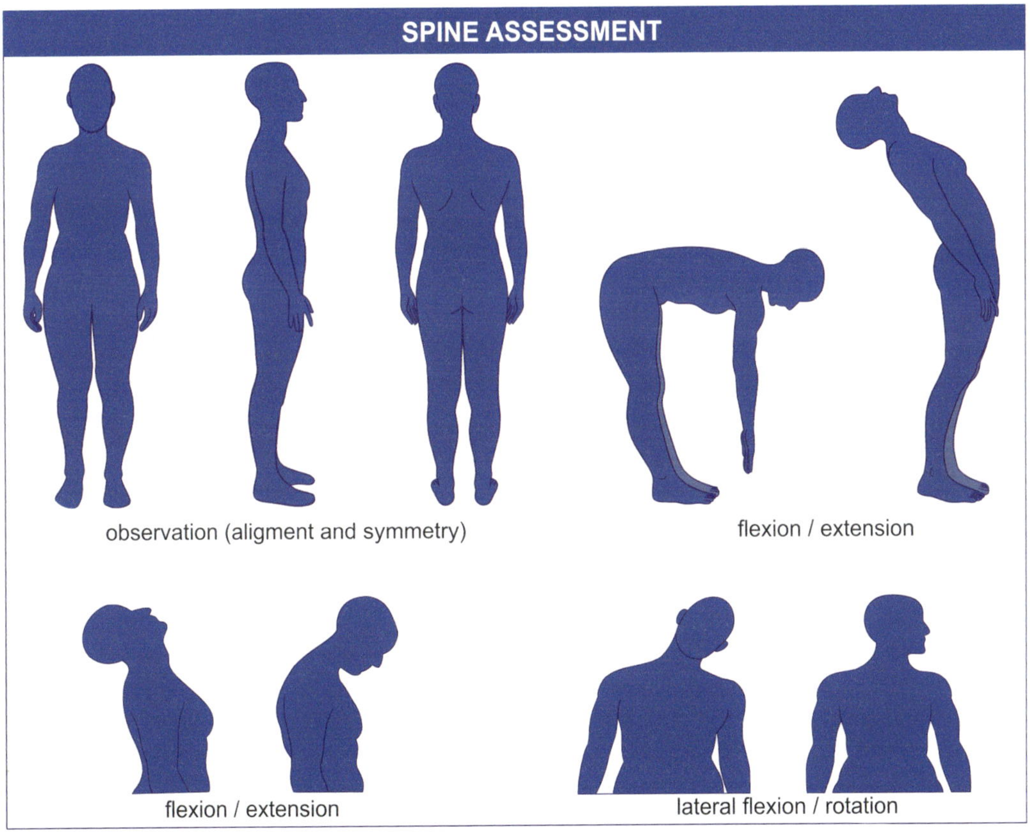

Fig. 17.2 Clinical assessment of spine. (Source: Mariana Percario Piedade)

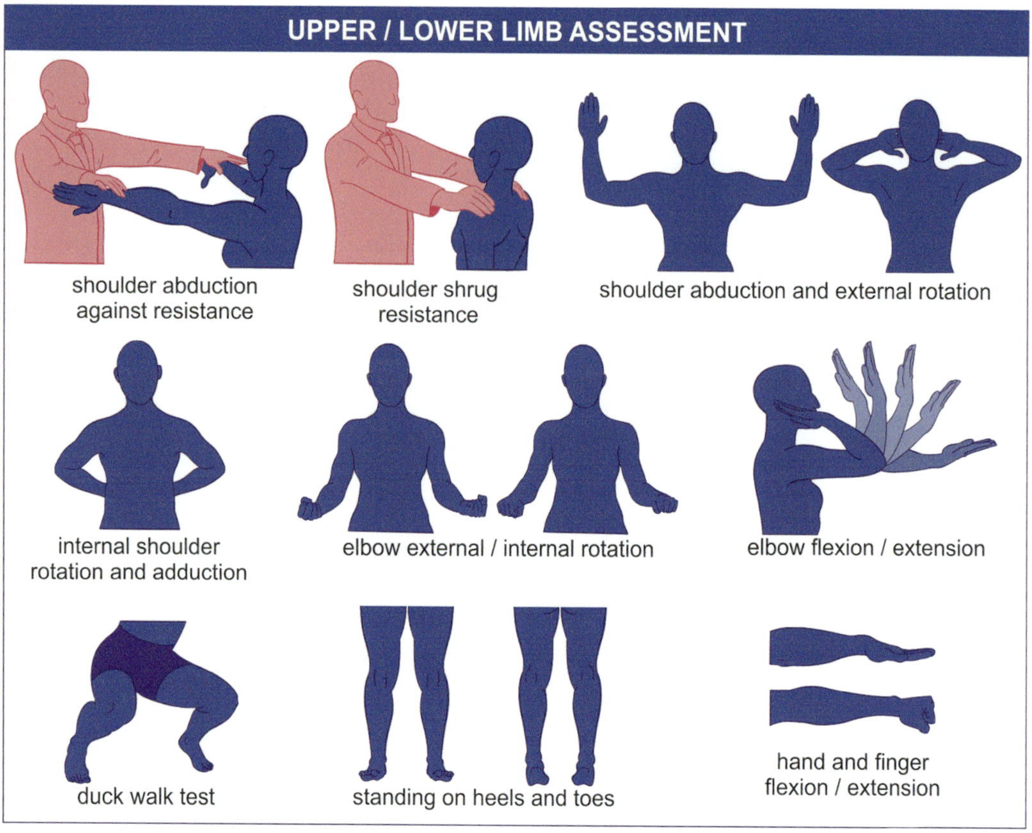

Fig. 17.3 Clinical assessment of upper and lower limbs. (Source: Mariana Percario Piedade)

17.5 PPE for Childhood and Adolescent Athletes

The sports medicine physician should remember that childhood and adolescence include individuals developing biological patterns and social behaviors that will manifest throughout their lives. Bone and muscle maturation is a lively process that involves biomechanical changes in the living tissues. In children, the bone structure is immature and consequently weaker (less mineralized) and ductile, whereas, in adolescents, the bone is more mineralized and, therefore, stiffer and more brittle until bone maturation occurs. Thus, this biological process and clinical patterns reinforce the concept that children cannot be considered small adults.

PPE helps screen unfavorable athletes' clinical conditions in some sports modalities allowing the physician to treat an athlete adequately, such as rhinitis or recurrent sinusitis or other clinical problem, such as the initial stages of Energy Deficiency in Sport (REDs)—low energy availability (involving eating disorders or not), low bone mineral density, and menstrual dysfunction, and therefore, should be carefully investigated [20, 21].

PPE guides whether a radiological assessment and laboratory test are needed based on the anamnesis and clinical findings in the physical examination, considering the practiced sports modality and physical demands involved. Moreover, psychological and mental distress should be assessed because young athletes go through a process of maturity involving more responsibility, obligations, and biological changes, which make them more vulnerable to social distress, overtraining conditions, and family pressure that may expose them to the inadequate social behavior of alcohol, smoking, and drug addiction [22–24].

17.6 Adulthood and Old Age

Life expectancy has contributed to many people starting regular physical activity and sports practice. In adulthood, the athlete reaches body maturity; however, this is the moment that the onset of musculoskeletal decline occurs, followed by progressive degenerative body changes involving joint degeneration and chronic diseases, such as obesity, hypertension, diabetes, hypercholesterolemia, arthrosis, and cardiovascular disorders.

This scenario reinforces the importance of PPE in the adults and elderly population because aging athletes are exposed to exercise-induced cardiovascular events related to undiagnosed coronary artery disease, which is the primary cause of sudden cardiac death in masters' athletes [25].

17.7 The Key Points of Pre-participation Physical Assessment

The sports physician must be aware of the major physical demands and potential risks of practiced sports. Close attention to the athlete's physical and psychological maturity is also important, particularly in athletes exposed to high mental stress due to their competition level [26].

Endurance sports, soccer, American football, cycling, basketball, volleyball, and MMA are examples of sports where the pre-participation assessment should be complemented by a periodic and careful cardiological evaluation, particularly in the case of the athlete's previous history of syncope, hypoglycemia, epilepsy, and heart problems. The cardiological assessment should include an electrocardiogram at rest and laboratory tests for triglyceride, cholesterol, and glycemia levels. A Doppler echocardiogram assesses the heart structure and function adapted to physical activity. An ergometric and cardiopulmonary test should be performed until exhaustion or stopped if the athlete presents adverse clinical signs or symptoms during the exam.

Moreover, laboratory exams are also required to evaluate kidney function, screen contagious and sexually transmitted diseases (hepatitis, AIDS), medical history of transfusion, and check the use of drugs, alcohol, and smoking, as shown in Table 17.3.

Table 17.3 Required laboratory exams by Premier League soccer teams for athletes' admission and clinical follow-up

Complete blood count (CBC)
Coagulation tests
Activated partial thromboplastin time
Prothrombin time and international normalized ratio (INR)
Platelet count
Bleeding time
Glucose
Kidney tests
Blood urea nitrogen, creatinine
Lipid profile
Total cholesterol, HDL, LDL, and triglycerides
Rheumatoid factor
C-reactive protein
Antinuclear factor (ANF)
Urinalysis
Serology
Hepatitis A, B, and C
Chagas disease serology
HIV serology
Liver tests
Alkaline phosphatase (ALP)
Alanine aminotransferase (ALT)
Aspartate aminotransferase (AST)
Creatine phosphokinase (CPK)
Lactate dehydrogenase (LDH)
Hormones
Thyroid profile: Thyroid stimulating hormone (TSH), T3, T4
Total and free testosterone
Dehydroepiandrosterone
Dihydrotestosterone
Uric acid

Take Home Messages

- The pre-participation evaluation (PPE) does not prevent an athlete from sports practice, but it is crucial in assessing underlying conditions that may be life-treating, causing sudden death.
- PPE should be performed 6–8 weeks before starting sports practice or a new program involving higher physical demands.

- Oral health assessment is essential in addressing oral hygiene and identifying indirect signs of an underlying disease and dietary deficiency.
- PPE helps screen unfavorable clinical conditions in young athletes, such as rhinitis or recurrent sinusitis, or other clinical problems, such as the initial stages of Energy Deficiency in Sport (REDs).
- Physicians must keep in mind that aging athletes are exposed to exercise-induced cardiovascular events related to undiagnosed coronary artery disease.

Acknowledgment We thank Ana Karina Piedade and Mariana Percario Piedade for preparing the figures.

References

1. Bianchi FP, Veneziani V, Cantalice MA, Notarnicola A, Tafuri S. Epidemiology of injuries among Italian footballers: the role of the playing field. Inj Prev. 2019;25:501–6.
2. Reissig J, Bitterman A, Lee S. Common foot and ankle injuries: what not to miss and how best to manage. J Am Osteopath Assoc. 2017;117:98–104.
3. Black AM, Eliason PH, Patton DA, Emery CA. Epidemiology of facial injuries in sport. Clin Sports Med. 2017;36:237–55.
4. Micieli JA, Easterbrook M. Eye and orbital injuries in sports. Clin Sports Med. 2017;36:299–314.
5. Scoggin JF 3rd, Brusovanik G, Izuka BH, Zandee van Rilland E, Geling O, Tokumura S. Assessment of injuries during Brazilian Jiu-Jitsu competition. Orthop J Sport Med. 2014;2:2325967114522184.
6. Čierna D, Lystad RP. Epidemiology of competition injuries in youth karate athletes: a prospective cohort study. Br J Sports Med. 2017;51:1285–8.
7. Čierna D, Barrientos M, Agrasar C, Arriaza R. Epidemiology of injuries in juniors participating in top-level karate competition: a prospective cohort study. Br J Sports Med. 2018;52:730–4.
8. Jones NS. Competitive diving principles and injuries. Curr Sports Med Rep. 2017;16:351–6.
9. Westermann RW, Giblin M, Vaske A, Grosso K, Wolf BR. Evaluation of men's and women's gymnastics injuries: a 10-year observational study. Sports Health. 2015;7:161–5.
10. Durstine J, Gordon B, Wang Z, Luo X. Chronic disease and the link to physical activity. J Sport Health Sci. 2013;2:3–11.
11. Dinas PC, Koutedakis Y, Flouris AD. Effects of exercise and physical activity on depression. Ir J Med Sci. 2011;180:319–25.
12. Sigal RJ, Kenny GP, Wasserman DH, Castaneda-Sceppa C, White RD. Physical activity/exercise and type 2 diabetes: a consensus statement from the American Diabetes Association. Diabetes Care. 2006;29:1433–8.
13. Moore GE. The role of exercise prescription in chronic disease. Br J Sports Med. 2004;38:6–7.
14. Nathanson AT, Young JMJ, Young C. Pre-participation medical evaluation for adventure and wilderness watersports. Wilderness Environ Med. 2015;26:S55–62.
15. Leischik R, Dworrak B, Foshag P, Strauss M, Spelsberg N, Littwitz H, Horlitz M. Pre-participation and follow-up screening of athletes for endurance sport. J Clin Med Res. 2015;7:385–92.
16. Sharma S, Merghani A, Gati S. Cardiac screening of young athletes prior to participation in sports: difficulties in detecting the fatally flawed among the fabulously fit. JAMA Intern Med. 2015;175:125–7.
17. Caswell SV, Cortes N, Chabolla M, Ambegaonkar JP, Caswell AM, Brenner JS. State-specific differences in school sports preparticipation physical evaluation policies. Pediatrics. 2015;135:26–32.
18. Zychowicz ME. Pre-participation physical evaluations for athletes. Nurse Pract. 2012;37:41–5.
19. Damasceno SMRP, Gonzalez MKS, Del Hoyo Fernandes RB, Gramuglia VL. In: Rocha Piedade S, Imhoff AB, Clatworthy M, Cohen M, Espregueira-Mendes J, editors. Oral health BT—the sports medicine physician. Cham: Springer International Publishing; 2019. p. 459–69.
20. Viner RT, Harris M, Berning JR, Meyer NL. Energy availability and dietary patterns of adult male and female competitive cyclists with lower than expected bone mineral density. Int J Sport Nutr Exerc Metab. 2015;25:594–602.
21. Mountjoy M, Sundgot-Borgen J, Burke L, et al. The IOC consensus statement: beyond the Female Athlete Triad—Relative Energy Deficiency in Sport (RED-S). Br J Sports Med. 2014;48:491–7.
22. Mirabelli MH, Devine MJ, Singh J, Mendoza M. The preparticipation sports evaluation. Am Fam Physician. 2015;92:371–6.
23. Sanders B, Blackburn TA, Boucher B. Preparticipation screening—the sports physical therapy perspective. Int J Sports Phys Ther. 2013;8:180–93.
24. Galanti G, Stefani L, Liverani L, Gensini GF. Pre-participation assessment in young athletes: a state affair. Intern Emerg Med. 2012;7:403–5.
25. Kim JH, Malhotra R, Chiampas G, et al. Cardiac arrest during long-distance running races. N Engl J Med. 2012;366:130–40.
26. Piedade SR, Ferreira DM, Filho MF, Zogiab RK, Martínez IC, Zayats V, Neyret P. In: Rocha Piedade S, Imhoff AB, Clatworthy M, Cohen M, Espregueira-Mendes J, editors. Pre-participation evaluation in sports practice BT—the sports medicine physician. Cham: Springer International Publishing; 2019. p. 13–25.

18 Respiratory (Shortness of Breath, Asthma, Dropped Lung)

Ricardo Siufi

18.1 Introduction

Symptoms and/or respiratory diseases may have a negative impact on elite athletes, regarding both their health context and performance. Upper respiratory tract symptoms (URTS) are the second most common symptom amongst these athletes, whereas injuries are in the first place (being only less frequent than injuries). Regarding Olympic and international competitions, URTS may compromise the athletes' performance by up to 10%. Due to this prevalence, upper respiratory tract infections (URTI) are thought to be the most frequent respiratory condition affecting elite athletes.

Nevertheless, there are other non-infectious conditions that may lead to URTS, such as respiratory allergies, bronchial asthma, airway hyperresponsiveness, exercise-induced vocal cord disfunction, including injury to the pulmonary epithelium, especially in athletes who practice sport in low air humidity environments (endurance—Fig. 18.1) and also those who are exposed to low temperatures, such as the Winter Olympics, for example (Fact Box 18.1).

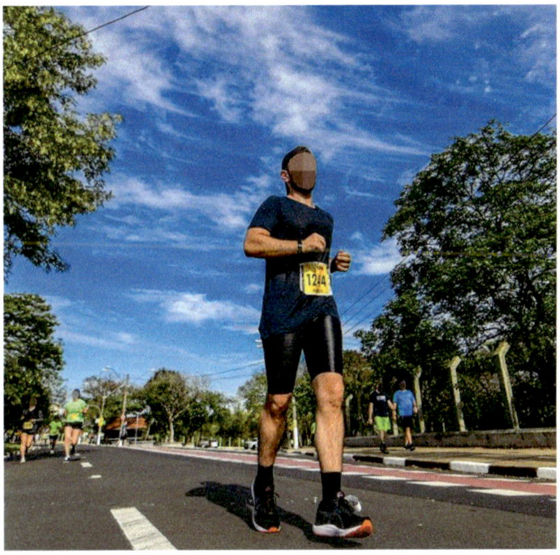

Fig. 18.1 Athlete practicing endurance. (Author's own collection)

> **Fact Box 18.1**
> Respiratory symptoms are the second most common symptom among athletes
>
> Among upper respiratory tract infections, viral infections are the most prevalent

R. Siufi (✉)
Internal Medicine, Pulmonology, Unicamp, Campinas, SP, Brazil

Healthcare Management, Hospital Israelita Albert Einstein, São Paulo, SP, Brazil

Pulmonology at São Leopoldo Mandic, Campinas, SP, Brazil

Pulmonology at the Universidade Santo Amaro (UNISA), São Paulo, SP, Brazil

S. Rocha Piedade et al. (eds.), *Sideline Management in Sports*,
https://doi.org/10.1007/978-3-031-33867-0_18

The prevalence of URTI in athletes is like the general population; however, the seasonal variation can be different

Known causes of respiratory tract inflammation in athletes are activation of the immune system, allergic response, asthma, and trauma to the respiratory epithelium

Although the incidence of URTS in athletes does not differ significantly from incidence in the general population, seasonal variations seem not to impact the professional competitors. The type of training as well as the various competitions throughout the year have a greater impact on their health—symptoms are more common when the training routines intensify, shortly before the event/tournament

Even though the URTS may represent a big concern for both athletes and their coaching staff, there are few studies which quantified the effects of the URTS on the performance outcomes. Various factors may contribute to the symptoms, such as bad quality of sleep, the journey, stress and low available energy, as well as dietetic changes (Flowchart 18.1).

Most of the URTI are viral; therefore, the sports medicine physician must be readily able to recognize this clinical condition, as well as its potential development to a bacterial infection, which represents a higher morbidity-mortality and greater impact on the athletes' health.

Other crucial concern is the recovery time after a disease, that means how long should the athlete reembark into his training routine. The time and necessity of complementary exams may vary depending on the kind of infection, its transmissibility window, the demand on the athlete, in conjunction with the severity spectrum of the condition itself. Decisions have to be made individually for each case, based on to the actual best available evidence, without compromising health of the athletes or the other involved participants.

Athletes can manifest different respiratory symptoms, which will be handled separately. The determination of the specific respiratory condition that the athlete may have will depend on the combination of these symptoms associated to the basis diagnosis, in addition to the clinical history and complementary exams. This will be described below.

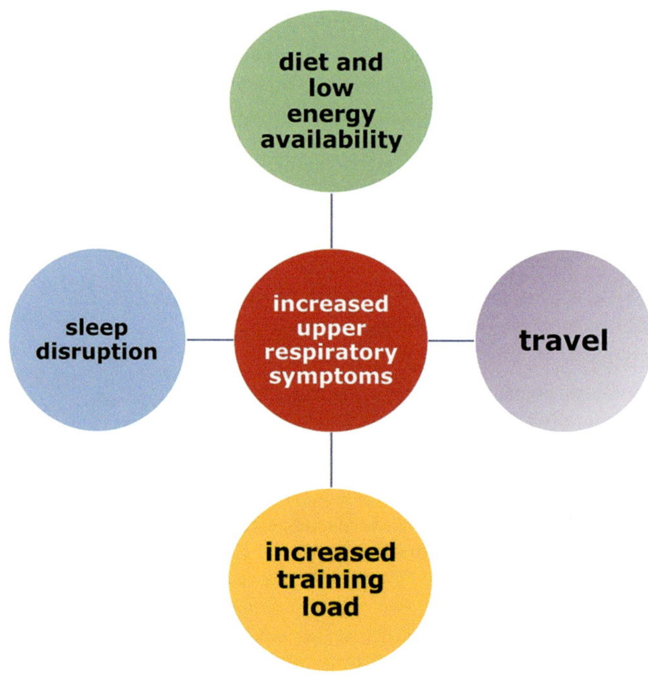

Flowchart 18.1 Factors contributing to URS in elite athletes. (Adapted from Sports Med, 2018)

18.2 Respiratory Symptoms

In the athletes' context, respiratory symptoms may represent an acute illness, lack of control, or exacerbation of an underlying illness.

18.2.1 Cough

It is a body reflex in response to the aspiration of irritating agents and various particles into the respiratory system and is an important defense mechanism, triggered by the activation of subepithelial nerve endings, which sense the presence of the foreign agent. Regarding athletes, as physical exercise significantly raises demand on the cardiorespiratory system, it leads to an increase not only in cardiac output, but also in volume-minute, which provokes airway mucosa dehydration. The physical factors that can induce cough during sports practice are, mainly, high ventilatory rates during intense physical exercise and predominantly mouth breathing—changes in the osmolarity of the airways mucus can trigger the cough reflex and stimulate coughing and mucus hypersecretion, regardless of airway caliber changes (Fact Box 18.2).

Fact Box 18.2

Cough is classified into acute (up to 3 weeks), subacute (3–8 weeks), and chronic (>8 weeks)

The main cause of acute cough is URTI

Regardless of the cough classification, always pay attention to the alarm sign or "red flags"

Consider tuberculosis in endemic countries and subacute/chronic cough

Cough can be secondary to an airway disease or it can be a physiological response to low relative (air) humidity or to low temperature. The prevalence of coughing in skiers can be up to three times higher in comparison to other athletes, whose cough reflex is caused particularly by the environmental exposure. Inhalation of irritating agents may cause acute cough or may occasionally trigger or exacerbate an underlying respiratory disease.

As for its duration, coughing can be classified as acute (<3 weeks), subacute (between 3 and 8 weeks), and chronic (>8 weeks), and the first healthcare approach, regardless of its duration, is to eliminate potentially life-threatening conditions (Fig. 18.2), such as pneumonia, severe asthma exacerbation, pulmonary thromboembolism, acute heart failure decompensation, among others.

In stable, non-life-threatening conditions, it should be considered as the main etiology of acute and subacute coughing, respectively, upper airway infection and post-infections coughing (Flowchart 18.2). However, it should always be taken into consideration the possibility of the exacerbation of a preexisting respiratory disease.

When it comes to coughing in athletes, the first step is a good case history and physical examination, followed by a pulmonary function test. An initial chest X-ray may be performed to rule out potential differential diagnoses or possible complications, though is often normal. Once alarming signs were excluded, upper airway cough syndrome, often secondary to rhinitis, should be considered as the first affection to be ruled out.

Further conditions will be addressed throughout the chapter.

18.2.2 Dyspnea

Dyspnea, a common cause of concern among athletes and physicians, is defined as a subjective experience of respiratory difficulty or discomfort, composed of qualitatively distinct sensations, of varying intensity, and that can be associated with multiple semiological findings. Nevertheless, concerning athletes, their physical examination may be normal.

When considering dyspnea as a response towards an increased physiological demand in exercise in high-performance athletes, all the main causes of dyspnea must have been ade-

Fig. 18.2 "Red flags"- cough. (Adapted from CHEST, 2017)

RED FLAGS

- hemoptysis
- smoker > 45 years of age with a new cough, change in cough or coexisting voice disturbance
- adults aged 55-80 years who 30 pack-year smoking history and currently smoke or who have quit within the past 15 years
- prominent dyspnea, especially at rest or at night
- hoarseness
- systemic symptoms - fever, weight loss
- trouble swallowing whet eating or drinking
- recurrent pneumonia
- history of abnormal respiratory exam and/or abnormal chest radiograph coinciding with the duration on cough

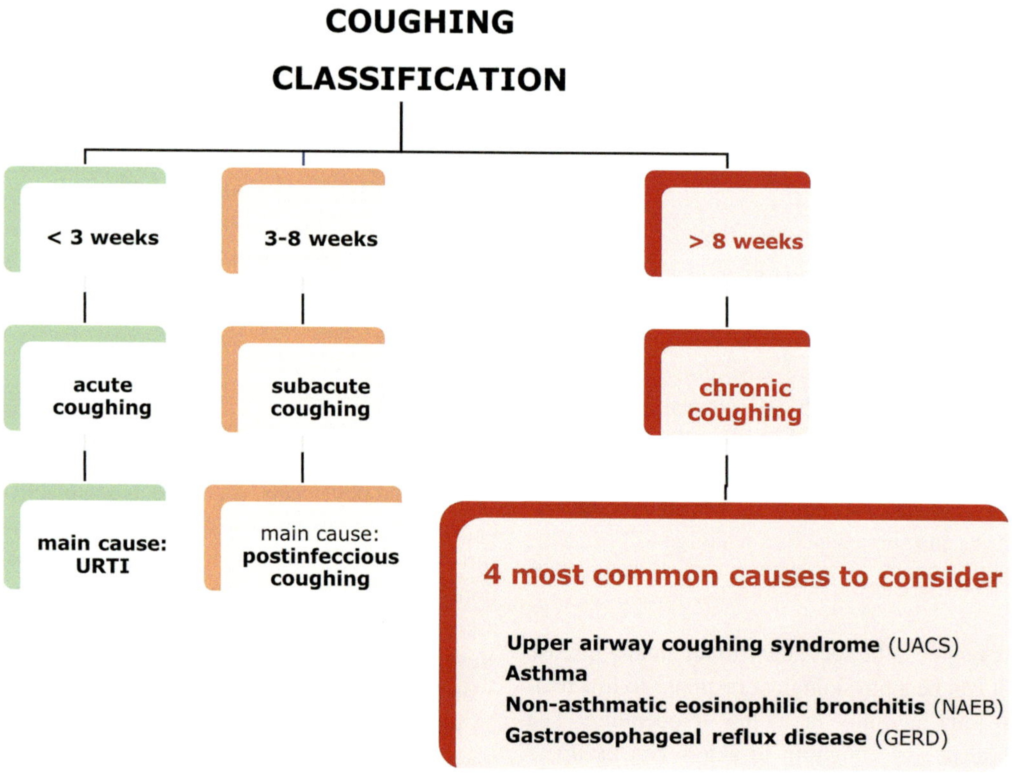

Flowchart 18.2 Cough classification. (Adapted from CHEST, 2017)

quately excluded beforehand—from the process of oxygen transport, to pneumological and cardiogenic causes.

It is not uncommon that athletes may complain of fatigue, intolerance to efforts or physical deconditioning. A detailed anamnesis must be carried out to assess the semiological details of the complaint. Furthermore, it is essential for the physician to keep the whole range of possibilities in mind. After all, as much as it is known that asthma is the most prevalent condition that causes dyspnea in individuals without other comorbidities, bronchodilator therapy will not work on those individuals with anemia, rib cage deformities, or infectious diseases.

More details on the topic will be covered in the specific diseases.

18.2.3 Wheeze

Wheezing, a commonly encountered complaint in the sports medicine context, refers to continuous lung sounds (present during inspiration and expiration), musical, better heard during expiration, and which are generated by a narrowing of the airway.

Although the main causes of wheezing are asthma and exercise-induced bronchoconstriction (EIB), the finding may also be present in other conditions such as vocal cord dysfunction, tonsil hypertrophy, upper airway cough syndrome, among others.

When assisting an athlete with a new complaint of wheezing, it is important, in the current context, to determine whether he or she has had a recent lower respiratory tract infection. It is also essential to investigate about past respiratory symptoms in childhood, rhinitis, and dermatitis, findings that favor the diagnosis of asthma. However, the most common etiology of wheezing among athletes who did not present it before is EIB, a condition that affects about 10% of the general population and up to 90% of patients with a previous diagnosis of asthma.

According to the current literature, asthma appears to be more prevalent in elite athletes (10%) than in the general population (6.9%). However, the studies used different diagnostic tests, which may compromise the prevalence.

If the wheezing is related to a previous lower respiratory tract infection, the athlete may experience reduced lung function. Such an entity can be secondary to a viral condition (which more commonly can be in the spectrum of post-COVID-19 syndrome and other acute viral infections) or bacterial (less common).

The diagnosis is based on the medical history and physical examination. If necessary, a pre- and post-bronchodilator pulmonary function test should be requested or, occasionally, we must perform the serial peak expiratory flow during physical activity.

18.3 Respiratory Diseases

18.3.1 Upper Respiratory Tract Infections

The common cold is the most frequent acute illness in the United States and the main cause that leads people to miss work and/or school days. An URTI tends to be a benign, self-limiting condition that typically lasts 5–14 days, manifested by runny nose, cough, and fever, caused by several families of viruses, including rhinovirus, coronavirus, and respiratory syncytial virus. Transmission is by direct contact, which englobes aerosol and droplets, as well as person-to-person contact, which depends on the time of contact and inherent aspects of the environment, such as ventilation.

The common cold may originate some complications, such as acute bacterial rhinosinusitis in 2.5% of patients with URTI and, to a lesser extent, pneumonia. It is worth to keep in mind that the main cause of exacerbation of asthma is URTI and, therefore, this etiology should always be taken into consideration in previously asthmatic patients with worsening of the condition.

The diagnosis is based on the clinical condition, and the etiologic diagnosis can be challenging sometimes. The incubation period for most viruses causing common cold is 24–72 h, up to

7 days for some viruses. Some risk factors are well established to predict worse outcome, such as immunosuppression, chronic diseases, and obesity.

Differential diagnoses include respiratory diseases with similar symptoms, such as flu syndrome, complications of acute nasopharyngitis (itself) such as acute otitis media, acute bacterial rhinosinusitis, and bacterial pneumonia, among others.

Treatment is symptomatic and antiviral therapy is not available for most viruses that cause URTIs. If the patient develops severe acute respiratory syndrome from COVID-19, the only medication that has shown an impact on mortality is corticosteroid therapy with dexamethasone for patients in need of supplemental oxygen therapy.

According to the American College of Sports Medicine, when an athlete presents suggestive symptoms of acute nasopharyngitis without fever or other systemic signs, physical activities can be resumed a few days after symptoms resolve. For moderate or severe cases, the assessment should be individual, depending on the spectrum of the disease and the athlete's baseline conditions.

18.3.2 Asthma

The regular practice of physical activity is one of the most recommended measures by doctors and pneumologists for controlled asthmatic patients, as it can improve asthma symptoms, quality of life, exercise tolerance, and lung function. Physical activity for elite athletes imposes an important demand on the cardiorespiratory system, with a significant increase in cardiac output and ventilation, which, in high-performance athletes, can reach 200 L/min, with a significant drop in temperature and humidity of the air flowing into the airways. In addition, due to predominant mouth breathing, there is a reduction in the ability to filter some particles, consequently increasing the penetration of allergens and pollutants, such as ozone and particulate matter, into the small airways. Therefore, it is not surprising that high-performance athletes and Winter game athletes have more respiratory complaints when compared to non-athletes (Fact Box 18.3).

Fact Box 18.3

Respiratory symptoms alone have a low predictive value for the diagnosis of asthma

Documentation of airway obstruction variability is required for diagnosis of asthma

EIB is different from airway hyperresponsiveness, which can be defined as a tendency for the airways to decrease in caliber more easily and more intensely than a normal airway

Inhaled corticosteroids are the mainstay of treatment in stable asthma

The main cause of exacerbation of bronchial asthma is a viral infection of the upper airways

The term exercise-induced bronchoconstriction (EIB) describes a transient obstruction of the airways after physical exercise—a common phenomenon among athletes who do not necessarily have asthma. Caution—EIB is different from airway hyperresponsiveness (AH), which can be defined as a tendency of the airways to narrow more easily and more intensely than a normal airway in response to various bronchoconstrictor stimuli.

High-intensity physical activity may contribute to the development of asthma, EIB, and AH, and early diagnosis of these conditions in athletes can prevent performance impairment. In athletes, the diagnosis of asthma can be made based on the clinical history and pattern of symptoms in addition to the presence of variable airflow obstruction documented by a positive bronchodilator response or another test, such as the bronchoprovocation test. Nonetheless, symptoms, in an isolated manner, have a low predictive value for the diagnosis of asthma and EIB in athletes; therefore, documentation of the variability of obstruction is required.

Special attention should be drawn to the identification of potentially misleading factors or possibly coexisting conditions, which may mimic or be associated with asthma in athletes.

Of these, one of the most common factors, for instance, is exercise-induced supraglottic or glottic obstruction, including focal cord dysfunction, a paradoxical closure of the vocal cords during inspiration. Other conditions such as rhinitis, gastroesophageal reflux, and hyperventilation syndrome are common among athletes, and if there is the diagnostic suspicion, complementary tests, as well as a specific treatment should be conducted.

The management of asthma and EIB consists in achieving the control of the disease, improving lung function, and preventing future risks such as disease exacerbations.

Non-pharmacological management involves measures such as adequate guidance on inhalation technique, environmental hygiene and advice on special situations, such as avoiding pollutants and, in some situations, encouraging the use of a mask, if well tolerated by the patient. It is important to avoid training in low relative humidity and in very low temperatures.

Regarding pharmacological treatment, inhaled corticosteroids are the main pharmacological class in the management of the disease and are released by the authorities. It is worth to keep in mind that the use of inhaled beta-2-agonist (SABA) does not improve the performance of asthmatic and non-asthmatic athletes. SABA are the preeminent pharmacological class for relief and are substantial when used 5–10 min before the practice of physical activity in patients with EIB, preferably via "Pressurized metered-dose inhalers" (pMDI) device. However, with frequent or regular use, it can develop tolerance, hence decreasing its bronchoprotective effect during exercise, possibly due to a "down regulation" of beta-2 receptors.

18.3.3 Pulmonary Thromboembolism

High-performance athletes, specifically marathon runners, are at risk of developing venous thromboembolism (VTE), a term that comprehends both deep vein thrombosis (DVT) and pulmonary thromboembolism (PTE).

The main clinical manifestations of pulmonary thromboembolism are sudden dyspnea and pleuritic chest pain, and its hypothesis should be considered in patients with such manifestations who present some risk factor.

Marathon runners have some conditions that put them in a risk group for thrombotic events, as shown in Table 18.1.

The preventive measures for athletes are the same as those for the non-athlete adult population and the assessment, if their activities may be resumed then it must be individualized, depending on the repercussion of the event as well as the presence or absence of residual pulmonary obstruction.

18.3.4 Acute Mountain Sickness (High Altitude Athletes)

High-altitude sports have become more popular in recent decades and range from regular rock climbing to endurance racing and team sports. However, such practices can have important health consequences.

Table 18.1 VTE: venous thromboembolism (Circulation, 2013)

Athlete-specific risk factor for VTE
Dehydration and hemoconcentration (decrease of the fluid content of the blood with increased concentration of red blood cells)
Injury and inflammation, including microtrauma to blood vessel walls
Immobilization during long-distance travel, including local car/coach journey and long-haul flights between events (e.g., the Boston [US], London [UK] and Paris [Europe] marathons)
Low heart rate (bradycardia) and blood pressure affecting the circulation and possibly exacerbating venous stasis
Thoracic outlet obstruction: an extra (cervical) rib or excess muscle/tendon tissue can compress the upper chest (subclavian) vein that drains the blood from the arm, obstruction and repeated trauma/strain to the vein can result in upper extremity deep vein thrombosis
May-Thurner syndrome (narrowing of the major left pelvic vein)
Narrowing or absence or the inferior vena cava (the main vein in the abdomen)

In acute exposure, the human body's first response to hypobaric hypoxia is an increase in the ventilatory response, triggered by the carotid body receptors. Acutely, the result is hypoxemia, desaturation, and increased ventilatory demand. Chronically, it progresses to hypoventilation, pulmonary hypertension, increased diffusing capacity and, in extreme cases, exacerbation of preexisting pulmonary diseases and, more rarely, high-altitude pulmonary edema.

A slow and gradual ascent is the major prevention that must be carried out, so that the athlete does not develop acute mountain sickness. The documents recommend that, once above 2500 m of altitude, we should climb from 600 to 1200 m every 24 h at most. The duration of acclimatization depends on whether the athlete resides on that altitude and what are the athlete's plans. Pharmacological prevention with acetazolamide and corticosteroid therapy should be considered as a complement to a slow and gradual ascent, when possible.

Take Home Messages

- Prompt recognition of the main respiratory conditions in elite athletes is crucial for the safety of the athlete as well as his/her team/staff.
- The individualization of specific clinical conditions is an important milestone in the treatment of each disease. After all, an URI may not respond to bronchodilation, whereas expectant treatment for bronchial asthma can be fatal.
- It is also essential, faced with a respiratory symptom or a previously diagnosed clinical condition, to know how to recognize the warning signs—those that potentially comprehend some life-threatening condition.
- Prevention and early recognition are, in fact, the way to go in the matter of respiratory diseases in elite athletes.

Bibliography

1. Vallerand JR, Weatherald J, Laveneziana P. Pulmonary hypertension and exercise. Clin Chest Med. 2019;40(2):459–69. https://doi.org/10.1016/j.ccm.2019.02.003.
2. Poussel M, Chenuel B. Bronchoconstriction induite par l'exercice sans asthme associé chez l'athlète: physiopathologie, diagnostic et prise en charge spécifique [Exercise-induced bronchoconstriction in non-asthmatic athletes]. Rev Mal Respir. 2010;27(8):898–906. French. https://doi.org/10.1016/j.rmr.2010.08.004. Epub 2010 Sep 28.
3. Dubé BP, Vermeulen F, Laveneziana P. Exertional dyspnoea in chronic respiratory diseases: from physiology to clinical application. Arch Bronconeumol. 2017;53(2):62–70. English, Spanish. https://doi.org/10.1016/j.arbres.2016.09.005. Epub 2016 Nov 4.
4. Weatherald J, Sattler C, Garcia G, Laveneziana P. Ventilatory response to exercise in cardiopulmonary disease: the role of chemosensitivity and dead space. Eur Respir J. 2018;51(2):1700860. https://doi.org/10.1183/13993003.00860-2017.
5. Fiorentino G, Esquinas AM, Annunziata A. Exercise and chronic obstructive pulmonary disease (COPD). Adv Exp Med Biol. 2020;1228:355–68. https://doi.org/10.1007/978-981-15-1792-1_24.
6. Padem N, Saltoun C. Classification of asthma. Allergy Asthma Proc. 2019;40(6):385–8. https://doi.org/10.2500/aap.2019.40.4253.
7. Ding S, Zhong C. Exercise and asthma. Adv Exp Med Biol. 2020;1228:369–80. https://doi.org/10.1007/978-981-15-1792-1_25.
8. Malaty J, Wu V. Vocal cord dysfunction: rapid evidence review. Am Fam Physician. 2021;104(5):471–5.
9. Khodaee M, Grothe HL, Seyfert JH, VanBaak K. Athletes at high altitude. Sports Health. 2016;8(2):126–32. https://doi.org/10.1177/1941738116630948.
10. Hartman-Ksycińska A, Kluz-Zawadzka J, Lewandowski B. High altitude illness. Przegl Epidemiol. 2016;70(3):490–9.
11. Côté A, Turmel J, Boulet LP. Exercise and asthma. Semin Respir Crit Care Med. 2018;39(1):19–28. https://doi.org/10.1055/s-0037-1606215. Epub 2018 Feb 10.
12. Boulet LP, Turmel J, Irwin RS, CHEST Expert Cough Panel. Cough in the athlete: CHEST guideline and expert panel report. Chest. 2017;151(2):441–54. https://doi.org/10.1016/j.chest.2016.10.054. Epub 2016 Nov 16.
13. Imray C, Wright A, Subudhi A, Roach R. Acute mountain sickness: pathophysiology, prevention, and treatment. Prog Cardiovasc Dis. 2010;52(6):467–84. https://doi.org/10.1016/j.pcad.2010.02.003.

14. Boulet LP, O'Byrne PM. Asthma and exercise-induced bronchoconstriction in athletes. N Engl J Med. 2015;372(7):641–8. https://doi.org/10.1056/NEJMra1407552.
15. Colbey C, Cox AJ, Pyne DB, Zhang P, Cripps AW, West NP. Upper respiratory symptoms, gut health and mucosal immunity in athletes. Sports Med. 2018;48(Suppl 1):65–77. https://doi.org/10.1007/s40279-017-0846-4.
16. Price OJ, Ansley L, Menzies-Gow A, Cullinan P, Hull JH. Airway dysfunction in elite athletes—an occupational lung disease? Allergy. 2013;68(11):1343–52. https://doi.org/10.1111/all.12265. Epub 2013 Oct 11.
17. Lin L, Decker CF. Respiratory tract infections in athletes. Dis Mon. 2010;56(7):407–13. https://doi.org/10.1016/j.disamonth.2010.05.001.
18. Hull JH, Dickinson JW, Jackson AR. Cough in exercise and athletes. Pulm Pharmacol Ther. 2017;47:49–55. https://doi.org/10.1016/j.pupt.2017.04.005. Epub 2017 Apr 12.
19. Page CL, Diehl JJ. Upper respiratory tract infections in athletes. Clin Sports Med. 2007;26(3):345–59. https://doi.org/10.1016/j.csm.2007.04.001.
20. Fields KB, Thekkekandam TJ, Neal S. Wheezing after respiratory tract infection in athletes. Curr Sports Med Rep. 2012;11(2):85–9. https://doi.org/10.1249/JSR.0b013e31824a78fc.
21. Boulet LP, Turmel J. Cough in exercise and athletes. Pulm Pharmacol Ther. 2019;55:67–74. https://doi.org/10.1016/j.pupt.2019.02.003. Epub 2019 Feb 13.
22. Carlsen KH, Hem E, Stensrud T. Asthma in adolescent athletes. Br J Sports Med. 2011;45(16):1266–71. https://doi.org/10.1136/bjsports-2011-090591.
23. Hull CM, Harris JA. Cardiology Patient Page. Venous thromboembolism and marathon athletes. Circulation. 2013;128(25):e469–71. https://doi.org/10.1161/CIRCULATIONAHA.113.004586.

19 Sudden Cardiac Arrest: Sideline Management

Clea Simone S. S. Colombo

19.1 Introduction

Sudden cardiac arrest (SCA) during sports is a rare but dramatic event that progresses to sudden death (SD) in most cases, unfortunately. Prompt and adequate care is critical to the success of SCA reversal and SD prevention. For each minute of delay in cardiopulmonary resuscitation (CPR), survival reduces by approximately 10% [1].

Frequently, SCA occurs due to arrhythmias secondary to underlying cardiac diseases, such as inherited structural cardiomyopathies and channelopathies or acquired myocarditis and obstructive coronary artery disease. However, arrhythmias can be triggered by exogenous factors such as stimulant substances, hyperthermia, and electrolyte disturbance.

Vigorous exercise, especially competitive sports, can lead to arrhythmia in predisposed individuals. Therefore, it is important to ensure that all athletes undergo preparticipation evaluation and receive proper guidance for competition. Weather conditions, routes, and specificities of the sport must be taken into account when assessing the risks during the event. In the field of play, any athlete who presents loss of consciousness and remains unconscious should be considered as a possible SCA.

19.2 Prevalence of Sudden Cardiac Death (SD) in Athletes

The incidence of SD in athletes is not accurate, as most of the available data come from non-academic sources (media records and claims from health insurance) and are captured from heterogeneous populations (different ages, sex, ethnicity, sports modalities) with different methodologies, what makes data analysis more difficult.

Studies show that 56–80% of SD in young athletes occur during exercise, with an incidence ranging from one per 1 million to one per 5000 athletes per year [2]. Some groups, such as males, Afro-descendants and basketball and soccer practitioners, seem to have a higher risk of SD. Male athletes are described as having a higher relative risk than females (3:1 versus 9:1, respectively), and African-Americans have a 3.2 times greater risk than whites. In basketball athletes, SD reports are one per 9000 per year in

Clea Simone S. S. Colombo (✉)
Sports Cardiology, St. George's University of London, London, UK

European Society of Cardiology, Sophia Antipolis, France

Sports Cardiology Clinics of São Leopoldo Mandic Medical School, Campinas, SP, Brazil

Sportscardio—Cardiology Clinic, Valinhos, SP, Brazil

S. Rocha Piedade et al. (eds.), *Sideline Management in Sports*,
https://doi.org/10.1007/978-3-031-33867-0_19

Table 19.1 Causes of sudden death in athletes

Cardiac			Non-cardiac
Inherited or congenital		Acquired	
Structural	Electric		
Hypertrophic cardiomyopathy	Wolff-Parkinson-White syndrome	Myocarditis	Heat stroke
Ventricular arrhythmogenic dysplasia	Long QT syndrome	Coronary artery disease (>35 yo)	Anabolic Androgenic Steroids
Anomalous origin coronary	Brugada syndrome		Stimulants
Marfan syndrome (aortic aneurysm)	Catecholaminergic polymorphic ventricular tachycardia		Electrolyte disturbance
Aortic stenosis			
Mitral valve prolapse			

white men, while in African-Americans, they reach one per 5300 per year in some American groups [3].

The causes of SD in athletes can be congenital or acquired, with genetic structural or "electrical" inherited heart diseases and viral myocarditis being the most common causes in young people (<35 years). In athletes aged 35 years or older, coronary artery disease is the most common cause of cardiac SD (>80% of the cases) (Table 19.1) [2]. Frequently, SCA is the first manifestation of these cardiac diseases.

SD in macroscopic structurally normal hearts (observed in autopsies) is called "sudden arrhythmic death syndrome" (SADS). It has been referred to as the most frequent cause of SD in young athletes in recent publications on the subject (United States of America, United Kingdom and Australia) [4]. However, hypertrophic cardiomyopathy (HCM) and arrhythmogenic ventricular dysplasia (AVD), both structural heart diseases with genetic causes, have been described as the main causes of SD in young athletes in the last decades [2].

Among the acquired ones, viral myocarditis has been shown to be an important and growing cause of malignant arrhythmias and SD in young athletes. Infection viruses such as Influenza, Coxsackie and Parvovirus are often neglected by the athlete and may lead to myocardial involvement. The acute phase is sometimes underdiagnosed but the myocardial injury can cause permanent sequelae [5]. Recently, **the SARS-CoV2 infection** (COVID-19 disease) raised attention to the occurrence of myocarditis in athletes, as it has emerged as a complication in infected individuals during the 2020 pandemic [6].

19.3 Prevention of Sudden Death

19.3.1 Pre-Participation Evaluation (PPE)

PPE is the fundamental tool for the prevention of SD in sports. The objective is to identify the silent pathologies that may predispose the athlete to SD during sports practice. The European Society of Cardiology (ESC), the Fédération Internationale de Football Association (FIFA), and the International Olympic Committee (IOC) recommend performing a medical assessment before starting sports practice, which includes personal and family medical history, physical examination, and 12-lead resting electrocardiogram (ECG) [7–9]. It should be repeated annually or sooner if they arise symptoms or abnormalities are found. Additional tests may be necessary and should be evaluated individually according to the initial findings.

Although it has already been demonstrated that the use of ECG in the PPE increases the sensitivity for detecting heart disease by more than four times, its practice is still a matter of controversy, mainly with discussions related to costs and the possible need to carry out additional complementary tests. The American Heart Association (AHA) does not include the ECG in the PPE, whereas in Europe, it is mandatory. The experience of more than two decades since the inclusion of the ECG in the PPE in Italy demonstrated a drop of 86% in the incidence rate of SD in young athletes [10]. This was mainly due to the fact that more than 80% of individuals with HCM and VAD have ECG abnormalities, even asymptomatic and with a normal physical examination, enabling the identification and disqualification of these athletes from sports. However, it is important to point out that the interpretation of the ECG must be performed by a physician who knows the pattern of the "athlete's ECG" since the physiological cardiac adaptations secondary to the practice of exercises cause alterations that can be confused with the initial manifestations of heart diseases, which could lead to unnecessary additional testing.

19.3.2 Medical Action Plan for Emergency Care

Prevention for SD must include an emergency care plan, with a well-defined "Medical Action Plan" (MAP), written and available to all present, including visitors.

The MAP should determine the responsible medical coordinator, the first responders, medical equipment, the level of care to be provided, the way of transportation and the post-SCA referral location [11].

The availability and distribution of an automated external defibrillator (AED) are one of the most important parts of the MAP. It is recommended an AED be within 3 min of any location in the arena, reaching a maximum of 5 min from emergency recognition and shock delivery. The AED should be easily visible and accessible, near the emergency phone number and ways of communication and response-team activation. It is recommended to check the device battery and leads periodically, as well as to have an extra set of pads. Other supplies to facilitate the action should be available, including towels, scissors and razors.

The emergency equipment depends on the level of care provided in the field and may include a sphygmomanometer, pulse oximetry, bag valve masks, advanced oropharyngeal airway insertion, supplemental oxygen, intravenous fluid and medications, such as aspirin and nitroglycerin [11].

All the staff (referees, coaches, physical trainers, physiotherapists, nurses, team doctors, administrators and others) must be educated in SCA recognition and AED use and trained in basic life support (BLS). It is recommended at least one physician is trained in ACLS [12].

Vehicles, hospital distance, routes and local medical facilities should be predetermined for appropriate transportation.

Periodic review of the MAP (recommended at least once a year) and regular practical training of the team are essential items for a good result in emergency care.

19.3.3 Planning Multiple Venues and Different Situations

Different sports modalities, events and multiple venues may require specific planning. Long races or large events should be carefully planned. We will address two examples as follows.

19.3.3.1 Marathons

The risk of death in a marathon is small, estimated to be one death per 149,968 participants (1 per 102,503 in males and one per 243,879 in females), but is higher in the best-studied marathons such as the London Marathon (1 per 71,933) [13]. Despite the recommendation of medical coverage distributed along the course of the running, it should be concentrated in the second half and the finish line because deaths tend to occur in the last quarter of the race.

It is recommended 1–5 first aid personnel for every 1000 runners, at least one medical doctor with ACLS certification for every 2500 runners, one basic and one advanced life support ambulance for every 500 runners and mobile responders along the route, aiming an AED less than 1 mile away from any athlete [11].

Other medical issues are not uncommon, being described at 25.3 per 1000, which include acute coronary syndrome, heat stroke and electrolyte disturbances [14].

19.3.3.2 Olympic Games

Multiple venue management may be challenging. Each venue should have its own MAP, considering the local and sports-specific characteristics. Prior visits to the venue and repeated training for the staff are crucial to be familiar with the emergency equipment and teamwork.

The host country is responsible to provide emergency care and medical staff in the venues. Therefore, if an SCA occurs during competition, the host emergency staff should be prepared to initiate CPR in the multivenue.

Visiting medical staff is allowed to assume care of their athletes in training areas. Foreign doctors must be aware of the conditions of permission to work in each country [11].

19.4 Current Treatment Recommendations for Emergency Care in Sudden Cardiac Arrest

Four factors are described as the main predictors of survival during an out-of-hospital cardiac arrest: witnessed cardiac arrest, early CPR, presence of a cardiac rhythm capable of defibrillation (tachycardia or ventricular fibrillation) and return to spontaneous circulation at the site. Figure 19.1 presents an algorithm for athlete's emergency care.

From this, the so-called "chain of survival" (Box 19.1) was established, which includes [15]:

Laypeople must not check for a pulse and healthcare providers should not spend more than 10s for this because it may delay the CPR and increase mortality.

> **Box 19.1 The Chain of Survival**
> – Immediate recognition of cardiac arrest
> – Rapid initiation of defibrillation
> – ACLS training
> – Good interaction with post-SCA care team

Agonal breathing, occasional gasping and myoclonic or seizure-like activity can occur within the first minutes of SCA and should be interpreted as SCA in a collapsed athlete,

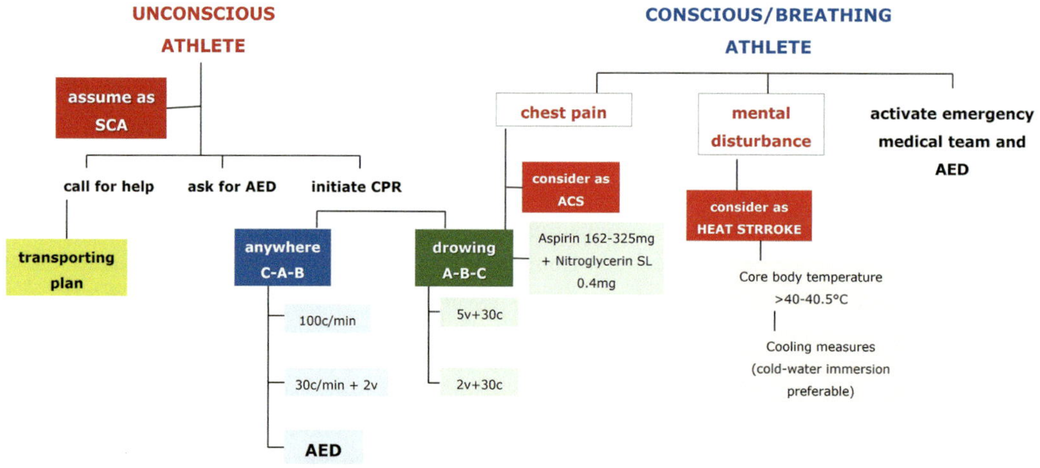

Fig. 19.1 Algorithm for athlete's emergency care. *Abbreviations*: *SCA* sudden cardiac arrest, *AED* automatic external defibrillator, *CPR* cardiopulmonary resuscitation, *C-A-B* chest compression before rescue breaths, *A-B-C* ventilation before chest compression, *c* chest compression, *v* ventilation, *min* minute, *ACS* acute coronary syndrome, *mg* milligrams, *SL* sublingual

avoiding delay in resuscitation. The emergency system must be activated and AED requested, which is essential for the success of the care [11].

In the case of an athlete with a decreased level of responsiveness who does not require immediate resuscitation, the use of the recovery position is recommended, monitoring signs of airway occlusion, inadequate breathing, and unresponsiveness. The recovery position is defined as lateral recumbent positioning, with the arm nearest the first aid provider at a right angle to the body and the elbow bent with palm up and far knee flexed (Fig. 19.2).

The presence or absence of signs of life should be determined and, if resuscitation is necessary, the person should be immediately positioned supine. The supine position is also recommended when the athlete is in positional asphyxia such as in neck and torso flexion positions.

The first responder should initiate CPR manoeuvres immediately (<1 min), with the "C-A-B" sequence (chest compressions before airway support) and defibrillation, when indicated, within a maximum of 3–5 min [16].

Hands-only (compression only) CPR is encouraged for the untrained lay rescuer and appears to achieve outcomes similar to those of conventional "A-B-C" CPR (compressions with rescue breathing). The correct chest compressions should be performed to a depth of 5 cm and wait for the complete return of the chest after each one. It is recommended to perform (Box 19.2):

Box 19.2 CPR

- Single responder = hands-only 100 compressions/min
- Trained personnel = 30 compressions/min followed by 2 bag-valve-mask-AMBU ventilations
- AED

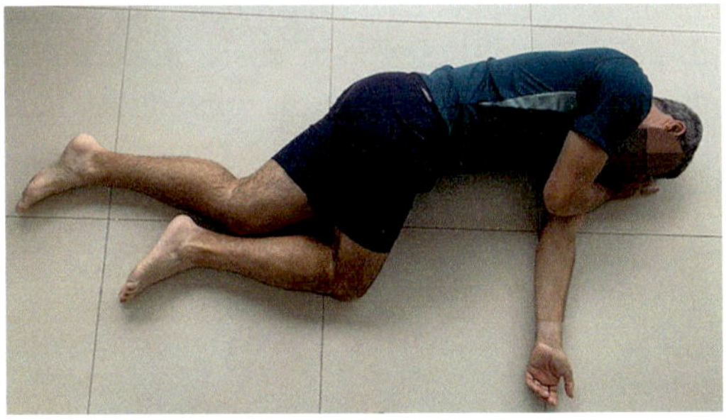

Fig. 19.2 Recovery position

Upon the arrival of the AED, chest compressions are interrupted to identify the heart rhythm and the need for a shock. The pause time between the interruption of chest compressions and the rhythm analysis by the AED should be as short as possible, minimizing the interval, with an immediate return after the shock because of the possibility of pulseless electric activity and asystole. The CPR time devoted to compressions is recommended to be at least 60%. Recently, some groups have advocated the hypothesis that AED should be used before chest compressions (if available) in-field-of-play SCA, given that most SCA during sports occurs due to arrhythmias [17].

Although current guidelines do not recommend transporting the victim during CPR because its efficiency decreases and the risk of injuries to providers increases, this do not apply to resuscitation of SCA in athletes. Resuscitative measures should continue until the athlete becomes responsive. If necessary, CPR should continue by air or road ambulance during transportation, performed by trained personnel during movement or with automated external chest compression devices [18].

After SCA, the comatose patient with mild hypothermia should not be actively warmed, aiming for the prevention of fever (target temperature ≤37.5 °C). The benefit of hypothermia at 32–34 °C is uncertain. Recent guidelines recommend against pre-hospital cooling with intravenous cold fluids because of rearrest and pulmonary oedema risk. Cooling devices with temperature control feedback are preferable [19].

19.5 Special Situations

19.5.1 Drowning

The "drowning chain of survival" is a little bit different from the one described previously. It includes preventive measures and a different approach for initiating CPR. Five steps recommended are as follows:

- Prevent drowning
- Recognize distress
- Provide flotation
- Remove from water
- Provide care (CPR if necessary)

Recognizing a person in distress in the water and knowing how to activate help is one of the most important steps to reduce mortality. Providing flotation is essential to prevent submersion and the use of an intermediary object (flotation device) may be necessary.

The drowning process leads first to unconsciousness and apnea, and if not interrupted, cardiac arrest may occur within minutes. Because of this, in-water resuscitation improves successful outcomes by more than three-fold. Usually, a few rescue breaths are enough for a person with isolated respiratory arrest (~0.5% of all rescues) to respond and if not, it should be assumed as SCA. However, in-water ventilation is only possible if highly trained personnel is in the rescue and chest compression is ineffective. So, transportation out of water is essential to initiate effective CPR, with the victim in a horizontal position but with the head above body level.

19.5.1.1 Treatment Recommendations

If the victim is unconscious but breathing, the rescuer should use the recovery position.

Vomiting is frequent (65–86%), and the attempt to expel water from the airway should be avoided because it increases the risk by more than five-fold.

If the victim is not breathing, a supine position with the trunk and head at the same level should be used, and CPR initiated. As the primary cause of SCA from drowning is the lack of oxygen, the CPR sequence is different from usual, starting with ventilation and following the "A-B-C" sequence.

It is recommended to perform [20]:

- 5 initial breaths followed by 30 chest compressions.
- 2 breaths to 30 compressions until recovery or ACLS is available. Use a face mask with supplemental oxygen or bag-mask ventilation with 15 L of oxygen until an orotracheal tube can be inserted. The orotracheal tube should not be aspirated and endotracheal administration of drugs is not recommended.
- AED available (Dry the skin before!).

Despite the most common rhythm in SCA following drowning being asystole, the AED must be available to check the presence of ventricular fibrillation and defibrillation when indicated. It may occur when the primary cause of SCA is a cardiac pathology, such as coronary artery disease or inherited underlying cardiac diseases, and in the presence of severe hypothermia.

19.5.2 Acute Coronary Syndrome

Some athletes may present acute coronary syndrome (ACS) before SCA. It should be suspected if an athlete presents chest pain or symptoms that may be related to ACS. The athlete's age and other risk factors must be taken into account. The use of stimulant substances and adrenaline surges during competition may trigger coronary plaque rupture in predisposed individuals. Recent viral infection, anabolic androgenic steroids use and other possible mechanisms that predispose to a hypercoagulable state, endothelial dysfunction and metabolic dysregulation should be considered.

Once ACS is suspected, it is recommended the following [11]:

- Remove the athlete from play, keep him seated or laid supine, and activate emergency medical staff.

– If hemodynamically stable, use oral aspirin 162–325 mg and sublingual nitroglycerin 0.4 mg (it can be repeated after every 5 min, 2-fold more).
– AED available.
– Transfer to a hospital that provides proper cardiologic treatment (coronary angiography).

19.5.3 Heat Stroke

Heat stroke is one of the most common life-threatening events during endurance sports (1–2 per 1000 participants) and the major non-cardiac cause of SCA. It is defined as a core body temperature >40–40.5 °C in an athlete with multiorgan dysfunction. The initial symptoms may be unrecognized because it ranges from chills, disorientation, loss of balance and aggressiveness to sudden collapse and SCA [21].

19.5.3.1 Treatment Recommendations [22]

– If suspected, core body temperature should be measured by inserting a standard thermometer into the rectum. The peripheral and tympanic temperature may be skewed after physical activity
– If confirmed, cooling measures must be initiated with ice packs to the axilla, groin and neck, cold towels and cooling blankets. If possible, cold-water immersion has been demonstrated to be faster and more effective
– Testing glucose and sodium blood levels, because other situations may be associated and represent confounding and aggravating factors
– AED available. Ventricular fibrillation may occur in some cases.

19.6 Conclusion

Sudden cardiac arrest during sports is rare but tragic because most cases progress to sudden death. Pre-participation evaluation can identify underlying cardiac disease and athletes at risk, playing a big role in prevention. Emergency care, according to "the chain of survival", especially the availability of AED, "hands-only"-CPR, medical action plan, and team training are essential for a good outcome after SCA. Some special situations may have different recommendations for CPR and specific care.

Take Home Messages

- An unconscious athlete in the arena must be considered an SCA.
- SCA = Call for help/AED and initiate CPR as C-A-B sequence (hands-only).
- SCA in Drowning SCA = CPR as A-B-C sequence (ventilation first).
- PPS is the key to SD prevention.
- Emergency care plan and training are part of SD preventive measures.
- AED availability for early defibrillation is essential for SCA good outcome.

References

1. Marenco JP, Wang PJ, Link MS, Homoud MK, Estes IIINAM. Improving survival from sudden cardiac arrest. JAMA. 2001;285(9):1193. Available from: http://jama.jamanetwork.com/article.aspx?doi=10.1001/jama.285.9.1193.
2. Harmon KG, Asif IM, Maleszewski JJ, Owens DS, Prutkin JM, Salerno JC, et al. Incidence, cause, and comparative frequency of sudden cardiac death in National Collegiate Athletic Association Athletes. Circulation. 2015;132(1):10–9. Available from: http://circ.ahajournals.org/lookup/doi/10.1161/CIRCULATIONAHA.115.015431.
3. Maron BJ, Haas TS, Murphy CJ, Ahluwalia A, Rutten-Ramos S. Incidence and causes of sudden death in U.S. college athletes. J Am Coll Cardiol. 2014;63(16):1636–43.
4. Finocchiaro G, Papadakis M, Robertus JL, Dhutia H, Steriotis AK, Tome M, et al. Etiology of sudden death in sports insights from a United Kingdom Regional Registry. J Am Coll Cardiol. 2016;67(18):2108–15.
5. Basso C, Carturan E, Corrado D, Thiene G. Myocarditis and dilated cardiomyopathy in athletes: diagnosis, management, and recommendations for sport activity. Cardiol Clin. 2007;25(3):423–9. Available from: http://linkinghub.elsevier.com/retrieve/pii/S0733865107000811.
6. Colombo CSSS, Leitão MB, Avanza Jr. AC, Borges SF, Silveira AD, Braga F, et al. Position Statement on Post-COVID-19 Cardiovascular Preparticipation

Screening: Guidance for Returning to Physical Exercise and Sports – 2020. Arq Bras Cardiol. 2021; 116(6):1213–26. https://doi.org/10.36660/abc.20210368.
7. Mont L, Pelliccia A, Sharma S, Biffi A, Borjesson M, Terradellas JB, et al. Pre-participation cardiovascular evaluation for athletic participants to prevent sudden death: position paper from the EHRA and the EACPR, branches of the ESC. Endorsed by APHRS, HRS, and SOLAECE. Europace. 2016;19(1):euw243. Available from: https://academic.oup.com/europace/article-lookup/doi/10.1093/europace/euw243.
8. FIFA pre-competition medical assessment. 2009 [cited 2018 May 7]. p. 1–15. Available from: http://resources.fifa.com/image/upload/fifa-pre-competition-medical-assessment-men-2835608.pdf?cloudid=mez1hpntbmzayhtzx3je.
9. International Ollympic Committee Medical Commission. Sudden cardiovascular death in sport—the Lausanne recommendations. 2004 [cited 2018 Feb 2]. p. 10–3. Available from: https://www.olympic.org/news/sudden-cardiovascular-death-in-sport-lausanne-recommendations-adopted.
10. Corrado D, Basso C, Pavei A, Michieli P, Schiavon M, Thiene G. Trends in sudden cardiovascular death in young competitive athletes after implementation of a preparticipation screening program. JAMA. 2006;296(13):1593. Available from: http://jama.jamanetwork.com/article.aspx?doi=10.1001/jama.296.13.1593.
11. Toresdahl B, Courson R, Börjesson M, Sharma S, Drezner J. Emergency cardiac care in the athletic setting: from schools to the Olympics. Br J Sports Med. 2012;46(Suppl. 1):i85.
12. Borjesson M, Dugmore D, Mellwig KP, Van Buuren F, Serratosa L, Solberg EE, et al. Time for action regarding cardiovascular emergency care at sports arenas: a lesson from the Arena study. Eur Heart J. 2010;31(12):1438–41.
13. Dayer MJ, Green I. Mortality during marathons: a narrative review of the literature. BMJ Open Sport Exerc Med. 2019;5(1):1–7.
14. Roberts WO. A 12-yr profile of medical injury and illness for the Twin Cities Marathon. Med Sci Sports Exerc. 2000;32(9):1549–55.
15. Berg RA, Hemphill R, Abella BS, Aufderheide TP, Cave DM, Hazinski MF, et al. Part 5: adult basic life support: 2010 American Heart Association guidelines for cardiopulmonary resuscitation and emergency cardiovascular care. Circulation. 2010;122(Suppl. 3):S685.
16. Field JM, Hazinski MF, Sayre MR, Chameides L, Schexnayder SM, Hemphill R, et al. Part 1: executive summary: 2010 American Heart Association guidelines for cardiopulmonary resuscitation and emergency cardiovascular care. Circulation. 2010;122(Suppl. 3):640–57.
17. Corrado D, Cipriani A, Zorzi A. Shocking insights on resuscitation after sports-related cardiac arrest. Eur Heart J. 2023;44:193–5.
18. Wilson MG, Drezner JA. IOC manual of sports cardiology. Wiley; 2016.
19. Wyckoff MH, Greif R, Morley PT, Ng K-C, Olasveengen TM, Singletary EM, et al. 2022 International consensus on cardiopulmonary resuscitation and emergency cardiovascular care science with treatment recommendations: summary from the basic life support; advanced life support; pediatric life support; neonatal life support; education, implementation, and teams; and first aid task forces. Circulation. 2022;146:e483.
20. Szpilman D, Orlowski JP. Sports related to drowning. Eur Respir Rev. 2016;25(141):348–59. https://doi.org/10.1183/16000617.0038-2016.
21. Yankelson L, Sadeh B, Gershovitz L, Werthein J, Heller K, Halpern P, et al. Life-threatening events during endurance sports: Is heat stroke more prevalent than arrhythmic death? J Am Coll Cardiol. 2014;64(5):463–9.
22. Sloan BK, Kraft EM, Clark D, Schmeissing SW, Byrne BC, Rusyniak DE. On-site treatment of exertional heat stroke. Am J Sports Med. 2015;43(4):823–9.

20 Neurologic Conditions: Stingers, Headaches, and Seizures

Phillip H. Yun and Ankur Verma

20.1 Stinger (Burner) [1–5]

A burner or stinger is a common upper extremity nerve injury that manifests as stinging or burning pain in one upper extremity after impact to the head, neck, and/or shoulder. Most stingers resolve spontaneously within seconds to minutes. However, some athletes experience symptoms that persist for weeks, become permanent neurological deficits, or become a recurrent issue limiting their ability to play collision or contact sports.

Injury occurs at the level of the brachial plexus or cervical nerve root through one of the proposed mechanisms:

1. **Traction injury**—brachial plexus or nerve root is stretched as the shoulder is depressed while the neck is forced away laterally from the involved shoulder.
2. **Compression injury**—nerve root is compressed in the neural foramen during extension and lateral flexion of the neck to the ipsilateral side.
3. **Direct injury**—brachial plexus is injured through direct impact at the supraclavicular fossa.

P. H. Yun (✉)
University of Chicago, Chicago, IL, USA
e-mail: phillip.yun@bsd.uchicago.edu

A. Verma
University of Illinois Chicago, Chicago, IL, USA
e-mail: averma28@uic.edu

20.1.1 Clinical Presentation [5–7]

- Acute pain radiating down the arm immediately following an inciting injury. Classically described as a burning pain by the athlete and generally in a circumferential, non-dermatomal pattern.
- Associated numbness, paresthesia, and/or weakness may be present as well.
- There is usually no associated neck pain or limitation in neck range of motion.
- Symptoms in bilateral upper extremities is a spinal cord injury until proven otherwise and not a stinger.
- History of previous stingers (number and laterality) should be ascertained as these influence return to play guidelines and diagnostic testing (Fact Box 20.1).

Fact Box 20.1
Red flag findings such as altered mental status, significant neck pain, decreased cervical range of motion, bilateral upper extremity findings, and/or lower extremity findings should prompt evaluation for an alternative diagnosis.

S. Rocha Piedade et al. (eds.), *Sideline Management in Sports*,
https://doi.org/10.1007/978-3-031-33867-0_20

20.1.2 Differential Diagnosis [4, 7, 8]

1. Cervical spine fracture
2. Cervical spine dislocation
3. Spinal cord contusion/injury
4. Cervical disc herniation
5. Cervical spine instability (i.e. atlantoaxial instability)
6. Vascular injury
7. Neck, shoulder, and/or arm muscle strain
8. Rotator cuff injury
9. Transient quadriplegia
10. Peripheral nerve injury
11. Thoracic outlet syndrome
12. Clavicle, acromion, or humeral fracture
13. Shoulder subluxation/dislocation/instability
14. Acromioclavicular sprain/dislocation

20.1.3 Discussion of Key Physical Examination Pearls and Findings [5, 7–9]

20.1.3.1 Rapid Evaluation

Assess for spinal cord or brain injury first. If any of the following are present along with stinger-like symptoms, the athlete should be withheld from the rest of the game, put in appropriate spine precautions, and should be considered for evaluation in the Emergency Department:

1. Altered mental status
2. Significant headache
3. Ataxia/incoordination
4. Presence of neurologic bilateral upper extremity findings
5. Presence of neurologic findings in lower and upper extremities
6. Significant neck pain, decreased cervical range of motion, and/or midline tenderness along cervical spinous processes

Otherwise, a focused evaluation can be conducted (Figs. 20.1, 20.2 and 20.3):

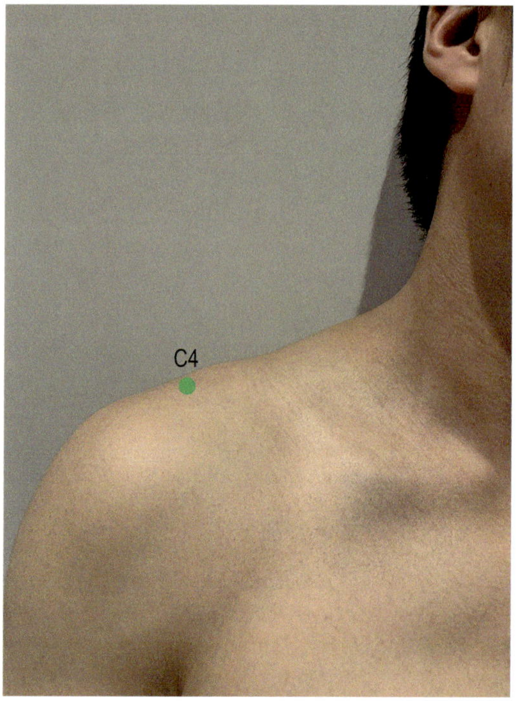

Fig. 20.1 C4 dermatome over the acromioclavicular joint

1. **Palpation**: Rule out fracture or dislocation and localize affected area
   (a) Cervical spine, sternoclavicular joint, clavicle, acromion, acromioclavicular joint, shoulder joint, humerus, elbow joint, radius/ulna, wrist, digits
2. **Strength testing**:
   (a) Ensure symmetric strength in neck and upper extremities with resisted movement testing
   (b) Special attention to muscles innervated by C5 and C6 as they are the most injured nerve roots
      - Deltoid—resisted shoulder abduction
      - Supraspinatus—empty can test
      - Infraspinatus—resisted shoulder external rotation
      - Biceps brachii—resisted elbow flexion and forearm supination
3. **Sensation testing**:

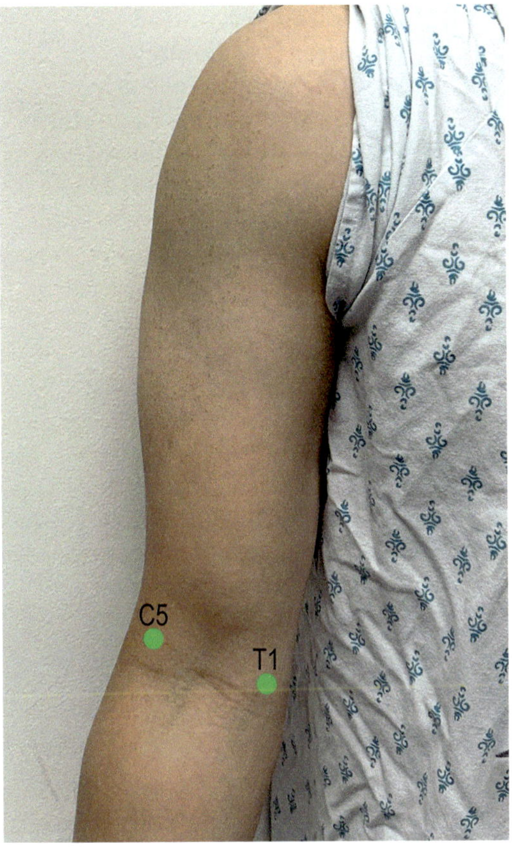

Fig. 20.2 C5 and T1 dermatomes over the antecubital fossa of the elbow

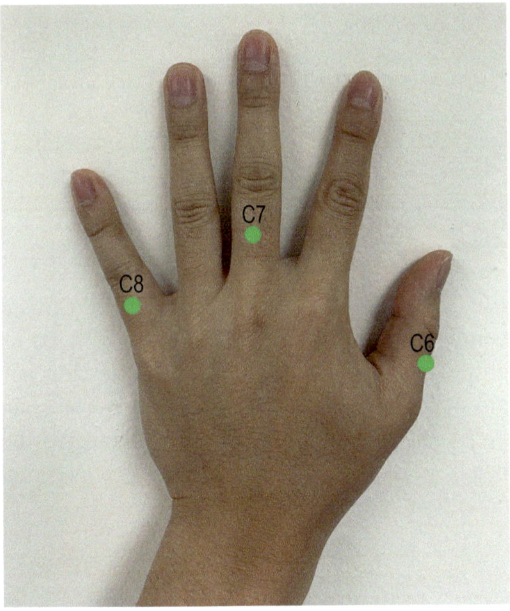

Fig. 20.3 C6, C7, and C8 dermatomes over the hand

   (a) C4—Over AC joint
   (b) C5—Radial side of the antecubital fossa just proximal to the elbow
   (c) C6—Dorsal surface of proximal phalanx of the thumb
   (d) C7—Dorsal surface of proximal phalanx of the third digit
   (e) C8—Dorsal surface of proximal phalanx of the fifth digit
   (f) T1—Ulnar side of the antecubital fossa, just proximal to the medial epicondyle
4. **Pulse testing**: Ensure symmetry by palpating radial pulses bilaterally
5. **Special maneuver**:
   (a) Spurling examination

20.1.4 Indications and Benefits of Additional Testing/Imaging (Point of Care or Referral) [4, 7, 8]

20.1.4.1 Point of Care Testing

None.

20.1.4.2 Referral

Immediate Emergency Department evaluation for the following:

1. Suspicion for intracranial bleed
2. Suspicion for cervical spine fracture, cervical spine dislocation/instability, or spinal cord injury
3. Suspicion for other unstable fracture

20.1.4.3 Outpatient Evaluation

Further evaluation on the outpatient basis is indicated for the following scenarios:

1. History of recurrent stingers (e.g., three or more episodes in lifetime, second-time stinger in same season)
2. Prolonged (>1 h) or persistent mild sensory deficits

Potential tests ordered on the outpatient basis include plain films, MRI, MRA/CTA, EMS/NCS (optimal time frame at least 3 weeks from date of injury).

20.1.5 Sideline Management Guidelines and Suggestions of the Specific Traumatic Injuries and Clinical Issues in Athletes [4, 7, 10]

There are no consensus guidelines on return to play. Below is a synthesis of expert opinions, favoring more conservative management.

20.1.5.1 Return to Play

No contraindications

- First-time stinger (seconds to minutes) with full resolution of symptoms and clinical manifestations
- Second-time stinger (seconds to minutes) not in the same game or season with full resolution of symptoms and clinical manifestations

Relative contraindications

- Second-time stinger in the same game or same season
- Some experts support return to same game if full resolution of symptoms and clinical manifestations within seconds to minutes

Absolute contraindication

- Unresolved neurologic deficits on clinical examination
- Neurologic deficits in bilateral upper extremities or any lower extremity
- Significant neck pain and/or lack of full cervical range of motion
- Third-time stinger regardless of timing

Full resolution of symptoms and clinical manifestations defined as the following:

1. No neurologic deficits on examination
2. Resolution of all symptoms per athlete history
3. Full cervical and shoulder range of motion without pain
4. Spurling's test negative
5. Ability to perform sport-specific skills without recurrent symptoms

20.1.6 Suggested Prevention Measures that Could be Implemented for Early Recognition or Risk Reduction (Altitude, Rules Modifications, Referee Instruction) [4, 11]

- Cervical collars may minimize risk of reinjury but may also increase the risk of overall cervical injuries due to the athlete's head in a more flexed position.
- Incorporation of strengthening exercises targeting cervical, thoracic, scapular, and core stabilizers.
- Review of proper tackling technique: (1) "head-up" technique and "see what you hit" concept and (2) initiating contact with the front of the shoulder and/or chest [11].

Take Home Messages

- Stingers (burners) present as a burning or stinging pain that radiate down one upper extremity following impact to the head, neck, and/or shoulder.
- Generally, most athletes report complete resolution of symptoms within seconds to minutes.
- Athletes may only return to play in the same game if there is full resolution of symptoms and clinical manifestations AND it is a first-time stinger OR second-time stinger but in a different season.

20.2 Headache [12, 13]

Headaches are one of the most common medical complaints and can be generally categorized as either primary or secondary. Primary headaches are conditions where the head pain is the main problem whereas in secondary headaches, the head pain is a symptom of an underlying condition.

Common examples of primary headaches are migraine, tension-type headache, trigeminal autonomic cephalalgia (e.g., cluster headache), and primary exercise headache. Common examples of secondary headaches are due to trauma, cranial/cervical vascular disorders, substance use or its withdrawal, infection, psychiatric disorders, disturbances to homeostasis, or referred pain from the cranium, neck, eyes, ears, nose, sinuses, teeth, mouth, or other facial or cervical structures.

In this chapter, we will focus on headaches that athletes may commonly experience and how to identify more worrisome secondary headaches.

20.2.1 Clinical Presentation [13–16]

- Tension headache
  - Most common primary headache characterized as being bilateral, non-throbbing, and of mild to moderate intensity without associated features.
  - Headache description: dull, pressure, head fullness, feels like a tight cap, band-like.
- Migraine
  - A common primary headache characterized as being generally unilateral and of moderate-to-severe intensity with several associated features.
  - Headache description: throbbing/pulsating, aggravated by physical activity, associated with nausea, vomiting, photophobia, and phonophobia. Duration lasting 4–72 h if untreated or unsuccessfully treated.
  - Some migraines are preceded by an aura of reversible focal neurologic symptoms including visual, sensory, speech, language, motor, brain stem, and/or retinal.
- Primary exercise headache
  - A headache that is brought on by and occurring only during or after strenuous physical exercise. Duration lasting up to 48 h.
  - Headache description: pulsating and bilateral. Not generally associated with nausea or vomiting.
  - Also previously known as primary exertional headache and benign exertional headache.
- Headache attributed to trauma or injury to the head and/or neck
  - A new headache that occurs for the first time in close temporal relation to trauma or injury to the head and/or neck.
  - Headache description: varied but can mimic tension headaches and migraines in quality.
  - The headache may be one of many symptoms including dizziness, fatigue, reduced ability to concentrate, psychomotor slowing, insomnia, anxiety, and irritability, at which point the athlete should be evaluated for post-concussion syndrome.
- External compression headache
  - A benign primary headache due to sustained compression of pericranial soft tissues. In sports, goggles and helmets are commonly implicated.
  - Headache description: constant and commonly at location of compression (Fact Box 20.2).

Fact Box 20.2 [17–19]
All headaches suspected to be primary exercise headaches need further evaluation with advanced imaging and a formal neurological evaluation. Previous studies have shown that up to 10–42% will have an intracranial abnormality, including cerebral aneurysm, arteriovenous malformation, intracranial hemorrhage, or a space occupying lesion.

20.2.2 Differential Diagnosis [6, 13]

As per the Headache Classification Committee of the International Headache Society, there are many classifications and subclassifications of headaches. The main goal is to differentiate between primary headaches, which are generally benign, from secondary headaches which can be more concerning.

- Headache attributed to cranial and/or vascular disorder: subarachnoid hemorrhage, stroke, vascular malformation, carotid dissection, vertebral dissection.
- Headache attributed to non-vascular intracranial disorder: intracranial hypertension, low cerebrospinal fluid pressure, aseptic meningitis, neoplasm, Chiari malformation.
- Headache attributed to a substance or its withdrawal: alcohol, phosphodiesterase inhibitor, cocaine, acetaminophen-overuse, non-steroidal anti-inflammatory drug-overuse, caffeine-withdrawal, estrogen-withdrawal.
- Headache attributed to infection: viral/bacterial/fungal meningitis or encephalitis, parasitic infection.
- Headache attributed to disorder of homeostasis: high-altitude, sleep apnea, cardiac cephalalgia, fasting, hypothyroidism, airplane travel, diving headache.
- Headache attributed to disorders of the cranium, neck, eyes, ears, nose, sinuses, teeth, mouth: acute angle-closure glaucoma, acute or chronic rhinosinusitis, temporomandibular disorder.

20.2.3 Discussion of Key Physical Examination Pearls and Findings [20, 21]

Red flag sign or symptom	Related secondary headaches
Systemic symptoms including fever	Infection, nonvascular intracranial disorders, carcinoid, pheochromocytoma
Neoplasm history	Neoplasm of the brain, metastasis
Neurologic deficit	Vascular and nonvascular intracranial disorders
Sudden onset headache with rapid peak (within seconds to a minute)	Subarachnoid hemorrhage, cervical or cranial vascular disorders (e.g., aneurysm)
New headache in older age (age 50)	Giant cell arteritis, neoplasms, cranial or cervical vascular disorders
Pattern change in headache	Neoplasms, cranial or cervical vascular disorders
Positional headache	Intracranial hypertension or hypotension
Precipitated by sneezing, coughing, or exercise	Posterior fossa malformations; Chiari malformation
Papilledema	Intracranial hypertension, neoplasms and other nonvascular intracranial disorders
Progressive headache and atypical presentations	Neoplasms and other nonvascular intracranial disorders
Pregnancy or puerperium	Cranial or cervical vascular disorders, postdural puncture headache, hypertension-related headaches (e.g., eclampsia), cerebral sinus thrombosis
Painful eye	Ophthalmic causes (e.g., acute angle glaucoma, orbital trauma), posterior fossa pathology, cavernous sinus pathology
Posttraumatic onset of headache	Post traumatic headache, subdural hematoma, vascular disorders
Immune system dysfunction (e.g., HIV)	Opportunistic infections
New medication or chronic analgesic use	Medication overuse headache, drug incompatibility
Chest pain, history of heart disease, exertional headache with relief upon rest	Cardiac cephalalgia

20.2.4 Indications and Benefits of Additional Testing/Imaging (Point of Care or Referral) [20, 22, 23]

All new headaches should be further evaluated to determine the diagnosis among the numerous primary and secondary headaches. Generally, workups can be conducted on an outpatient basis; however, if worrisome symptoms or signs are present that would indicate a potentially life-threatening or highly morbid condition, the athlete should be sent to the Emergency Room for immediate evaluation and management.

Specific scenarios that would warrant an Emergency Room visit would be:

1. Fever, neck stiffness, altered mental status → concern for meningitis/encephalitis
2. Focal neurologic deficits → vascular or nonvascular intracranial disorders
3. Sudden thunderclap headache with rapid peak within seconds to a minute → subarachnoid hemorrhage
4. New visual disturbance, eye pain, trauma to the eye → ophthalmologic emergencies
5. Chest pain, shortness of breath → referred pain from coronary artery disease

20.2.5 Sideline Management and Suggestions of the Specific Traumatic Injuries and Clinical Issues in Athletes [24]

Athletes who develop headaches during games or practice should be withheld from play until further evaluation. Initial evaluation should include the following:

- Detailed history and physical examination including vital signs, orthostatic blood pressure readings, oculomotor examination, musculoskeletal examination of the head and neck, neurologic examination
- Concussion evaluation if indicated

If red flag symptoms or signs are present, Emergency Room evaluation is indicated as noted above. For nonemergent cases, close follow-up should be arranged until symptoms resolve and headache etiology and management have been determined. If the athlete is cleared to go home, athletes should keep a headache diary to bring to their outpatient appointments.

No medications should be given in the initial evaluation on the sidelines as they may mask symptoms or exacerbate underlying conditions (e.g., giving NSAIDs to those with subarachnoid hemorrhages). If the headache is confirmed to be typical for the athlete and another concomitant process has been ruled out, the athlete may take their usual medication regimen (e.g., migraines with triptans and NSAIDs).

20.2.6 Suggested Prevention Measures that Could be Implemented for Early Recognition or Risk Reduction (Altitude, Rules Modification, Referee Instruction) [13, 25]

- *Athletes with pre-existing primary headaches*: Work with their primary care physicians or neurologists in establishing a preventative and acute management plan for their headaches.
- *External compression headache*: Ensure proper fit and positioning of sporting equipment including goggles and helmets. Headache typically resolves within an hour of relieving external compression.
- *Medication overuse headache*: Athletes who frequently take analgesics for their headaches (more than 10–15 days per month) are at increased risk of developing medication overuse headaches. These athletes should be considered for preventative medications. Ensure preventative medications are allowed for each athlete's sporting event (e.g., beta-blockers).
- *Primary exercise headache*: Activity modification. Indomethacin 25–150 mg daily prior to exercise.

Take Home Messages

- Athletes that develop headaches during games or practice should be withheld from play until further evaluation on the sidelines or at a higher level of care if indicated.
- Athletes with suspected primary exercise headaches should undergo advanced imaging as studies show 10–42% have an intracranial abnormality.
- Athletes with red flag signs or symptoms that suggest a life-threatening or highly morbid condition should be evaluated in the Emergency Room promptly. A few of these include: (1) thunderclap headache with rapid peak within seconds to a minute, (2) unresolving visual disturbance with eye trauma, and (3) focal neurologic deficits and/or altered mental status.

20.3 Seizure [26–29]

A seizure is defined as "a transient occurrence of signs and/or symptoms due to abnormal excessive or synchronous neuronal activity in the brain." Seizures can either be (1) unprovoked or (2) an acute symptomatic seizure that occurs at the time of a systemic insult or close temporal association with a documented brain insult, such as a traumatic brain injury. Epilepsy, on the other hand, is defined as a pathologic tendency to have recurrent unprovoked seizures.

Seizures can be further classified by level of brain involvement: (1) focal onset (previously known as partial) involving a particular region of the brain or (2) generalized onset involving both hemispheres. A third classification exists called unknown onset where the onset of seizure was unobserved.

20.3.1 Clinical Presentation [29, 30]

Seizures have a diverse array of manifestations based on which part of the brain is affected, as noted below. Most seizures spontaneously end within 2–3 min. Following the end of seizure activity, the postictal period is often noted by altered awareness and/or function, where athletes may appear groggy or confused. Full recovery to an athlete's pre-seizure baseline may take seconds, minutes, or even longer.

- Focal onset: level of consciousness can either be fully intact or impaired. Athletes can manifest with motor findings, sensory findings, or both. Focal onset seizures can progress to becoming generalized seizures.
  - Motor findings: automatisms, epileptic spasms, atonic, clonic, hyperkinetic, myoclonic, or tonic seizures
  - Nonmotor findings: autonomic, behavior arrest, cognitive, emotional, or sensory seizures (Fact Box 20.3)
- Generalized onset:
  - Motor findings: tonic-clonic, clonic, tonic, myoclonic, myoclonic-tonic-clonic, myoclonic-atonic, atonic, or epileptic spasms
  - Nonmotor findings: typical absence, atypical absence, myoclonic, or eyelid myoclonic (Fact Box 20.4)

Seizure classification	Clinical manifestations
Automatisms	Repetitive, purposeless motor activities—lip smacking, head nodding, and patting
Epileptic spasms	Flexion at waist with either flexion or extension of the arms
Atonic	Loss of tone
Clonic	Repeated, regularly spaced jerking movements
Hyperkinetic	Thrashing motion
Myoclonic	Irregular, not rhythmic jerking movements
Tonic	Increased tone or stiffening of limbs and/or neck
Behavior arrest	Cessation of movement—blank stare, not moving, and not speaking
Autonomic, cognitive, emotional, sensory	Clear emotional changes such as dread/fear/pleasure, hallucinations, déjà vu, jamais vu, paresthesias, changes in heart-rate, piloerection, diaphoresis, visual or auditory disturbances
Tonic-clonic	Initial stiffening with subsequent rhythmic jerking of all limbs. Tongue biting may occur initially and incontinence subsequently
Myoclonic-tonic-clonic	Initial irregular jerking movements followed by a tonic-clonic seizure
Myoclonic-atonic	Initial irregular jerking movements followed by loss of tone bilaterally
Absence	Sudden cessation of activity sometimes followed by automatisms followed by immediate recovery
Eye myoclonic	Eyelid jerks and upward deviation of the eyes

Fact Box 20.3 [31]

Convulsive status epilepticus is a medical emergency, and the operational diagnosis is defined as either (1) a convulsive seizure lasting >5 min or (2) two or more seizures without a return to the baseline level of consciousness between seizures.

Fact Box 20.4 [32–34]
Concussive convulsions and tonic posturing may occur immediately after head trauma and are not considered seizures. The pathophysiology is unknown, but some suggest it may be due to transient disinhibition of the brainstem resulting in the recurrence of neonatal reflexes and cortical disturbance from mechanical forces. Concussive convulsions are marked by initial tonic posturing followed by either clonic or myoclonic jerks. In other instances, only tonic posturing may be seen. On average, these episodes last for 30s but can go on for minutes.

20.3.2 Differential Diagnosis [35]

- Syncope
- Transient ischemic stroke or stroke
- Migraine aura
- Panic attack
- Concussive convulsions or tonic posturing (fencing position, bear hug position, and righting movement)
- Psychogenic nonepileptic seizure

20.3.3 Discussion of Key Physical Examination Pearls and Findings [36]

The postictal state may include a variety of sensory, motor, and/or cognitive manifestations. Duration of postictal state ranges, but typically after a generalized seizure, most patients begin to recover with 10–20 min and show consistent improvement:

- Cognitive: declined alertness, delirium, speech disturbances (i.e., dysphasia), psychiatric disturbances (i.e., violent behavior, anxiety, depression)
- Sensory: headache, visual disturbances, paresthesia
- Motor: weakness, paresis, catatonia
- Others: incontinence, tongue laceration, shoulder dislocation

20.3.4 Indications and Benefits of Additional Testing/Imaging (Point of Care or Referral) [5, 35]

20.3.4.1 Point of Care Testing

- Glucose check for hypoglycemia

20.3.4.2 Referral to the Emergency Room

Generally, there should be a low threshold for sending athletes to the Emergency Room after seizure-like activity. The following are the specific reasons for Emergency Room referral:

- First-time seizures
- Convulsive status epilepticus
- Prolonged seizure activity
- Concern for respiratory compromise
- Incomplete return to baseline mental status or neurologic function
- Injuries sustained during seizure activity that cannot be managed on the sidelines

20.3.5 Sideline Management and Suggestions of the Specific Traumatic Injuries and Clinical Issues in Athletes [5, 37, 38]

20.3.5.1 Management During Seizure Activity

- *Athlete specific*: Monitor athlete's airway, breathing, and circulation. Assists athlete to the ground safely. Remove or loosen restrictive equipment if possible. Cushion head if possible. Do not restrain the athlete. Do not place anything in the athlete's mouth.
- *Environment specific*: Move athlete to safe environment if needed—away from water, onto even surface, away from harmful objects.
- If concerned for convulsive status epilepticus:

- Assess and maintain airway, breathing, and circulation
- Call EMS
- Check for hypoglycemia if possible
- Abortive therapy with a benzodiazepine if seizures continue for >3 min

Benzodiazepine	Children and adults
IM Midazolam (first line)	• 13–40 kg: 5 mg • >40 kg: 10 mg
IV Lorazepam (first line)	• 0.1 mg/kg/dose, max: 4 mg/dose
IV Diazepam (first line)	• 0.15–0.2 mg/kg/dose, max: 10 mg/dose
Rectal diazepam	• 0.2–0.5 mg/kg, max: 20 mg/dose
IN Midazolam	• Infants, children, and adolescents: 0.2 mg/kg as a single dose • Ages 12 years and above: 5 mg dose as a single dose

Buccal midazolam may also be used—dosing and delivery varies based on age and/or weight

20.3.5.2 Management After Seizure Activity

- Once seizure activity has ceased, roll athlete to the side in case of postictal emesis
- Assess and maintain airway, breathing, and circulation
- Full neurologic evaluation (multiple evaluations over time to assess for improvement)
- Fracture and dislocation evaluation
- Skin and oral laceration evaluation
- If available, fundoscopic evaluation to assess for papilledema, a sign of elevated intracranial pressure

20.3.6 Suggested Prevention Measures that Could be Implemented for Early Recognition or Risk Reduction (Altitude, Rules Modification, Referee Instruction) [27, 39, 40]

- The International League Against Epilepsy Task Force on Sports and Epilepsy offers general guidance for participation in sports in those with seizure history/epilepsy who have been evaluated and managed by neurology.
- In addition, traumatic brain injury likely represents a substantial percentage of preventable epilepsy, and sports-specific guidelines to minimize risk of traumatic brain injury is crucial.
- Pre-participation evaluation is important to assess risk for preventable causes of seizures including metabolic derangements (hypoglycemia, hyponatremia, hypocalcemia, hypomagnesemia, uremia) and drugs/toxic substances related (alcohol, cocaine, hallucinogens, phencyclidine/PCP). For children, febrile seizures are also well described but rare after the age of 5.

Group 1 sports (no significant additional risk)	Group 2 sports (moderate risk to athlete but not to bystanders)	Group 3 sports (high risk for athlete, and for some sports, also for bystanders
• Athletics (except for sports in Group 2) • Bowling • Most collective contact sports (e.g., judo, wrestling) • Collective sports on the ground (e.g., baseball, basketball, cricket, field hockey, football, rugby, volleyball) • Cross-country skiing • Curling • Dancing • Golf • Racquet sports (e.g., squash, table tennis, tennis)	• Alpine skiing • Archery • Athletics (pole vault) • Biathlon, triathlon, modern pentathlon • Canoeing • Collective contact sports involving potentially serious injury (e.g., boxing, karate) • Cycling • Fencing • Gymnastics • Horse riding (e.g., Olympic equestrian events) • Ice hockey • Shooting • Skateboarding • Skating • Snowboarding • Swimming • Water skiing • Weightlifting	• Aviation • Climbing • Diving • Horse racing • Motor sports • Parachuting • Rodeo • Scuba diving • Ski jumping • Solitary sailing • Surfing, wind-surfing

	Group 1 sports	Group 2 sports	Group 3 sports
One or more symptomatic seizures	Permitted	Permitted at neurologist's discretion, with restrictions	Permitted at neurologist's discretion, with restrictions
Single unprovoked seizure	Permitted	Permitted after 12 months of seizure freedom	Permitted after 12 months of seizure freedom
Seizure-free (12 months or longer)	Permitted	Permitted	Permitted
Sleep-related seizures only	Permitted	Permitted at neurologist's discretion, with restrictions	Generally barred
Seizures without impaired awareness	Permitted	Permitted at neurologist's discretion, with restrictions	Generally barred
Seizures with impaired awareness	Permitted at neurologist's discretion applies when seizures are precipitated by specific activities	Permitted at neurologist's discretion, with restrictions	Generally barred
Epilepsy resolved (no seizures >10 years and off AED >5 years)	Permitted	Permitted	Permitted
Medication withdrawal	Permitted at neurologist's discretion applies when seizures are precipitated by specific activities	Permitted after appropriate periods following AED cessation	Permitted after appropriate periods following AED cessation

Take Home Messages

1. Seizures have a wide range of manifestations spanning from cognitive, sensory, and motor findings, and for some, residual symptoms and physical examination findings remain in the postictal period.
2. Medical providers should have a low threshold for having athletes be evaluated in the Emergency Room following seizure like activity.
3. Concussive convulsions and tonic posturing can occur immediately following head trauma and are not generally considered to be true seizures.

References

1. Levitz CL, Reilly PJ, Torg JS. The pathomechanics of chronic, recurrent cervical nerve root neurapraxia: the chronic burner syndrome. Am J Sports Med. 1997;25:73. https://doi.org/10.1177/036354659702500114.
2. Markey KL, Di Benedetto M, Curl WW. Upper trunk brachial plexopathy. Am J Sports Med. 1993;21:650. https://doi.org/10.1177/036354659302100503.
3. Feinberg JH. Burners and stingers. Phys Med Rehabil Clin N Am. 2000;11:771.
4. Bowles DR, Canseco JA, Alexander TD, Schroeder GD, Hecht AC, Vaccaro AR. The prevalence and management of stingers in college and professional collision athletes. Curr Rev Musculoskelet Med. 2020;13:651. https://doi.org/10.1007/s12178-020-09665-5.
5. Dimberg EL, Burns TM. Management of common neurologic conditions in sports. Clin Sports Med. 2005;24:637. https://doi.org/10.1016/j.csm.2005.04.002.
6. Brukner P, Khan K, Clarsen B, et al. In: Brukner P, Clarsen B, Cook J, et al., editors. Brukner & Khan's clinical sports medicine: injuries, vol. 1. 5th ed. McGraw Hill; 2017. https://csm.mhmedical.com/content.aspx?bookid=1970&sectionid=168688260.
7. Standaert CJ, Herring SA. Expert opinion and controversies in musculoskeletal and sports medicine: stingers. Arch Phys Med Rehabil. 2009;90:402. https://doi.org/10.1016/j.apmr.2008.09.569.
8. Safran MR. Nerve injury about the shoulder in athletes, part 2: long thoracic nerve, spinal accessory nerve, burners/stingers, thoracic outlet syndrome. Am J Sports Med. 2004;32:1063. https://doi.org/10.1177/0363546504265193.
9. Rupp R, Biering-Sørensen F, Burns SP, et al. International standards for neurological classification of spinal cord injury. Top Spinal Cord Inj Rehabil. 2021;27:1. https://doi.org/10.46292/sci2702-1.
10. Hsu WK, Jenkins TJ. Spinal conditions in the athlete: a clinical guide to evaluation, management and controversies. Springer; 2019.
11. Heck JF, Clarke KS, Peterson TR, Torg JS, Weis MP. National Athletic Trainers' Association position statement: head-down contact and spearing in tackle football. J Athl Train. 2004;39:101.
12. Seifert T. Headache in sports. Curr Pain Headache Rep. 2014;18 https://doi.org/10.1007/s11916-014-0448-x.
13. Olesen J. Headache classification committee of the International Headache Society (IHS) the International Classification of Headache Disorders, 3rd edition. Cephalalgia. 2018;38:1. https://doi.org/10.1177/0333102417738202.
14. Jensen RH. Tension-type headache—the normal and most prevalent headache. Headache. 2018;58:339. https://doi.org/10.1111/head.13067.
15. Ashina M, Terwindt GM, Al-Karagholi MAM, et al. Migraine: disease characterisation, biomarkers, and precision medicine. Lancet. 2021;397:1496. https://doi.org/10.1016/S0140-6736(20)32162-0.
16. Krymchantowski AV. Headaches due to external compression. Curr Pain Headache Rep. 2010;14:321. https://doi.org/10.1007/s11916-010-0122-x.
17. Sands GH, Newman L, Lipton R. Cough, exertional, and other miscellaneous headaches. Med Clin North Am. 1991;75:733. https://doi.org/10.1016/S0025-7125(16)30446-1.
18. Pascual J, Iglesias F, Oterino A, Vazquez-Barquero A, Berciano J. Cough, exertional, and sexual headaches: an analysis of 72 benign and symptomatic cases. Neurology. 1996;46:1520. https://doi.org/10.1212/WNL.46.6.1520.
19. Rooke ED. Benign exertional headache. Med Clin North Am. 1968;52:801. https://doi.org/10.1016/s0025-7125(16)32870-x.
20. Do TP, Remmers A, Schytz HW, et al. Red and orange flags for secondary headaches in clinical practice: SNNOOP10 list. Neurology. 2019;92:134. https://doi.org/10.1212/WNL.0000000000006697.
21. Lima V, Burt B, Leibovitch I, Prabhakaran V, Goldberg RA, Selva D. Orbital compartment syndrome: the ophthalmic surgical emergency. Surv Ophthalmol. 2009;54:441. https://doi.org/10.1016/j.survophthal.2009.04.005.
22. Edlow JA. Managing patients with nontraumatic, severe, rapid-onset headache. Ann Emerg Med. 2018;71:400. https://doi.org/10.1016/j.annemergmed.2017.04.044.
23. Schut ES, de Gans J, van de Beek D. Community-acquired bacterial meningitis in adults. Pract Neurol. 2008;8:8. https://doi.org/10.1136/jnnp.2007.139725.
24. Smith ED, Swartzon M, McGrew CA. Headaches in athletes. Curr Sports Med Rep. 2014;13:27. https://doi.org/10.1249/JSR.0000000000000021.

25. Diamond S. Prolonged benign exertional headache: its clinical characteristics and response to indomethacin. Headache J Head Face Pain. 1982;22:96. https://doi.org/10.1111/j.1526-4610.1982.hed2203096.x.
26. Fisher RS, Van Emde BW, Blume W, et al. Epileptic seizures and epilepsy: definitions proposed by the International League Against Epilepsy (ILAE) and the International Bureau for Epilepsy (IBE). Epilepsia. 2005;46:470. https://doi.org/10.1111/j.0013-9580.2005.66104.x.
27. Beghi E, Carpio A, Forsgren L, et al. Recommendation for a definition of acute symptomatic seizure. Epilepsia. 2010;51:671. https://doi.org/10.1111/j.1528-1167.2009.02285.x.
28. Fisher RS, Acevedo C, Arzimanoglou A, et al. ILAE official report: a practical clinical definition of epilepsy. Epilepsia. 2014;55:475. https://doi.org/10.1111/epi.12550.
29. Fisher RS, Cross JH, French JA, et al. Operational classification of seizure types by the international league against epilepsy: position paper of the ILAE Commission for Classification and Terminology. Epilepsia. 2017;58:522. https://doi.org/10.1111/epi.13670.
30. Pack AM. Epilepsy overview and revised classification of seizures and epilepsies. Contin Lifelong Learn Neurol. 2019;25:306. https://doi.org/10.1212/CON.0000000000000707.
31. Trinka E, Cock H, Hesdorffer D, et al. A definition and classification of status epilepticus—report of the ILAE Task Force on Classification of Status Epilepticus. Epilepsia. 2015;56:1515. https://doi.org/10.1111/epi.13121.
32. McCrory PR, Berkovic SF. Video analysis of acute motor and convulsive manifestations in sport- related concussion. Neurology. 2000;54:1488. https://doi.org/10.1212/WNL.54.7.1488.
33. Tényi D, Gyimesi C, Horváth R, et al. Concussive convulsions: a YouTube video analysis. Epilepsia. 2016;57:1310. https://doi.org/10.1111/epi.13432.
34. McCrory PR, Eerkovic SF. Concussive convulsions incidence in sport and treatment recommendations. Sport Med. 1998;25:131. https://doi.org/10.2165/00007256-199825020-00005.
35. Smith PEM. Initial management of seizure in adults. N Engl J Med. 2021;385:251. https://doi.org/10.1056/nejmcp2024526.
36. Pottkämper JCM, Hofmeijer J, van Waarde JA, van Putten MJAM. The postictal state — what do we know? Epilepsia. 2020;61:1045. https://doi.org/10.1111/epi.16519.
37. Glauser T, Shinnar S, Gloss D, et al. Evidence-based guideline: treatment of convulsive status epilepticus in children and adults: report of the guideline committee of the American epilepsy society. Epilepsy Curr. 2016;16:48. https://doi.org/10.5698/1535-7597-16.1.48.
38. Mctague A, Martland T, Appleton R. Drug management for acute tonic-clonic convulsions including convulsive status epilepticus in children. Cochrane Database Syst Rev. 2018;2018:CD001905. https://doi.org/10.1002/14651858.CD001905.pub3.
39. Capovilla G, Kaufman KR, Perucca E, Moshé SL, Arida RM. Epilepsy, seizures, physical exercise, and sports: a report from the ILAE Task Force on Sports and Epilepsy. Epilepsia. 2016;57:6. https://doi.org/10.1111/epi.13261.
40. Thurman DJ, Begley CE, Carpio A, et al. The primary prevention of epilepsy: a report of the Prevention Task Force of the International League Against Epilepsy. Epilepsia. 2018;59:905. https://doi.org/10.1111/epi.14068.

Psychological Disorders

21

Jessica Bartley and Amber Donaldson

21.1 Introduction

According to the Center for Disease Control and Prevention (CDC), psychological disorders are among the most common health conditions in the United States and more than half of Americans will experience a psychological disorder in their lifetime and one-fifth of American adults will experience a psychological disorder annually [1]. According to the Global Burden of Disease Study in 2017, psychological disorders are one of the leading causes of functional impairment worldwide and it was also estimated that 13% of adults worldwide experience some form of a psychological disorder annually [2].

While sport has numerous benefits, including but not limited to, learning to build relationships and social connections, improved time and stress management, increased concentration and confidence, and regular physical activity and fitness, studies still suggest that one in three athletes might experience psychological symptoms during or immediately after their career. For elite athletes, a 2019 meta-analysis found that 33.6% of elite athletes and 26.4% of former athletes reported symptoms of anxiety and depression [3].

Athletes may have previously been diagnosed with a psychological disorder and are under the care of a provider, but they may also be unaware of an underlying diagnosis and what may lead to a diagnosable psychological disorder. Therefore, it is critical for medical providers to be prepared to manage an acute psychological injury. The purpose of this chapter is to provide clinical presentation and differential diagnoses for psychological disorders common in elite athletes and how they may present in a sports setting. This will be followed by a description of how to develop and execute a Mental Health Emergency Action Plan (MHEAP) which may require sideline management within a sports setting.

21.2 Description of Psychological Disorders

The World Health Organization has characterized psychological disorders as "a clinically significant disturbance in an individual's cognition, emotional regulation, or behavior" and it is often accompanied by distress or impairment in functioning [4]. Psychological disorders are included in the International Classification of Diseases (ICD) as well as the Diagnostic and Statistical Manual of Mental Disorders, also known as the

J. Bartley
Department of Sports Medicine, United States Olympic and Paralympic Committee, Colorado Springs, CO, USA
e-mail: jessica.bartley@usopc.org

A. Donaldson (✉)
U.S. Coalition for the Prevention of Illness and Injury in Sport, Colorado Springs, CO, USA
e-mail: amber.donaldson@usopc.org

S. Rocha Piedade et al. (eds.), *Sideline Management in Sports*,
https://doi.org/10.1007/978-3-031-33867-0_21

DSM [5]. In the United States, the DSM was created to help identify psychological disorders as well as resources for World War II servicemen and veterans and has become the standard classification of psychological disorders in our country. The latest edition, the Diagnostic and Statistical Manual of Mental Disorders, Fifth Edition, Text Revision (DSM-5-TR), was published in 2022 and aligns closely with the tenth version of the ICD (ICD-10).

In the following sections, descriptions of each psychological disorder a clinical provider may encounter will be detailed along with information on prevalence, possible manifestations of these disorders in athletes (where known), as well as the most common validated screening tools. Note, there are no athlete-specific stand-alone assessments/screeners for any psychological disorder, except for sleep, feeding and eating disorders, as well as competitive anxiety, which will be noted.

21.2.1 Anxiety Disorders

In the United States, anxiety disorders are the most common psychological disorder with nearly 30% of adults in the United States impacted at some point in their life [6]. In a large systematic review and meta-analysis, they found no difference in anxiety profiles between athletes and non-athletes though there may be some slightly different sources of anxiety which are sport participation related [7]. The most recognized anxiety disorder, Generalized Anxiety Disorder or GAD is characterized by clinically significant anxiety and this anxiety occurs more than half of the days for at least 6 months [5]. In addition, a person experiencing GAD might find it difficult to control anxiety while experiencing three or more of the following symptoms: restlessness, fatigue, difficulty concentrating, irritability, muscle tension, or sleep disturbance. It is also important to note that if another psychological disorder, such as Depressive Disorders, Psychotic Disorders, Personality Disorders, or others is a more accurate diagnosis and is causing anxiety, then those would be considered the primary diagnosis. Other common anxiety disorders are Panic Disorder and/or Panic Attack as well as Social Anxiety Disorder, Agoraphobia, and other Specific Phobias. In addition to generalized anxiety, athletes might experience anxiety related to competition or performance and according to the DSM-5-TR, they could meet criteria for a Specific Phobia that could be situational to competition.

In October 2022, the U.S. Preventive Services Task Force suggested that adults should regularly be screened for anxiety even if they are not experiencing symptoms due to the prevalence of the disorder [8]. The most common assessment is the Generalized Anxiety Disorder-7 or GAD-7,which is a self-report questionnaire for ages 12 and older that includes seven questions related to the frequency of anxiety-related behaviors in the preceding 2 weeks [9]. The Generalized Anxiety Disorder Severity Scale (GADSS) is similar to the GAD-7, but it measures the intensity of anxiety-related symptoms for adults ages 18 and older [10]. The Beck Anxiety Inventory (BAI) is also a self-report questionnaire for ages 17 and older that can be administered to assess the severity of anxiety symptoms [11]. Alternatively, the Sport Competition Anxiety Scale (SCAT) measures anxiety levels before or during competition or performance situations [12].

21.2.2 Obsessive-Compulsive and Related Disorders

Obsessive-Compulsive Disorder or OCD was previously considered an anxiety disorder but was recently shifted into its own category because OCD is distinguished by obsessive thoughts resulting in compulsive actions while in contrast, an individual with generalized anxiety will experience anxious thoughts without necessarily engaging in compulsive actions [13]. To diagnose OCD, an individual would be experiencing unwanted and distressing thoughts, urges, or images and there is an attempt to ignore or suppress these thoughts with another thought or action (e.g., compulsion). OCD is only diagnosed if the psychological disorder is not better accounted for by one of the following: Generalized Anxiety Disorder, Feeding and Eating Disorders, Schizophrenia Spectrum and Other Psychotic Disorders, Paraphilic Disorders, or related Obsessive-Compulsive Disorders such as Trichotillomania or Excoriation [13].

Currently, the lifetime prevalence of OCD among US adults is 2.3% with subthreshold obsessive-compulsive symptoms occurring in 28.2% of adults [14]. Competitive athletes' traits (e.g., perfectionism, being highly disciplined and overly responsible, and secrecy) often mask OCD. Calorie obsession, a hyper-focus on the body, superstitions, and rituals are also normative for athletes. There is a recent study completed on collegiate athletes that suggests that 5.2% would meet the criteria for OCD; double the rate of the general population [15].

The Yale-Brown Obsessive-Compulsive Scale or the Y-BOCS is the best assessment tool to identify Obsessive-Compulsive Disorder in adults with a version, the Children's Yale-Brown Obsessive-Compulsive Scale for ages 6–17 [16]. It is designed to rate the severity and type of symptoms with individuals struggling with obsessions and compulsions. There are currently no assessments that identify OCD in sports settings.

21.2.3 Trauma- and Stressor-Related Disorders

Trauma- and stressor-related disorders are a new category of psychological disorders in the DSM-5 that involve exposure to a traumatic or stressful event. Two of the most common trauma-related disorders are Acute Stress Disorder and Post-Traumatic Stress Disorder (PTSD). These two disorders are essentially the same except Acute Stress Disorder typically begins immediately after the trauma and lasts from 3 days to 1 month and PTSD lasts for more than a month and can be the continuation of an Acute Stress Disorder [17]. Previously, trauma- and stressor-related disorders were considered anxiety disorders but were recently recategorized because individuals were experiencing anxiety as well as other symptoms such as anger, aggression, dissociation, or anhedonia. Acute Stress Disorder and PTSD are often confused and when diagnosing, it is also important to rule out Adjustment Disorder and Brief Psychotic Disorder. Other disorders might also be diagnosed along with Acute Stress Disorder or PTSD such as Depressive Disorders, Anxiety Disorders, Obsessive Compulsive Disorders, and Dissociative Disorders. An estimated 3.6% of US adults have experienced PTSD in the past year. A recent study suggested that elite athletes might experience PTSD at rates much higher than the general population—anywhere from 13 to 25% [18].

PTSD can be assessed by several measures used to diagnose or better understand the severity of symptoms. The Post-Traumatic Stress Disorder Checklist for DSM-5 or the PCL-5 is a 20-item self-report measure that is reflective of the DSM-5 symptoms while the Post-Traumatic Stress Diagnostic Scale for DSM-5 or the PDS-5 is a 24-item self-report measure that assesses the severity in the last month according to the DSM-5 [19, 20]. The Brief Trauma Questionnaire or the BTQ is a self-report questionnaire derived from the Brief Trauma Interview and helps to understand the types of trauma that an individual has experienced [21]. More recently, the Adverse Childhood Experiences (ACE) Questionnaire is being utilized more to gain a better understanding of trauma that occurred during childhood (ages 0–17) that may impact an athlete later in life, but can be completed at any age [22].

21.2.4 Depressive Disorders

According to the National Institute of Mental Health, depression impacts 8.4% of adults in the United States with around 17% of young adults (18–25 years of age) being impacted [23]. The most common depressive disorder is Major Depressive Disorder (MDD). Major depression is characterized by a period of more than 2 weeks with at least five of the following: depressed mood, loss of interest or pleasure in activities, weight fluctuations, sleep disturbance, psychomotor agitation or retardation, fatigue, feelings of worthlessness or excessive/inappropriate guilt, decreased concentration, or thoughts or death/suicide. These symptoms must cause clinically significant distress or impairment and not be attributable to substances or a medical condition. The following disorders must also be ruled out to diagnose MDD: Schizoaffective Disorder, Schizophrenia, Schizophreniform Disorder, Delusional Disorder, or other Unspecified Schizophrenia Spectrum or Psychotic Disorders and there cannot be a manic or hypomanic episode [24].

One of the most utilized mental health screeners for depression is the Patient Health Questionnaire-9 or the PHQ-9. The PHQ-9 is a diagnostic tool to screen individuals aged 12 and older in primary care settings for the presence and severity of depression [25]. The Beck Depression Inventory or the BDI is another widely used screen for depression and measures the behavioral manifestations and severity of depression [11]. The Hamilton Rating Scale for Depression (HRSD) measures depression in individuals before, during, and after treatment. The scale is often administered by healthcare providers and scored based on 17 items [26].

21.2.5 Bipolar and Related Disorders

There are two types of bipolar disorder—Bipolar I Disorder and Bipolar II Disorder. Bipolar I Disorder involves episodes of severe mania while Bipolar II Disorder involves depressive episodes and episodes of hypomania. Manic episodes often include increased energy, racing thoughts, a decreased need for sleep, and feeling wired, while hypomanic episodes are characterized by elation and hyperactivity. An estimated 4.4% of US adults experience bipolar disorder at some point in their lives. It can occur at any age, but it often develops between the ages of 15 and 19 years of age and rarely develops after the age of 40 [27]. Notably, the typical age of onset coincides with average peak performance in elite athletes—although the known prevalence in elite athletes is limited [28].

The most widely used screening for bipolar disorder is the Mood Disorder Questionnaire or the MDQ. The MDQ is a self-report questionnaire that can be quickly scored by a healthcare provider to better understand mania and hypomania [29]. The Young Mania Rating Sale or the YMRS is a helpful assessment to evaluate manic symptoms over time with individuals who experience mania [30].

21.2.6 Feeding and Eating Disorders

Feeding and eating disorders address a number of psychological disorders that often range from anorexia nervosa to bulimia and binge eating disorder. Around 9% of US adults will experience an eating disorder in their lifetime [31]. To be diagnosed with Anorexia Nervosa, the following criteria must be met: restriction of energy intake relative to requirements leading to a significantly low body weight in the context of age, sex, developmental trajectory, and physical health. This is coupled with an intense fear of gaining weight or becoming fat and a disturbance in the way in which one's body weight, shape, or size is experienced. Binge Eating Disorder was recently added to the diagnostic manual and must include recurrent episodes of binge eating during a discrete period of time while experiencing a sense of lack of control. The binge eating episodes must also be associated with three of the following: eating much more rapidly than normal, eating until feeling uncomfortably full, eating large amounts of food when not feeling physically hungry, eating alone due to embarrassment about the quantity of food, or feeling disgusted, depressed, or guilty afterwards. Bulimia Nervosa would be diagnosed if an individual engages in binge eating episodes, but also completes compensatory behaviors following the binge eating episodes (e.g., obsessively or compulsively exercising, vomiting or laxative use). Concerns about weight, shape, or size are necessary for the Anorexia Nervosa and Bulimia Nervosa diagnosis while it is not necessarily present with a Binge Eating Disorder diagnosis [31].

A comprehensive analysis was completed by the International Olympic Committee (IOC) Mental Health Working Group suggesting that athletes struggle with disordered eating more often (0–19% of male athletes and 6–45% of female athletes) [32]. Also related to feeding and eating disorders commonly seen in athletes is Relative Energy Deficiency in Sport or REDS. REDS describes "a syndrome of poor health and declining athletic performance that happens when athletes do not get enough fuel through food to support the energy demands of their daily lives and training" [33, 34]. The management of athletes with REDS requires a multidisciplinary team and a comprehensive evaluation to ensure a treatment plan is in place and regularly reviewed with these athletes. These athletes will be key to identifying as they may present with stress fractures or other physical findings that will negatively impact both their health and performance and may require modified training or time away from training [34].

One of the shortest and most impactful screening tools for eating disorders is the SCOFF (derived from questions around Sick, Control, One, Fat, and Food) [35]. The Eating Attitudes Test-26 or EAT-26 is the most widely used standardized self-report measure of symptoms and concerns characteristic of eating disorders [36]. The Eating Disorder Inventory-3 consists of consists of 91 items organized into 12 primary scales: Drive for Thinness, Bulimia, Body Dissatisfaction, Low Self-Esteem, Personal Alienation, Interpersonal Insecurity, Interpersonal Alienation, Interoceptive Deficits, Emotional Dysregulation, Perfectionism, Asceticism, and Maturity Fears [37]. The only athlete-specific eating disorder questionnaire is the Brief Eating Disorder in Athletes Questionnaire or BEDA-Q, which is a brief questionnaire comprising nine items and was developed to identify symptoms of eating disorders in athletes [38].

21.2.7 Substance-Related and Addictive Disorders

The DSM-5-TR recognizes substance-related disorders in ten separate classes of drugs: alcohol, caffeine, cannabis, hallucinogens, inhalants, opioids, sedatives, hypnotics/anxiolytics, stimulants, and tobacco. Across all of these substances, there are 11 different criteria: taking the substance in larger amounts or for longer than prescribed; wanting to cut down or stop using the substance but not managing to; spending a lot of time getting, using, or recovering from use of the substance; cravings and urges to use the substance; not managing to do what you should at work, home, or school because of substance use; continuing to use, even when it causes problems in relationships; giving up important social, occupational, or recreational activities because of substance use; using substances again and again, even when it puts you in danger; continuing to use, even when you know you have a physical or psychological problem that could have been caused or made worse by the substance; needing more of the substance to get the effect you want (tolerance); and development of withdrawal symptoms, which can be relieved by taking more of the substance. If combining all of the substances above, the prevalence of all Substance Use Disorders is approximately 36% in the United States [39]. According to the 2019 IOC Consensus Statement on Mental Health in Elite Athletes, the most commonly used and misused substances by elite athletes are alcohol, caffeine, nicotine, cannabis/cannabinoids, and stimulants including anabolic-androgenic steroids [40].

For drug and alcohol use and abuse screening, there are a few very brief measures that can be used to identify a problem with drugs or alcohol, and none of which are specific to athletes. The Alcohol Use Disorders Identification Test or the AUDIT-C is a three-question screener that helps identify individuals who might be considered hazardous drinkers or have active alcohol use disorders [41]. The CAGE—which stands for questions that address the following: Cutting Down, Annoyed, Guilty, and Eye-Opener—is utilized to better understand alcohol use [42]. The CAGE-AID is an adaptation of the CAGE and conjointly screens for alcohol and drugs [43]. Finally, the Drug Abuse Screen Test-10 or the DAST-10 is a measure consisting of 10 binary self-report questions around the quantity and frequency of drug use [44].

21.2.8 Sleep–Wake Disorders

Insomnia is the most common Sleep–Wake Disorder and is essentially an inability to initiate or maintain sleep. Approximately one-third of adults in the United States report symptoms related to insomnia at some point in the year with short-term insomnia impacting around 10% and one in five cases of short-term insomnia transitioning to long-term insomnia [45]. Unfortunately, a recent study completed by the IOC categorized nearly 49% of Olympic athletes as "poor sleepers" [46]. The other common Sleep–Wake Disorders are Narcolepsy, Restless Leg Syndrome, and Sleep Apnea.

There are countless assessments to identify sleep concerns with some assessments measuring a single sleep disorder (e.g., the Insomnia Severity Index or the ISI, the Berlin Questionnaire for Sleep Apnea, the STOP Questionnaire, or the Snore, Tired, Observed, Pressure Questionnaire for Sleep Apnea, the International Restless Legs Syndrome Rating Scale or the IRLS, and the Epworth Sleepiness Scale or the EPS) while other assessments measure sleep more globally. The most common global sleep scale is the Pittsburgh Sleep Quality Index or the PSQI—which measures sleep quality and sleep disturbance over the past month [47]. Finally, the Athlete Sleeping Screening Questionnaire or the ASSQ is a sleep screening tool that assesses sleep disturbance and daytime dysfunction based on the types and severity of sleep difficulties for athletes [48].

21.2.9 Schizophrenia Spectrum and Other Psychotic Disorders

To diagnose Schizophrenia Spectrum Disorder, two of the following must be present for a significant period of time during a 1-month period: delusions, hallucinations, disorganized speech, grossly disorganized or catatonic behavior, or negative symptoms (e.g., diminished emotional expression or avolition) with at least one of the symptoms to include psychosis (e.g., delusions, hallucinations, or disorganized speech). Continuous signs of the disturbance must persist for at least 6 months. The following psychological disorders must also be ruled out: Schizoaffective Disorder and Depressive or Bipolar Disorder with Psychotic Features and the symptoms cannot be attributable to substance use or a medical condition [49].

If Schizophrenia Spectrum Disorder is suspected, it is important for an individual to complete a physical exam, including brain imaging, to rule out medical conditions that could be leading to psychosis. Drugs that lead to psychosis should also be ruled out or polypharmacy interactions which may be present, particularly in Paralympic athletes who are potentially taking multiple medications. Following these evaluations, the Positive and Negative Syndrome Scale or the PANSS is the best measure to identify the positive and negative symptoms associated with Schizophrenia or Other Psychotic Disorders [50].

21.2.10 Traumatic Brain Injury/Concussion

Though not a psychological disorder, concussion and head injuries are a significant portion of many sports [51, 52]. Current evidence suggests a possible link between sports-related concussion and depression as well as suicidal ideation in elite and pediatric athletes, thus an important topic to include in this chapter. Further discussion regarding the assessment and management of sport-related concussions will be discussed in other chapters within this text and thus will only briefly be addressed here. There remains controversy of whether head injuries may exacerbate underlying psychological disorders or whether head trauma can contribute to the development of mental health concerns [51, 53]. Continued study in this area is important to help parse this out.

Evidence supports the idea that exercise can be a protective factor in regard to psychological well-being [54]. As more evidence is emerging about the potential impacts of concussions on self-reported cognitive function it is important to ensure proper management is provided to the athlete at the time of injury, including psychological support [55]. This emerging evidence supports the importance of collecting a baseline of both psychological statuses through a tool such as the Sport Mental Health Assessment Tool (SMHAT), which will be detailed below, as well as baseline concussion assessments such as the Sport Concussion Assessment Tool (SCAT-V, soon to be released SCAT-VI) to be able to identify any changes that may occur during an athlete's season [56].

21.3 Screening and Assessment for Psychological Disorders in Athletes

Screenings and assessments for psychological disorders are often used to identify symptoms and can lead to the diagnosis of psychological disorders. These screenings and assessments are often deployed in primary care settings to help medical providers connect patients to the most appropriate resources. The results of these screenings and assessments can provide these providers with critical information for the management of psychological disorders on the sidelines.

In 2019, the IOC formed a consensus group to review mental health in athletes which was the first group to review the research in this area and develop subsequent guidelines and recommendations for the management of elite athletes and mental health [40]. In this consensus, it was reiterated that mental and physical health cannot be separated, and athletes should be treated in a comprehensive manner. This includes relevant past and current history related to injury related pain, concussion, trauma, abuse, etc. [57, 58]. Discussion on ways of positively influencing the environments in which athletes participate, such as rule changes and equipment, were also discussed which are important aspects of sideline coverage for medical providers to be advocates around. In 2020, the consensus group went on to develop the Sport Mental Health Assessment Tool 1 (SMHAT-1) which is a standardized assessment tool intended to identify elite athletes potentially at risk for or already experiencing psychological symptoms or disorders [59].

The goal of the SMHAT-1 is to identify areas where athletes may need additional support and can help with the facilitation of timely referrals to mental health providers and/or resources for support and/or treatment. As outlined in Figure, the SMHAT-1 begins with the completion of the Athlete Psychological Strain Questionnaire (APSQ) and based on the outcomes of this screen, it guides medical providers to complete six associated validated screens, all of which have previously been discussed. These include the General Anxiety Disorder-7 (GAD-7); Patient Health Questionnaire-9 (PHQ-9); Athlete Sleep Screening Questionnaire (ASSQ); Alcohol Use Disorders Identification Test Consumption (AUDIT-C); Cutting Down, Annoyance by Criticism, Guilty Feeling, and Eye Openers Adapted to Include Drugs (CAGE-AID); and the Brief Eating Disorder in Athletes Questionnaire (BEDA-Q).

When working with any athletes or sports teams' medical providers should ensure psychological screening questions, such as the SMHAT, are included in the annual Pre-Participation Physicals (PPEs) for all athletes. A system should also be in place to flag any athlete who endorses suicidality, self-harm, or harm to others from the PHQ-9. A licensed mental health provider, who is part of the interdisciplinary team, should immediately contact any athlete who flags to ensure an appropriate safety plan is in place.

As the provider is reviewing the results with the athlete, they should create an environment in which the athlete feels safe to discuss any concerns that may have arisen during the screening. At this time the provider should review any relevant emergency action plan steps that will be taken if exacerbation of any symptoms arises at any time, including during training or competition so the athlete is aware. Providers should ensure that anytime they inquire about medical conditions and they also inquire about psychological symptoms. The providers must also be vigilant in noting any changes in cognitive, function, emotional state, and behavioral changes in daily functioning. It is also important to ensure there is a safe environment and availability of a confidential hotline or process for fellow teammates or friends to submit concerns for an athlete.

21.4 Definition of Problem, Crisis, and Emergency

Prior to creating a mental health emergency action plan (MHEAP), it is important to distinguish the difference between a mental health problem, a crisis, and an emergency [60]. As seen in Table 21.1 they differ regarding response time and associated safety risk.

A problem is a matter or situation that is often unsolicited and needs to be addressed. While a problem may create stress and be difficult to solve, the athlete can often find a solution. Consequently, a problem that can be resolved by an athlete is not a crisis and does not require immediate care.

A crisis is an upset in a steady mental state that may create a disruption or breakdown in a person's normal or usual pattern of functioning. The upset, or disequilibrium, is typically acute. A crisis constitutes circumstances or situations which cannot be resolved by one's customary problem-solving resources. If a situation can wait 24–72 h for a response, without placing an athlete or their family in jeopardy, it is a crisis and not an emergency. An example of a mental health crisis can include, but is not limited to, self-harming or maladaptive coping behaviors such as cutting. These are not life-threatening and do not cause serious property damage. This may also include challenges coping with academic concerns, medical concerns, legal concerns, a significant loss, or death directly or indirectly impacting the athlete, rapid mood swings, increased agitation, isolation, medication non-compliance, and substance use and/or abuse.

An emergency is a sudden, pressing necessity, such as when a life is in danger because of an accident, a suicide attempt or potential imminent suicide attempt, or interpersonal violence. It requires immediate attention from law enforcement, Child Protective Services (CPS) or other providers trained to respond to life-threatening events. Some examples of emergent situations include managing suicidal and/or homicidal ideation, managing victims of sexual assault, including mandatory SafeSport reporting, managing highly agitated or threatening behavior, acute psychosis (often involving hallucinations and/or delusions), or paranoia, managing acute delirium/confusion state, and managing acute intoxication or drug overdose.

Table 21.1 Distinguishing aspects of problem, crisis, and emergent psychological situations

	RESPOND IMMEDIATELY	GET CONNECTED WITH MENTAL HEALTH PROVIDER	MAKE REFERRAL (see non-emergency referral process)
Situation	Emergency	Crisis	Problem
Response Time	Minutes	Today	Days or more
Physical Safety	Imminent Danger	High Risk	Low to Moderate Risk
Behavior Change	Dramatic or Sudden	Noticeable Change	Gradual Change
Coping Options & Hope	Very limited or None	Limited	Some Coping & Options

21.5 Mental Health Emergency Action Plan (MHEAP)

Creating a mental health emergency action plan (MHEAP) is a critical step to ensure there is a comprehensive plan for the management of mental health crises as well as mental health emergencies. Early identification of an impending or evolving crisis or emergency is key to a successful emergency action plan to ensure all members of the team are aware and comfortable in the execution of their role.

As a sports medicine provider, there will be times in which athletes may display symptoms or behaviors that could cause concern or discomfort or that may interfere with team dynamics. Without appropriate intervention, the athlete or others' safety may be jeopardized and/or the athlete's symptoms may persist. Some signals distressed athletes might exhibit could go unnoticed for a variety of reasons, and even when noticed, it can be difficult to intervene. Providers may feel unsure of how to respond or may have competing demands on their time when overseeing the care of many athletes. It is important to know that without intervention, the problem most likely will not go away. Part of an effective intervention requires knowing how to act during these incidents and what resources to call upon.

A provider interacting daily with athletes is in an excellent position to recognize behavior changes that characterize a psychological disorder. An athlete's behavior, especially if it is inconsistent with previous observations, could constitute a "cry for help." The MHEAP provides a standard of care to ensure the health and safety of the athlete and the organization, as well as a systematic approach to identify, assess, and refer emotionally distressed athletes.

Another important aspect of the emergency response process is to ensure that providers have access to the most accurate contact details for the athlete as well as emergency contact numbers so that critical time is not lost tracking that information down in the middle of a crisis or emergent situation. As a reminder confidentiality is critical in these cases and only those who have a role to play in the response should be provided with any details around the case. Figure 21.1 is an example of an MHEAP Action Plan which details steps to take in various situations and who should be communicated with along the way.

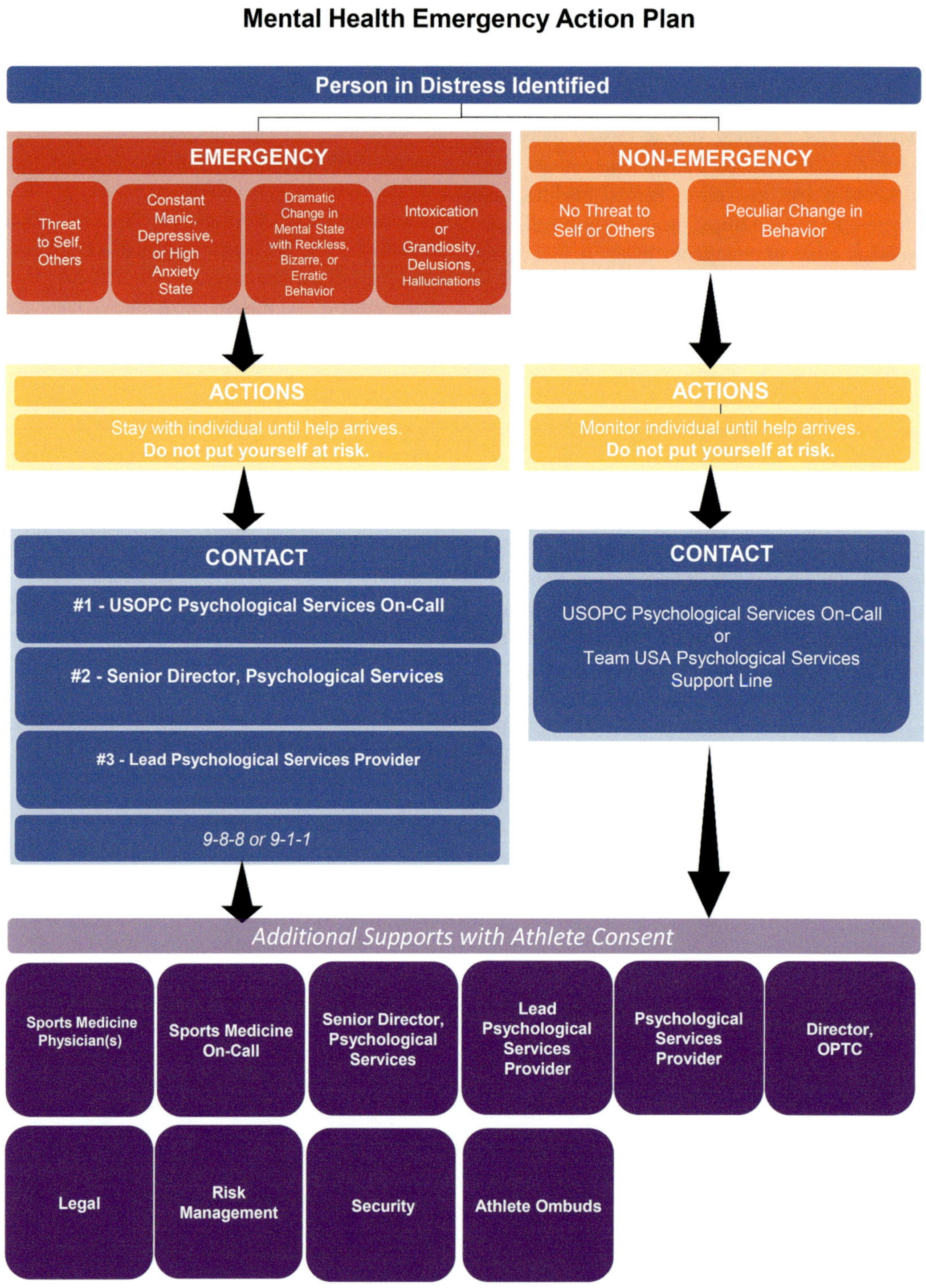

Fig. 21.1 Mental Health Emergency Action Plan flowsheet example (Commander, C and Bartley, J. USOPC Mental Health Emergency Action Plan Flowsheet. United States Olympic & Paralympic Committee, 2021)

21.6 Development of the Mental Health Emergency Care Team

An emergency team must be created to ensure there is a multidisciplinary approach to the care of any athlete's psychological needs during a crisis or emergency. This team may vary depending on the resources available, but should include:

- Chief Medical Officer/Head Team Physician/ Lead Clinical Provider
- Licensed Mental Health Provider
- First Responder
- Director of Security, where applicable

This emergency team should also be very aware of the other stakeholders in the greater multidisciplinary team who interact and care for an athlete as illustrated in Fig. 21.2. There should also be sufficient redundancy in the system to allow for someone else to step in if the licensed mental health provider is not available. All members of the crisis care team and any others who may be involved in the MHEAP, including fellow athletes, should have gatekeeper training, such as Mental First Aid or QPR training that is renewed every 3 years.

The team must be aware of the local resources and behavioral health services in the locations where the athletes will be training and competing. These include emergency hotlines, behavioral health specialists within law enforcement, 24/7 centers, psychiatry access, and the process for involuntary hospitalization in the state if that became necessary.

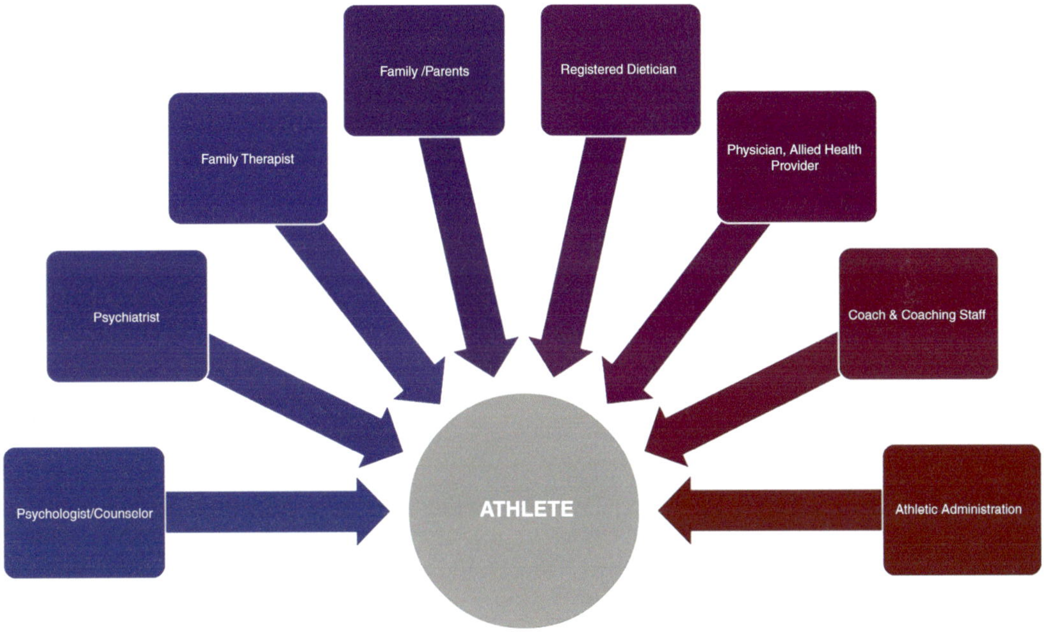

Fig. 21.2 The multidisciplinary team involved in the psychological care of an athlete

21.7 Sideline Management of Psychological Disorders

As has been detailed above, a great deal of preparation needs to be in place before getting to the sideline. It is critical to lay the groundwork and ensure the appropriate information is collected regarding the psychological history and current concerns of the athlete. Ensuring a multidisciplinary team is identified as the response team and all are aware of their roles is also important. This should be practiced regularly just as situational practice is done for cardiac or spinal injuries.

21.8 Removal/Return to Play

There may be times when an athlete is deemed unsafe or not psychologically sound to engage in training or competition. In those instances, an athlete may be removed from participating in sport if they exhibit:

1. Unsafe behaviors of self-harm or harm to others; and/or
2. Participating in sport significantly negatively affects MH functioning and/or safety.

After MH evaluations, the athlete will receive treatment recommendations that are commensurate with their needed level of care. To return to play, athletes must demonstrate they no longer meet the criteria to be removed. The athlete will then be returned to play in a graduated return to play in accordance with their treatment plan. At times this may require a contract with the athlete to ensure all guidelines are clearly detailed and the athlete understands their responsibility in the process as well.

21.9 Conclusion

As a medical provider tasked with keeping athletes safe and on the field of play, it is critical to ensure psychological and behavioral health is considered at all times. Treatment of the athlete as a whole individual, both physical and mental, is important to providing the most appropriate and comprehensive care to the athletes. This chapter has provided information on each psychological disorder and what to be on the lookout for in athletes as well as ways to screen for this information thus enabling the identification of the most appropriate resources and support. The development of an MHEAP was also discussed and is critical to have in place, shared and regularly practiced so this becomes as common practice as the management of any other emergencies. With these practices in place, the athletes' health and safety can be prioritized. This can ultimately lead to maximizing performance and enjoyment in sport.

Fact Box

One in three athletes might experience psychological symptoms during or immediately after their career [3].

Fact Box

Approximately one-third of adults in the United States report symptoms related to insomnia at some point in the year [45] with nearly 49% of Olympic athletes categorized as "poor sleepers" [46].

Take Home Messages

In summary, key takeaways for sideline management of a psychological disorder include

- Ensure comprehensive screening is completed on all athletes utilizing information from a variety of validated tools.
- Create an MHEAP including a multidisciplinary emergency response team and practice it regularly.
- Normalize the inclusion of psychological and behavioral health within the discussions of total health with athletes and all stakeholders.

References

1. Centers for Disease Control and Prevention (CDC). Mental health. Atlanta, GA, USA. 2022. https://www.cdc.gov/mentalhealth/.
2. GBD 2017 Disease and Injury Incidence and Prevalence Collaborators. Global, regional, and national incidence, prevalence, and years lived with disability for 354 diseases and injuries for 195 countries and territories, 1990–2017: a systematic analysis for the Global Burden of Disease Study 2017. Lancet. 2018;392(10159):1789–858.
3. Gouttebarge V, Castaldelli-Maia JM, Gorczynski P, Hainline B, Hitchcock ME, Kerkhoffs GM, et al. Occurrence of mental health symptoms and disorders in current and former elite athletes: a systematic review and meta-analysis. Br J Sports Med. 2019;53(11):700–6.
4. World Health Organization (WHO). Mental disorders. World Health Organization; 2022. https://www.who.int/health-topics/mental-health#tab=tab_1
5. American Psychiatric Association. Diagnostic and statistical manual of mental disorders. 5th ed. American Psychiatric Association Publishing; 2022.
6. Bandelow B, Michaelis S. Epidemiology of anxiety disorders in the 21st century. Dialogues Clin Neurosci. 2015;17(3):327–35.
7. Rice SM, Gwyther K, Santesteban-Echarri O, Baron D, Gorczynski P, Gouttebarge V, et al. Determinants of anxiety in elite athletes: a systematic review and meta-analysis. Br J Sports Med. 2019;53(11):722–30.
8. U.S. Preventive Services Task Force. Screening for anxiety in adults. 2022.
9. Spitzer RL, Kroenke K, Williams JB, Löwe B. A brief measure for assessing generalized anxiety disorder: the GAD-7. Arch Intern Med. 2006;166(10):1092–7.
10. Shear K, Belnap BH, Mazumdar S, Houck P, Rollman BL. Generalized anxiety disorder severity scale (GADSS): a preliminary validation study. Depress Anxiety. 2006;23(2):77–82.
11. Beck AT, Steer RA, Brown G. Beck Depression Inventory-II. Washington, DC: American Psychological Association; 1996. https://doi.org/10.1037/t00742-000.
12. Martens R. Sport competition anxiety test, vol. 5. Champaign: Human Kinetics Publishers; 1977. p. 150–5.
13. American Psychiatric Association. Diagnostic and statistic manual of mental disorders. In: Obsessive-compulsive and related disorders. 5th ed; 2022. https://doi.org/10.1176/appi.books.9780890425787.x06.
14. Harvard Medical School. National Comorbidity Study (NCS) Harvard Medical School. 2017. https://www.hcp.med.harvard.edu/ncs/index.php.
15. Cromer L, Kaier E, Davis J, Stunk K, Stewart SE. OCD in college athletes. Am J Psychiatry. 2017;174(6):595–7.
16. Goodman WK, Price LH, Rasmussen SA, Mazure C, Fleischmann RL, Hill CL, et al. The Yale-Brown Obsessive Compulsive Scale. I. Development, use, and reliability. Arch Gen Psychiatry. 1989;46(11):1006–11.
17. American Psychiatric Association. Diagnostic and statistical manual of mental disorders. In: Trauma and stressor-related disorders. 5th ed. American Psychiatric Association Publishing; 2022. https://doi.org/10.1176/appi.books.9780890425787.x07.
18. Aron CM, Harvey S, Hainline B, Hitchcock ME, Reardon CL. Post-traumatic stress disorder (PTSD) and other trauma-related mental disorders in elite athletes: a narrative review. Br J Sports Med. 2019;53(12):779–84.
19. Blevins CA, Weathers FW, Davis MT, Witte TK, Domino JL. The posttraumatic stress disorder checklist for DSM-5 (PCL-5): development and initial psychometric evaluation. J Trauma Stress. 2015;28(6):489–98.
20. Foa EB, Cashman L, Jaycox L, Perry K. The validation of a self-report measure of posttraumatic stress disorder: the Posttraumatic Diagnostic Scale. Psychol Assess. 1997;9:445–51.
21. Schnurr P, Vielhauer M, Weathers F, Findler M. Brief Trauma Questionnaire (BTQ). American Psychological Association; 1999. https://doi.org/10.1037/t07488-000.
22. Murphy A, Steele H, Steele M, Allman B, Kastner T, Dube SR. The Clinical Adverse Childhood Experiences (ACEs) Questionnaire: implications for trauma-informed behavioral healthcare. In: Briggs RD, editor. Integrated early childhood behavioral health in primary care: a guide to implementation and evaluation. Cham: Springer International Publishing; 2016. p. 7–16.
23. National Institutes of Mental Health. Depression. National Institute of Mental Health; 2022. https://www.nimh.nih.gov/health/statistics/major-depression
24. American Psychiatric Association. Diagnostic and statistical manual of mental disorders. 5th ed. American Psychiatric Association Publishing; 2022. https://doi.org/10.1176/appi.books.9780890425787.
25. Kroenke K, Spitzer RL. The PHQ-9: a new depression diagnostic and severity measure. Psychiatr Ann. 2002;32:509–15.
26. Hamilton M. Hamilton Depression Rating Scale (HDRS). J Neurol Neurosurg Psychiatry. 1960;23:56–62.
27. American Psychiatric Association. Diagnostic and statistical manual of mental disorders. 5th ed. American Psychiatry Association Publisher; 2022. https://doi.org/10.1176/appi.books.9780890425787.x03.
28. Currie A, Gorczynski P, Rice SM, Purcell R, McAllister-Williams RH, Hitchcock ME, et al. Bipolar and psychotic disorders in elite athletes: a narrative review. Br J Sports Med. 2019;53(12):746–53.

29. Hirschfeld RM. The mood disorder questionnaire: its impact on the field [corrected]. Depress Anxiety. 2010;27(7):627–30.
30. Young RC, Biggs JT, Ziegler VE, Meyer D. A Young Mania Rating Scale. American Psychological Association; 1978. https://doi.org/10.1037/t20936-000.
31. American Psychiatric Association. Diagnostic and statistical manual of mental disorders. In: Feeding and eating disorders. 5th ed. American Psychiatry Association Publishing; 2022. https://doi.org/10.1176/appi.books.9780890425787.x10.
32. Sundgot-Borgen J, Torstveit MK. Prevalence of eating disorders in elite athletes is higher than in the general population. Clin J Sport Med. 2004;14(1):25–32.
33. Statuta SM, Asif IM, Drezner JA. Relative energy deficiency in sport (RED-S). Br J Sports Med. 2017;51(21):1570–1.
34. Mountjoy M, Sundgot-Borgen JK, Burke LM, Ackerman KE, Blauwet C, Constantini N, et al. IOC consensus statement on relative energy deficiency in sport (RED-S): 2018 update. Br J Sports Med. 2018;52(11):687–97.
35. Hill LS, Reid F, Morgan JF, Lacey JH. SCOFF, the development of an eating disorder screening questionnaire. Int J Eat Disord. 2010;43(4):344–51.
36. Orbitello B, Ciano R, Corsaro M, Rocco PL, Taboga C, Tonutti L, et al. The EAT-26 as screening instrument for clinical nutrition unit attenders. Int J Obes. 2006;30(6):977–81.
37. Garner DM. Eating disorder inventory-3 (EDI-3). Int J Eat Disord. 2004;35(4):478–9.
38. Martinsen M, Holme I, Pensgaard AM, Torstveit MK, Sundgot-Borgen J. The development of the brief eating disorder in athletes questionnaire. Med Sci Sports Exerc. 2014;46(8):1666–75.
39. American Psychiatric Association. Diagnostic and statistical manual of mental disorders. 5th ed. American Psychiatry Association Publisher; 2022. https://doi.org/10.1176/appi.books.9780890425787.x16.
40. Reardon CL, Hainline B, Aron CM, Baron D, Baum AL, Bindra A, et al. Mental health in elite athletes: International Olympic Committee consensus statement (2019). Br J Sports Med. 2019;53(11):667–99.
41. Bradley KA, DeBenedetti AF, Volk RJ, Williams EC, Frank D, Kivlahan DR. AUDIT-C as a brief screen for alcohol misuse in primary care. Alcohol Clin Exp Res. 2007;31(7):1208–17.
42. Ewing JA. Detecting alcoholism. The CAGE Questionnaire. JAMA. 1984;252(14):1905–7.
43. Brown RL, Rounds LA. Conjoint screening questionnaires for alcohol and other drug abuse: criterion validity in a primary care practice. Wis Med J. 1995;94(3):135–40.
44. Villalobos-Gallegos L, Pérez-López A, Mendoza-Hassey R, Graue-Moreno J, Marín-Navarrete R. Psychometric and diagnostic properties of the Drug Abuse Screening Test (DAST): comparing the DAST-20 vs. the DAST-10. Salud Mental. 2015;38:89–94.
45. Dopheide JA. Insomnia overview: epidemiology, pathophysiology, diagnosis and monitoring, and nonpharmacologic therapy. Am J Manag Care. 2020;26(4 Suppl):S76–84.
46. Drew M, Vlahovich N, Hughes D, Appaneal R, Burke LM, Lundy B, et al. Prevalence of illness, poor mental health and sleep quality and low energy availability prior to the 2016 Summer Olympic Games. Br J Sports Med. 2018;52(1):47–53.
47. Klingman KJ, Jungquist CR, Perlis ML. Questionnaires that screen for multiple sleep disorders. Sleep Med Rev. 2017;32:37–44.
48. Bender AM, Lawson D, Werthner P, Samuels CH. The clinical validation of the Athlete Sleep Screening Questionnaire: an instrument to identify athletes that need further sleep assessment. Sports Med Open. 2018;4(1):23.
49. American Psychiatric Association. Diagnostic and statistical manual of mental disorders. In: Schizophrenia spectrum and other psychotic disorders. American Psychiatric Association Publisher; 2022. https://doi.org/10.1176/appi.books.9780890425787.x02.
50. Kay SR, Opler LA, Lindenmayer JP. The Positive and Negative Syndrome Scale (PANSS): rationale and standardisation. Br J Psychiatry Suppl. 1989;7:59–67.
51. Ziminski D, Szlyk HS, Baiden P, Okine L, Onyeaka HK, Muoghalu C, et al. Sports- and physical activity-related concussion and mental health among adolescents: findings from the 2017 and 2019 Youth Risk Behavior Survey. Psychiatry Res. 2022;312:114542.
52. Rice SM, Parker AG, Rosenbaum S, Bailey A, Mawren D, Purcell R. Sport-related concussion and mental health outcomes in elite athletes: a systematic review. Sports Med. 2018;48(2):447–65.
53. Gouttebarge V, Kerkhoffs G. Sports career-related concussion and mental health symptoms in former elite athletes. Neurochirurgie. 2021;67(3):280–2.
54. Leddy JJ, Haider MN, Ellis M, Willer BS. Exercise is medicine for concussion. Curr Sports Med Rep. 2018;17(8):262–70.
55. Cunningham J, Broglio SP, O'Grady M, Wilson F. History of sport-related concussion and long-term clinical cognitive health outcomes in retired athletes: a systematic review. J Athl Train. 2020;55(2):132–58.
56. McCrory P, Meeuwisse W, Dvořák J, Aubry M, Bailes J, Broglio S, et al. Consensus statement on concussion in sport-the 5(th) international conference on concussion in sport held in Berlin, October 2016. Br J Sports Med. 2017;51(11):838–47.
57. Hainline B, Derman W, Vernec A, Budgett R, Deie M, Dvořák J, et al. International Olympic Committee consensus statement on pain management in elite athletes. Br J Sports Med. 2017;51(17):1245–58.
58. Mountjoy M, Brackenridge C, Arrington M, Blauwet C, Carska-Sheppard A, Fasting K, et al. International

Olympic Committee consensus statement: harassment and abuse (non-accidental violence) in sport. Br J Sports Med. 2016;50(17):1019–29.
59. Gouttebarge V, Bindra A, Blauwet C, Campriani N, Currie A, Engebretsen L, et al. International Olympic Committee (IOC) Sport Mental Health Assessment Tool 1 (SMHAT-1) and Sport Mental Health Recognition Tool 1 (SMHRT-1): towards better support of athletes' mental health. Br J Sports Med. 2021;55(1):30–7.
60. Medicine USOPCS. United States Olympic and Paralympic Committee Mental Health Emergency Action Plan (MHEAP). 2022.

Genitourinary Disorders 22

Ricardo Miyaoka

22.1 Introduction

Genitourinary disorders in sports may result from either physical injury as a consequence of direct abdominal trauma or secondary to functional disturbances derived from abusive use of supplements, such as creatine or steroid agents.

Bagga et al. consulted the American National Electronic Injury Surveillance System (NEISS) and reported a yearly incidence of >14,500 sporting-related genitourinary injuries, approximately 2/3 of which were within the pediatric population [1]. In fact, sports-related trauma causes about 10% of all abdominal injuries [2].

In children, renal damage in blunt abdominal trauma is the most common urologic injury and may vary from 1% [3] up to 20% [4]. There have been nearly three million children treated in US emergency departments between 1990 and 2014 because of soccer-related injuries [5], although the risk of internal abdominal injury is estimated to be low, varying from 2.3 to 6/1,000,000 being more common in females than males [6, 7]. The abdomen has a large surface area unprotected by bony support. Protective gear in this area can affect athletic performance and is not often worn, which makes this area prone to potentially serious injury [2]. The most common sport to cause abdominal injury is cycling [2], but a wide range of sports both recreational and organized, contact and noncontact, have been associated with renal injury, although injury is rare overall. Almost all sports-related injuries are blunt and are either abdominal or flank directed, rapid deceleration, or high-velocity impacts provoked either by objects that are part of the sport or high-speed sports [3].

Bagga et al. also reported on product-related genitourinary injuries after analyzing an American National database that was validated to provide a probability sample of injury-related emergency department presentations. Sixty-nine percent of the cases occurred in men. The most common categories of products involved were sporting items in 30.2% of cases and exercise equipment with bicycles the most frequently associated product [8].

Although infrequent, urologic damage secondary to blunt abdominal trauma deserves proper diagnosis and immediate attention to avoid complications that could lead to temporary or permanent loss of organ function or even death. In this sense, the athletic sideline is a unique clinical setting. The physician has the advantage of witnessing the mechanism of injury but is challenged by the potential disadvantage of patients who might consciously ignore or withhold information and symptoms in hopes of returning to play. Most commonly, orthopedic surgeons provide sideline medical services as

R. Miyaoka (✉)
Division of Urology, State University of Campinas-UNICAMP, Campinas, SP, Brazil
e-mail: rmiyaoka@unicamp.br

S. Rocha Piedade et al. (eds.), *Sideline Management in Sports*,
https://doi.org/10.1007/978-3-031-33867-0_22

team physicians in all types of sports and levels of competition. Forty-five percent of sports-related emergency department visits diagnoses are either fractures or sprains/strains [9]. Orthopedic surgeons manage musculoskeletal conditions daily and are well prepared to triage them rapidly. However, as athletic team physicians, they must be able to deal with non-musculoskeletal just as well. They include cerebral/neurologic, ocular, dental, respiratory/pulmonary, cardiac, gastrointestinal, and genitourinary systems. Sideline preparedness can be defined as "the identification and planning for medical services to promote the safety of the athlete, to limit injury, and to provide medical care at the site of practice or competition" [10].

This chapter reviews the causes of sports-related genitourinary disorders, tools for proper diagnosis, and insights for better sideline management when facing non-traumatic kidney disturbances and traumatic genitourinary injuries.

22.2 Clinical Disorders

22.2.1 Creatine-Related Kidney Function Damage

Creatinine is nowadays one of the most used oral supplements by professional athletes to enhance their strength and muscle mass. Creatine is not an essential nutrient. It is naturally produced in the liver from two amino acids: glycine and arginine (*N*-[aminoiminomethyl]-*N*-methyl piturglycine). Creatine can also be found in meat and fish [11, 12]. Creatine enters the muscle from blood circulation and is converted to a compound named phosphocreatine by the action of creatine kinase. Phosphocreatine can generate energy by releasing adenosine triphosphate (ATP). As such, creatine supplementation increases storage in muscles and ultimately leads to more phosphocreatine and ATP formation. High loads of ATP can improve muscle gain and performance, mainly in extensive exercise [11].

The fact that the kidney plays a key role in body hemostasis, metabolizing and excreting exogenous compounds, such as creatine raises the question of whether creatine overload may correlate with kidney damage in short- and long-term athlete users. Creatine can convert into creatinine in the skeletal muscles and liver by non-enzymatic hydrolysis [13]. Serum creatinine has historically been adopted as a classic marker of kidney function.

The first reports addressing the possible effects of creatine consumption on kidney function in the literature were published around 30 years ago. In 1998, nephrologists reported a decrease of approximately 60% in creatinine clearance after a 25-year-old male athlete took creatine for 7 weeks [14], and he fully recovered after 1 month of creatine discontinuation.

Short-term creatine use is defined as the use of this agent for less than 1 month. An experimental study by Edmunds et al. [15] showed that creatine supplementation (loading dose of 2.0 g/kg for 1 week followed by 1/5 of loading dose for 5 weeks) exacerbated disease progression indexes (e.g., serum urea concentration and creatinine clearance) in an animal model of cystic renal disease.

The low-dose regimen is considered as daily creatine supplementation under 20 g. Clinical studies do not show a significant negative impact on kidney function following short-time creatine ingestion. However, its real effects on the body content of creatinine are equivocal. Poortmans and Francaux reported that 20 g/day of creatine supplementation for 5 days in healthy men did not significantly change the amount of creatinine in both the urine and serum, neither in creatinine excretion rate nor in creatinine clearance [16]. A randomized, double-blind placebo-controlled trial on both sexes using the same creatine regimen did not affect either plasma creatinine or creatinine clearance, but increased total body mass and free fat mass [17].

On the other hand, other clinical studies suggested that short-time creatine administration could affect the concentration of creatinine level and creatinine clearance. Hultman et al. described the use of 20 g/day of creatine supplementation for 6 days, which increased total creatine concentration in the muscle. They followed with a maintenance dose of 2 g/day, which elevated serum creatinine and urinary excretion [12]. Along with these findings, Kreider et al. [18] reported the effect of 28 days of creatine administration (15.75 g/day) in football players in a randomized double-blinded trial. They showed an increase in total body weight, fat and bone free mass, and serum creatinine content [18]. Finally, a study by Robinson et al. demonstrated that ingestion of 20 g/day of creatine for either 5 days or 9 weeks resulted in an increase in serum creatinine concentration by 25% and 40%, respectively [19].

In another chemical pathway, creatine may convert to sarcosine, which, in turn, may form other cytotoxic agents, including methylamine [20]. Formaldehyde can also be derived from methylamine by means of semicarbazide-sensitive amine oxidase [21]. Formaldehyde and methylamine can potentially damage the integrity of epithelium, endothelial cells, and the kidney [21, 22]. As demonstrated by Poortmans et al., creatinine homeostasis may not reveal creatine overload. Consumption of 21 g of creatine monohydrate daily for 14 days in healthy volunteers elevated the content of plasma creatine by about 7.2-fold and creatine urine excretion rate by about 141-fold with no change in plasma creatinine level as well as creatinine output. Additionally, creatine supplementation significantly increased the 24-h urine level of methylamine and formaldehyde by about 9.2 and 4.5-fold, respectively. However, there was no correlation between creatine serum and urine methylamine or formaldehyde [23]. Sale et al. studied the use of creatine as a single dose or a fractioned intake (20 g/day q.d. versus 5 g/dose t.i.d. for 5 days). Single-dose regimen caused lower excretion of creatine, leading to a greater creatine retention in the body and probably in the muscles. However, lowering the peak plasma creatine concentration by spreading its dose evenly throughout the day decreased methylamine urinary output [24]. Finally, in a double-blind, randomized study by Nasseri et al. [25], creatine supplementation induced an elevation in formaldehyde urinary excretion more than two times lower in individuals under resistance training.

Daily creatine supplementation that exceeds 20 g/day is considered a high-dose regimen. Volek et al. reported an elevation in serum creatinine content after 7 days of creatine supplementation (0.3 g/kg per day) in 20 healthy men. No significant changes were observed in the urinary sodium, potassium, and creatine excretion rates [26].

The consumption of creatine for months or years is described as long-term supplementation. The results of a randomized placebo-controlled study (induction dose of 21 g/day for 5 days and maintenance dose of 3 g/day for 58 days) showed that long-term creatine use in healthy men had no significant effect on creatinine clearance, urea clearance, and albumin excretion rate compared with control group [27]. Accordingly, a study performed in the American College of Football Players demonstrated that consumption of 5–20 g/day of creatine for 0.25–5.6 years had no long-term detrimental effects on studied kidney function parameters including serum urea, creatinine, and creatine clearance [28]. In fact, in support of the aforementioned studies, a consistent review of the literature showed that both acute ingestion (4–5 days) of large amounts of creatine as well as longer creatine supplementation (up to 5.6 years) minimally affected creatinine concentrations and kidney function in healthy young adults. Recently, a randomized double-blinded placebo-controlled trial confirmed no harmful effects on kidney function after high-dose creatine supplementation (about 10 g/day) use over 3 months in healthy males undergoing aerobic training [29].

There is, however, at least one case report suggesting a possible association between kidney dysfunction and creatine supplementation. Taner et al. reported on an 18-year-old man with a chief complaint of nausea, vomiting, and gastric pain. He was a bodybuilder and had been using creatine supplementation with the initial dose of 20 g/day for 5 days followed by 1 g/day for the following 6 weeks. Serum creatinine was 201.55 nmol/L at admission. Urinalysis revealed proteinuria. Imaging with renal ultrasound was normal, and renal biopsy suggested acute tubular necrosis. During hospitalization, creatine was discontinued, and fluids were administered intravenously. Laboratory normalization occurred after 25 days [30].

In conclusion, creatine supplementation seems to have no clinically significant side effects or adverse effects when given appropriately. Additionally, although short-term (5 days–2 weeks) high-dose oral creatine supplementation (from 20 g/day to 0.3 g/kg/day) stimulates the production of methylamine and formaldehyde (as potential cytotoxic metabolites of creatine) in the urine of healthy humans, there is no definite clinical evidence on their deleterious effect on kidney function. There seems to be no major clinical concern on the use of both short- and long-term (5 days–5 years) with different doses of creatine (5–30 g/day) on different studied indexes of kidney function at least in healthy athletes and bodybuilders with no baseline renal diseases. Finally, there is insufficient data about the effects of creatine supplementation on renal function and creatinine serum in elderly patients, those with baseline renal function impairment, or individuals with other comorbidities. Until more clarifying data are available, it is advisable to suggest that creatine supplementation not be used by sportsmen or women with pre-existing renal disease or those with a potential risk for kidney dysfunction, including diabetes mellitus, hypertension, and proteinuria [31].

22.2.1.1 Sideline Management

The diagnosis of acute renal failure secondary to creatine depends on a high suspicion index based on nonspecific symptoms, including sudden nausea, vomiting, and gastric pain. Hospitalization should be considered for diagnostic purposes and treatment. In the event of hospitalization of an athlete under the use of creatine and diagnosis of acute renal insufficiency, it is recommended discontinuation of creatine use; administration of intravenous fluids in abundance as tolerated by cardiac and renal parameters; attention not to prescribe any potentially renal harmful drugs that include especially non-steroidal anti-inflammatory agents, antibiotics such as aminoglycosides, among others. Full recovery may take several weeks, and regular laboratory follow-up is needed to monitor its development.

22.2.1.2 Prevention

Creatine supplementation should be avoided in those individuals in whom kidney dysfunction seems more likely to develop, including elderly patients, individuals with known kidney diseases, and those who possess a potential kidney-related injury pathology including diabetes, hypertension, autoimmune diseases, proteinuria, severe stone disease, and so on.

Creatine dosages should be kept within commonly prescribed regimens as their functional and/or adverse effects are likely predictable.

22.2.2 Steroids Abuse

Anabolic–androgenic steroid abuse has become prevalent in regions, such as Scandinavia, the United States, Brazil, and British Commonwealth countries [32]. Unfortunately, literature data on these drugs' effects on renal function are scarce and limited to experimental studies and anecdotal case reports. Regular, long-term use of anabolic–androgenic steroids can induce various renal disorders directly or indirectly through different mechanisms [33]. Some mild renal abnormalities, such as an increase in serum creatinine, blood urea nitrogen, or uric acid, without sclerotic/fibrotic morphological alteration or decrease in cystatin C clearance, can be recovered after discontinuing anabolic–androgenic steroids [34], which is the only recommended measure at first.

22.2.3 Hematuria

Sports-associated hematuria is common and has been reported in up to 95–100% of cases after exercise [35, 36]. Significant hematuria that requires further investigation is defined as the presence of more than five red blood cells per high-powered field. Most cases present with microscopic hematuria while only 2–3% have macroscopic or frank hematuria [37].

Previous research has suggested multiple potential mechanisms of urinary tract injury, including direct urinary tract trauma, hypoxic renal injury and ischemia, the release of a hemolyzing factor during exercise, non-steroidal anti-inflammatory drug use, dehydration, hemolysis due to tissue impact trauma, myoglobinuria release, and peroxidation of red blood cells [38]. Many cases remain idiopathic whatsoever.

Sports-associated hematuria can be divided into sports that directly cause the phenomenon, broadly divided into contact sports that may cause direct injury to the urinary tract (boxing, football, and rugby) and non-contact sports that may result in non-traumatic physiological changes and subsequent hematuria (rowing, running, and swimming).

The presence of hematuria was demonstrated in 27% urine analysis of 82 boxers after 150 fights over a 3-year period. When assessing a control group of boxers with strenuous exercise but no boxing contact, Kleiman found a rate of significant hematuria in only 4% [37].

A rate of 24.4% of hematuria was seen in a group of 30 elite Rugby Union players following five matches throughout the season. In comparison, rates of hematuria following non-contact training sessions were lower at 7.7%. All cases were microscopic and spontaneously resolved within 48 h [39].

In non-contact activities, the well-documented phenomenon "March" hematuria or hemoglobinuria produces discoloration of the urine after prolonged bouts of weight-bearing exercises. One study involving Candombe drummers, who usually march and drum for 2–4 h each time, showed urine discoloration in 23% with microscopic hematuria in an additional 30%. Blood film examination in those with urine discoloration showed fragmented red cells associated with increased serum total bilirubin, suggesting that red cell hemolysis plays a role in exercised-induced hematuria [40]. The source of hematuria following exercise has evidence suggesting both glomerular and non-glomerular sources, possibly attributed to extrarenal microtraumas [41, 42].

22.2.3.1 Sideline Management

If macroscopic hematuria occurs following an obvious kidney trauma, clinical support with hemodynamic resuscitation and referral for immediate abdominal imaging should be attempted (see sideline management for kidney injuries further ahead in this chapter). Apart from this situation, there is no current specific recommendation for hematuria management following sports.

Additional investigation with computerized tomography may lead to the diagnosis of incidental abnormalities/malignancies. Given the prevalence of both urological (up to 22.6%) and non-urological (6.8–56%) clinically significant findings, it is important to investigate all persistently noted hematuria lasting over 48 h [43–45] (Table 22.1).

Table 22.1 Degree of hematuria with grades of renal trauma

Author	Trauma	Macroscopic hematuria	Microscopic hematuria	Absent hematuria	Total
Stein et al. (1994)	Significant injury > grade 2	8	17	–	25
	Grade 1–2	6	13	4	23
	Total	14	30	4	48
Ishida et al. (2017)	Significant injury > grade 2	9	25	1	35
	Grade 1–2	5	21	7	33
	Total	14	46	8	68

(Reproduced from Akiboye RD, Sharma DM. Haematuria in sport: a review. Eur Urol Focus 2019; 5: 912–6)

22.3 Traumatic Disorders

22.3.1 Kidney and Ureteric Injuries

Kidneys are located in the retroperitoneum of the abdomen at the level of the 12th rib bilaterally, protected posteriorly by the back muscles and anteriorly by abdominal organs. They are involved by Gerota's fascia and cushioned perirenal fat, which offers a quite protected situation against external trauma [46]. Nevertheless, intense direct impact on the abdomen or flank can still lead to parenchymal laceration; subtle rapid deceleration can transmit great forces to the fixed renal hilum leading to pedicle or pyeloureteral junction injury [46, 47].

Ureters are much less likely to suffer injury following blunt abdominal trauma as they are malleable and loose structures. Less mobile sections of the ureter as the ureteropelvic junction and proximal segment are more exposed to injury.

22.3.1.1 Overview

Children are believed to be more susceptible to renal trauma than their adult counterparts. Reasons include greater size of the kidney compared with the body, less perirenal fat to cushion the kidney, weaker abdominal muscles, and less protection from ribs resulting in transmission of greater forces [46–48].

Wan and colleagues [49] assessed the National Pediatric Trauma Registry from 1990 to 1999 and described injuries related to contact sports. Only 5439 (6.64%) out of 81,923 trauma cases were due to sports in school-aged children, and only 459 were abdominal or testicular (0.56%) injuries. Sixty-two percent of kidney injuries were related to football, but other sports included baseball, basketball, hockey, and soccer. McAleer and colleagues [50] reported only six renal injuries caused by team sports after reviewing their trauma registry of 16 years period. Bicycling (Fig. 22.1) was the most common cause (27.6%), while team sports accounted for 6.1%, followed by skateboarding (6.1%), rollerblading (6.1%), playing ball (4.1%), equestrian sports (4.1%), and trampoline jumping (1%).

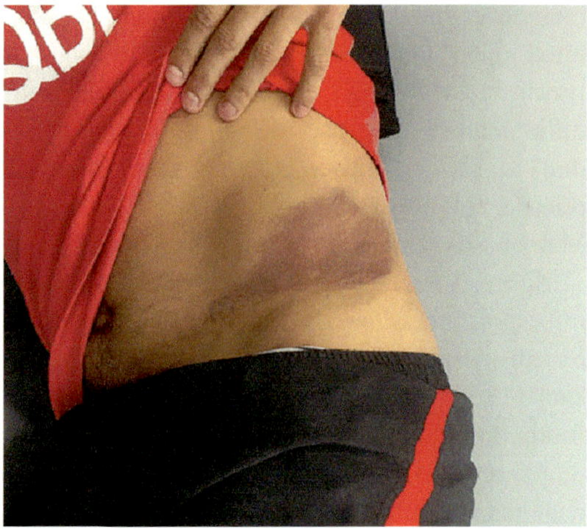

Fig. 22.1 Flank ecchymosis

A 30-year review of abdominal injuries in Sweden showed that of 136 sports-related abdominal injuries, 59 were renal. This was only second to abdominal contusion [51].

Renal injuries may be classified based on their severity. They may be termed minor, major, or catastrophic, or alternatively, they may be classified as Grade I through V according to the American Association for the Surgery of Trauma (AAST) (Table 22.2). Grade I injuries are the most common accounting for approximately 80% of cases. This grade includes hematuria with normal imaging studies, contusion, and nonexpanding subcapsular hematoma without parenchymal laceration. Grade II injuries include nonexpanding perinephric hematoma confined to the retroperitoneum and renal parenchymal lacerations less than 1 cm in depth and without collecting system rupture or urinary extravasation. Grade III injuries include renal parenchymal lacerations more than 1 cm in depth and without collecting system rupture or urinary extravasation. Grade IV injuries are characterized by corticomedullary laceration involving the renal collecting system and by damage to the main renal vessels that can lead to segmental infarctions. Grade V injuries include shattered or devascularized kidneys, ureteropelvic junction avulsion, and complete laceration or thrombosis of the main renal artery or vein. A shattered kidney is the most severe form of renal laceration, which is

Table 22.2 Kidney injury scale by the American Association for the surgery of trauma

Grade	Type of injury	Description of injury
I	Contusion	Microscopic or gross hematuria, urologic studies normal
	Hematoma	Subcapsular, non-expanding without parenchymal laceration
II	Hematoma	Nonexpanding perirenal hematoma confined to Gerota's fascia
	Laceration	<1 cm parenchymal depth of renal cortex without urinary extravasation
III	Laceration	>1 cm parenchymal depth of renal cortex without urinary extravasation or collecting system rupture
IV	Laceration	Parenchymal laceration extending through the renal cortex, medulla, and collecting system
	Vascular	Main renal artery or vein injury contained hemorrhage
V	Laceration	Completely shattered kidney
	Vascular	Avulsion of renal hilum that devascularizes the kidney

(Reproduced with permission of Wolters Kluwer from Moore EE, Shackford SR, Pachter HL, McAninch JW, Browner BD, Champion HR, Flint LM, Gennarelli TA, Malangoni MA, Ramenofsky ML, Trafton PG. J Trauma. 1989 Dec;29(12):1664–6)

fractured in three or more segments with associated injury to the collecting system [52].

Although most sports related renal injuries are low-grade (AAST grades I–II), isolated blows to the flank sustained during sports related activities can also produce high-grade renal injury (AAST III–V) [53, 54]. Patel et al. evaluated the incidence of high-grade renal injuries at four large trauma centers in the United States to determine differences in clinical characteristics and management for these two mechanistic groups of blunt renal trauma [55]. They retrospectively reviewed and identified 320 cases of AAST grades III–V from 2005 through 2014. Of these, 18% were sports-related injuries mainly caused by snowboarding (25%), skiing (25%), and contact sports (24%). Isolated kidney injury was more common in sports-related cases than non-sports related injuries (69% vs 39%, respectively, $p < 0.001$) where concomitant pelvic fracture or thoracic injury were more likely ($p < 0.001$ and $p = 0.004$, respectively). Additionally, 24% of cases presented as an isolated renal injury without associated hypotension or tachycardia [55].

In a series reported by Kakhimov et al. [56], kidney injuries were the second most common (after spleen injuries) in young male soccer players. The most common cause of trauma was a direct impact of the elbow/knee/foot to the flank. All cases were managed conservatively, although two of them were grade IV renal injuries. Management included hemoglobin and vital signs monitoring, and supportive measures including intravenous fluids, analgesia, and antiemetics.

Kim et al. recently reported on a systematic review of genitourinary injuries arising from football and rugby [57]. Included studies were all retrospective series or case reports. In the pediatric population, the proportion of football-related kidney injuries is less than 1% of all football-related injuries and total sports-related injuries. In adults, no proportion could be determined from the existing studies. However, the only reported injury per exposure was 0.000012 per exposure [57].

Trauma to the ureter is significantly less common than renal trauma, with ureteric injury accounting for 1–2% of all urological traumas [58]. Unfortunately, ureteric and bladder injuries are poorly documented in the literature [45].

22.3.1.2 Clinical Presentation

Physical examination usually presents as diffuse abdominal pain and less often as acute abdomen [56]. Symptoms and signs will depend on the severity of renal injury, including flank bruising, rib pain and/or fracture, abdominal tenderness, hematuria, hypotension, and tachycardia. However, significant renal injury can be present without pain, particularly if the injury to the kidney is within the substance of the kidney, resulting in bleeding into the renal collecting system only and not the surrounding tissues. Besides, a review of 2500 traumatic renal injuries over a 20-year period found hematuria to be absent in 4% [59]. Immediate medical assistance in sports-derived abdominal trauma does not differ from trauma derived from other causes and must include the ABCDE algorithm (airway, breathing, and circulation with pulse and blood pressure measurements; followed by neurological and physical assessment). Interestingly, in adults, blood pressure is an adequate assessment of volume status, whereas, in children, it can be misleading as normotension can coexist with hypovolemia [4, 47].

On physical examination, attention should be taken to signs indicating renal injury. Objective signs include hematuria, flank hematoma, flank or abdominal ecchymosis (Fig. 22.2) or tenderness, pelvic pain, rib fractures or pain, transverse process pain, penetrating injuries, or abdominal examination with peritoneal signs (rebound tenderness and guarding) [60].

Microscopic hematuria is the most common laboratory finding in renal trauma [47]. In fact, 80–95% of adults with significant renal trauma present with hematuria [46, 61]. If microscopic hematuria is detected, quantification can help determine if further imaging is indicated. In adults, microscopic hematuria and hypotension are predictors of significant renal injury. In children, hematuria of more than 50 red blood cells (RBC) per high-power field is indicative of additional imaging [4, 46, 47]. However, the presence or absence and number of RBCs do not necessarily correlate with injury severity. For example, a deceleration injury can result in renal vascular pedicle avulsion and not provoke hematuria.

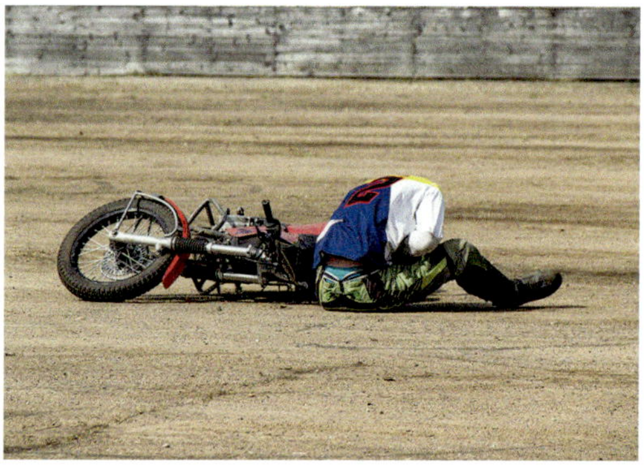

Fig. 22.2 Bicycle-related trauma represents almost 1/3 of sports-related blunt abdominal trauma

22.3.1.3 Sideline Management

Management of the athlete with renal trauma depends on the severity of the injury, and the ultimate goal is to preserve the greatest function with the least morbidity. Most sports-related renal trauma involves contusion and can be managed conservatively with observation, bed rest, and supportive therapy [62].

Initial aid should focus on the athlete's vital signs following the trauma's ABC principles (airway, breathing, and circulation). Once the patient is secured to be well oxygenated and hemodynamically stable, a urine dipstick test should be performed. If hematuria is present, hospital admission for abdominal imaging (contrast-enhanced computerized tomography would be the first choice) and laboratory blood work to assess acute anemia and renal function should be considered. In addition, if the kinetics involved in the trauma mechanism or if the athlete shows signs of flank bruising or hematoma, rib fracture, or intense flank pain, which are highly suspicious for renal trauma, hospital admission must be considered as well. Since sports-related mechanisms of renal injury are often less pronounced, a significant injury could be easily overlooked. The series reported by Patel et al. verified that 7% of sports related renal injuries required any renal specific procedural/ surgical intervention [55].

According to Sandler et al. [63], indications for imaging in renal trauma settings differ in adults and children. In adults, it would be recommended if there is penetrating injury, gross hematuria, microscopic hematuria with shock, or suspicion of major associated intra-abdominal injury. Stable adult athletes with microscopic hematuria can be observed without imaging. On the other hand, all children with blunt abdominal trauma and any degree of hematuria, regardless of blood pressure, should be imaged, although this is not a consensus [64].

Conservatively, managed athletes with renal contusion should be observed until hematuria disappears and removed from contact sports for 6 weeks [62]. More severe injuries may take 6–8 weeks to heal completely [65]. As such, return to contact or collision sports may require

6–12 months in athletes with extensive renal injuries and some may even choose not to return to these sports at all [62].

22.3.1.4 Prevention

The American Academy of Pediatrics Committee on Sports Medicine and Fitness has recommended that those with a solitary kidney be given a "qualified yes" on a case-by-case basis involving appropriate counseling for contact, collision, and limited-contact sports [4]. Pre-existing renal abnormalities, such as pelvic, iliac or multicystic kidneys, hydronephrosis, and ureteropelvic junction obstruction pose a higher risk to kidneys and should be advised as such. Although the loss of a solitary kidney is certainly catastrophic, Psooy et al. published an article that puts risk in perspective [66]. Sports that carry a risk of renal injury have five times the risk of a head injury; yet, having only one brain does not deter participation in sports. For children who have a higher risk of renal injury, either because of a solitary kidney or an abnormal one, counseling of the patient and parents is important and should include information on protective equipment (rib protectors, blocking vest, and kidney belt, although there is no existing data on efficacy) and possible long-term consequences (including renal insufficiency, dialysis, and renal transplant) [67]. Nonetheless, protective gear may negatively affect the athlete's performance, and this should be discussed (Fig. 22.3). Guidelines provided by the American Academy of Pediatrics do not restrict any sporting activity for those with a solitary kidney or testicle. Instead, protective equipment is encouraged for athletes with a solitary kidney to participate in contact and collision sports [68].

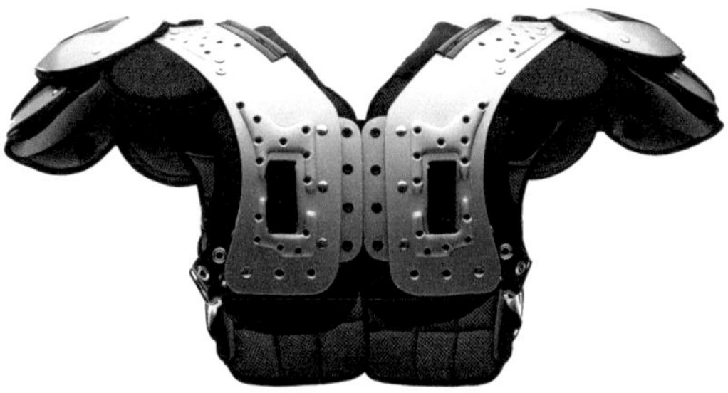

Fig. 22.3 Football gear for thoraco-abdominal protection_protective gear is often avoided since it may negatively impact performance

22.3.2 Bladder Injuries

The bladder is located deep within the pelvic bony structure, offering a well-protected condition from blunt sports-related trauma. Especially when it is empty, the bladder is almost completely safe from injury behind the pubic rami. However, if sufficiently intense kinetic force causes pelvic fracture, it may result in bladder perforation. As the bladder fills, it rises above the protective bony structures, exposing itself to the unprotected abdomen and making it more vulnerable to blunt injury. In infants and young children, the urinary bladder is in the abdomen even when empty, and it usually descends into the pelvis by the age of 20 years [69].

Nevertheless, bladder injury occurs in only 1.6% of all blunt abdominal trauma cases [70].

22.3.2.1 Overview

Bladder rupture in blunt abdominal trauma is uncommon because of its position but is associated with a mortality rate as high as 22% [71]. Trauma injuries may result from either macro or micro traumatic mechanisms.

Macrotraumatic mechanisms include high-energy blunt trauma that disrupts the bony pelvis, such as a direct blow to the distended bladder. Of all bladder injuries, 60–85% result from blunt trauma. Sports that incorporate high-velocity contact and collision are the ones under higher risk. Martial arts, softball, snowboarding, football, rugby, gymnastics, and hockey are examples and involve acceleration, deceleration, and spearing.

Microtraumatic injury to the bladder can result from repetitive jolting, which can occur in long-distance running, generating transient bladder contusions. A combination of exertional forces and intra-abdominal pressure can produce a repeated impact of the flaccid wall onto the bladder base. The bladder may be empty or nearly empty while the runner is competing, and this permits apposition of the bladder surfaces, which can manifest as transient hematuria. Partial filling of the bladder could prevent this type of insult [69].

Bladder injuries can be defined as contusions or bladder ruptures. Bladder ruptures following blunt abdominal trauma may be classified as either extraperitoneal (70–90% of cases), with urine leakage limited to the perivesical space, or intraperitoneal (15–25%), in which the peritoneal surface disrupts and urine extravasates into the abdominal cavity [72].

Extraperitoneal lesions are more commonly associated with pelvic fractures. Eighty-three percent of bladder ruptures have pelvic fractures, but only 10% of patients with pelvic fractures have bladder ruptures [73].

Intraperitoneal bladder rupture usually results from a blunt lower abdominal force on a full bladder and is thus related to the degree of bladder distention and the magnitude of pelvic injury.

22.3.2.2 Clinical Presentation

Although the nonspecific, clinical presentation of bladder injury often consists of a triad of symptoms: gross hematuria, suprapubic or abdominal pain/tenderness, and difficulty or inability to void. Hematuria may be transient and even microscopic, but although grossly clear urine without a pelvic fracture practically excludes a bladder rupture, the absence of hematuria does not rule out a bladder injury, and if the history and physical examination strongly suggest a possible intra-abdominal injury, the diagnosis must be endured [74].

Bladder contusion can present with transient hematuria but may also be clinically silent, making its incidence truly unknown. The amount of hematuria does not indicate the degree of severity of bladder injury. Nor does the ability to urinate exclude bladder injury or perforation.

Although bladder perforation is considerably rare in athletes, a delay in diagnosis can increase the mortality rate. Understanding the trauma mechanism and whether the athlete could have sustained a pelvic fracture is essential for accurate and timely diagnosis [69]. The immediate assessment of the athlete with an abdominal injury must take into account the potential for the evolution of critical injuries [75].

In general, bladder rupture will present with signs of peritoneal irritation, including distention, guarding, and rebound tenderness. The rectal examination will help exclude rectal injury and allow for evaluation of the prostate position. If the prostate is "high riding" or elevated, it suggests a possible associated urethral disruption.

22.3.2.3 Sideline Management

Basic life support with vital signs assessment and resuscitation maneuvers as needed is the fundamental aspect of initial sideline management.

If pelvic fracture is suspected, immobilization for immediate transportation is mandatory.

If acute urinary retention develops and a tender full bladder globe can be palpable in the lower abdomen, and if hospital assistance cannot be offered soon enough, a suprapubic relief puncture can be executed using an intravenous 14/16 gauge catheter (Abbocath) at 1–2 cm above the pubic bone. The needle should enter perpendicular to the abdominal wall straight into the bladder. Urine can be aspirated with the aid of a syringe until definitive urine derivation with a cystostomy can be executed.

22.3.2.4 Prevention

Prevention would be key, and using padding to prevent injury is ideal. However, padding is not practical in most contact sports, which would put athletes at risk of blunt abdominal injury and may negatively impact competitive performance. Therefore, protective gear should be worn when possible, and the bladder should be kept empty during exercise and before engaging in any competitive event [69].

22.3.3 Testicle Injuries

Testicle injuries are rare in children who play team and individual contact and collision sports. Wan et al. reported only one testicle injury during a 10-year period, and none was lost [49]. The low incidence of testicular injuries may be attributed to the cremasteric reflex, strength of the tunica albuginea, and the position of the testicles being free and mobile, perhaps making them less vulnerable to crush injury and disruption [49]. Despite being relatively uncommon compared with other sports injuries, more than half of all testicular injuries are sustained during sports [76]. Ninety percent of blunt testicular injuries are isolated; 5% are associated with penile injury, and less than 2% are bilateral [77].

22.3.3.1 Clinical Presentation

The most common sign of testicle injury is scrotal swelling, pain, erythema, and discoloration. Systemically, there can be nausea, emesis, and even syncope [78]. If the mechanism of trauma is suspected to be excessively intense, or pain and/or local swelling is unusually persistent or overwhelming, referral for hospitalization and image assessment with scrotal ultrasound is recommended. Rupture of the tunica albuginea with exposure to seminiferous tubules, if diagnosed, demands immediate surgical repair. A hemiscrotal hematocele is often apparent as a tender mass larger than a baseball and causing loss of rugae of the scrotal skin. Such hematocele is common in association with testicular rupture and will not transilluminate [78].

22.3.3.2 Sideline Management

Most testicle traumas are minor and limited to contusion, which is conservatively treated with analgesics and anti-inflammatory agents, icing, and rest [76]. Testicular support with an athletic supporter or compression shorts can reduce local pain and swelling. If a testicular rupture is suspected either because of clinical presentation or mechanism of trauma, the athlete must be referred to a center where immediate ultrasound is available. Ultrasound is highly sensitive for detecting testicular rupture and avulsion [79]. Sensitivity, specificity, positive predictive value, and negative predictive value are, respectively, 50, 76, 67, and 62% when only ultrasound signs of heterogeneous parenchyma and loss of contour with direct tunica albuginea breach are found. However, when testis rupture is evidenced, sensitivity, specificity, PPV, and NPV are 100, 65, 73, and 100%, respectively [79].

22.3.3.3 Prevention

Testicles are recognized as an organ vulnerable to injury, and specific protective cups have been designed to guard them. The immediate cause of this type of injury involves kicking, gouging, punching, and kneeing, usually during tackles, but in some cases due to intentional twisting and grabbing leading to traumatic torsion or disruption. As such, there should be more strict enforcement of rules concerning these flagrant fouls [49]. However, in a survey among high school and college male athletes, only 12.9% indicated that they wore a cup, and rates for each individual sport, other than baseball and lacrosse, were less than 10% [80]. In addition, education could bring more awareness by the players to seek immediate assistance when injured.

22.3.4 Penile Injuries

The male genitalia are seldom injured during athletic activity. The nonerect penis is highly mobile. When erect, however, the penis is susceptible to acute trauma with resultant fracture of the tunica albuginea. The area of the fracture is acutely swollen or ecchymotic. This is a true urologic emergency necessitating evacuation of the clot and repair of the tunical tear. The patient usually neglects to mention the sexual activity that caused the fracture and reports it as a consequence of work- or sports-related trauma.

Direct blows to the flaccid penis or perineum may lead to vascular injuries and potency abnormalities. Vascular injuries are more likely to be caused by straddle-type injuries or direct blows to the pubis, such as spearing with football helmets. The injury is classically within Buck's fascia, and patients have butterfly-type ecchymosis on the perineum [81].

Long-distance cyclists may experience paresthesia and numbness in the perineum and phallus following prolonged cycling. Bicycler's penis resolves spontaneously with no apparent sequelae [81].

22.3.4.1 Sideline Management

If there is no ecchymosis formation and just local pain, analgesics and local ice may relieve immediate trauma, and the athlete may probably resume playing after the pain is controlled. However, immediate hospitalization is needed if there is ecchymosis formation or penile frank hematoma. Early surgical repair may prevent loss of erectile function.

22.3.4.2 Prevention

Using genital padding for contact sports such as football or Martial Art may offer protection from a direct blow to the genitalia.

Altering the angle of the bicycle seat to decrease perineal pressure may help avoid bicycler's penis occurrence [81].

22.3.5 Urethral Injuries

Urethral injuries following sport are poorly reported, although they represent 4% of all trauma to the genitourinary tract. "Straddle-type" injuries, commonly caused by cycling or motorcycle trauma to the perineal region, confer a high risk of urethral injury with or without the presence of pelvic fracture [82]. Men are five times more likely to have urethral injuries due to longer length and reduced mobility of the male urethra [83].

Table 22.3 synthetizes recommended sideline approaches to genitourinary trauma situations.

Table 22.3 Sideline management of abdominal and genitourinary injuries

Structure	Description	Hallmark signs/symptoms	Sideline management	Return to play
Diaphragm	Spasm (commonly described as "getting the wind knocked out"); most common injury in collision sports	Sudden shortness of breath immediately after abdominal impact that resolves quickly	Hip flexion and removal of constrictive equipment can relieve dyspnea	After breathing has normalized
Muscular abdominal wall	Contusion or rectus sheath hematoma	Hematoma can mimic acute abdomen—sudden pain, rapid swelling, rebound and/or guarding, with or without nausea/vomiting; tender mass inferior to umbilicus	Keep abdomen in a supported/flexed position: avoid active abdominal flexion and stretching of the muscles	As symptoms allow
Liver	Most commonly injured organ Injury can result from deceleration or direct blow Hepatic injury scale: I–VI (I most common/least severe; VI fatal) 50–80% of liver injuries stop bleeding spontaneously	Right upper quadrant pain with radiation to shoulder or neck, rib tenderness, with or without guarding	Transport the patient to the emergency department	No RTP General surgery clearance necessary for RTP

Table 22.3 (continued)

Structure	Description	Hallmark signs/symptoms	Sideline management	Return to play
Spleen	Most commonly injured organ in sports Most common cause of death via abdominal trauma in athletes Injury is six times more common in snowboarding than in skiing Increased risk in children and in patients with splenomegaly, infection (e.g., mononucleosis), pregnancy, portal hypertension Delayed rupture in up to 8% of adults	Examination findings can be unreliable because of splenic capsule containing initial bleeding and delaying symptoms Initial sharp left-sided pain (10th, 11th, and 12th ribs) transitioning to a dull ache Generalized abdominal tenderness and distension, with or without rebound and guarding Radiating pain to shoulder secondary to diaphragmatic irritation from free intraperitoneal blood	Transport the patient immediately to the emergency department. Hemodynamic status can change quickly	No RTP Postsplenectomy patients should be vaccinated against *Haemophilus influenzae* type B, *Neisseria meningitidis* serogroups, and pneumococcus
Stomach/ intestine/ pancreas	Rare; results from direct trauma	Abdominal pain and tenderness that diminishes within the first 2 h and increases again over the next 6–8 h	Transport the patient to the emergency department	No guidelines—dependent on disease process and symptoms
Kidney	Most common genitourinary injury; more common in children than in adults Sports-related mechanism (blow to the flank) is likely an isolated injury Low (I or II) and high (III–V) grade (American Association for the Surgery of Trauma Classification) injuries can be seen in sports	Hematuria and hypotension are the most important indicators of severity Hemodynamic instability is absent in nearly 25% when sports-related	Monitor vital signs. Transport the patient to the emergency department	No RTP until hematuria has completely resolved
Bladder	More common in children than in adults Increased risk with full/ distended bladder Incidence is approximately 1%. 22% mortality after blunt trauma Macrotrauma: associated with pelvic fractures (83%), collision/high energy sports Microtrauma: repetitive self-impact of empty bladder walls in long-distance runners Injury can be extraperitoneal, intraperitoneal, or combined	May be similar to acute abdomen Triad: gross hematuria, suprapubic or abdominal pain or tenderness, and difficulty or inability to void Elevated prostate on rectal exam Transient hematuria with microtrauma or contusion	Transport patient to emergency department if rupture is suspected or the clinical triad is present	No RTP

(continued)

Table 22.3 (continued)

Structure	Description	Hallmark signs/symptoms	Sideline management	Return to play
Testicle	More common than penile injury Rupture is rare, but sports are the most common cause (football) Protected by testicular mobility, the cremasteric reflex, and the strength of the tunica albuginea Rupture involves tunica albuginea and extravasation of seminiferous tubules Torsion: 4–8% trauma related	Severe pain, nausea, emesis, with or without syncope; swelling, ecchymosis, and tenderness to palpation Examination technique: grasp neck of scrotum with three fingers posterosuperiorly to the involved testis and the thumb anteriorly. Swelling below the thumb suggests testicular or epididymal injury or hydrocele. Swelling above the thumb suggests an incarcerated hernia or spermatic cord injury Hemiscrotal hematocele: large tender mass causing loss of scrotal rugae; does not transilluminate (hydrocele does); associated with rupture Torsion: absent cremasteric reflex, high/horizontal testicular line, small area of cyanosis on the scrotal skin (blue dot sign, torsion of the appendix testis)	Manual detorsion: turn involved testis laterally, (two thirds of torsions involve medial rotation); if symptoms and tactile feel suggest necessity, attempt medial rotation secondarily. Successful (reduction in pain) in 26–80% of patients Transport patient for surgical exploration; outcomes are better with early surgery	RTP when injury symptoms and surgical and traumatic wounds have resolved[a]
Penis, urethra, and ureter	Rare (<1% of genitourinary injuries) Posterior urethra is most at risk for crush injury (immobile and close to the pelvis) Membranous urethra is most at risk in patients with pelvic fracture (crosses the urogenital diaphragm 2–3 cm posterior to the symphysis pubis)	Urethral injury: blood at meatus, perineal ecchymosis, hematocele, urinary retention, and high-riding prostate	Do not attempt Foley catheter placement Transport patient for surgical exploration	RTP when injury symptoms and surgical and traumatic wounds have resolved

(From Chen AW, Archbold CS, Hutchinson M, Domb BG. Sideline Management of Nonmusculoskeletal injuries by the orthopaedic team physician. J Am Acad Orthop Surg 2019; 27: e146-e155)
RTP return to play
[a]The American Academy of Pediatrics supports sports participation for children with a single or undescended testicle but recommends protective equipment in high-risk sports

Take Home Messages

- There is no current solid evidence associating creatine use with renal failure, except for anecdotal case reports.
- Creatine seems safe to be used in predetermined dosages and for long periods of time (up to 5 years).
- Athletes with renal impairment or at higher risk of developing renal dysfunction not be encouraged to take creatine.
- Evidence linking steroid abuse and renal failure is scarce; however, if suspected, steroids should be interrupted immediately with high chances of renal recovery.
- In any sports-related genitourinary suspected trauma, basic life support with trauma ABC protocol should be prioritized.
- Gross hematuria, microscopic hematuria with hypotension, and hematuria in children should prompt transport for hospital admission and immediate imaging; renal trauma should be suspected.
- Bladder injury is usually associated with blunt abdominal trauma; if a pelvic fracture occurs, the suspicion index should be elevated.
- If urinary retention develops after pelvic fracture and/or urethra disruption, a suprapubic percutaneous puncture may be performed to alleviate bladder fullness until a definitive cystostomy can be performed.
- Testicular injuries with tunica albuginea tear demand immediate hospitalization and surgical repair within 72 h.
- Penile injuries are rare but also demand immediate hospitalization for surgical repair.
- Urethral injuries are unusual and demand imaging for adequate diagnosis; men are five more times likely to present it.

References

1. Bagga HS, Fisher PB, Tasian GE, Blaschko SD, McCulloch CE, McAninch JW, Breyer BN. Sports-related genitourinary injuries presenting to United States Emergency Departments. Urology. 2015;85:239–45.
2. Brown DL. Genitourinary problems in the athlete. In: Birrer RB, O'Connor FG, editors. Sports medicine for the primary care physician. 3rd ed. Boca Raton: CRC Press; 2004. p. 751–60.
3. Kuan JK, Wright JL, Nathens AB, et al. American Association for the Surgery of Trauma Organ Injury Scale for kidney injuries predicts nephrectomy, dialysis, and death in patients with blunt injury and nephrectomy for penetrating injuries. J Trauma. 2006;60(2):351–6.
4. Bernard JJ. Renal trauma: evaluation, management, and return to play. Curr Sports Med Rep. 2009;8(2):98–103.
5. Smith NA, Chounthirath T, Xiang H. Soccer-related injuries treated in emergency departments: 1990–2014. Pediatrics. 2016;138:e20160346.
6. Kucera KL, Currie DW, Wasserman E, et al. Incidence of sport-related internal organ injuries due to direct contact mechanisms among high school and collegiate athletes across 3 national surveillance systems. J Athl Train. 2019;54:152–64.
7. Grinsell MM, Butz K, Gurka MJ, et al. Sport-related kidney injury among high school athletes. Pediatrics. 2012;130:e40–5.
8. Bagga HS, Tasian GE, Fisher PB, McCulloch CE, McAninch JW, Breyer BN. Product related adult genitourinary injuries treated at emergency departments in the United States from 2002 to 2010. J Urol. 2013;189(4):1362–8.
9. Burt CW, Overpeck MD. Emergency visits for sports-related injuries. Ann Emerg Med. 2001;37:301–8.
10. Chen AW, Archbold CS, Hutchinson M, Domb BG. Sideline management of nonmusculoskeletal injuries by the orthopaedic team physician. J Am Acad Orthop Surg. 2019;27:e146–55.
11. Davani-davari D, Karimzadeh I, Ezzatzadegan-Jahromi S, Sagheb MM. Potential adverse effects of creatinne supplements on the kidney in athletes and bodybuilders. IJKD. 2018;12:253–60.
12. Hultman E, Soderlund K, Timmons J, Cederblad G, Greenhaff P. Muscle creatine loading in men. J Appl Physiol. 1996;81:232–7.
13. Ropero-Miller JD, Paget-Wilkes H, Doering PL, Goldberger BA. Effect of oral creatine supplementation on random urine creatinine, pH, and specific gravity measurements. Clin Chem. 2000;46:295–7.
14. Pritchard N, Kalra P. Renal dysfunction accompanying oral creatine supplements. Lancet. 1998;351(9111):1252–3.

15. Edmunds JW, Jayapalan S, DiMarco NM, Saboorian H, Aukema HM. Creatine supplementation increases renal disease progression in Han: SPRD-cy rat. Am J Kidney Dis. 2001;37:73–8.
16. Poortmans J, Francaux M. Renal dysfunction accompanying oral creatine supplements. Lancet. 1998;352:234.
17. Mihic S, MacDonald JR, McKenzie S, Tarnopolsky MA. Acute creatine loading increases free-fat mass, but does not affect blood pressure, plasma creatinine, or CK activity in men and women. Med Sci Sports Exerc. 2000;32:291–6.
18. Kreider RB, Ferreira M, Wilson M, et al. Effects of creatine supplementationon body composition, strength, and sprint performance. Med Sci Sports Exerc. 1998;30:73–82.
19. Robinson TM, Sewell DA, Casey A, Steenge G, Greenhaf PL. Dietary creatine supplementation does not affect some haematological indices, or indices of muscle damage and hepatic and renal function. Br J Sports Med. 2000;34:284–8.
20. Wyss M, Kaddurah-Daouk R. Creatine and creatinine metabolism. Physiol Rev. 2000;80:1107–213.
21. Yu P, Zuo D. Formaldehyde produced endogenously via deamination of methylamine. A potential risk factor for initiation of endothelial injury. Atherosclerosis. 1996;120:189–97.
22. Yu PH, Wright S, Fan EH, Lun ZR, Gubisne-Harberle D. Physiological and pathological implications of semicarbazide-sensitive amine oxidase. Biochem Biophys Acta. 2003;1647:193–9.
23. Poortmans JR, Kumps A, Duez P, Fofonka A, Carpentier A, Francaux M. Effect of oral creatine supplementation on urinary methylamine, formaldehyde, and formate. Med Sci Sports Exerc. 2005;35:1717.
24. Sale C, Harris RC, Florance J, Kumps A, Sanvura R, Poortmans JR. Urinary creatinend methylamine excretion following 4 × 5 g × day^{-1} or 20 × 1 g × day^{-1} of creatine monohydrate for 5 days. J Sports Sci. 2009;27:759–66.
25. Nasseri A, Jafari A. Effects of creatine supplementation along with resistance training on urinary formaldehyde and serum enzyme in wrestlers. J Sports Med Phys Fitness. 2016;56:458–64.
26. Volek JS, Mazzetti SA, Farquhar WB, Barnes BR, Gomez AL, Kraemer WJ. Physiological responses to short-term exercise in the heat after creatine loading. Med Sci Sports Exerc. 2001;33:1101–8.
27. Poortmans JR, Francaux M. Long-term oral creatine supplementation does not impair renal function in healthy athletes. Med Sci Sports Exerc. 1999;31:1108–10.
28. Mayhew DL, Mayhew JL, Ware JS. Effects of long-term creatine supplementation on liver and kidney functions in American college football players. Int J Sport Nutr Exerc Metab. 2002;12:453–60.
29. Pline KA, Smith CL. The effect of creatine intake on renal function. Ann Pharmacother. 2005;39:1093–6.
30. Taner B, Aysim O, Abdulkadir U. The effects of the recommended dose of creatine monohydrate on kidney function. NDT Plus. 2011;4:23–4.
31. Davani-Davari D, Karimzadeh I, Ezzatzadegan-Jahromi S, Sagheb MM. Potential adverse effects of creatine supplement on the kidney in athletes and bodybuilders. IJKD. 2018;2:253–60.
32. Kanayama G, Pope HG. History and epidemiology of anabolic androgens in athletes and non-athletes. Mol Cell Endocrinol. 2017;464:4–13.
33. Luciano RL, Castano E, Moeckel G, Perazella MA. Bile acid nephropathy in a bodybuilder abusing an anabolic androgenic steroid. Am J Kidney Dis. 2014;64:473–6.
34. Turilazzi E, Perilli G, Di Paolo M, Neri M, Riezzo I, Fineschi V. Side effects of AAS abuse: an overview. Mini Rev Med Chem. 2011;11:374–89.
35. Gilli P, Vitali ED, Tataranni G, Farinelli A. Exercise-induced urinary abnormalities in long-distance runners. Int J Sports Med. 1984;5:237–40.
36. Mousavi M, Sanavi S, Afshar R. Effects of continuous and intermittent trainings on exercise-induced hematuria and proteinuria in untrained adult females. NDT Plus. 2011;4:217–8.
37. Kleiman A. Hematuria in boxers. JAMA. 1958;168:1633–40.
38. Jones GR, Newhouse I. Sports-related hematuria: a review. Clin J Sports Med. 1997;7:119–25.
39. Strickland C, Greenwell J, Strauss D. Urinalysis for detecting post-game haematuria in elite rugby union: a screening tool for renal trauma? Leeds: University of Leeds; 2013.
40. Tobal D, Olascoaga A, Moreira G, et al. Rust urina after intense hand drumming is caused by extracorposcular haemolysis. Clin J Am Soc Nephrol. 2008;3:1022–7.
41. Fasset RG, Owen JE, Fairley J, Birch DF, Fairley KF. Urinary red-cell morphology during exercise. Br Med J (Clin Resid Ed). 1982;285:1455–7.
42. Mydlik M, Derzsiová K, Bohus B. Renal function abnormalities after marathon run and 16-kilometre long-distance run. Przegl Lek. 2012;69:1–4.
43. Song JH, Beland MD, Mayo-Smith WW. Incidental clinically important extraurinary findings at MDCT urography for hematuria evaluation: prevalence in 1209 consecutive examinations. Am J Roentgenol. 2012;199(3):616–22.
44. Bromage SJ, Liew MP, Moore KC, Raju B, Shackley DC. The economic implications of unsuspected findings from CT urography performed for haematuria. Br J Radiol. 2012;85(1017):1303–6.
45. Akiboye RD, Sharma DM. Haematuria in sport: a review. Eur Urol Focus. 2019;5:912–6.
46. Santucci RA, Wessells H, Bartsch G, et al. Evaluation and management of renal injuries: consensus statement of the renal trauma subcommittee. BJU Int. 2004;93(7):937–54.
47. Buckley KJC, McAninch JW. The diagnosis, management and outcomes of pediatric injuries. Urol Clin N Am. 2006;33:33–40.

48. Brown SL, Elder JS, Spirnak JP. Are pediatric patients more susceptible to major renal injury from blunt trauma? A comparative study. J Urol. 1998;160:38–40.
49. Wan J, Corvino TF, Greenfield SP, et al. Kidney and testicle injury in team and individual sports: data from the national pediatric trauma registry. J Urol. 2003;70:1528–31.
50. McAleer IM, Kaplan GW, LoSasso BE. Renal and testis injuries in team sports. J Urol. 2002;168:1805–7.
51. Berqvist D, Hedelin H, Karlsson G, et al. Abdominal injury from sporting activities. Br J Sports Med. 1982;16:76–9.
52. Lee YJ, Oh SN, Rha SE, Byun JY. Renal trauma. Radiol Clin N Am. 2007;45:581–92.
53. Lloyd GL, Slack S, McWilliams KL, Black A, Nicholson TM. Renal trauma from recreational accidents manifests different from injury patterns than urban renal trauma. J Urol. 2012;188:163–8.
54. Fanning DM, Forde JC, Mohan P. A simple football injury leading to a grade 4 renal trauma. BMJ Case Rep. 2012;2012:bcr1020114959.
55. Patel DS, Redshaw JF, Breyer BN, Smith TG, Erickson BA, Majercik SD, et al. High-grade renal injuries are often isolated in sports-related trauma. Injury. 2015;46:1245–9.
56. Kakhimov S, Zaki P, Hess J, Hennrikus W. Abdominal organ injuries in youth soccer: a case series and review of literature. Curr Sports Med Rep. 2021;20(2):69–75.
57. Kim JK, Koyle MA, Lee MJ, Nason GJ, Ren LY, O'Kelly F. A systematic review of genitourinary injuries arising from rugby and football. J Pediatr Urol. 2020;16(2):130–48.
58. McGeady JB, Breyer BN. Current epidemiology of genitourinary trauma. Urol Clin N Am. 2013;40:323–34.
59. Santucci R, McAninch J. Diagnosis and management of renal trauma: past, present and future. J Am Coll Surg. 2000;191:443–51.
60. Brophy RH, Gamradt SC, Barnes RP, et al. Kidney injuries in professional American football. Am J Sports Med. 2008;36:85–90.
61. Alonso RC, Nacenta SB, Martinez PD, et al. Kidney in danger: CT findings of blunt and penetrating renal trauma. Radiographics. 2009;29(7):2033–53.
62. Cianflocco AJ. Renal complications of exercise. Clin Sports Med. 1992;11:437–51.
63. Sandler CM, Amis ES, Bigongiari LR, et al. Diagnostic approach to renal trauma. Radiology. 2000;215(Suppl):727–31.
64. Kawashima A, Sandler CM, Corl FM, et al. Imaging of renal trauma: a comprehensive review. Radiographics. 2001;21:557–74.
65. Petterson E. Genitourinary trauma. In: Feliciano DV, Moore EE, Mattox KL, editors. Trauma. 3rd ed. Stanford: Appleton and Lange; 1996. p. 691–3.
66. Psooy K. Sports and the solitary kidney: how to counsel parents. Can J Urol. 2006;13(3):3120–6.
67. Viola TA. Closed kidney injury. Clin Sports Med. 2013;32:219–27.
68. Rice SG. Medical conditions affecting sports participation. American Academy of pediatrics council on sports medicine and fitness. Pediatrics. 2008;121:841–8.
69. Guttman I, Kerr HA. Blunt bladder injury. Clin Sports Med. 2013;32:239–46.
70. Gomez RG, Ceballos L, Coburn M, et al. Consensus statement on bladder injuries. BJU Int. 2004;94(1):27–32.
71. Iverson AJ, Morey AF. Radiographic evaluation of suspected bladder rupture following blunt trauma: critical review. World J Surg. 2001;25(12):1588–91.
72. Jonhson M. Genitourinary. In: O'Connor FG, editor. Sports medicine: just the facts. Columbus: McGraw-Hill; 2005. p. 157–61.
73. Zacharias C, Robinson JD, Linnau KF, et al. Blunt urinary bladder trauma. Curr Probl Diagn Radiol. 2012;41(4):140–1.
74. Brandes S, Borrelli J Jr. Pelvic fracture and associated urologic injuries. World J Urol. 2001;25(12):1578–87.
75. Ryan JM. Abdominal injuries and sport. Br J Sports Med. 1999;33(3):155–60.
76. Styn NR, Wan J. Urologic sports injuries in children. Curr Urol Rep. 2010;11(2):114–21.
77. Cass AS, Luxenberg M. Testicular injuries. Urology. 1991;37(6):528–30.
78. Wasko R, Goldstein AG. Traumatic rupture of the testicle. J Urol. 1966;95(5):721–3.
79. Guichard G, El Ammari J, Del Coro C, et al. Accuracy of ultrasonography in diagnosis of testicular rupture after blunt scrotal trauma. Urology. 2008;71(1):52–6.
80. Bieniek JM, Sumfest JM. Sports-related testicular injuries and the use of protective equipment among young male athletes. Urology. 2014;84:1485–9.
81. York JP. Sports and the male genitourinary system. Phys Sportsmed. 1990;18(10):92–100.
82. Nichols TW. Bicycle-seat haematuria. N Engl J Med. 1984;311:1128.
83. Lowe MA, Mason JT, Luna GK, Maier RV, Copass MK, Berger RE. Risk factors for urethral injuries in men with traumatic pelvic fractures. J Urol. 1988;140(3):506–7.

23 Gastrointestinal Disorders

Gustavo Henrique Kujavo,
Bruno Paula Leite Arruda,
and Sérgio Rocha Piedade

23.1 Introduction

On the sideline, the sports physician should be aware of clinical signs and athletes' complaints after a sports energy and trauma mechanism is involved. Nevertheless, they should also be very attentive to the athlete's health and any clinical complaint presented in training or competing. Sports practice involves high-demand physical activity, and it does not matter if the competition is against an adversary or a personal physical challenge; the sports' dark side may occur in both, with a price to be paid.

They constantly search to win, fight against body limits, offer outstanding dedication and hard training, and sometimes accept abstinence from moments with friends and family, believing the winner takes all! However, sports practice is not just a fairy tale; injuries happen, and the treatment and recovery may account for the high physical and mental demands to get back on the sports scene.

Recently, with the spread of high-resistance activities, interest in research on the subject has increased considerably. Participation in marathons and ultramarathons has risen dramatically over the last 25 years, drawing attention to deleterious symptoms resulting from intense physical exertion during training and competitions [1, 2].

Gastrointestinal Tract Disorders (GIT) are common in endurance and ultra-endurance activities, especially in long-term activities (>1 h), reducing sports performance and offering health risks. Research from the 1980s already documented the presence of these symptoms, which were called "*Runner's Trots*" [3], and also included nausea, vomiting, heartburn, abdominal pain, fecal urgency, and bloody diarrhea in athletes from various types of sports [4–8].

Riddoch et al. in a questionnaire applied to 471 participants of the Belfast Marathon in 1986 showed that 83% of the competitors presented one or more GI symptoms (53% suffered from fecal urgency and 38% from diarrhea) during or immediately after the race [9]. The intensity and severity of symptoms vary significantly from mild discomfort and belching to severe intestinal bleeding [10]. In all cases, these problems affect not only the result but also the recovery of the athletes. A recent report of the 161 km ultramarathon "Western States Endurance Run" in the United States showed that GI disorders caused

G. H. Kujavo (✉)
Departament of Anesthesiology, Hospital Unimed Campinas, Campinas, SP, Brazil

B. P. L. Arruda
Nucleo de estudos do Instituto Willson Mello, Campinas, Brazil

S. R. Piedade
Exercise and Sports Medicine, Department of Orthopedics, Rheumatology, and Traumatology, University of Campinas-UNICAMP, Campinas, SP, Brazil
e-mail: piedade@unicamp.br

S. Rocha Piedade et al. (eds.), *Sideline Management in Sports*,
https://doi.org/10.1007/978-3-031-33867-0_23

approximately 35% of withdrawals [11]. Marathon legend Bill Rodgers, with four Boston Marathon and New York City Marathon wins in the late 1970s, said in an interview, "More marathons are decided in the bathroom than at the dinner table."

The etiology of these GIT disorders is complex and not fully understood, but it certainly involves multiple factors, such as reduced intestinal blood flow, the release of gastrointestinal hormones, mechanical stress on the GIT, dehydration, psychological factors, environmental factors, and previous intestinal pathologies [12]. The clinical approach of the sports doctor will be based on the exclusion of differential diagnoses of pathologies that offer a greater health risk and, finally, to offer the different options of therapies presented in the literature.

This chapter aims to discuss the prevalent factors for gastrointestinal disorders in athletes, upper and lower gastrointestinal symptoms, differential diagnosis, the impact of stress on the gastrointestinal tract, anamnesis, and clinical history, and call attention to potential red flags, treatment, and nutritional strategies.

23.2 Athlete Gastrointestinal Tract

It is well-known that sports and regular physical activity cause natural physiological stress to our body, playing a vital role in homeostasis, performance, and survival [13]. Allostasis is the stress of maintaining stability, or homeostasis, through a network of interacting mediators [14]. Acute allostasis promotes adaptations in the body; however, when these adaptations are either insufficient or the chronic stressor is kept (e.g., intense training program followed by competition), the allostatic system becomes overloaded and, consequently, can damage tissues and the immune, cardiovascular and nervous system systems [14]. An example of this is seen in high-performance athletes, who constantly challenge their physical limits and may push them to the "dark side" of physical exercises, predisposing clinical and musculoskeletal disorders.

23.3 Neurophysiology of Physical Exercises

Physical exercises activate the sympathetic and parasympathetic autonomic nervous system (ANS). The sympathetic axis represents the classic "fight or flight," resulting from increased adrenaline and noradrenaline levels, heart rate, contractile force, and vasoconstriction. On the other hand, the parasympathetic opposes the sympathetic system [15]. Furthermore, this stress activates two distinct but interconnected pathways, the sympathetic adrenomedullary system (SAM) and the hypothalamus pituitary adrenal axes (HPA), which are responsible for maintaining homeostasis during stress (e.g., allostasis) [14].

The hypothalamus pituitary adrenal axis is significant for the allostasis process. Its main mediators are the hormones of this axis, particularly catecholamines [norepinephrine (N.E.) and epinephrine] and cytokines, as well as the paraventricular nucleus (PVN) of the hypothalamus that are also activated in the presence of a stressor, which acts on the anterior pituitary gland and finally on the adrenal cortex, initiating the synthesis and release of glucocorticoids in the body, such as cortisol [15]. The amygdala and hippocampus interpret stressors and regulate appropriate responses. Furthermore, the amygdala plays a vital role in the HPA axis.

23.4 Training and Competition

Thorough training and competition (e.g., maintenance of allostatic overload), mainly endurance sports, such as swimming, cycling, long-distance running, and triathlon, demand an intense workout and competition routine. The body recognizes it as a stressor. The responses generated by the HPA axis and the adaptation of the amygdala can become insufficient, and as a result, catecholamines (N.E. and epinephrine) are released into the bloodstream and peripheral tissues, including the cardiovascular system and the gastrointestinal tract (GIT) [14].

Although a clear relationship between stress induced by exercise and the alteration of the intestinal microbiota still needs to be improved [16], literature has shown that there is a connection between the central nervous system (CNS) and the enteric nervous system (ENS) in the gastrointestinal tract (GIT), known as the gut–brain axis.

Bi-directional communication between the central nervous system (CNS) and the enteric nervous system (ENS) occurs under normal conditions, and the brain–gut axis is stimulated by various CNS- and gut-directed stressors [17].

These events involve the CNS, the neuroimmune and neuroendocrine systems, the autonomic nervous system and its arms (sympathetic and parasympathetic), and the intestinal microbiota [18]. This connection is primarily via the vagus nerve, which runs from the brainstem to the digestive tract and regulates almost every aspect of the passage of digestive material through the intestine. Some authors have found the influence of the vagus nerve on the intestinal microbiota in the production of metabolic precursors, neurotransmitters, and active metabolites and on the GIT in brain neurochemistry and the HPA axis [19, 20].

In this bidirectional system, the intestinal microbiota, in turn, can also influence the vagus nerve and the HPA axis due to its connection with the endocrine system because of the action of certain specific intestinal populations. Hormones, such as GABA, neuropeptides, and intestinal microbiota are forms of communication between the intestine–brain axis and can influence intestinal motility and permeability [15, 21]. Intestinal permeability is a barrier to control molecular exchanges of ions, water, and leukocytes. Lamprecht et al. [22] demonstrated increased intestinal permeability as an acute effect of exercise, which allows the passage of lipopolysaccharides (LPS) in the GIT.

Reactions to lipopolysaccharides (LPS) trigger an inflammatory response, such as cytokines and interleukins [23], demonstrating that physical activity with an effort above 60% and 80% of the maximum oxygen consumption (VO_{2max}) are stimuli for the release of hormones such as cortisol, and when above 80% of the VO_{2max}, there is an increase in the levels of ACTH. The rise in body temperature, and blood flow directed away from the intestine, caused by intense and prolonged exercise can disrupt this intestinal barrier and increase hormonal and immune stress by increasing pro-inflammatory cytokines and their permeability [22, 24].

23.5 Epidemiology

A substantial proportion of endurance athletes are affected by GIT symptoms, and the incidence, generally, is 20–50% in athletes during training and competitive events. However, these acute symptoms are transient and do not harm the athlete's long-term health. The difference between the beneficial effects of physical activity and the onset of harmful effects on the GIT is mainly based on the intensity of the practice [25].

Mild lower intestinal tract symptoms are more predominant, and there is a higher incidence among young people and females, especially in the menstrual period, as presented in Table 23.1. Fecal urgency and diarrhea were experienced in 74% and 68% of women, respectively, during and after competitions [5, 9]. Likewise, the severity of symptoms is directly proportional to the athlete's performance. For example, runners with better times (below 3 h and 34 min in a marathon race) suffered significantly more vomiting than the others [9]. Psychological factors involving pre-competition anxiety and environmental changes, such as high temperatures during competitions, also interfere with the onset of symptoms [26–29] (Table 23.1).

Kinetic energy acts in different ways on athletes in the practice of each modality. Positions during sporting activity are important components in developing GIT symptoms and affect the upper and lower GIT differently. In a cyclist, abdominal pressure can increase when leaning forward and affect the GI tract's upper part. On the other hand, repetitive trunk impacts during running can cause an extra mechanical load on the GIT, which apparently affects the lower part more than the upper part, confirming the theory that the intensity of friction of the psoas muscle directly on the colon affects the damage of the

Table 23.1 Prevalence factors for gastrointestinal disorders in athletes

Linked to the individual	Linked to the intensity of the competition	Nutritional	Life habits/use of medication	Environment
Sex/menstrual cycle	Duration	Fatty food	Aspirin, NSAIDs	Temperature
Age (young>)	Intensity	Carbohydrate solution	Vitamin C	
Physical fitness	Type of sport	Food rich in fibers	Smoking	
Years of training	Competition speed	Time of fasting	Alcohol abuse	
Previous gastrointestinal pathologies	Dehydration	Lactose, fructose, and sorbitol intolerance	Consumption of fizzy drinks	
Anxiety/psychiatric disorders		Liquids: orange juice, coffee		
Immunomediated hypersensibility		Eating during exercise		

Table 23.2 Upper and lower gastrointestinal symptoms during competition

Gastrointestinal disorders	Comparative prevalence level		
	Runners	Cyclists	Triathletes
Upper (reflux, gastritis, nausea, and vomiting)	++	+++	+
Lower (diarrhea, abdominal pain, and bleeding)	++++	++	+

intestinal mucosa in a complementary way. Runners and marathoners suffer more from flatulence and diarrhea than athletes from other sports. In these, the major cause of race abandonment is fecal urgency [8].

Additionally, nutritional aspects play a decisive role in the onset and prevalence of symptoms in different modalities, for example, triathletes manage to ingest more fluids and food than runners during competition. Perhaps, this explains why they are the modality that is less affected by these disorders [29] (Table 23.2).

23.6 Pathophysiology

Four critical factors have been put forward to contribute to the pathophysiology of gastrointestinal complaints in athletes, which will be discussed below: TGI blood flow reduction, mechanical forces/mechanical stress, neuroendocrine changes, and psycho-emotional involvement. Other interferences fall into the hydric/nutritional aspects of the athletes during the competition period [12].

23.6.1 Reduction of Intestinal Blood Flow

The GIT and splanchnic organs are supplied with arterial blood through three pathways: Celiac Trunk, Superior, and Inferior Mesenteric Artery. These arteries branch out into a dense vascular, serous, submucosal, and mucosal plexus, which subsequently flows into a capillary microcirculatory network that irrigates the entire intestinal mucosa. At rest, splanchnic blood flow accounts for approximately 25% of cardiac output and serves as the main reservoir of blood for the circulatory system [30].

Reduced intestinal blood flow during exercise is the predominant factor in GI disorders during endurance and ultra-endurance activities. It results from the vasoconstriction of the splanchnic vascular bed due to the action of catecholamines on α-adrenergic receptors and/or activation of the renin–angiotensin system by hypovolemia induced by exercise resulting from dehydration. This type of reduction can reach critical levels and be aggravated during hyperthermia, dehydration, hypoglycemia, hypoxia, changes in blood viscosity, deformability, and aggregation of erythrocytes or by a combination of these factors. Rehrer et al. found that the loss of 3.5–4.0% of body weight caused by dehydration during exercise is associated with increased gastrointestinal symptoms [31, 32].

At rest, 90% of blood flow to the intestine is directed to the mucosa. Therefore, this region is the most likely to present changes as a result of reduced intestinal blood flow during exercise. As previously mentioned, the GIT mucosa acts as a barrier between the external and internal environments, preventing the penetration of antigenic, carcinogenic, and toxic compounds from the intestinal lumen into the interstitial fluid. On the other hand, the impairment of the mucosa due to the reduction in blood flow caused by exercise increases intestinal permeability through communicating junctions (protein structures that allow the passage of ions and molecules between juxtaposed cells).

The passage of aggressive compounds through gap junctions stimulates the migration of neutrophils, which, when activated, trigger a local immune response with the production of free radicals and the release of lysosomal enzymes, which further damage the intestinal epithelium.

This sequence of events enhances intestinal permeability and inflammatory response, leading to gastrointestinal symptoms and, in some cases, even endotoxemia (Fig. 23.1). Athletes, who do long-term activities, especially ultra-marathoners, may experience intestinal bleeding during and after exercise. This injury is due to a decrease in the supply of oxygen and intestinal nutrients, which produces a morphological and functional disarrangement of the mucosa, and consequent necrosis of gastric cells, hepatocytes, and intestinal cells. Although such blood loss is transient, it can cause clinically important repercussions of serum iron and anemia [33].

23.6.2 Mechanical Factors

Continuous friction on the GI tract produced by repetitive impact exercise releases vasoactive intestinal peptide (VIP) and prostaglandins, causing increased intestinal secretion and diarrhea. This is supported by the fact that the frequency of these symptoms is approximately twice as high during running compared to cycling and swimming, where impact and mechanical vibration are lower. Furthermore, it has been shown that psoas muscle hypertrophy can cause pressure against the colon/cecum and stimulate increased motility and defecation (cecal-slap syndrome) [34].

Esophageal motility is also affected during exercise. Transient lower esophageal sphincter (LES) relaxation, increased pressure gradient between the stomach and esophagus, and

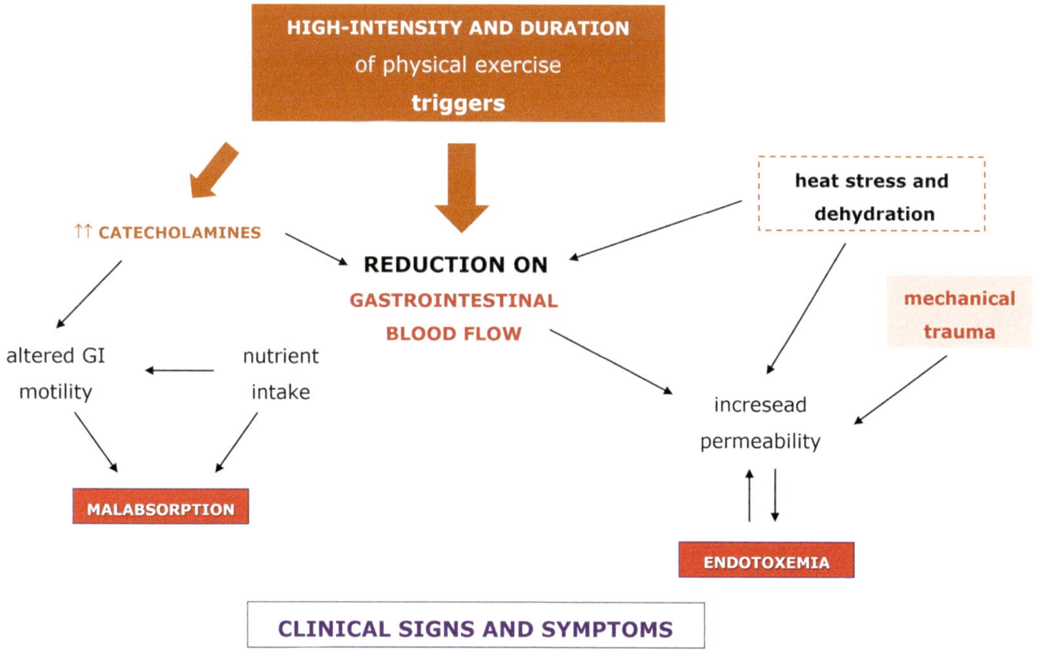

Fig. 23.1 The impact of the stress on the gastrointestinal tract

decreased esophageal clearance have all been associated with physical exertion and are all factors in the production of GERD symptoms [35].

23.6.3 Gastrointestinal Hormones

Many hormones associated with GIT function at rest, responsible for secretion, absorption, and motility, suffer from an alteration of plasma concentrations during exercise and may contribute to the development of gastrointestinal symptoms. These include cholecystokinin, vasoactive intestinal peptide (VIP), secretin, pancreatic polypeptide, somatostatin, histidine–methionine peptide (PHM), peptide YY, gastric inhibitory peptide, gastrin, glucagon, motilin, catecholamines, endorphins, and prostaglandins.

Vasoactive intestinal peptide, PHM, gastrin, and motilin are released in high amounts by the ischemic bowel. These peptides decrease the absorption of sodium ions and increase the intestinal content, promoting diarrhea. In addition, secretin, glucagon, gastric inhibitory peptide, and prostaglandins are also released into the bloodstream as a result of strenuous exercise and are known to increase intestinal secretion and thereby cause diarrhea.

Diarrhea can also result from colon relaxation caused by a drop in plasma insulin concentration and an increase in pancreatic polypeptide levels. Concomitantly, there is a decrease in the pressure exerted by the lower esophageal sphincter and gastric emptying, resulting from the rise in PHM and VIP [33].

23.6.4 Psycho-Emotional Involvement

The physiology of the digestive tract and the subjective experience of symptoms are strongly affected by psychosocial factors. Brain–gut interactions are increasingly recognized as underlying pathomechanisms of functional gastrointestinal disorders. Bi-directional communication between the central nervous system (CNS) and the enteric nervous system (ENS) occurs in health and disease. Various CNS- and gut-directed stressors stimulate the brain–gut axis. Processes modulating responsiveness to stressors along the brain–gut axis involve neural pathways and immunological and endocrinological mechanisms [36]. Disturbances such as stress can affect the modulation of gastrointestinal motility and secretion and may trigger neuroimmune and neuroendocrine reactions via the brain–gut [37–39].

Natural anxiety toward any important competition is exacerbated by the constant search for better results and challenges that this population commonly faces, such as long journeys; sleep deprivation; "JET LAG"; routes never before attempted; strong adversaries, opposing fans; and the overcoming of physical limits. Mental stress can also trigger psychiatric diseases, such as phobias and depression, and can be linked to worsening pre-existing GI pathologies, such as irritable bowel syndrome and gastritis. According to Sullivan and Wong, 32% of athletes who complained of gastrointestinal symptoms had emotional stress [40, 41].

23.6.5 Clinical Approach

Most athletes' gastrointestinal disorders are mild and occasional [11]. However, due to their wide range of symptoms, they can be the first sign of numerous pathologies. The peculiarities of high-performance athletes and their adaptation to stress confuse the traditional semiotics of abdominal complaints [42]. For example, a young marathon runner of childbearing age can remain amenorrheic for several months without suspecting pregnancy. Furthermore, this population's lifestyle and metabolic profile cannot "blind" us to differential cardiological diagnoses that must be immediately discarded in the face of retrosternal pain or abdominal discomfort during exertion.

Recent injuries or other socio-emotional factors interfere with the expectation of test results. After a long recovery period, athletes can raise anxiety levels, triggering the onset of psychiatric disorders. Finally, we must direct our attention to

Table 23.3 Prevalence of symptoms and differential diagnosis

Gastrointestinal disorders	Symptoms	Differential diagnosis	Diagnosis test
Upper git	**Heartburn**	Angina, myocardial infarction (MI), anxiety	Electrocardiogram (EKG) Serial troponin, cardiac stress testing + follow-up Based on concerning findings
		GERD	Upper endoscopy, 24-h pH monitoring, and manometry
		Anxiety	
	Belching	Dyspepsia, GERD, and psychiatric disorders	Upper endoscopy
	Nausea/vomiting	GERD, dehydration, electrolyte disorders, gastritis, gastroenteritis, pregnancy, anxiety, and panic syndrome	Complete blood count (CBC), electrolytes, upper endoscopy, and pregnancy test
	Side stitch/ abdominal cramps	Exercise-related transient abdominal pain (ETAP), rib stress fractures, sports hernia, cholecystitis, symptomatic gallstones, gastritis, peptic ulcers, hepatitis, pancreatitis, bacterial gastroenteritis, food intolerance, cecal volvulus (cecal slap syndrome), and gastrointestinal ischemia	Complete blood count (CBC), erythrocyte sedimentation rate (ESR), hepatic and pancreatic function markers, ultrasound, upper endoscopy, computed tomography angiography (CTA), X-ray, and bone scan
Lower git	Rectal bleending/ melena	Gastrointestinal bleeds, inflammatory bowel disease (IBD), colon cancer, diverticular disease, acute gastroenteritis (AGE), cecal slap syndrome, and anorectal diseases	Complete blood count (CBC), complete metabolic profile, fecal occult blood (FOB), iron studies and ferritin levels, colonoscopy, and computed tomography (CT)
	Flatulence	Endometriosis	Magnetic resonance
	Acute gastroenteritis (AGE) and food intolerance	Complete blood count (CBC) and lactose activity assay by jejunal biopsy	Acute gastroenteritis (AGE) and food intolerance
	Urge for defecation	Acute gastroenteritis (AGE), irritable bowel syndrome (IBS), and hyperthyroidism	Complete blood count (CBC) and thyroid-stimulating hormone (TSH)
	Diarrhea	Cecal slap syndrome, irritable bowel syndrome (IBS), inflammatory bowel disease (IBD), acute gastroenteritis (AGE), parasitic diseases, food intolerance, and hyperthyroidism	Complete blood count (CBC) and thyroid-stimulating hormone (TSH)

hemorrhagic gastritis, hematochezia, melena, and intestinal ischemia, which present more significant medical challenges.

As a priority, the clinical consultation of the sports physician should assess the onset of symptoms, their frequency, and their correlation with periods of greater physical and mental stress, such as in previous training sessions and competitions. Semiology should primarily follow the differentiation between upper and lower GIT complaints, as they will facilitate requesting complementary exams (Table 23.3).

The persistence of symptoms, as well as nutritional aspects of improvement or worsening, should be looked into. On trips to races, it is not uncommon to observe bacterial gastroenteritis (traveler's diarrhea), toxic colitis, or other food intolerances due to changes in food consumption. The approach initially excludes higher-risk organic pathologies such as malignant GI tumors, peptic ulcer disease, aortic vascular disease, pulmonary embolism, hepatitis, and pancreatitis. All patients should be asked about red-flag symptoms, such as weight loss, dysphagia, black or

Table 23.4 Anamnesis: clinical history and potential red flags

Clinical history		Red flags
Family history	Dysmenorrhea	Sudden retrosternal pain
Onset and symptoms recurrence	Endometriosis	**Syncope**
Physical exercises and emotional triggers	Radiotherapy	Weight loss
Injuries and surgeries	Chemotherapy	Dysphagia
Nutritional interferences	Drug addiction	Palpable abdominal mass
Food intolerance	Chronic use of NSAIDs	Vomiting bloody
Allergies	Alcohol abuse	Bloody hematochezia
Orofacial diseases	Gastroesophageal reflux disease	Melena

bloody stools, and abdominal masses, and a full physical examination should be performed with these etiologies in mind [35] (Table 23.4).

The sports doctor should also question the health history, looking for possible previous pathologies, surgeries, inherited diseases, or another else under treatment, such as lactose malabsorption and intolerance [43], endometriosis, inflammatory bowel diseases, irritable bowel syndrome, gastrointestinal reflux disease, obstructive cholecystopathy, familial polyposis, diverticular disease, chemotherapy, and radiotherapy that can interfere with the functioning of the GIT. The use of medications, hormone replacement, and recreational drugs should be researched. The abuse of non-steroidal anti-inflammatory drugs (NSAID), aspirin, alcohol consumption, and smoking both favor the appearance of direct gastric lesions and potentiate reflux symptoms.

23.6.6 Gastroesophageal Reflux Disease (GERD)

GERD is a common cause of upper GI symptoms in endurance athletes. As mentioned earlier, it worsens with increased exercise intensity, is more commonly associated with belching, heartburn, or chest pain, and is worse with postprandial exercise. Activities with large increases in intra-abdominal pressure contribute to symptoms as well. Since GERD may respond to changes in eating habits alone, one treatment strategy for athletes with exertional GERD is to initiate a trial of lifestyle and training modifications for 4–6 weeks before considering acid-suppressive medications and proton pump inhibitors (PPI) [44, 45].

The American College of Gastroenterology has recommended lifestyle modification to include elevation of the head of the bed, decreased fat intake in the diet, smoking cessation, and avoiding recumbency for 3 h postprandially [44, 46]. Simons [47] also has recommended avoiding solid food and high carbohydrate drinks before strenuous activity and rather trying liquid meals with lower carbohydrate content and being sure to keep well hydrated around the time of the activity. When carbohydrate intake is a priority during exercise, drinks containing up to 10% glucose are thought to be the safest and tend to cause the fewest upper GI symptoms [48]. If symptoms persist or if the history and physical examination suggest GERD in the athlete, a 2-week trial of a once-daily PPI, such as 20-mg omeprazole or 30-mg lansoprazole, should be used (Table 23.5). Before any therapy, medical evaluation to exclude cardiac causes is mandatory when the athlete complains of heartburn or chest pain.

23.6.7 Nausea and Vomiting

Athletes commonly experience episodes of nausea and vomiting with strenuous or prolonged exercise. These symptoms, however, are not limited to training or competing, as many athletes will have symptoms even at rest when not training. Preventing nausea and vomiting can be difficult because the etiology is not always clear [29]. In addition, data on fluid and carbohydrate intake symptoms during activity are often contradictory. The official American College of Sports Medicine (ACSM) nutritional guidelines state that during exercise, the primary goals for nutri-

Table 23.5 Clinical conditions and treatment

Clinical conditions	Sports-related involvement	Treatment
Reflux	Potentially due to decreased esophageal motility and decreased blood flow, also may be due to decreased lower esophageal sphincter tone and delayed gastric emptying	• Standard GERD therapy • Medicaments 4 h before exercise (e.g., H2 blocker or PPI) • No eating 3 h before exercise • Dietary modification (especially limiting carbs before exercise, glucose is considered less irritating) • PPI (once or twice daily) if there is no improvement with nomed treatments • Decreased fat and protein to improve gastric emptying
Nausea/vomiting	As noted above	• Avoid psychological stress • Avoid eating 3 h before sports • Avoid NSAID • Trial H2 blocker or PPI • Avoid dehydration
Eructation	As noted above	• As noted above
Gastritis (including UGI bleed and peptic ulcer disease)	Often hemorrhagic; due to decreased blood flow, motion effect, or NSAID effect	• H2 blocker, PPI, antacid • Avoid NSAID
Exercise-induced abdominal pain (side stitch)	May be due to diaphragm spasm, peritoneal irritation, thoracic intercostal nerve compression, or gas trapped in hepatic/splenic circulation. No definitive cause	• Rhythmic breathing (coordinate with footfall)
Diarrhea	Anxiety, altered GI hormone secretion increases motility (motilin, gastrin), high fiber diet, lactose intolerance, sorbitol or fructose intolerance, immune-mediated hypersensitivity, endotoxins, and cecal slap syndrome	• Avoid NSAID • Avoid psychological stress • Nutritional strategies
Lower GI bleed gross or microscopic	Bleeding due to necrosis from decreased blood flow and ischemia (especially with a longer duration of activity) cecal slap syndrome (mechanical)	

ent consumption are to replace fluid losses and provide carbohydrates for maintaining blood glucose levels (Table 23.5). For events shorter than 1 h, carbohydrate replenishment in amounts currently found in popular sports drinks (6–8%) is optimal for performance, whereas rates of 30–60 g/h should be used for events lasting longer than 1 h [49].

23.6.8 Upper and Low GI Bleeding/Gastritis/Ulcers

Perhaps, the most dramatic digestive disorder associated with exercise is gastrointestinal hemorrhage. While a few case reports document acute massive upper and low GI bleeding, the majority of exercise-associated GI hemorrhages have been hidden [50]. While 'runner's anemia' may often represent a pseudoanemia from expanded plasma volume, intravascular hemolysis may be present, and iron may be lost with hematuria. Runners may develop hematemesis or melena after competitive or training events or present only symptoms of profound iron deficiency and anemia [51].

While cases of presumed ischemic colitis occur and anorectal sources of bleeding have been identified, the most frequently reported lesion of running-associated bleeding has been, by far, hemorrhagic gastritis. The lesion is transient, is quickly solved with rest, and is not recognized if endoscopy is not carried out within

72 h of the event. While exercise-associated intestinal bleeding is common, individual cases must be evaluated clinically [10].

A 2-week prophylactic regimen of oral proton pump inhibition was shown to decrease the incidence of gastrointestinal bleeding in ultramarathon runners successfully. Because of the widespread use of aspirin and NSAID to relieve pain related to training, athletes may be at an increased risk of damage to the GI mucosa. If a patient continuously uses NSAID, despite symptoms or previous ulceration or bleeding, it would be beneficial to add a PPI for GI protection (Table 23.5) [52–54].

23.6.9 Side Stitch/Exercise-Related Transient Abdominal Pain

Exercise-related transient abdominal pain (ETAP), or its more common name, a "side stitch," is a common complaint in runners and is characterized as an acute, sharp, cramping, or pulling sensation in the abdomen, occasionally radiating to the shoulder, that occurs during exercise and solves itself spontaneously. Patients will often have to decrease their level of exercise when they experience pain. A retrospective report by Morton and Callister indicates that over 60% of runners have experienced ETAP within the past year. ETAP is commonly experienced by runners starting a new or increased running routine [55]. They have also observed that well-trained runners are less likely to experience the side stitch, which was reported significantly more frequently in women than in men (8.2% vs 1.8%).

Despite its very characteristic symptomatology, the etiology of the pain remains unclear. Theories for the cause of pain include a lack of blood flow to the diaphragm during exercise leading to pain from ischemia, pain from stress on subdiaphragmatic ligaments, and irritation of the parietal peritoneum. All proposed treatments are anecdotal, with no proven effective way to prevent or treat a painful episode. One proposed treatment method is the practice of rhythmic breathing, which involves the coordination of inhalation and exhalation with foot strikes while running (Table 23.5) [35, 56].

23.6.10 Intestines/Diarrhea

Management of lower GI disturbances focuses on dietary manipulations, timing, and pharmacologic means (Table 23.5). Antidiarrheal medications such as loperamide are used cautiously for frequent diarrhea episodes, although there are concerns about central nervous system depression. Concerns about interfering with sweating mitigate the use of anticholinergic medications [47].

23.6.11 Nutritional Strategies for Gastrointestinal Problems

The habitual diet has a central role in developing some of the GI symptoms experienced by endurance athletes. Dietary practices that are very rich in fiber, such as vegetarian and vegan diets, fundamentally impact gut microbiota composition. There are several mechanisms by which ingested food may lead to the development of GI symptoms, including autoimmune responses, malabsorption, or even a potential placebo effect. Consumption of gluten-free diets and restrictions on foods high in fermentable oligosaccharides, disaccharides, monosaccharides, and polyols (FODMAP) have been reported in athletes. While potential dietary 'triggers' may be one nutritional factor responsible for exercise-associated GI symptoms, it is important to consider nutrient timing in and around exercise. For example, while daily consumption of fat, protein, and fiber is crucial to athletes' wider health and well-being, ingestion <90 min before exercise has been shown to increase the risk of GI distress (Table 23.6) [32, 33, 35, 57].

23.6.12 Carbohydrates—"*Training the Gut*"

Carbohydrate (CHO) ingestion during endurance exercise has regularly been shown to be ergogenic, but it has also been associated with GI symptoms [12]. Greater CHO intakes during

Table 23.6 Nutritional strategies

Nutritional strategies	
Avoid dehydration	Start physical exercise well hydrated, so they should drink 5–7 mL/kg body weight gradually in the 4 h before. If they do not produce dark or highly concentrated urine, they should drink an additional 3–5 mL/kg body weight about 2 h before the event Avoid dehydration throughout the competitive event; therefore, an intake of 0.5 L/h of sports drinks is recommended During the competitive event, drink beverages or solutions containing 4–8% HC (g/100 mL) and 0.5–0.7 g/L sodium content
Dietary changes	Avoid eating foods rich in fiber, fat, and protein and with high amounts of FODMAPs on the day of the race, including during and on the days before the competition Avoid consumption of foods rich in fructose, especially drinks that contain this HC in free form Ingest 30/60 g/h of HC if the event is 1–2.5 h. If it lasts more than 2.5 h, the athlete must ingest 90 g/h of HC in a 2:1 ratio of glucose and fructose, respectively Eating food at frequent and regular intervals avoids a total intake at once Never consume any food within 90 min of competitions Avoid introducing new foods or drinks on race days without testing them in training
Training the gut	Regular intake of CHO during exercise training for 2 weeks before a competition
Dietary supplements	Probiotics >8 billion CFU 2–8 weeks Zinc carnosine 37.5/day 2 weeks Colostrum 1.7 g/kg/day 1–2 weeks Glutamine 20–50 g 2 h per-exercise Vitamin C 1000 mg 2 h pré-exercise Prebiotics? Betaine?

exercise have typically resulted in increased GI symptom prevalence and/or severity. Incidences of bloating, urge to defecate, nausea, and flatulence were all higher when participants consumed 108 g/h CHO compared to 72 g/h during 120 min cycling at 63% VO_{2max} [58]. Within these studies, it is important to consider that some differences may be related to the composition of the ingested CHO (osmolality, type of carbohydrate, etc.). Additionally, when athletes ingest CHO during endurance competition, there appears to be an increase in GI symptom prevalence when they are unaccustomed to taking on fuel caloric replacement during training [59]. However, regular intake of CHO during exercise training ("**training the Gut**") causes adaptations that reduce the incidence of GI symptoms [60]. Indeed, Costa et al. have shown that, following a period of gut training for 2 weeks, there were reductions in the severity of GI symptoms compared to athletes who consumed a non-CHO-containing placebo (Table 23.6) [61].

23.6.13 Dietary Supplements

Several dietary supplements have been investigated for their potential therapeutic effect on the GI tract during endurance exercise. For example, acute supplementation with glutamine [62], bovine colostrum [63], zinc carnosine [64], vitamin C [65], L-citrulline [66], probiotics [67], have all shown positive outcomes in attenuating indirect markers of GI permeability and/or damage following a single bout of endurance exercise compared to a placebo. In this context, other supplements like prebiotics [68], betaine [69], and polyphenol curcumin may also be promising in diet supplementation. Many prebiotics, such as oligosaccharides in human breast milk or plant-based carbohydrates like inulin and oligofructose, are well known to improve gut barrier function and reduce LPS translocation. Betaine and polyphenol curcumin act by reducing pro-inflammatory cytokines and have essential anti-oxidant properties (Table 23.6).

23.7 Final Considerations

Gastrointestinal symptoms are very common in the athletic population, occurring in up to 70% of elite athletes. They usually seek medical help because such complaints interfere with personal performance. The most common GI symptoms experienced by athletes are eructation, heartburn, nausea, vomiting, ETAP, flatulence, and diarrhea. The four main factors in the pathophysiology of these UGI symptoms are mechanical forces, altered GI blood flow, neuroendocrine changes, and emotional disorders. The physician taking care of athletes must be able to recognize these common entities and be able to rule out more serious pathological conditions. Once identified, there are prevention and treatment guidelines in place that the sports medicine physician should become familiar with in order to provide the highest quality care to the athletes he or she treats.

Take Home Messages

- Gastrointestinal disorders are common in endurance sports, especially in long-term activities (>1 h), reducing sports performance and offering health risks.
- The etiology of these disorders is complex and not fully understood but involves TGI blood flow reduction, mechanical forces/mechanical stress, neuroendocrine changes, and psycho-emotional involvement.
- Positions during sporting activity are important components in developing GIT symptoms and affect the upper and lower GIT differently.
- Although most GI symptoms are mild and occasional, the medical assessment should consider the exclusion of differential diagnoses that offer a greater health risk.
- Exercise-related transient abdominal pain ("side stitch') is characterized as an acute, sharp, cramping, or pulling sensation in the abdomen, occasionally radiating to the shoulder that occurs during exercise and solves itself spontaneously.
- The current therapy is focused on a nutritional strategy based on avoiding dehydration, dietetic changes, training the gut, and dietary supplements.

References

1. Knechtle B, Knechtle P, Lepers R. Participation and performance trends in ultra-triathlons from 1985 to 2009. Scand J Med Sci Sports. 2011;21(6):e82–90. https://doi.org/10.1111/j.1600-0838.2010.01160.x.
2. Scheer V. Participation trends of ultra endurance events. Sports Med Arthrosc Rev. 2019;27(1):3–7. https://doi.org/10.1097/JSA.0000000000000198.
3. Fogoros R. 'Runner's trots': gastrointestinal disturbances in runners. JAMA. 1980;243(17):1743–4.
4. Sullivan S. The gastrointestinal symptoms of running. N Engl J Med. 1981;304(15):915.
5. Keeffe E, Lowe D, Goss J, Wayne R. Gastrointestinal symptoms of marathon runners. West J Med. 1984;141:481–4.
6. Priebe WM, Priebe J. Runners diarrhoea prevalence and clinical symptomatology. Am J Gastroenterol. 1984;79:827–8.
7. Worobetz L, Gerrard D. Gastrointestinal symptoms during exercise in enduro athletes: prevalence and speculations on the aetiology. N Z Med J. 1985;98:644–6.
8. Sullivan SN. Exercise-associated symptoms in triathletes. Physician Sports Med. 1987;15(9):105–10.
9. Riddoch C, Trinick T. Gastrointestinal disturbances in marathon runners. Br J Sports Med. 1988;22(2):71–4. https://doi.org/10.1136/bjsm.22.2.71.
10. Moses FM. The effect of exercise on the gastrointestinal tract. Sports Med. 1990;9(3):159–72. https://doi.org/10.2165/00007256-199009030-00004.
11. Stuempfle KJ, Hoffman MD. Gastrointestinal distress is common during a 161-km ultramarathon. J Sports Sci. 2015;33(17):1814–21. https://doi.org/10.1080/02640414.2015.1012104.
12. de Oliveira EP, Burini RC, Jeukendrup A. Gastrointestinal complaints during exercise: prevalence, etiology, and nutritional recommendations. Sports Med. 2014;44(Suppl 1):S79–85. https://doi.org/10.1007/s40279-014-0153-2.
13. Galley JD, Nelson MC, Yu Z, et al. Exposure to a social stressor disrupts the community structure of the colonic mucosa-associated microbiota. BMC Microbiol. 2014;14:189. https://doi.org/10.1186/1471-2180-14-189.
14. McEwen BS, Wingfield JC. The concept of allostasis in biology and biomedicine. Horm Behav. 2003;43(1):2–15. https://doi.org/10.1016/s0018-506x(02)00024-7.
15. Ulrich-Lai YM, Herman JP. Neural regulation of endocrine and autonomic stress responses. Nat Rev Neurosci. 2009;10(6):397–409. https://doi.org/10.1038/nrn2647.
16. Clark A, Mach N. Exercise-induced stress behavior, gut–microbiota–brain axis and diet: a systematic review for athletes. J Int Soc Sports Nutr. 2016;13:43. https://doi.org/10.1186/s12970-016-0155-6.
17. Arneth BM. Gut–brain axis biochemical signalling from the gastrointestinal tract to the central nervous system: gut dysbiosis and altered brain function.

Postgrad Med J. 2018;94(1114):446–52. https://doi.org/10.1136/postgradmedj-2017-135424.
18. Wang Y, Kasper LH. The role of microbiome in central nervous system disorders. Brain Behav Immun. 2014;38:1–12. https://doi.org/10.1016/j.bbi.2013.12.015.
19. Sampson TR, Mazmanian SK. Control of brain development, function, and behavior by the microbiome. Cell Host Microbe. 2015;17(5):565–76. https://doi.org/10.1016/j.chom.2015.04.011.
20. Saulnier DM, Ringel Y, Heyman MB, Foster JA, Bercik P, Shulman RJ, Versalovic J, Verdu EF, Dinan TG, Hecht G, Guarner F. The intestinal microbiome, probiotics and prebiotics in neurogastroenterology. Gut Microbes. 2013;4(1):17–27. https://doi.org/10.4161/gmic.22973.
21. Eisenstein M. Microbiome: bacterial broadband. Nature. 2016;533(7603):S104–6. https://doi.org/10.1038/533S104a.
22. Lamprecht M, Bogner S, Schippinger G, Steinbauer K, Fankhauser F, Hallstroem S, Schuetz B, Greilberger JF. Probiotic supplementation affects markers of intestinal barrier, oxidation, and inflammation in trained men; a randomized, double-blinded, placebo-controlled trial. J Int Soc Sports Nutr. 2012;9(1):45. https://doi.org/10.1186/1550-2783-9-45.
23. Brown WM, Davison GW, McClean CM, Murphy MH. A systematic review of the acute effects of exercise on immune and inflammatory indices in untrained adults. Sports Med Open. 2015;1(1):35. https://doi.org/10.1186/s40798-015-0032-x.
24. Lambert GP. Stress-induced gastrointestinal barrier dysfunction and its inflammatory effects. J Anim Sci. 2009;87(14 Suppl):E101–8. https://doi.org/10.2527/jas.2008-1339.
25. Peters HP, De Vries WR, Vanberge-Henegouwen GP, Akkermans LM. Potential benefits and hazards of physical activity and exercise on the gastrointestinal tract. Gut. 2001;48(3):435–9. https://doi.org/10.1136/gut.48.3.435.
26. Gill SK, Hankey J, Wright A, Marczak S, Hemming K, Allerton DM, Ansley-Robson P, Costa RJ. The impact of a 24-h ultra-marathon on circulatory endotoxin and cytokine profile. Int J Sports Med. 2015;36(8):688–95. https://doi.org/10.1055/s-0034-1398535.
27. Snipe RMJ, Khoo A, Kitic CM, Gibson PR, Costa RJS. The impact of exertional-heat stress on gastrointestinal integrity, gastrointestinal symptoms, systemic endotoxin and cytokine profile. Eur J Appl Physiol. 2018;118(2):389–400. https://doi.org/10.1007/s00421-017-378-z.
28. Brock-Utne JG, Gaffin SL, Wells MT, Gathiram P, Sohar E, James MF, Morrell DF, Norman RJ. Endotoxaemia in exhausted runners after a long-distance race. S Afr Med J. 1988;73(9):533–6.
29. Peters HP, Bos M, Seebregts L, Akkermans LM, van Berge Henegouwen GP, Bol E, Mosterd WL, de Vries WR. Gastrointestinal symptoms in long-distance runners, cyclists, and triathletes: prevalence, medication, and etiology. Am J Gastroenterol. 1999;94(6):1570–81. https://doi.org/10.1111/j.1572-0241.1999.01147.x.
30. Gelman S, Mushlin PS. Catecholamine-induced changes in the splanchnic circulation affecting systemic hemodynamics. Anesthesiology. 2004;100(2):434–9. https://doi.org/10.1097/00000542-200402000-00036.
31. Rehrer NJ, Janssen GM, Brouns F, Saris WH. Fluid intake and gastrointestinal problems in runners competing in a 25-km race and a marathon. Int J Sports Med. 1989;10(Suppl 1):S22–5. https://doi.org/10.1055/s-2007-1024950.
32. Rehrer NJ, Beckers EJ, Brouns F, ten Hoor F, Saris WH. Effects of dehydration on gastric emptying and gastrointestinal distress while running. Med Sci Sports Exerc. 1990;22(6):790–5. https://doi.org/10.1249/00005768-199012000-00010.
33. Smith KA, Pugh JN, Duca FA, Close GL, Ormsbee MJ. Gastrointestinal pathophysiology during endurance exercise: endocrine, microbiome, and nutritional influences. Eur J Appl Physiol. 2021;121(10):2657–74. https://doi.org/10.1007/s00421-021-04737-x.
34. Porter AM. Marathon running and the caecal slap syndrome. Br J Sports Med. 1982;16(3):178. https://doi.org/10.1136/bjsm.16.3.178.
35. Waterman JJ, Kapur R. Upper gastrointestinal issues in athletes. Curr Sports Med Rep. 2012;11(2):99–104. https://doi.org/10.1249/JSR.0b013e318249c311.
36. Mulak A, Bonaz B. Irritable bowel syndrome: a model of the brain–gut interactions. Med Sci Monit. 2004;10(4):RA55–62.
37. Cannon WB. The movements of the intestines studied by means of the Röntgen rays. J Med Res. 1902;7(1):72–5.
38. O'Brien JD, Thompson DG, Day SJ, Burnham WR, Walker E. Perturbation of upper gastrointestinal transit and antroduodenal motility by experimentally applied stress: the role of beta-adrenoreceptor mediated pathways. Gut. 1989;30(11):1530–9. https://doi.org/10.1136/gut.30.11.1530.
39. Barone FC, Deegan JF, Price WJ, Fowler PJ, Fondacaro JD, Ormsbee HS 3rd. Cold-restraint stress increases rat fecal pellet output and colonic transit. Am J Physiol. 1990;258(3 Pt 1):G329–37. https://doi.org/10.1152/ajpgi.1990.258.3.G329.
40. Sullivan SN, Wong C, Runners' diarrhea. Different patterns and associated factors. J Clin Gastroenterol. 1992;14(2):101–4. https://doi.org/10.1097/00004836-199203000-00005.
41. Sullivan SN, Wong C, Heidenheim P. Does running cause gastrointestinal symptoms? A survey of 93 randomly selected runners compared with controls. N Z Med J. 1994;107(984):328–31.
42. Viola TA. Evaluation of the athlete with exertional abdominal pain. Curr Sports Med Rep. 2010;9(2):106–10. https://doi.org/10.1249/JSR.0b013e3181d4086d.
43. Usai-Satta P, Scarpa M, Oppia F, Cabras F. Lactose malabsorption and intolerance: what should be the best clinical management? World J Gastrointest Pharmacol Ther. 2012;3(3):29–33. https://doi.org/10.4292/wjgpt.v3.i3.29.
44. DeVault KR, Castell DO, American College of Gastroenterology. Updated guidelines for the diagnosis and treatment of gastroesophageal reflux disease.

Am J Gastroenterol. 2005;100(1):190–200. https://doi.org/10.1111/j.1572-0241.2005.41217.x.
45. Simons SM, Kennedy RG. Gastrointestinal problems in runners. Curr Sports Med Rep. 2004;3(2):112–6. https://doi.org/10.1249/00149619-200404000-00011.
46. Parmelee-Peters K, Moeller JL. Gastroesophageal reflux in athletes. Curr Sports Med Rep. 2004;3(2):107–11. https://doi.org/10.1249/00149619-200404000-00010.
47. American Dietetic Association; Dietitians of Canada; American College of Sports Medicine, Rodriguez NR, Di Marco NM, Langley S. American College of Sports Medicine position stand. Nutrition and athletic performance. Med Sci Sports Exerc. 2009;41(3):709–31. https://doi.org/10.1249/MSS.0b013e31890eb86.
48. Schwartz AE, Vanagunas A, Kamel PL. Endoscopy to evaluate gastrointestinal bleeding in marathon runners. Ann Intern Med. 1990;113(8):632–3. https://doi.org/10.7326/0003-4819-113-8-632.
49. Stewart JG, Ahlquist DA, McGill DB, Ilstrup DM, Schwartz S, Owen RA. Gastrointestinal blood loss and anemia in runners. Ann Intern Med. 1984;100(6):843–5. https://doi.org/10.7326/0003-4819-100-6-843.
50. Thalmann M, Sodeck GH, Kavouras S, Matalas A, Skenderi K, Yannikouris N, Domanovits H. Proton pump inhibition prevents gastrointestinal bleeding in ultramarathon runners: a randomised, double blinded, placebo controlled study. Br J Sports Med. 2006;40(4):359–62. https://doi.org/10.1136/bjsm.2005.024463.
51. Peura DA. Prevention of nonsteroidal anti-inflammatory drug-associated gastrointestinal symptoms and ulcer complications. Am J Med. 2004;117(Suppl 5A):63S–71S. https://doi.org/10.1016/j.amjmed.2004.07.010.
52. Yeomans ND, Tulassay Z, Juhász L, Rácz I, Howard JM, van Rensburg CJ, Swannell AJ, Hawkey CJ. A comparison of omeprazole with ranitidine for ulcers associated with nonsteroidal anti-inflammatory drugs. Acid Suppression Trial: Ranitidine versus Omeprazole for NSAID-associated Ulcer Treatment (ASTRONAUT) Study Group. N Engl J Med. 1998;338(11):719–26. https://doi.org/10.1056/NEJM199803123381104.
53. Morton DP, Callister R. Factors influencing exercise-related transient abdominal pain. Med Sci Sports Exerc. 2002;34(5):745–9. https://doi.org/10.1097/00005768-200205000-00003.
54. Eichner ER. Stitch in the side: causes, workup, and solutions. Curr Sports Med Rep. 2006;5(6):289–92. https://doi.org/10.1097/01.csmr.0000306432.46908.b3.
55. Kondo T, Nakae Y, Mitsui T, Kagaya M, Matsutani Y, Horibe H, Read NW. Exercise-induced nausea is exaggerated by eating. Appetite. 2001;36(2):119–25. https://doi.org/10.1006/appe.2000.0391.
56. Jentjens RL, Moseley L, Waring RH, Harding LK, Jeukendrup AE. Oxidation of combined ingestion of glucose and fructose during exercise. J Appl Physiol (1985). 2004;96(4):1277–84. https://doi.org/10.1152/japplphysiol.00974.2003.
57. ter Steege RW, Van der Palen J, Kolkman JJ. Prevalence of gastrointestinal complaints in runners competing in a long-distance run: an internet-based observational study in 1281 subjects. Scand J Gastroenterol. 2008;43(12):1477–82. https://doi.org/10.1080/00365520802321170.
58. Jeukendrup AE. Training the gut for athletes. Sports Med. 2017;47(Suppl 1):101–10. https://doi.org/10.1007/s40279-017-0690-6.
59. Costa RJS, Snipe RMJ, Kitic CM, Gibson PR. Systematic review: exercise-induced gastrointestinal syndrome-implications for health and intestinal disease. Aliment Pharmacol Ther. 2017;46(3):246–65. https://doi.org/10.1111/apt.14157.
60. Pugh JN, Sage S, Hutson M, Doran DA, Fleming SC, Highton J, Morton JP, Close GL. Glutamine supplementation reduces markers of intestinal permeability during running in the heat in a dose-dependent manner. Eur J Appl Physiol. 2017;117(12):2569–77. https://doi.org/10.1007/s00421-017-3744-4.
61. Morrison SA, Cheung SS, Cotter JD. Bovine colostrum, training status, and gastrointestinal permeability during exercise in the heat: a placebo-controlled double-blind study. Appl Physiol Nutr Metab. 2014;39(9):1070–82. https://doi.org/10.1139/apnm-2013-0583.
62. Davison G, Marchbank T, March DS, Thatcher R, Playford RJ. Zinc carnosine works with bovine colostrum in truncating heavy exercise-induced increase in gut permeability in healthy volunteers. Am J Clin Nutr. 2016;104(2):526–36. https://doi.org/10.3945/ajcn.116.134403.
63. Ashton T, Young IS, Davison GW, Rowlands CC, McEneny J, Van Blerk C, Jones E, Peters JR, Jackson SK. Exercise-induced endotoxemia: the effect of ascorbic acid supplementation. Free Radic Biol Med. 2003;35(3):284–91. https://doi.org/10.1016/s0891-5849(03)00309-5.
64. van Wijck K, Wijnands KA, Meesters DM, Boonen B, van Loon LJ, Buurman WA, Dejong CH, Lenaerts K, Poeze M. L-Citrulline improves splanchnic perfusion and reduces gut injury during exercise. Med Sci Sports Exerc. 2014;46(11):2039–46. https://doi.org/10.1249/MSS.0000000000000332.
65. Jäger R, Mohr AE, Carpenter KC, Kerksick CM, Purpura M, Moussa A, Townsend JR, Lamprecht M, West NP, Black K, Gleeson M, Pyne DB, Wells SD, Arent SM, Smith-Ryan AE, Kreider RB, Campbell BI, Bannock L, Scheiman J, Wissent CJ, Pane M, Kalman DS, Pugh JN, Ter Haar JA, Antonio J. International Society of Sports Nutrition Position Stand: probiotics. J Int Soc Sports Nutr. 2019;16(1):62. https://doi.org/10.1186/s12970-019-0329-0.
66. Huaman JW, Mego M, Manichanh C, Cañellas N, Cañueto D, Segurola H, Jansana M, Malagelada C, Accarino A, Vulevic J, Tzortzis G, Gibson G, Saperas

E, Guarner F, Azpiroz F. Effects of prebiotics vs a diet low in FODMAPs in patients with functional gut disorders. Gastroenterology. 2018;155(4):1004–7. https://doi.org/10.1053/j.gastro.2018.06.045.
67. Willingham BD, Ragland TJ, Ormsbee MJ. Betaine supplementation may improve heat tolerance: potential mechanisms in humans. Nutrients. 2020;12(10):2939. https://doi.org/10.3390/nu12102939.
68. Szymanski MC, Gillum TL, Gould LM, Morin DS, Kuennen MR. Short-term dietary curcumin supplementation reduces gastrointestinal barrier damage and physiological strain responses during exertional heat stress. J Appl Physiol (1985). 2018;124(2):330–40. https://doi.org/10.1152/japplphysiol.00515.2017.

24 Hematologic and Endocrine Conditions: Exercise Collapse-Associated with Sickle Cell Trait, Exertional Rhabdomyolysis, Hyperglycemia, and Hypoglycemia

Phillip H. Yun and Kaleigh Suhs

24.1 Exercise Collapse Associated with Sickle Cell Trait: [1, 2]

Sickle cell trait is present in approximately 9% of African Americans in the United States and is generally a benign carrier condition without the usual symptoms of sickle cell disease. However, exercise-related deaths seen in warfighters and athletes with sickle cell trait have led to a new clinical presentation being defined called exercise collapse associated with sickle cell trait (ECAST). ECAST may occur if a "perfect storm" of factors come together that leads to the sickling of red blood cells in working muscles and other organ systems.

24.2 Clinical Presentation: [1, 3, 4]

- Common scenario: preseason athletic training where an athlete exercises at near maximal exertion, either repeated or sustained, without adequate interval rest periods.
- Onset: can occur as early as 2 min into exercise but also can manifest after an hour of exercise.
- ECAST presents as a clinical spectrum from mild weakness to fulminant disease.
  - Early: alert and oriented ×3; more weakness than pain; slumps to ground rather than collapsing or hobbling; normal muscular tone; tachypneic but moving air well
  - Late: disoriented; fulminant rhabdomyolysis; end-organ failure

Fact Box
Consider a diagnosis of ECAST if weakness is a predominant early symptom rather than pain in an athlete with sickle cell trait.

24.2.1 Differential Diagnosis: [4]

1. Exercise-associated muscle cramps
2. Acute cardiac event (arrhythmia, sudden cardiac arrest)
3. Heat exhaustion
4. Exertional and non-exertional heat stroke
5. Exercise-associated postural hypotension
6. Sudden cardiac arrest
7. Exercise-associated hyponatremia
8. Acute hypoglycemia
9. Anaphylaxis
10. Respiratory collapse (asthma)
11. Sickle cell crisis

P. H. Yun (✉)
University of Chicago, Chicago, IL, USA
e-mail: phillip.yun@bsd.uchicago.edu

K. Suhs
Orthopaedic Surgery and Rehabilitation Medicine, University of Chicago, Chicago, IL, USA

Banner Health, Phoenix, AZ, USA

S. Rocha Piedade et al. (eds.), *Sideline Management in Sports*,
https://doi.org/10.1007/978-3-031-33867-0_24

Discussion of key physical examination pearls and findings: [4–6]

	ECAST	Cardiac	Heat stroke	Muscle cramps	Asthma
General appearance	Slumps to ground	Falls suddenly	Ataxia, confused	Alert, limping	Tachypnea
Defining characteristic	Weakness > pain	Unresponsive	Confusion and >104 °F	Intense muscle pain lasting seconds to minutes	Shortness of breath
Mental status	Can talk at first	Unconscious	Disoriented	Alert and oriented ×3	Difficulty speaking
Timing	Can occur early or late	No warning	Usually occurs late	Can occur early or late	Can occur early or late
Temperature	<104 °F	Irrelevant	>104 °F	<104 °F	<104 °F
Muscles	Normal tone	Seizing, limp	Varied	Increased tone	Normal tone

Indications and benefits of additional testing/imaging (point of care or referral): [1]

- There are no readily available point-of-care tests that can be done on the sidelines that confirm a diagnosis of sickle cell trait or ECAST. ECAST is a clinical diagnosis.
- Laboratory testing often begins with a sickle cell solubility test which has approximately a 1% false negative rate. A definitive diagnosis of sickle cell trait can be made by (1) hemoglobin separation and quantitation methods or (2) analysis of β-globin genes. Beginning August 2022, all incoming NCAA athletes must have sickle cell testing.
- Referral to the Emergency Room or management on an outpatient basis is based on their clinical status as noted below.

Sideline management guidelines and suggestions of the specific traumatic injuries and clinical issues in athletes: [1, 6]

- No evidence-based guidelines exist for managing an ECAST event. However, the ACSM and CHAMP Summit group and the National Athletic Trainers' Association have made recommendations on emergent management, which are summarized below:
  1. Assess athlete responsiveness (circulation, airway, and breathing)
  2. Brief history and assess vital signs including rectal temperature
  3. Cool athlete if needed, rest, hydrate (orally or intravenously), and apply high-flow oxygen if available
  4. If no immediate improvement, transport the athlete to the Emergency Department
     (a) It is important to communicate with the Emergency Department about the following: ECAST as a potential diagnosis, aggressive fluid and electrolyte management, blood gas monitoring, and cardiac monitoring
  5. If the athlete becomes completely asymptomatic with minimal intervention on the sidelines, outpatient consultation with a physician is recommended for further evaluation and discussion on a graded return to activity.
     (a) Athletes should not be allowed to return to practice or play if ECAST is suspected

Suggested prevention measures that could be implemented for early recognition or risk reduction (altitude, rules modifications, referee instruction): [1, 6]

- There are no evidence-based guidelines on return to play following an ECAST event. However, the ACSM and CHAMP have made joint recommendations that can be followed:
  1. Must be asymptomatic at rest and have normal end-organ function
  2. Full history and physical examination (comorbidities, drug use, supplements, family, and environmental risk factors)
  3. Graded return to play under close supervision by medical personnel
  4. Education on the importance of proper hydration and the possibility of subsequent ECAST events with high heat stress and exercise intensity

- The National Athletic Trainers' Association has made recommendations on mitigating risk in athletes with sickle cell trait, which are summarized below:
  1. Allow athletes to build up slowly in training with paced progressions with adequate rest and recovery periods.
  2. Athletes should be excluded from participation in performance tests such as mile runs and serial sprints.
  3. Cessation of activity with the onset of symptoms such as muscle cramping, pain, swelling, weakness, tenderness, and inability to catch breath with early reporting.
  4. Allow athletes with sickle cell trait to set their own pace.
  5. Adjust work/rest cycles based on environmental heat, emphasize hydration, control asthma, no workout if an athlete is ill, and monitor closely if an athlete is new to altitude.

Take Home Messages

- ECAST can occur in athletes with sickle cell trait who exercise at near maximal intensity without adequate intervals of rest.
- The clinical presentation can mimic other potentially severe conditions such as rhabdomyolysis but is distinguished early on by disproportional weakness rather than pain in an athlete with a normal mental status.
- Prevention of ECAST is crucial and includes allowing athletes to build up slowly in training with adequate rest periods.

24.3 Exertional Rhabdomyolysis: [7, 8]

Rhabdomyolysis is a clinical syndrome characterized by muscle necrosis leading to the release of intracellular components such as myoglobin, potassium, and creatinine kinase into the systemic circulation. There are three categories of rhabdomyolysis which include: (1) trauma or muscle compression, (2) nontraumatic and exertional, and (3) nontraumatic and nonexertional. Exertional rhabdomyolysis can be seen in athletes who overexert themselves during unaccustomed strenuous exercise that is intense, prolonged, and/or involving repetitive muscle overload (in particular, eccentric loading). Risk factors for developing rhabdomyolysis are many including the following: inadequate conditioning, poor hydration, exercise in high heat/humidity, medications (stimulants, NSAIDS), sickle cell trait, and ongoing infection.

24.3.1 Clinical Presentation: [7, 9–11]

- Exertional rhabdomyolysis presents as a clinical spectrum from mild pain to fulminant disease. Muscular symptoms are most commonly present in the proximal upper and lower extremities, calves, and/or lower back depending on the type of exercise.

Fact Box

An athlete can present during exercise or within the first 24–72 h after exercising. Consider exertional rhabdomyolysis when pain is out of proportion to what would be expected for muscle soreness.

- Early:
  - Musculoskeletal: muscle pain, swelling, stiffness, and cramping. May also complain of weakness in affected muscle groups
  - Nonspecific: malaise, fever, abdominal pain, nausea, vomiting
- Late:
  - Delirium
  - Compartment syndrome (tense muscles with out-of-proportion pain)

- Loss of consciousness or exercise-associated collapse secondary to cardiac arrhythmia/arrest
- Oliguria
- Other presentations: acute renal failure, disseminated intravascular coagulation

24.3.2 Differential Diagnosis: [1, 12–14]

1. Exercise-associated muscle cramps
2. Delayed onset muscle soreness
3. Exercise collapse associated with sickle cell trait
4. Nontraumatic myopathies
5. Heat exhaustion
6. Exertional and non-exertional heat stroke
7. Muscle strain
8. Elevated serum creatine kinase without exertional rhabdomyolysis muscle symptoms

24.3.3 Discussion of Key Physical Examination Pearls and Findings: [8, 10, 15]

- Musculoskeletal: muscle tenderness, weakness, and/or swelling. Swelling may become more present after hydration
- Kidneys: dark colored urine (tea or cola colored), decreased urinary output, and oliguria
- Skin: discoloration or blistering (secondary to ischemic tissue injury)
- Mental status: ranges from alert and oriented ×3 to delirium/obtundation
- Other: signs of hypovolemia, hypothermia/hyperthermia

Indications and benefits of additional testing/imaging (point of care or referral): [11, 16]

- Point-of-care testing:
  1. Urine dipstick: positive for blood
  2. Basic metabolic panel (i-STAT): hyperkalemia, metabolic acidosis, acute kidney injury with an elevated BUN and/or Cr
- Indications for referring to the Emergency Room:
  1. Severe muscle symptoms including pain, stiffness. and/or weakness despite resting
  2. Metabolic and electrolyte abnormalities (hyperkalemia, metabolic acidosis)
  3. Acute kidney injury (an increase in serum creatinine of ≥0.3 mg/dL within 48 h, a serum creatinine ≥1.5 times baseline level within previous 7 days, or urine output of <0.5 mL/kg/h for 6–12 h)
  4. Dark urine (tea or cola colored) or confirmed urine blood
  5. Concern for compartment syndrome, arrhythmia, or mental status declines
- Considerations for expedited outpatient testing:
  1. If concerned for mild rhabdomyolysis without enough concern to send to the Emergency Room, consider expedited outpatient laboratory testing including: CBC, BMP, creatinine kinase, and urinalysis.
  2. Refer to the Emergency Room for the following findings: creatine kinase >10,000–20,000 U/L, acute kidney injury, myoglobinuria, and metabolic/electrolyte abnormalities.
  3. May consider outpatient monitoring with creatine kinase, BMP, and urinalysis every 24–72 h until creatinine kinase consistently downtrend and below 5000 U/L. Inform athlete of the following: (1) ensure adequate oral hydration (1 L every 6 h with no more than 4 L per 24 h), (2) ensure consistent urine flow, and (3) no nephrotoxic medications such as non-steroidal anti-inflammatory medications.

Sideline management guidelines and suggestions of the specific traumatic injuries and clinical issues in athletes: [16]

- Sideline evaluation:
  1. Vital signs and focused neurologic evaluation

2. History and physical examination
   Localize and quantify the level of pain
   Evaluate for compartment syndrome
   Evaluate for cardiac arrhythmia
3. Evaluate for alternative diagnoses as noted above and manage appropriately For example, provide rapid cooling for athletes with heat stroke
4. Allow the athlete to rest with adequate oral hydration
5. Point of care testing if available (urine dipstick, point of care basic metabolic panel)
6. Re-evaluate at subsequent time points to monitor the trajectory of symptoms
7. Consider transportation to the Emergency Room or expedited outpatient work-up as noted above

- A diagnosis of exertional rhabdomyolysis if the following criteria are met:
  1. Severe muscle symptoms (pain, stiffness, and/or weakness)
  2. Laboratory evidence of myonecrosis (creatine kinase ≥5× upper limit of normal)
  3. Recent exercise/exertion
- Given that sideline creatine kinase measurements are not feasible, consider a diagnosis of rhabdomyolysis if an athlete presents with severe muscle symptoms that persist despite rest. Point of care testing and other findings as noted above would also support a diagnosis of exertional rhabdomyolysis.
- Athletes should not return to play or practice if exertional rhabdomyolysis is suspected based on clinical and/or point-of-care testing.

Suggested prevention measures that could be implemented for early recognition or risk reduction (altitude, rules modifications, and referee instruction) [15–17]

The NCAA have identified ten factors that increase the risk of exertional rhabdomyolysis. Athletes, athletic trainers, coaches, strength and conditioning personnel, and healthcare professionals should be aware of these factors and take precautions. In addition, special attention should be given to those with sickle cell trait with regard to the heat and humidity levels of the exercise environment.

1. The hardest-working athletes who consistently push their performance
2. Workouts that are not part of a periodized, progressive exercise program
3. Novel workouts or exercises immediately following a transitional period
4. Irrationally intense workouts with the intent to punish or intimidate a team
5. Performing exercises to muscle failure with eccentric activity
6. Focusing on an intense drill or exercise on one muscle group with progressive overload and fast repetitions to failure
7. Increasing the number of exercise sets and reducing the time needed to finish
8. Increasing the amount of weight lifted solely based on the percentage of body weight
9. Trying to condition athletes into shape in a single day or over a few days
10. Conducting an unduly intense workout following a game loss or perceived poor practice performance

Athletes diagnosed with exertional rhabdomyolysis should gradually return to play or practice in a formalized structure (Figs. 24.1 and 24.2).

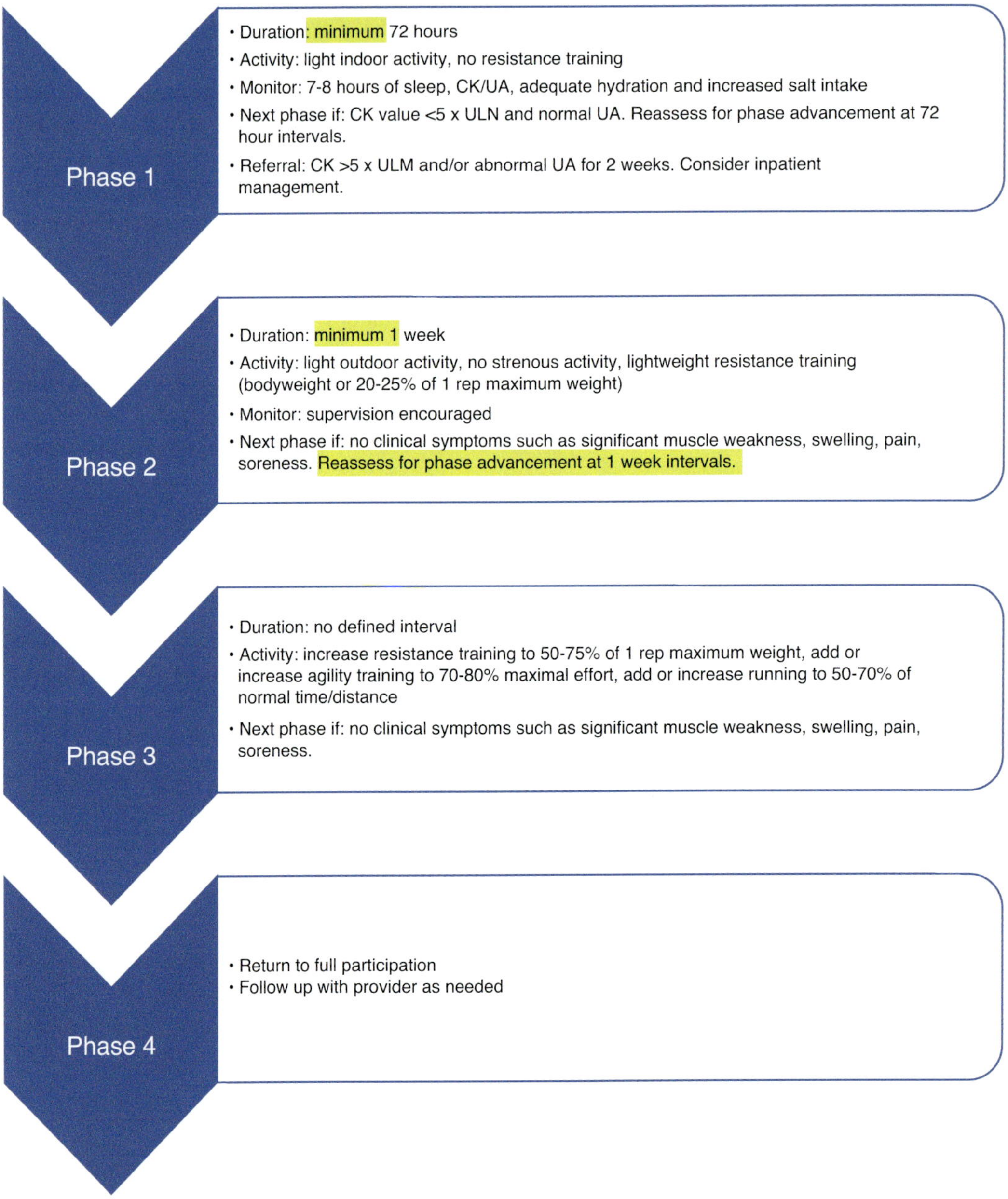

Fig. 24.1 A multiphase return to play guidelines after an episode of exertional rhabdomyolysis initially outlined by the Consortium for Health and Military Performance. (Modified with permission of Wolters Kluwer Health from "Nye NS, Kasper K, Madsen CM, Szczepanik M, Covey CJ, Oh R, et al. Clinical Practice Guidelines for Exertional Rhabdomyolysis: A Military Medicine Perspective. Curr Sports Med Rep. 2021.")

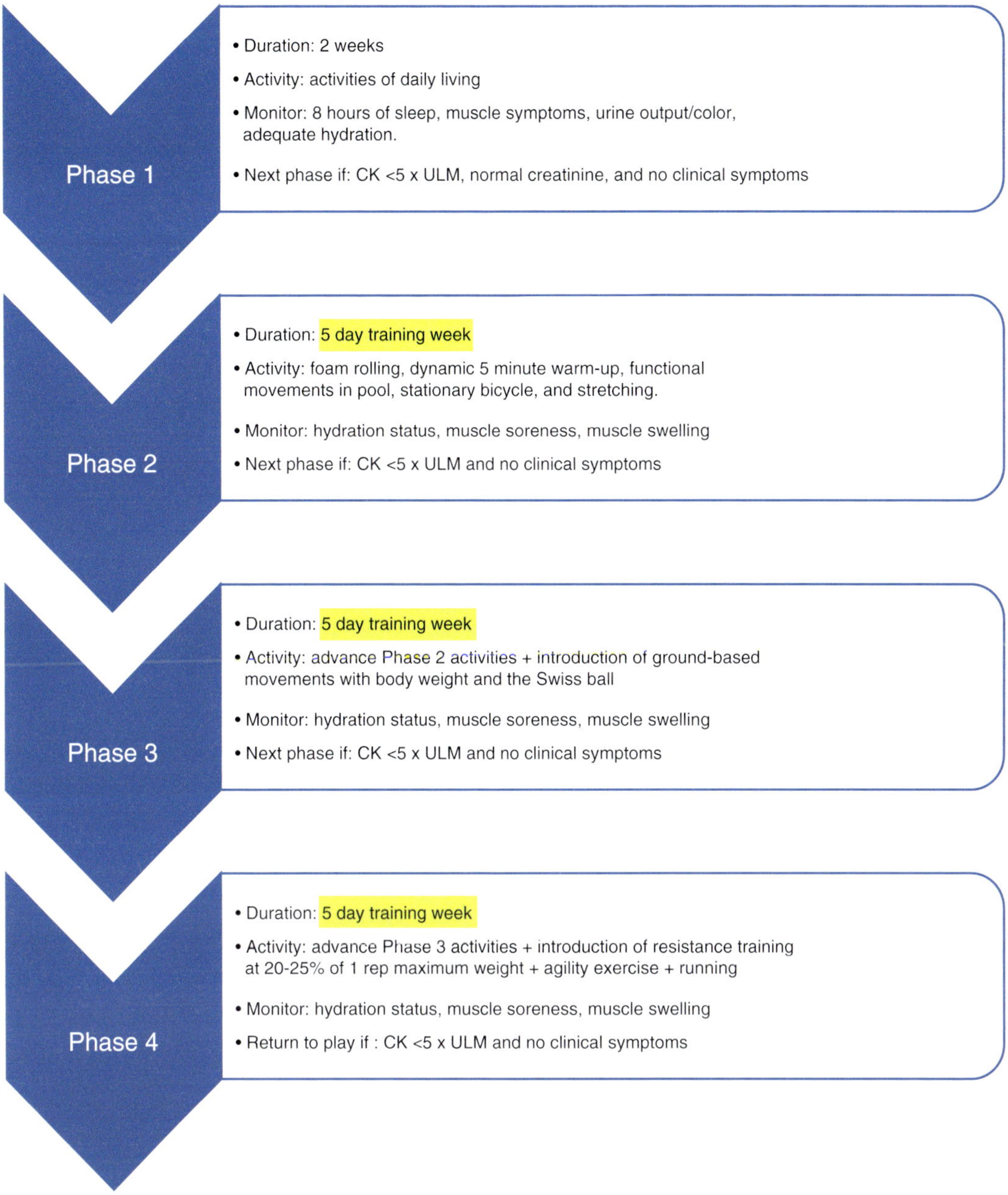

Fig. 24.2 A multiphase return to play guidelines after an episode of exertional rhabdomyolysis outlined by the National Athletic Trainers' Association. (Modified with permission of the National Athletic Trainers' Association from "Schleich K, Slayman T, West D, Smoot K. Return to play after exertional rhabdomyolysis. J Athl Train. 2016.")

Take Home Messages

- Exertional rhabdomyolysis is a clinical syndrome that occurs in athletes who overexert themselves and should be suspected in those with pain out of proportion to general muscle soreness from activity.
- In athletes with significant symptoms or signs, point-of-care testing is recommended to test for urine blood, hyperkalemia, and acute kidney injury.
- Athletes with suspected rhabdomyolysis should not return to exercise and should be allowed to rest and hydrate while getting evaluated by the medical team.

24.4 Hypoglycemia and Hyperglycemia: [18]

Hypoglycemia can be seen in athletes with or without diabetes mellitus. Exercise-induced hypoglycemia can occur during, shortly after, or many hours after exercise. While hypoglycemia is frequently defined as a serum glucose level ≤70 mg/dL, symptoms of hypoglycemia can occur above this value. Hypoglycemic episodes should be carefully monitored as severe hypoglycemia can lead to obtundation and seizures in athletes. On the other hand, hyperglycemia is typically only a concern in athletes with diabetes mellitus. The primary concern for hyperglycemic diabetic athletes is that they are at an increased risk of developing diabetic ketoacidosis or hyperosmolar hyperglycemic state.

24.4.1 Clinical Presentation: [19, 20]

24.4.1.1 Hypoglycemia

Non-diabetic athletes generally experience symptoms at serum glucose levels ≤55 mg/dL although this varies among and within individuals over time. Diabetic athletes generally experience symptoms at serum glucose levels ≤65 mg/dL although this varies among and within individuals over time as well. Severe hypoglycemia is defined as a hypoglycemic event requiring the assistance of another person to actively administer carbohydrates, glucagon, or other resuscitative actions.

There are two categories of hypoglycemic symptoms as noted below

1. Autonomic symptoms: tremor, palpitations, anxiety, sweating, hunger, and paresthesia
2. Neuroglycopenic symptoms: dizziness, weakness, drowsiness, delirium, confusion, seizures, and coma.

24.4.1.2 Hyperglycemia

The classic symptoms of hyperglycemia are polyuria, polydipsia, nocturia, blurred vision, and weight loss. Diabetic ketoacidosis and hyperosmolar hyperglycemic state have additional symptoms that should be screened for if concerned for hyperglycemia:

1. Diabetic ketoacidosis: anorexia, nausea, vomiting, abdominal pain, lethargy, mental obtundation, coma
2. Hyperosmotic hyperglycemic state: lethargy, mental obtundation, coma, hemiparesis, hemianopsia

24.4.2 Differential Diagnosis

1. Heat exhaustion
2. Heat stroke
3. Seizure
4. Hyponatremia
5. Cardiac: arrhythmia, symptomatic valvular disease, acute cardiac event
6. Dehydration
7. Side effects or overdose from medications or recreational drugs
8. Intra-abdominal processes: acute appendicitis and acute pancreatitis
9. Pulmonary processes: asthma/respiratory collapse and anaphylaxis

24.4.3 Discussion of Key Physical Examination Pearls and Findings: [20]

24.4.3.1 Hypoglycemia

- Abnormal vital signs
- Altered mental status
- Slurred or slow speech
- Autonomic findings including tremor, tachycardia, and diaphoresis

24.4.3.2 Hyperglycemia

- Abnormal vital signs
- Hyperventilation (Kussmaul ventilation)
- Smell of ketones
- Abdominal tenderness
- Altered mental status
- Nausea and vomiting
- Signs of dehydration

Indications and benefits of additional testing/imaging (point of care or referral): [21]

Point of care testing

- Fingerstick blood glucose testing is the most important sideline test to perform. All athletes with a history of diabetes and athletes with signs and symptoms of hypoglycemia should be tested.
- Basic metabolic panel (i-STAT): electrolyte abnormalities, metabolic acidosis, acute kidney injury
- Urine dipstick: the presence of ketones

Fact Box

Do not rely solely on continuous glucose monitoring in an acute event as these devices measure interstitial glucose, which can lag behind circulating blood glucose levels by 15 min or more.

Referral

- All athletes with findings concerning for diabetic ketoacidosis or hyperosmotic hyperglycemic state should be referred to a higher level of care.
- All athletes with critical lab findings on point of care testing
- All athletes with persistent altered mental status
- All athletes with loss of consciousness or seizures

Sideline management guidelines and suggestions of the specific traumatic injuries and clinical issues in athletes: [21–24]

Hypoglycemia

- If conscious and able to swallow:
  1. Give 0.3 g/kg fast-acting carbohydrate (~9 g of glucose for 30 kg child, 15 g for ≥50 kg)
  2. If on an insulin pump, suspend until blood glucose >70 mg/dL
  3. Recheck blood glucose in 15 min
     – If <70 mg/dL, repeat step 1–3 until >70 mg/dL
  4. Once blood glucose >70 mg/dL, follow up with a 10–15 g carbohydrate snack

Fact Box

Fast acting carbohydrates:	*10–15 g carbohydrate snack (slower acting)*
1. Glucose tablets (generally 5 g/tablet)	1. 1 piece of fruit (tennis ball size)
2. 8 ounces of apple or grape juice (~30–40 g)	2. 1 slice of bread
3. Regular soda (not sugar-free)	3. 1 small tub yogurt (100 g)
4. Honey	4. 1 cup milk (200 mL)
5. Hard candies	5. 5 × water crackers
6. 8 ounces of Gatorade (~14 g)	

- If unconscious or unable to swallow:
  1. Position on side and maintain airway
  2. Administer glucagon
     (a) SC or IM: <25 kg → 0.5 mg/L; >25 kg → 1 mg
     (b) Intranasal: ≥4 years → 3 mg
  3. If on insulin pump, suspend until blood glucose >70 mg/dL
  4. Recheck blood glucose in 15 min

(a) If unresponsive, repeat steps 1–4 in addition to re-evaluation
(b) If responsive, follow conscious and able to swallow pathway
5. Recommend transferring to a higher level of care as soon as possible

Hyperglycemia

- If concerned for diabetic ketoacidosis or hyperosmotic hyperglycemic state: recommend transferring to a higher level of care
- If blood glucose 250–299 mg/dL: check urine ketones
  - If negative urine ketones, ok to exercise and recheck blood glucose every 15–30 min
  - If positive, postpone exercise and evaluate for DKA
- If blood glucose >300 mg/dL: postpone exercise. Evaluate for DKA and HHS. Check blood glucose every 15–30 min.

Suggested prevention measures that could be implemented for early recognition or risk reduction (altitude, rules modifications, and referee instruction) [24, 25]

Glucose monitoring

- Check blood glucose 60 min prior to exercise. Below are the general guidelines for participation in sports:
  - <70 mg/dL: postpone exercise, consume 15–30 g of carbohydrates, repeat blood glucose check
    If severe hypoglycemia, do not return to sports on that day.
  - 70–99 mg/dL: consume 15–30 g of carbohydrates prior to exercise
  - 100–199 mg/dL: optional to consume 15–30 g of carbohydrates prior to exercise
  - 200–249 mg/dL: discourage pre-exercise carbohydrates
  - 250–299 mg/dL: check urine ketones
    If negative urine ketones, ok to exercise but no pre-exercise carbohydrates.
    If positive, postpone exercise and evaluate for DKA.
  - >300 mg/dL: postpone exercise. Evaluate for DKA/HHS and manage hyperglycemia

Insulin regimen

- Ensure athletes have an established insulin regimen before, during, and after exercise.
- Adjustments to the athlete's baseline insulin regimen may be necessary based on the intensity of exercise, duration, and type of insulin used.
- Insulin pumps should be removed during swimming or contact/collision sports.

Preventative measures

- In addition to two blood glucose checks prior to exercise (establish trend), recommend checking blood glucose every 30 min during exercise and as needed if the athlete or medical staff notice signs or symptoms of hypo/hyperglycemia.
- There is a risk of delayed hypoglycemia that usually occurs 6–12 h after exercise. This occurs due to depleted glycogen stores and an inadequate replacement of carbohydrates.
- Recommend checking glucose levels at least twice in the 4-h window post-exercise to monitor for delayed hypoglycemia (i.e., 2 h and 4 h post-exercise blood glucose checks).
- Fluid intake recommendations for diabetics are the same as for nondiabetic athletes.
- Carbohydrate intake:
  - A few hours before exercise: carbohydrate rich, low glycemic index meal.
  - For exercise routines longer than 1 h, 30–100 g of carbohydrate for each hour of exertion, based on intensity of exercise.
  - Post-exercise: 1.2–1.5 g of carbohydrate/kg/h during the first 4–5 h. Ideally, this meal is carbohydrate rich and has a high glycemic index.

Take Home Messages

- Hypoglycemia and hyperglycemia are important endocrine conditions to monitor for in athletes, especially those with diabetes mellitus.
- Hypoglycemic episodes can be life threatening and should be managed with the cessation of activity, blood glucose check, oral carbohydrates, and/or glucagon. It is important not to administer anything orally if the athlete has altered mental status.
- Hyperglycemia generally occurs in those with diabetes mellitus and requires close attention once blood glucose levels reach 250 mg/dL or above, which should trigger the medical staff to consider DKA or HHS.

References

1. O'Connor FG, Bergeron MF, Cantrell J, Connes P, Harmon KG, Ivy E, et al. ACSM and CHAMP summit on sickle cell trait: mitigating risks for warfighters and athletes. Med Sci Sports Exerc. 2012;44(11):2045–56.
2. Connes P, Reid H, Hardy-Dessources MD, Morrison E, Hue O. Physiological responses of sickle cell trait carriers during exercise. Sport Med. 2008;38(11):931–46.
3. Quattrone RD, Eichner ER, Beutler A, Adams WB, O'Connor FG. Exercise collapse associated with sickle cell trait (ECAST): case report and literature review. Curr Sports Med Rep. 2015;14(2):110–6.
4. Eichner ER. Sickle cell trait in sports. Curr Sports Med Rep. 2010;9(6):347–51.
5. Maughan RJ, Shirreffs SM. Muscle cramping during exercise: causes, solutions, and questions remaining. Sport Med. 2019;49(Suppl 2):115–24.
6. National Athletic Trainers' Association. Consensus statement: sickle cell trait and the athlete. Annu Meet Natl Athl. 2007.
7. Tietze DC, Borchers J. Exertional rhabdomyolysis in the athlete: a clinical review. Sports Health. 2014;6(4):336–9.
8. Rawson ES, Clarkson PM, Tarnopolsky MA. Perspectives on exertional rhabdomyolysis. Sport Med. 2017;47(Suppl 1):33–49.
9. Hummel K, Gregory A, Desai N, Diamond A. Rhabdomyolysis in adolescent athletes: review of cases. Phys Sportsmed. 2016;44(2):195–9.
10. Khan FY. Rhabdomyolysis: a review of the literature. Neth J Med. 2009;67(9):272–83.
11. Scalco RS, Snoeck M, Quinlivan R, Treves S, Laforét P, Jungbluth H, et al. Exertional rhabdomyolysis: physiological response or manifestation of an underlying myopathy? BMJ Open Sport Exerc Med. 2016;2(1):e000151.
12. Cleak MJ, Eston RG. Delayed onset muscle soreness: mechanisms and management. J Sports Sci. 1992;10(4):325–41.
13. Schwellnus MP, Drew N, Collins M. Muscle cramping in athletes-risk factors, clinical assessment, and management. Clin Sports Med. 2008;27(1):183–94.
14. Armstrong LE, Casa DJ, Millard-Stafford M, Moran DS, Pyne SW, Roberts WO. Exertional heat illness during training and competition. Med Sci Sports Exerc. 2007;39(3):556–72.
15. Manspeaker S, Henderson K, Riddle D. Treatment of exertional rhabdomyolysis in athletes: a systematic review. JBI Database Syst Rev Implement Rep. 2016;14(6):117–47.
16. Nye NS, Kasper K, Madsen CM, Szczepanik M, Covey CJ, Oh R, et al. Clinical practice guidelines for exertional rhabdomyolysis: a military medicine perspective. Curr Sports Med Rep. 2021;20(3):169–78.
17. Schleich K, Slayman T, West D, Smoot K. Return to play after exertional rhabdomyolysis. J Athl Train. 2016;51(5):406–9.
18. Younk LM, Mikeladze M, Tate D, Davis SN. Exercise-related hypoglycemia in diabetes mellitus. Expert Rev Endocrinol Metab. 2011;6(1):93–108.
19. Hepburn DA, Deary IJ, Frier BM, Patrick AW, Quinn JD, Fisher BM. Symptoms of acute insulin-induced hypoglycemia in humans with and without IDDM: factor-analysis approach. Diabetes Care. 1991;14(11):949–57.
20. Maletkovic J, Drexler A. Diabetic ketoacidosis and hyperglycemic hyperosmolar state. Endocrinol Metab Clin N Am. 2013;42(4):677–95.
21. Kirk SE. Hypoglycemia in athletes with diabetes. Clin Sports Med. 2009;28(3):455–68.
22. Abraham MB, Jones TW, Naranjo D, Karges B, Oduwole A, Tauschmann M, et al. ISPAD clinical practice consensus guidelines 2022: assessment and management of hypoglycemia in children and adolescents with diabetes. Pediatr Diabetes. 2022;19:178–92.
23. Glaser N, Fritsch M, Priyambada L, Rewers A, Cherubini V, Estrada S, et al. ISPAD clinical practice consensus guidelines 2022: diabetic ketoacidosis and hyperglycemic hyperosmolar state. Pediatr Diabetes. 2022;23:835–56.
24. Shugart C, Jackson J, Fields KB. Diabetes in sports. Sports Health. 2010;2(1):29–38.
25. MacDonald MJ. Postexercise late-onset hypoglycemia in insulin-dependent diabetic patients. Diabetes Care. 1987;10(5):584–8.

25 Breast and Gynecological Disorders in Sport

Amanda T. Wise and Melody R. Hrubes

25.1 Introduction

Sideline evaluations for breast and gynecological conditions in the female athlete are infrequent, but important to consider when evaluating an athlete with complaints of the anterior chest wall and abdominopelvic pain. The most common sports-related breast and gynecologic conditions are non-emergent; however, it is of utmost importance for the sideline clinician to be aware of breast and gynecologic emergencies requiring a higher level of care. Without recognition and with delay of treatment, athletes may sustain significant lifelong issues such as breast deformity or infertility with associated psychosocial impact [1]. While we recognize that breast and gynecological conditions can impact all genders, the focus of this chapter is on the sideline management of breast and gynecologic injuries in cis-gendered females.

25.2 Clinical Presentation and Initial Assessment

Obtaining a succinct history of the athlete is vital to any sideline evaluation. Most commonly, athletes will present with breast or abdominopelvic pain. Paying particularly close attention to the onset (traumatic versus atraumatic; sudden versus insidious) and the location of the injury or symptoms will help the clinician hone in on the differential diagnosis. Gathering collateral information from witnesses if missed by the sideline clinician may also be helpful. The astute clinician should also assess the severity of symptoms and alleviating and aggravating factors. Given the proximity to the chest wall and abdomen, it is imperative to obtain a review of systems in order to rule out cardiopulmonary conditions and an acute abdomen. It is also important to confirm the athlete's past medical and surgical history and elucidate whether they have experienced similar symptoms in the past.

The age of the female athlete should be considered when interviewing and performing a physical examination for a breast or gynecological condition, considering the Tanner stage of development in young female athletes. In the youth athlete, special questions the sideline clinician should ask are age at onset of menarche, if the athlete has regular monthly menstruation, abnormal menstrual bleeding, and their last known menstrual period. In female athletes of child-bearing age, the clinician should assess their menstrual history as above, gravidity and parity (if or when applicable), and consider breast history such as history of or current breast-feeding, or breast implantation. When assessing

A. T. Wise
University of Texas Southwestern Medical Center, Dallas, TX, USA

M. R. Hrubes (✉)
Non-operative Sports Medicine, Rothman Orthopaedics, New York, NY, USA

S. Rocha Piedade et al. (eds.), *Sideline Management in Sports*,
https://doi.org/10.1007/978-3-031-33867-0_25

the mature athlete, it can be helpful to ask about their menopausal status. Post-menopausal women have an increased risk of acute coronary syndrome which can mimic breast pain [2]. For all athletes with abdominopelvic pain with the potential for gynecological etiology, the clinician should also obtain a recent sexual history, accounting for behaviors that may increase the risk of contracting of a sexually transmitted infection or pelvic inflammatory disease such as unprotected intercourse or multiple partners.

25.3 Physical Examination

25.3.1 Breast Injuries

When a sudden, traumatic injury to the anterior chest wall occurs, or an athlete complains of breast or chest discomfort, a thorough physical examination should include the following

- Prompt assessment of airway, breathing, and circulation (ABCs) given its location overlying vital cardiopulmonary structures
- Obtaining vitals such as heart rate, blood pressure, respiratory rate, and oxygen saturation may be helpful, but can also be time consuming on the sideline
- Cardiopulmonary examination, including cardiac and lung auscultation with a stethoscope, assessment of distal pulses, as well as chest wall percussion if there is high suspicion for a pneumothorax
- Brief neck examination to assess for signs of tracheal deviation to rule out tension pneumothorax
- Skin examination, observing for ecchymosis, erythema, rashes, abrasions, or lacerations of the chest wall
- Breast and chest wall examination including observation for deformity, palpation of the chest wall along the rib cage, breast tissue, and axilla to assess for tenderness or masses, and assessment for nipple discharge or bleeding

25.3.2 Gynecological Injuries

Acute lower abdominal quadrant pain may also be mistaken for pelvic pain or vice versa. Distinguishing pelvic versus intraperitoneal injuries with history alone can be challenging, and a comprehensive examination should include the following to obtain a differential diagnosis:

- As above, a quick evaluation of the ABCs and vitals is helpful in determining the acuity of the athlete's condition
- Abdominal examination while laying supine including observation, light and deep palpation of all quadrants, assessing for rebound tenderness or guarding, auscultation of bowel sounds and vascular bruits, and an evaluation for costovertebral angle tenderness
- An assessment of urinary excretion and whether the athlete has hematuria, dysuria, or is anuric, can help rule out urinary tract issues
- Gynecologic examination on the sideline may include asking the athlete if they are experiencing vaginal discharge or bleeding, and while lying supine assessing for suprapubic tenderness or fullness and enlarged inguinal lymph nodes

With both breast and gynecologic examinations, privacy and discretion are paramount. At least one chaperone should be present if the examination is necessary to clear an athlete to return to play. Invasive gynecologic examinations are rarely necessary on the sideline. If an urgent bimanual or speculum examination is warranted, the clinician should send the athlete to urgent or emergent care for evaluation to avoid unnecessary repetition of an invasive examination. This allows for simultaneous diagnostic testing or treatment at the next level of care. For underage athletes, clinicians should obtain consent from their guardian for a breast or gynecologic examination unless there is a clear, life-threatening emergency and a guardian cannot be reached in a timely manner.

25.4 Breast Injuries and Conditions

25.4.1 Anatomy of the Breast

Breast tissue largely consists of mammary glands and subcutaneous fat. Its borders extend transversely from the lateral edge of the sternum to the midaxillary line, and vertically from the second to the sixth ribs with a tail extending up into the axillary fossa. The tissue and mammary glands are supported by suspensory ligaments which are anchored to the dermis. Superficially, the breast has a round and pigmented areola with a projecting nipple at its prominence connected to a system of mammary ducts. Deep to the breast underlies the retromammary space or bursa, which allows for relative movement, followed by the pectoralis major and serratus anterior fascia [3]. Injury to the breast or anterior chest wall can affect any of the above or surrounding structures.

25.4.2 Breast Trauma

Traumatic breast injuries from a direct blow have a reported prevalence of 29% and 47.9% in elite and collegiate female athletes, respectively, but are largely underreported to medical or team personnel. Only 10% of these athletes seek evaluation or treatment [1, 4]. Findings on physical examination include skin changes such as ecchymosis, laceration or abrasion, and tenderness on palpation. It is important to rule out acute cardiopulmonary conditions that may mimic breast discomfort due to location but should prompt emergent evaluation.

Most breast-related traumatic injuries are nonemergent. Treatment should include ice, compression, and oral or topical analgesics or anti-inflammatories for symptom control. Abrasions should be cleaned with sterile saline and covered with a clean, dry dressing. Lacerations may be closed with topical skin adhesives or sutures that should be removed 10–14 days later. Tetanus prophylaxis should be considered for any open wound [5]. The athlete should rest for 3–7 days to allow for scar tissue healing and strengthening, followed by mobilization of the upper extremities and chest wall and return to play as tolerated [6]. Adequate breast support during this time will optimize tissue healing. The sideline clinician should follow up in 1–2 weeks following injury, monitoring closely for infection, and should counsel the athlete on possible sequela of a traumatic breast injury.

With enough force, a breast hematoma or fat necrosis may develop. Some large hematomas may require a diagnostic breast ultrasound if unresolved after 6–8 weeks from the initial injury and may benefit from ultrasound-guided aspiration. Fat necrosis can eventually lead to scarring, deformity, skin tethering, nipple retraction, and calcification of breast tissue that may mimic malignancy. If any of these changes occur and there is a concern for breast cancer depending on the athlete age and risk factors, a workup to rule out malignancy should be done. Advanced diagnostic imaging including mammography with or without breast ultrasound or breast magnetic resonance imaging (MRI) is appropriate [4–6]. Depending on these results, a biopsy may be required to rule out malignancy.

Prevention of breast trauma may reduce the need for extensive and expensive workups, as well as the emotional and mental anguish that may come with it. In the youth athlete, traumatic injury to the breast bud can cause significant breast asymmetry and result in psychological distress [7]. Although all jewelry is prohibited in most contact sports, sports medicine clinicians should also consider screening for nipple piercings that may predispose athletes to nipple trauma or irritation. Instructing athletes to remove nipple piercings prior to competition may prevent further breast injury. Strategies to reduce breast trauma remain limited due to significant underreporting of the injury [8]. Wearing breast or chest padding in contact sports may be protective, however only 2.1% of collegiate athletes report wearing protective equipment in addition to a sports bra [4]. One study on Australian football and rugby female athletes found that the majority do not wear protective breast equipment due to the lack of awareness of its existence, discomfort, and poor fit despite it being perceived as being protective against contact injury [9]. Mandating the wear of well-fitted breast or chest protective equipment in contact sports may be a future consideration for prevention.

25.4.3 "Runner's Nipple"

Also referred to as "jogger's nipple," this friction-induced injury typically results from repetitive clothing contact and is commonly associated with long-distance running. Other associations include high BMI and infrequent sports bra use [1]. Approximately 2–16.3% have reported jogger's nipples on marathon day, and friction-related breast injuries have been reported to be 20% in elite female athletes [1, 10]. Athletes may present with nipple discomfort or bleeding through their clothing. On examination, the nipples and surrounding areola may have erythema, pain, and cracked lesions and fissures with crusting and bloody discharge.

Treatment of this condition on the sideline includes cleaning skin with soap and water, applying petroleum jelly, or an antibiotic ointment like erythromycin if available, and covering with a clean bandage [5, 6, 10]. These injuries do not typically prevent return to sport participation as long as bleeding is controlled and lesions are contained to prevent spread to other athletes. Red flags to assess for include fever or other systemic symptoms. Advanced workup or imaging is not indicated unless the lesions are noted to be from an atraumatic, non-infectious etiology. This may suggest a diagnosis of malignancy and mammography is warranted.

"Runner's nipple" can be prevented by applying lubricants such as petroleum jelly or adhesive tapes or bandages prior to running. Regular sports bra use that is well fitted with optimal cushioning and support may prevent this injury from occurring. Wearing dry clothing made from synthetic materials that are moisture-wicking and well-fitted, instead of loose or too-tight fitting clothing made from rougher organic materials like cotton, may also be protective and prevent these friction injuries [5, 6, 10].

25.4.4 Exercise-Induced Breast Pain

This condition occurs as a result of significant breast movement relative to the trunk resulting in breast pain during physical activity. Exercise-induced breast pain (EIBP) is associated with increased breast mass, larger cup size, and sports that may increase overall breast motion such as the magnitude of movement, rate of breast bounce, and duration of physical activity [11–14]. Though hormonal variations in the menstrual cycle can cause generalized breast pain, also known as mastalgia, and can also make EIBP worse, the two conditions should be distinguished from each other. EIBP has been reported in 40–44% of female athletes with significantly higher severity in running, jumping, or landing activities, and can negatively affect levels of activity in the general population and performance of highly skilled athletes [11, 13, 15, 16].

The athlete may present with a history of insidious onset, atraumatic, and symmetric breast discomfort recurring with physical activity. On sideline evaluation, it is important to rule out exertional angina or acute coronary syndrome. Tenderness to palpation of bilateral breasts may be present without other significant findings. Though EIBP will rarely render the athlete unable to train or play, it has been perceived by athletes to negatively affect performance [11]. Further workup is usually not necessary, but mammography should be considered if symptoms are unilateral, persist despite preventive measures, or there is high clinical suspicion for malignancy.

Prevention strategies are largely focused on wearing proper-fitting sports bras and educating females on how to assess their own bra fit [17–20]. One study in 2012 found a statistically significant difference between the bra size women wear based on traditional bra fitting criteria compared to a bra size recommended by professional bra fitting criteria [17]. Having larger breast and band size increases the inaccuracy of traditional bra fittings and, in this case, women should seek professional bra fitting for optimal comfort and protection [17, 21]. The type of activity should also be considered when selecting a sports bra as this can determine specific design features to look for such as encapsulation or compression designs, band size, strap length, width, and orientation, material, and closure types. Higher levels of impact or activities that increase breast motion require increasing amounts of support [13, 14, 22]. Durability and frequent replacement of sports bras should also be considered, as one recent study has demonstrated reduced sports bra support and increased breast motion after repeated wear and 25 washes [23]. Sports bra prescription by a clinician may be at the forefront of EIBP prevention and further research into this is warranted [14, 23].

25.4.5 Postpartum Mastitis

Mastitis is an inflammatory condition of breast tissue with or without infection. Studies have reported 2.5–20% of all lactating females experience mastitis [24]. Though mastitis can also be seen after trauma, the highest incidence of lactational mastitis occurs within 4 weeks postpartum and is significantly associated with nipple damage [24, 25]. Postpartum athletes may present with breast pain, fevers, chills, or myalgias. On breast examination, the patient will present with unilateral breast swelling and erythema. There may be associated tenderness with palpation and the clinician should assess for a hard or fluctuant mass that may be concerning for abscess. Treatment largely consists of supportive therapy including cold compresses, analgesics, anti-inflammatories, massage, increased fluid intake, and continued lactation to maintain adequate breast drainage. For symptoms lasting 12–24 h with fever or other systemic symptoms, prescribe antibiotics with coverage for *Staphylococcus aureus*. Antibiotic treatment may offer more rapid relief of symptoms [26]. If symptoms persist despite 2–3 days of antibiotic therapy, a diagnostic breast ultrasound may be helpful to evaluate for a breast abscess that may require drainage [25, 27].

25.4.6 Breast Implant Rupture

Though exceedingly rare, breast implant rupture should be considered in the adult or mature athlete who sustained direct, high-velocity trauma to the breast. There are limited studies assessing the prevalence of sports-related breast implant rupture, but there has been at least one reported case in a female boxer after sustaining breast trauma in a fight [28, 29]. Risk factors increasing the risk of rupture include increasing implant age and severe capsular contracture after implantation [29, 30]. Though most implant ruptures are asymptomatic, physical exam findings may include breast pain, swelling, asymmetry or deformity, palpable masses in the breast, axilla, or anterior chest wall, enlarged lymph nodes, capsular contracture, or a palpable implant shell on the affected breast. Patients with silicone implants are more likely to experience the above symptoms with extracapsular ruptures compared to intracapsular ruptures, which may present with only subtle breast changes. In those with saline implants, patients may experience breast deflation more acutely within a few days without other exam findings, whereas those with silicone implants may notice a more gradual onset of symptoms due to the viscosity of silicone gel. MRI breast is the study of choice to confirm diagnosis [29, 31, 32].

Treatment of breast implant rupture is nonemergent. The athlete should be referred to their primary surgeon once the diagnosis is confirmed. In asymptomatic or minimally symptomatic patients, a watch-and-wait approach without definitive treatment may be taken. Implant removal and capsulectomy may be necessary for extracapsular ruptures, if there is a high risk of silicone spread, or the patient is highly symptomatic [29, 30, 33]. Athletes may return to sport as tolerated with minimal symptoms and without fever or other B symptoms. If surgery is required, the athlete may return to light activity 2 weeks postoperatively, with a full return to activity at 6–8 weeks. To prevent this injury from occurring, some local governing bodies for combat sports have implemented competition rules that prevent athletes with breast implants from competing. To reduce patient morbidity associated with implant rupture, the U.S. Food and Drug Administration recommends that patients with silicone gel implants undergo MRI screening 3 years postoperatively and every 2 years thereafter [29].

25.4.7 Other Chest Conditions

The sideline clinician should take care to rule out the conditions of surrounding structures. An athlete presenting with anterior chest wall pain may instead have a cardiopulmonary emergency, such as acute coronary syndrome, aortic dissection, unstable arrhythmia, cardiopulmonary contusion, pneumothorax, or pulmonary embolism. It is important to ask whether the athlete is experiencing shortness of breath, palpitations, pre-syncopal symptoms, radiating chest pain, and a family history of sudden cardiac death. If any of these symptoms are present, the sideline clinician should obtain a set of vitals and perform a thorough cardiopulmonary examination to make sure the patient is stable. Ensure the automated external defibrillator (AED) is in proximity. If any of the above symptoms are present with abnormal vital signs, the patient should be sent to the emergency department (ED) for further workup and treatment including an EKG, troponin and electrolytes on lab work, chest X-ray, echocardiogram, and potentially advanced workup with computed tomography (CT) of the chest as well as cardiac or chest MRI. The athlete can return to sport once the workup has been completed and negative.

Athletes experiencing chest wall pain with pleuritic symptoms may also have a musculoskeletal condition. In the setting of trauma, rib or sternal fractures should be considered on the differential and on physical exam may have reproduced pain with palpation or compression of these structures. Costochondritis may also present with these same exam findings. If a fracture is suspected, the patient should be removed from play and sent for emergent evaluation with chest X-ray, ultrasound, or CT chest. Rib fractures can be treated with pain management with analgesics, rest, and incentive spirometry to prevent atelectasis and infection. Athletes may return to play as tolerated after 6 weeks of rest and healing. Sternal fractures are treated similarly but may require surgical fixation if displaced. Return to play may occur 8–12 weeks after rest and symptom resolution. Given the pectoralis major (PM) underlies the majority of breast tissue, PM strain or rupture should be considered with breast or pain that begins after excessive eccentric loading. Physical examination may reveal ecchymosis and swelling in the axilla, localized pain at its insertion on the humerus, and weakness with shoulder adduction. Diagnosis should be confirmed with ultrasound, MRI of the shoulder if toward PM insertion, or MRI of the chest wall if located more proximally. Treatment depends on the severity of the injury and may range from conservative treatment with analgesia and immobilization to surgical repair.

25.5 Gynecological Injuries and Conditions

25.5.1 Anatomy of the Female Reproductive System

The female reproductive system is made of external and internal genitalia. Externally, the mons pubis lies anterior to the pubic bones and with typical development becomes covered in pubic hair. Posterior to the mons pubis are prominent skin folds, the labia majora and labia minora, that cover the clitoris and vestibule. The vestibule is inferior to the clitoris and contains the external urethral orifice, vaginal orifice, which are arranged, respectively, from anterior to posterior, as well as the greater vestibular glands (Bartholin glands) and lesser vestibular glands. The urethra runs in parallel with the vagina through the pelvic diaphragm. Collectively, these structures make up the female vulva. The rectum is positioned posteriorly to the vulva. The internal female genitalia consists of the vagina, uterus, uterine or fallopian tubes, and ovaries. The vaginal canal extends upward and is connected to the cervix of the uterus. The uterus lays between the urinary bladder and the rectum and is made of three layers: the outermost perimetrium, myometrium, and innermost endometrium, the last of which is shed during menstruation or maintained with the implantation of an embryo after conception. The uterine horns then extend bilaterally into uterine tubes that ascend and arch over with distal fimbriae that spread over the superomedial aspect of each ovary and open into the peritoneal cavity [3].

25.5.2 Vulvar and Vaginal Injuries

In the female athlete, injuries to this region are usually traumatic or friction induced. Vulvar and vaginal injuries in sport, also known as "straddle" or "saddle" injuries, usually result in hematomas, lacerations, and tears and are uncommon. Non-obstetric vulvar injuries have an estimated incidence of 3.7% [34]. Vulvar and vaginal injuries have been reported in cycling, snowboarding, skating, and water sports to name a few [35–39]. Athletes will present with exquisite pain in the vulvar or perineal region and may also present with bleeding. Additionally, the clinician should screen for gynecological piercings that may not have been removed prior to competition. It is important to rule out recent sexual assault on the differential diagnosis. Physical exam may reveal a hematoma with significant labia majora or minora swelling, laceration, tears, or bleeding. The clinician should palpate the surrounding pubic and pelvic bones to rule out fracture.

Treatment should begin with rest, ice, compression, and analgesia and bleeding should be controlled with applied pressure [34]. Simple lacerations can be repaired by the team physician, but complex lacerations or tears should be presented to an ED for evaluation and repair. Some complex lacerations or tears may require anesthesia due to pain and psychological distress. Small and stable hematomas can be treated with conservative measures. Red flags that absolutely warrant emergent evaluation include increasing hematoma expansion, uncontrolled or unidentifiable bleeding unexplained by menses, inability to urinate due to the size of the hematoma or swelling causing urethral obstruction, as well as signs of hemodynamic instability from severe blood loss anemia, and concerns for sexual assault. Radiographs should be ordered to rule out pelvic fracture as well as a cystourethrogram if concerned for urethral injury [40]. Acutely increasing vulvar hematomas will require surgical intervention or embolization due to risks of necrosis and urinary obstruction. Athletes may return to play after treatment and symptom resolution. There is limited research on the prevention of these injuries given how uncommon they are in female athletes. Applying barrier cream, reducing layers of clothing while riding, and using equipment such as bicycle seat cushions as well as bicycle and seat modifications may prevent these injuries in cyclists [41].

25.5.3 Ovarian Torsion

Ovarian, or adnexal, torsion is a gynecologic emergency the sideline clinician should consider when an athlete complains of pelvic pain. This condition occurs when the ovary twists over supporting ligaments, resulting in obstructed blood flow and swelling that can then lead to necrosis, hemorrhage, autoamputation, and potentially reduced fertility [42, 43]. This condition occurs most commonly in females of child-bearing age with over half of cases associated with an ovarian mass. Other cases are associated with pregnancy, in vitro fertilization, and trauma [40, 42, 44, 45]. Athletes may present with sudden onset constant or intermittent sharp, unilateral pelvic pain with or without abdominal or adnexal tenderness on exam.

If there is any suspicion of ovarian torsion, the athlete should be immediately referred to the ED for further evaluation. Pregnancy should be ruled out, as ectopic pregnancies may have a similar presentation. Transvaginal pelvic ultrasound with Doppler is the diagnostic test of choice to assess for reduced blood flow to the ovary. CT abdomen and pelvis should also be done to rule out other causes of an acute abdomen such as appendicitis or bowel obstruction. Treatment is emergent surgery for attempted ovarian salvage and reduction, or salpingo-oophorectomy if unsalvageable [42, 46, 47]. Cases associated with an ovarian mass may require a malignancy workup. Return to sport may occur at 6–8 weeks post-operatively. Oophoropexy, a controversial procedure that fixes the ovary in position, has been used to prevent recurrence and could potentially be indicated for individuals of child-bearing age with a single ovary. Evidence remains limited to support its widespread use [42, 48].

25.5.4 Abnormal Uterine Bleeding (AUB)

AUB is a clinical diagnosis based on patient history and refers to heavy menstrual bleeding or intermenstrual bleeding, also known as menorrhagia and metrorrhagia, respectively. AUB can have multiple causes and the etiology may depend on the individual's age. Some common causes include endometriosis, uterine fibroids, coagulopathy, and malignancy [49]. It is important to obtain a detailed history when assessing abnormal uterine bleeding. Key pieces of information to obtain are the date of the last menstrual period, frequency and regularity of menstruation, frequency of changing tampons or pads, personal or family history of coagulopathy, sexual history, history of pregnancies, as well as symptoms of anemia such as lightheadedness, palpitations, shortness of breath, or fatigue. Physical examination may be limited, but athletes may have tachycardia, hypotension, hypoxia, and copious amounts of bleeding. With any signs of hemodynamic instability, symptoms or anemia, or persisting bleeding, the athlete must be removed from play and sent to the ED for further evaluation and appropriate treatment [50].

Workup in the ED should include a CBC and coagulation studies to assess for severe blood loss anemia and coagulopathy, and a pregnancy test to rule out abortion. A gynecologic speculum and bimanual exam are necessary to rule out an identifiable source of focal bleeding and test for sexually transmitted infections and pelvic inflammatory disease that can cause AUB [47]. Diagnostic imaging is primarily with transvaginal ultrasound but may also benefit from a CT abdomen/pelvis [51, 52]. To treat AUB, patients may require blood transfusion, reversal of coagulopathy, ablation, uterine artery embolization, or even hysterectomy. After they have been stabilized and discharged, the athlete should be referred to gynecology to complete outpatient workup and treatment if indicated. They may be able to return to play as soon as their symptoms have resolved. Screening for risks of AUB should be done as part of the athlete's preparticipation examination [53]. Prevention of AUB or its recurrence can be met with hormonal medications such as combination of oral contraceptives or an intrauterine device [50, 54].

25.5.5 Pelvic Inflammatory Disease (PID)

An estimated 4.4% of females of child-bearing age have been treated for PID in their lifetime [55]. PID results from ascending bacterial infection from the lower to the upper female reproductive tract that leads to inflammation. When PID is suspected, it is important to elicit sexual history as more than 85% of cases are due to sexually transmitted infections and the remaining 15% are due to enteric bacteria and respiratory pathogens [56]. Athletes typically present with pelvic pain, fever, purulent vaginal discharge, and may also have AUB. To meet diagnostic criteria for PID, the athlete must have direct abdominal, cervical, and adnexal tenderness, commonly known as the "chandelier" sign. All three must be present with at least one additional finding of fever, leukocytosis, high inflammatory markers, positive gram stain or culture, purulent cervical discharge, and pelvic abscess to make the diagnosis [47].

Athletes should be held from play and immediately sent to the ED for evaluation and treatment. A comprehensive infectious workup and pregnancy rule-out will be necessary since ectopic pregnancies can have a similar presentation. A gynecologic bimanual and speculum exam must be done along with cultures and gram stain of cervical fluid. Diagnostic imaging includes transvaginal and pelvic ultrasound and CT abdomen/pelvis to assess for a tubo-ovarian abscess and inflammation. Treatment is based on complications. Uncomplicated PID can be treated with one-time intramuscular ceftriaxone for gonorrhea and a 14-day course of doxycycline for chlamydia, and the athlete may return to play after completing the antibiotic course. If complicated by a tubo-ovarian abscess, pregnancy, or severe PID, the athlete will require hospital admission and IV antibiotics. Some cases may require drainage and approximately 25% of cases will require surgical intervention [40, 47]. Athletes can expect a full return to play about 6–8 weeks post-operatively. Prevention of PID in athletes starts with the preparticipation examination, counseling on safe sex practices, and encouraging consistent condom use with sexual activity [57].

25.5.6 Bartholin's Cyst or Abscess

The greater vestibular gland, or Bartholin's gland, assists with vulval and vaginal lubrication during sexual arousal and activity. The gland's ducts can be obstructed by mucus, trauma, or edema which can lead to cyst formation. Secondary infection of these cysts most commonly results in infection or abscess. These conditions have an estimated prevalence of 2–3% in women and risk factors are single women, multiple sexual partners, and lower socioeconomic status [58, 59]. Athletes may present with complaints of vulvar swelling and/or pain with rest and fever, and have a history of pain with sexual activity. If the athlete is presenting with fever and hemodynamic instability on the sideline, the athlete should be removed from play and sent to the ED for further evaluation. On physical exam, there may be asymmetrical swelling with a fluctuant and painful mass between the vestibule and labia minora at the 4 o'clock or 8 o'clock position. Abscesses may have purulent drainage from the ducts.

Treatment largely depends on symptoms. If a cyst is present and there are no signs concerning infection, it can be managed with rest, cold or warm compress, and analgesics if there are no signs of fever or hemodynamic instability. Athletes may return to play once symptoms resolve. If an abscess is present, the athlete may require drainage and placement of a Word catheter that will need to stay in place for 3–4 weeks. In cases of recurrence, athletes may require marsupialization or the creation of a surgical pouch to allow ongoing drainage. Excision can be considered for refractory cases [59]. Antibiotics should be prescribed for cases with overlying cellulitis, pregnancy, or systemic involvement, but should be tailored to the culture sensitivities. Amoxicillin–clavulanic acid can be initiated until culture results [60]. Return to play after treatment of a Bartholin's abscess may depend on the treatment above but will be at least 3–4 weeks before the athlete can be cleared. Emphasis on proper gynecological hygiene and safe sex practices may reduce the occurrence of this condition.

25.5.7 Other Abdominopelvic Conditions

Conditions that cause an acute abdomen can occur concomitantly or present similarly to the above gynecologic emergencies. The clinician should recall the other structures and vital organs in the intraabdominal cavity to rapidly build a differential diagnosis. From the gastrointestinal system, an athlete with acute abdominopelvic pain may also have appendicitis and should be considered in athletes with right lower quadrant pain with tenderness at McBurney's point. Contralaterally, an athlete with left lower quadrant pain may also have diverticulitis or severe constipation with ileus. From the renal system, kidney stones passing through the ureter can also radiate to the groin and are commonly associated with dysuria or hematuria. An ascending urinary tract infection causing pyelonephritis may also present similarly with the addition of fever, chills, and diaphoresis. While the above conditions typically present without inciting trauma, they should not be glossed over when an athlete associates the onset of pain with a traumatic event. If there is concern for any of the above conditions or signs of hemodynamic instability, the athletes should be sent to the ED for further evaluation and treatment. The workup includes a complete blood count, metabolic panel, lactate, urinalysis, and reflex urine culture. CT abdomen and pelvis may be necessary to rule out the conditions above.

After ruling out acute emergent conditions, musculoskeletal conditions that may mimic acute gynecological or abdominopelvic conditions should be considered. Given its proximity, groin-related injuries should remain high on the differential and include adductor or iliopsoas strain, core muscle injury or athletic pubalgia, and osteitis pubis. In the youth athlete, groin or pelvic pain may be a result of an avulsion fracture of the anterior superior iliac spine, anterior inferior iliac spine, iliac crest, or ischial tuberosity. In these cases, hip and pelvis radiographs and musculoskeletal ultrasound may assist with diagnosis. Traumatic pelvic fractures are rare in sports without high-energy impact, but stress fractures should be considered in endurance athletes at high risk for relative energy deficiency in sports or rapid increase in physical activity. CT or MRI of the pelvis or hip may be helpful to make this diagnosis.

25.6 Summary

The astute sideline clinician should be able to distinguish between an acute cardiopulmonary or abdominopelvic condition and from acute breast or gynecologic conditions. Though rare, it is important to be proactive when evaluating for breast or gynecological disorders. Athletes may underreport these conditions on the sideline due to their discomfort discussing the location of pain or injury; so, the physician should have a low threshold to screen, and comfortably ask straightforward questions. Athletes may feel more comfortable reporting it to medical professionals of the same gender [8, 61]. Preventing or providing evidence-based treatment for these conditions may improve athletic performance and reduce long-term healthcare consequences for the athlete.

Fact Boxes [2–3]

- Sports medicine physicians should consider professional prescription of a sports bra to reduce EIBP in female athletes.
- Athletes found to have ovarian torsion should be referred for malignancy workup since over half of the cases in females of child-bearing age are associated with an ovarian mass.
- Red flags that should prompt emergent evaluation include radiating chest pain, hemodynamic instability, fever, and intractable pain.

References

1. Brisbine BR, Steele JR, Phillips EJ, McGhee DE. The occurrence, causes and perceived performance effects of breast injuries in elite female athletes. J Sports Sci Med. 2019;18(3):569–76.
2. El Khoudary SR, Aggarwal B, Beckie TM, Hodis HN, Johnson AE, Langer RD, et al. Menopause transition and cardiovascular disease risk: implications for timing of early prevention: a scientific statement from the American Heart Association. Circulation. 2020;142(25):e506–e32.
3. Agur AMR, Dalley AF, Moore KL, Moore KL. Moore's essential clinical anatomy. 6th ed. Philadelphia: Wolters Kluwer; 2019.
4. Smith LJ, Eichelberger TD, Kane EJ. Breast injuries in female collegiate basketball, soccer, softball and volleyball athletes: prevalence, type and impact on sports participation. Eur J Breast Health. 2018;14(1):46–50.
5. Greydanus DE, Omar H, Pratt HD. The adolescent female athlete: current concepts and conundrums. Pediatr Clin N Am. 2010;57(3):697–718.
6. Obourn PJ, Benoit J, Brady G, Campbell E, Rizzone K. Sports medicine-related breast and chest conditions-update of current literature. Curr Sports Med Rep. 2021;20(3):140–9.
7. Jansen DA, Spencer Stoetzel R, Leveque JE. Premenarchal athletic injury to the breast bud as the cause for asymmetry: prevention and treatment. Breast J. 2002;8(2):108–11.
8. Smith LJ, Miller E, Eichelberger T, Kane EJ. Breast injury during sport participation. Int J Sports Exerc Med. 2018;4(112):1.
9. Brisbine BR, Steele JR, Phillips EJ, McGhee DE. Use and perception of breast protective equipment by female contact football players. J Sci Med Sport. 2020;23(9):820–5.
10. Mailler EA, Adams BB. The wear and tear of 26.2: dermatological injuries reported on marathon day. Br J Sports Med. 2004;38(4):498–501.
11. Brisbine BR, Steele JR, Phillips EJ, McGhee DE. Breast pain affects the performance of elite female athletes. J Sports Sci. 2020;38(5):528–33.
12. Brisbine BR, Steele JR, Phillips EJ, McGhee DE. Can physical characteristics and sports bra use predict exercise-induced breast pain in elite female athletes? Clin J Sport Med. 2021;31(6):e380–e4.
13. Burbage J, Cameron L. An investigation into the prevalence and impact of breast pain, bra issues and breast size on female horse riders. J Sports Sci. 2017;35(11):1091–7.
14. McGhee DE, Steele JR. Biomechanics of breast support for active women. Exerc Sport Sci Rev. 2020;48(3):99–109.
15. Brown N, Burnett E, Scurr J. Is breast pain greater in active females compared to the general population in the UK? Breast J. 2016;22(2):194–201.
16. Norris M, Blackmore T, Horler B, Wakefield-Scurr J. How the characteristics of sports bras affect their performance. Ergonomics. 2021;64(3):410–25.

17. White J, Scurr J. Evaluation of professional bra fitting criteria for bra selection and fitting in the UK. Ergonomics. 2012;55(6):704–11.
18. Rizzone KH, Edison B, Coleman N, Carter C, Ichesco I, Cassidy P, et al. Sports bra preferences by age and impact of breast size on physical activity among American females. Int J Environ Res Public Health. 2021;18(23):12732.
19. Bowles KA, Steele JR, Munro B. What are the breast support choices of Australian women during physical activity? Br J Sports Med. 2008;42(8):670–3.
20. Haworth L, Aitkenhead R, Grecic D, Chohan A. Understanding experience, knowledge and perceived challenges related to bra fit for sports participation: a scoping review Res Sports Med. 2022.
21. McGhee DE, Steele JR. Optimising breast support in female patients through correct bra fit. A cross-sectional study. J Sci Med Sport. 2010;13(6):568–72.
22. Milligan A, Mills C, Corbett J, Scurr J. The influence of breast support on torso, pelvis and arm kinematics during a 5 km treadmill run. Hum Mov Sci. 2015;42:246–60.
23. Wakefield-Scurr J, Hamilton C, Reeves K, Jones M, Jones B. The effect of washing and wearing on sports bra function. Sports Biomech. 2022.
24. Wilson E, Woodd SL, Benova L. Incidence of and risk factors for lactational mastitis: a systematic review. J Hum Lact. 2020;36(4):673–86.
25. Barbosa-Cesnik C, Schwartz K, Foxman B. Lactation mastitis. JAMA. 2003;289(13):1609–12.
26. Jahanfar S, Ng CJ, Teng CL. Antibiotics for mastitis in breastfeeding women. Sao Paulo Med J. 2016;134(3):273.
27. Spencer JP. Management of mastitis in breastfeeding women. Am Fam Physician. 2008;78(6):727–31.
28. Krajcova A, Hurt K, Kufa R, Molitor M. Breast implant rupture: a sports trauma report. Ceska Gynekol. 2020;85(2):116–9.
29. Handel N, Garcia ME, Wixtrom R. Breast implant rupture: causes, incidence, clinical impact, and management. Plast Reconstr Surg. 2013;132(5):1128–37.
30. Holmich LR, Friis S, Fryzek JP, Vejborg IM, Conrad C, Sletting S, et al. Incidence of silicone breast implant rupture. Arch Surg. 2003;138(7):801–6.
31. Expert Panel on Breast Imaging, Lourenco AP, Moy L, Baron P, Didwania AD, diFlorio RM, et al. ACR Appropriateness Criteria® breast implant evaluation. J Am Coll Radiol. 2018;15(5S):S13–25.
32. Everson LI, Parantainen H, Detlie T, Stillman AE, Olson PN, Landis G, et al. Diagnosis of breast implant rupture: imaging findings and relative efficacies of imaging techniques. AJR Am J Roentgenol. 1994;163(1):57–60.
33. Hillard C, Fowler JD, Barta R, Cunningham B. Silicone breast implant rupture: a review. Gland Surg. 2017;6(2):163–8.
34. Jones IS, O'Connor A. Non-obstetric vulval trauma. Emerg Med Australas. 2013;25(1):36–9.
35. Virgili A, Bianchi A, Mollica G, Corazza M. Serious hematoma of the vulva from a bicycle accident. A case report. J Reprod Med. 2000;45(8):662–4.
36. Kanai M, Osada R, Maruyama K, Masuzawa H, Shih HC, Konishi I. Warning from Nagano: increase of vulvar hematoma and/or lacerated injury caused by snowboarding. J Trauma. 2001;50(2):328–31.
37. Herrmann B, Crawford J. Genital injuries in prepubertal girls from inline skating accidents. Pediatrics. 2002;110(2 Pt 1):e16.
38. Gauthier I, Clancy AA, Lipson J, Pascali D. Water-related vaginal injury: a case report and review of the literature. J Obstet Gynaecol Can. 2018;40(7):926–30.
39. Bagga HS, Fisher PB, Tasian GE, Blaschko SD, McCulloch CE, McAninch JW, et al. Sports-related genitourinary injuries presenting to United States emergency departments. Urology. 2015;85(1):239–44.
40. McWilliams GD, Hill MJ, Dietrich CS 3rd. Gynecologic emergencies. Surg Clin N Am. 2008;88(2):265–83. vi
41. Puleo RM, Barreveld A, Rice S, Althausen Plante AM, Kotler DH. Unique concerns of the woman cyclist. Phys Med Rehabil Clin N Am. 2022;33(1):61–79.
42. ACOG Committee. Adnexal torsion in adolescents: ACOG Committee opinion no. 783. Obstet Gynecol. 2019;134(2):e56–63.
43. Habek D, Marton I, Luetic AT, Prka M. Adnexal autoamputation after torsion. Arch Gynecol Obstet. 2022;305(5):1377.
44. Huang HJ, Huang YC, Kuo HC, Chang CY. A rare cause of acute abdomen after a sport-related blunt abdominal trauma—torsion of a normal ovary in a pre-pubertal girl. JACME. 2014;4(4):157–60.
45. Littman ED, Rydfors J, Milki AA. Exercise-induced ovarian torsion in the cycle following gonadotrophin therapy: case report. Hum Reprod. 2003;18(8):1641–2.
46. Anders JF, Powell EC. Urgency of evaluation and outcome of acute ovarian torsion in pediatric patients. Arch Pediatr Adolesc Med. 2005;159(6):532–5.
47. Mahonski S, Hu KM. Female nonobstetric genitourinary emergencies. Emerg Med Clin N Am. 2019;37(4):771–84.
48. Fuchs N, Smorgick N, Tovbin Y, Ben Ami I, Maymon R, Halperin R, et al. Oophoropexy to prevent adnexal torsion: how, when, and for whom? J Minim Invasive Gynecol. 2010;17(2):205–8.
49. Munro MG, Critchley HO, Broder MS, Fraser IS, FIGO Working Group on Menstrual Disorders. FIGO classification system (PALM-COEIN) for causes of abnormal uterine bleeding in nongravid women of reproductive age. Int J Gynaecol Obstet. 2011;113(1):3–13.
50. American College of Obstetricians and Gynecologists. ACOG Committee Opinion no. 557: management of acute abnormal uterine bleeding in nonpregnant reproductive-aged women. Obstet Gynecol. 2013;121(4):891–6.
51. Doubilet PM. Diagnosis of abnormal uterine bleeding with imaging. Menopause. 2011;18(4):421–4.
52. Shi AA, Lee SI. Radiological reasoning: algorithmic workup of abnormal vaginal bleeding with endovaginal sonography and sonohysterography. AJR Am J Roentgenol. 2008;191(6 Suppl):S68–73.

53. Parmigiano TR, Zucchi EV, Araujo MP, Guindalini CS, Castro Rde A, Di Bella ZI, et al. Pre-participation gynecological evaluation of female athletes: a new proposal. Einstein (Sao Paulo). 2014;12(4):459–66.
54. Lethaby A, Wise MR, Weterings MA, Bofill Rodriguez M, Brown J. Combined hormonal contraceptives for heavy menstrual bleeding. Cochrane Database Syst Rev. 2019;2(2):CD000154.
55. Kreisel K, Torrone E, Bernstein K, Hong J, Gorwitz R. Prevalence of pelvic inflammatory disease in sexually experienced women of reproductive age—United States, 2013–2014. MMWR Morb Mortal Wkly Rep. 2017;66(3):80–3.
56. Brunham RC, Gottlieb SL, Paavonen J. Pelvic inflammatory disease. N Engl J Med. 2015;372(21):2039–48.
57. Daly P, Gustafson R. Public health recommendations for athletes attending sporting events. Clin J Sport Med. 2011;21(1):67–70.
58. Illingworth B, Stocking K, Showell M, Kirk E, Duffy J. Evaluation of treatments for Bartholin's cyst or abscess: a systematic review. BJOG. 2020;127(6):671–8.
59. Long N, Morris L, Foster K. Bartholin gland abscess diagnosis and office management. Prim Care. 2021;48(4):569–82.
60. Bhide A, Nama V, Patel S, Kalu E. Microbiology of cysts/abscesses of Bartholin's gland: review of empirical antibiotic therapy against microbial culture. J Obstet Gynaecol. 2010;30(7):701–3.
61. Drummond JL, Velasquez BJ, Cross RS, Jones ML. Self-reported comfort in athletic training of gender-specific and non-gender-specific injuries and issues. J Athl Train. 2005;40(3):211–7.

Dermatological Disorders Associated with Sports

26

Renata Ferreira Magalhães, Paulo Eduardo Neves Ferreira Velho, Elisa Nunes Secamilli, Thaís Helena Buffo, Juliana Yumi Massuda Serrano, Tiago Almeida Santos Costa, and Hamilton Ometo Stolf

26.1 Standard Description of Skin Lesions in Dermatology

The dermatological examination is part of the dermatologist's routine, but it should be part of the general practitioner's general physical examination, including in the evaluation of athletes, since many complaints or dermatological findings are common in this group. The dermatological assessment should be carried out with the person not dressed; in an environment with good natural lighting, the entire skin and mucous membranes should be inspected, lesions should be palpated, and complementary techniques such as dermoscopy may be used, mainly to assess lesions suspected of malignancy. Knowing the elementary lesions (Table 26.1) is essential to elaborate diagnostic hypotheses and monitor the evolution of dermatoses [1, 2].

R. F. Magalhães (✉) · Paulo Eduardo Neves Ferreira Velho · E. N. Secamilli T. H. Buffo · J. Y. M. Serrano · T. A. S. Costa · H. O. Stolf
Dermatology Division, Faculty of Medical Science, University of Campinas, Sao Paulo, Brazil
e-mail: renatafm@unicamp.br

S. Rocha Piedade et al. (eds.), *Sideline Management in Sports*,
https://doi.org/10.1007/978-3-031-33867-0_26

Table 26.1 Description of skin lesions

Color change	Macule	Flat, non-palpable lesions <1 cm in diameter
	Erythema	Blanchable redness stain
	Petechiae/purpura/ecchymosis	Non-blanchable, deep red to purple color of varying sizes
	Hyperpigmentation	Darkening of skin color
	Hypopigmentation	Lightening of skin color
Solid lesions	Patch	Flat, non-palpable lesion >1 cm in diameter
	Papule	Solid, elevated, superficial, palpable lesion <1 cm in diameter
	Plaque	Solid, elevated, superficial, palpable lesions >1 cm in diameter
	Nodule	Solid, elevated, deep, palpable lesion >1 cm in diameter
	Tumor	Solid, larger, exophytic, than a nodule >3 cm
Thickness changes	Lichenification	Thickened area of epidermis with accentuated normal skin markings
	Keratosis	Increased thickness of the corneal layer
	Atrophy	Decreased thickness of the epidermis
Liquid content lesions	Abscess	Nodule or tumor with free pus (purulent material)
	Vesicle	Elevated, superficial, clear fluid-filled lesions <1 cm in diameter
	Bullae	Elevated, superficial, clear fluid-filled lesions >1 cm in diameter
	Pustule	Cavitary injury filled with pus
Secondary lesions (caused by outside factors)	Maceration	Area of hyperkeratosis with moisture, with a whitish appearance
	Ulcer	Deep loss and depressed area of epidermis And dermis
	Erosion	Superficial loss of epidermis
	Excoriation	Traumatized, linear or wedge-shaped erosion as a result of scratching, rubbing, and picking
	Scale	Flakes representing heaped-up
	Fissure	Linear crack in skin, which extends into the dermis
	Crust	Scab with dried serum, blood, or pus

Adapted from: Emer et al. [2]

26.2 Introduction

Dermatological disorders resulting from various sports modalities are frequent. The practice of sports can cause skin lesions of various origins, acute or chronic, by repeated mechanical trauma, infectious, or allergic, besides the environmental risk of exposure to various physical and chemical agents and weather conditions, such as cold and ultraviolet radiation. The involvement of the skin can have a significant impact on the athlete's performance. Treatments can also influence the course of physical activity, topical or systemic, causing local and systemic adverse events, absorption, and even doping risk. Chronic skin diseases such as atopic dermatitis or psoriasis may interfere with exercise as well [2, 3].

26.3 Traumatic Injuries

Chronic trauma, friction, and pressure may induce changes in the affected skin acutely or chronically, even leaving sequelae. It commonly occurs on the feet of runners and impact sports players, skaters, and on the hands of sports practitioners such as tennis, hockey, golf, Olympic gymnastics, rowers, and wrestlers [2] (Figs. 26.1, 26.2 and 26.3). The various manifestations of chronic trauma caused by exercise are shown in Table 26.2.

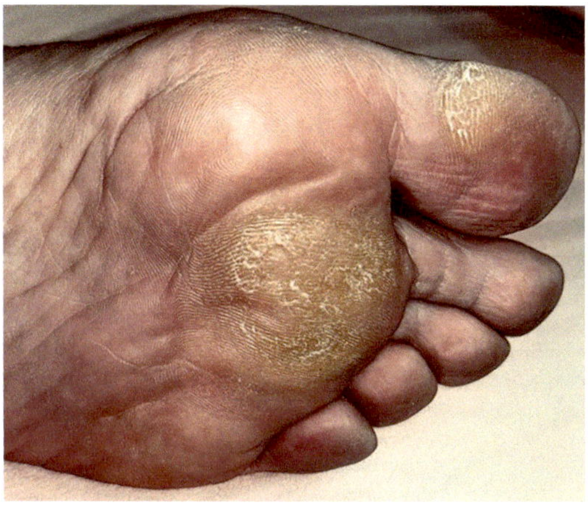

Fig. 26.1 Calluses in the support areas of the runner's foot. (Courtesy: Prof. Dr. Renata Magalhães, Faculty of Medical Sciences, Unicamp)

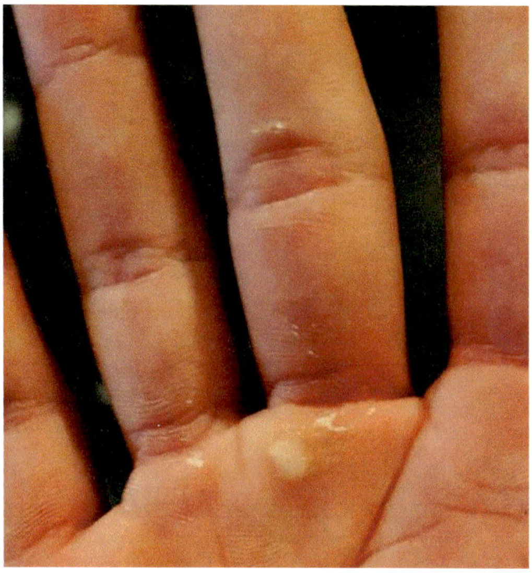

Fig. 26.2 Blistering and peeling due to trauma on training equipment. (Courtesy: Dr. Renata Magalhães, Faculty of Medical Sciences, Unicamp)

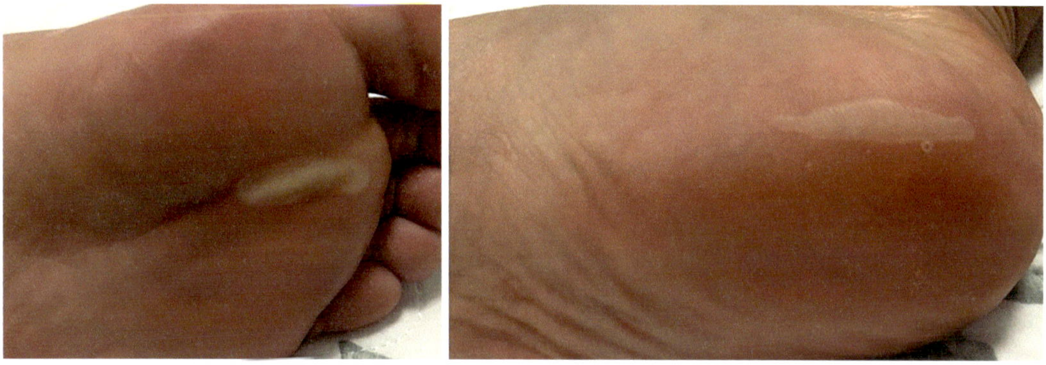

Fig. 26.3 Blisters in the plantar region of the runner. (Courtesy: Dr. Juliana Yumi Massuda Serrano, Faculty of Medical Sciences, Unicamp)

Table 26.2 Cutaneous lesions due to trauma associated with exercising

Type of injury	Mechanism and clinical presentation	Observations
Friction blisters	Continuous friction, even slight, may generate epidermal necrosis or detachment in the dermoepidermal region, forming blisters with clear or hemorrhagic content, more common on the feet, where humidity and heat facilitate its occurrence This is more problematic in skating, where the skates are hard and tight	Prevention with the use of absorbent socks and talcum powder, and use of two socks, one of cotton in contact with the skin and the other of acrylic, besides appropriate footwear according to the athlete's anatomy and the sports activity For established lesions, drain the contents with a needle and leave the roof, three times in 24 h, which accelerates healing; or cover the roofless exulceration with hydrocolloid dressing, which decreases pain and re-epithelialization time

(continued)

Table 26.2 (continued)

Type of injury	Mechanism and clinical presentation	Observations
Callosities	Calluses occur in areas of repeated traumas, usually from previous blisters. They result from defense of bony and tendon prominences to friction. In the feet, they are located on the calcaneus, the metatarsal support, the lateral aspect of the fifth polydactyl, and the interdigital spaces, called soft callus. Most are asymptomatic	Appropriate and comfortable footwear is recommended; keratolytics such as salicylic acid or abrasives may promote temporary benefit The use of orthoses and protection for trauma areas are recommended
Friction dermatitis	Chronic repeated friction in the same area Erythema, papules, or plaques with hyperkeratosis and scaling or lichenification in an area of chronic attrition	It has been described in sumo wrestlers located in the knee/leg or knuckles, in baseball pitchers in the ankle and knee, known as "baseball pitcher's friction" and in the rower's gluteal region, known as "rower's hip," which is due to friction on an unpadded seat or metal machine training
Piezogenic papules	Bilateral 1–5 mm nodules, which form on the sides of the heels by herniation of the subcutaneous tissue, sometimes painful, pressure being an aggravating factor and showing up more evident in the orthostatic position. It may prevent exercise due to pain	Found in long-distance runners, on the feet. On the wrists and palms, where the constant pressure around the hand can cause herniation of subdermal fat, such as gymnastics
Broken ear of judo fighters	Acute inflammatory process with erythema, pain and edema, then liquefaction of the cartilage of the pinna and the deformity of the ear, due to friction and impact on the kimono and tatami	
Artificial turf athlete's hallux (turf toe)	The hallux becomes painful, swollen, and erythematous, resembling acute gout or paronychia. It is an acute tendonitis of the extensor and flexor tendons by the effort in the fast start and stop. Seen in athletes who run on artificial turf, such as football or American football	The treatment is rest and proper footwear for artificial turf
Joggers' nipples	Painful, erythematous nodules on the nipples that crack and may ulcerate. They occur due to friction with synthetic and tight clothing. More commonly seen in women, long-distance runners	Treatment is based on topical cream antibiotics and protection with a soft cotton bandage
Athlete's nodes	Asymptomatic, hypertrophic, skin-colored or erythematous or brownish nodules of 0.5–4 cm, located on the feet, ankles, and hand joints, due to repeated trauma and friction and possibly to foreign bodies with sand and tissue. They are seen in football players, boxers, surfers, and wrestlers, but may appear in any sport Sports-related connective tissue nevi of the collagen type (collagenomas), molecular metabolism of collagen resulting in enhanced synthesis, and/or accumulation of collagen may have a contributory role	Treatment options include conservative measures or surgical intervention. Recurrent trauma and friction to the involved location
Swimmers shoulders	Slightly edematous erythematous plaques on the shoulders of male swimmers from friction with the beard	It is recommended to shave before practicing the sport
Rowers' gluteus	Erythematous, lichenified, and hyperkeratotic plaques in the sacral region, as chronic simple lichen. From prolonged friction with inadequate seating	It is recommended to improve seating comfort
Runners' gluteus	Bruising in the upper intergluteal region in long-distance runners, perhaps due to friction	Disappears spontaneously after a period without training. Use of drying substances may be useful

Table 26.2 (continued)

Type of injury	Mechanism and clinical presentation	Observations
Dancer's cysts	Inflammatory, erythematous, edematous, and painful nodules in the sacral region. They occur due to the practice of exercises on hard surfaces such as platform, mat, and tatami	Differential diagnosis with pilonidal cyst
Ping pong patches	Erythematous patches of 2–3 cm, associated with the high-velocity impact caused by the ball on the forearms and hands	

Adapted from: Emer et al., Levine et al., Mailler-Savage et al., Basler et al., Herring et al., Brennan et al., Singh et al., Dickens et al., Hame et al., Cohen et al., Pharis et al., André et al., Laffitte et al., Koehn et al. [2–16]

26.3.1 Intertrigo

It is an inflammatory condition of the skin folds induced by friction from skin-to-skin friction and aggravated by heat, moisture, and infection. Friction may cause inflammation with maceration and erosion. The condition is often aggravated by secondary infection by bacterial, fungal, or viral agents. It affects intertriginous areas such as the groin, armpits, inframammary and abdominal folds, and the interdigital spaces of the hands and feet. It makes differential diagnosis from other causes of erythema of the folds (inverse psoriasis, seborrheic dermatitis, contact dermatitis, candidiasis, erythrasma, dermatophytosis, histiocytosis, dermatitis due to zinc deficiency, acantholytic dermatoses, etc.) [17].

Dyshidrosis is another frequent cause, mainly in the feet, and can affect the spaces between the toes, associated with hyperhidrosis, atopy, or stress. The diagnosis is clinical, and direct examination with (KOH), culture of skin scrapings, and biopsy can be used to rule out other diagnoses. Treatment is preventive to eliminate friction, heat, and maceration taking precautions to keep skin folds cool and dry. In the installed lesion, drying agents, barrier creams, topical corticosteroids, antifungals, and antibacterials may be needed [2, 18, 19].

26.4 Hemorrhagic Disorders

Seen on the feet of athletes in sports with sudden stops and starts and on the hands of athletes in sports that require a lot of pressure and force, as shown in Table 26.3 (Figs. 26.4 and 26.5).

The treatment consists of avoiding trauma and exaggerated pressure, correcting the technique of movement, using appropriate equipment and proper footwear, and cutting the nails close. Subungual painful hematoma should be treated with drainage, perforating the nail with a needle or scalpel blade 11. X-ray is recommended due to the possibility of associated bone fracture if the pain is intense.

Table 26.3 Hemorrhagic disorders due to the practice of physical exercise

Type of injury	Mechanism and clinical presentation	Observations
Black stitches on ankles (black heel or talon noir)	Petechiae with bilateral linear distribution that forms on the upper portion of the ankle or plantar region, dorsum of the hands and wrists, asymptomatic. The lesions start erythematous and become dark and may be confused with melanoma. Dermatoscopy helps in the diagnosis	Seen in athletes in sports with sudden stops and starts, such as football, basketball, and tennis Treatment consists of superficial excoriation of the skin, removing the superficial layers and hematoma
Blackheads on the hands (black palm or tache noir)	Similar to the previous one but occurs in the palms	Seen on weightlifters, gymnasts, golfers, basketball and tennis players, and mountain climbers
Bruising of the toe of tennis users (tennis toe or jogger's toenail)	Painful subungual hematomas, unilateral or bilateral, which may cause nail dystrophies when long-lasting or recurrent. More common in the hallux and second toe. The differential diagnosis is with melanoma	Seen on tennis players, marathon runners, skiers, climbers, hikers
Skiers' bruises	Stains on the hypothenar region or even the entire palm from pressure due to the grip of the ski pole	
Purple by paintball	Purplish and annular stains at the impact sites of the paintball from the paintball	

Adapted from: Schneider et al., Wilkinson et al., Ayres et al., Dissemomnd et al. [20–23]

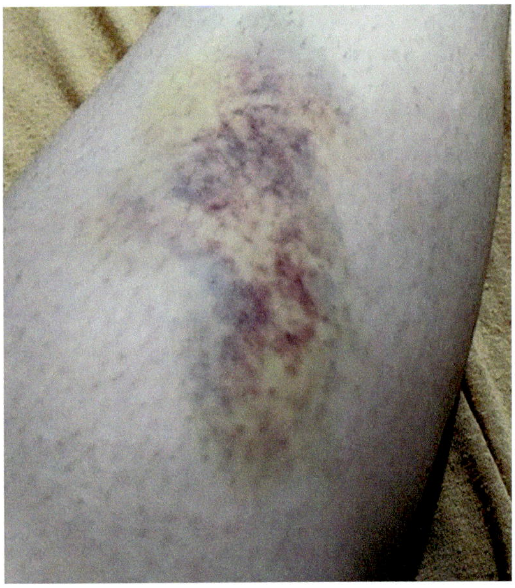

Fig. 26.4 Ecchymosis due to trauma on the leg of a judo fighter. (Courtesy: Dra. Ariany Denofre, Faculty of Medical Sciences, Unicamp)

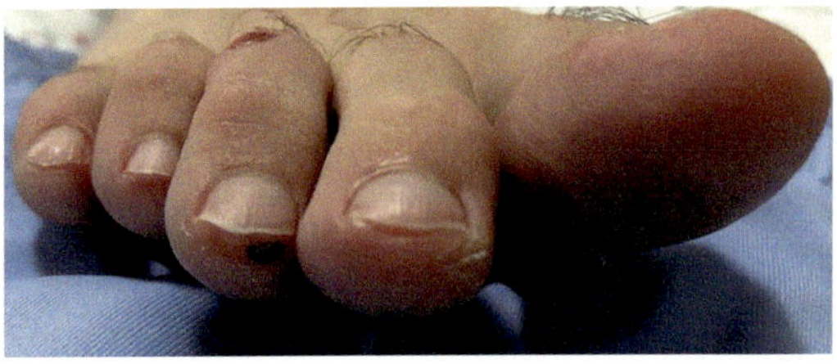

Fig. 26.5 Hemorrhagic blisters on the jogger's toe. (Courtesy: Dr. Juliana Yumi Massuda Serrano, Faculty of Medical Sciences, Unicamp)

26.5 Nails Disorders

Nails are often affected in impact sports such as running, soccer, volleyball, basketball, and ballet, due to external trauma and pressure. The injuries cause pain and make training impossible (Figs. 26.6, 26.7 and 26.8). Table 26.4 shows these main nail alterations (Figs. 26.9, 26.10, 26.11, 26.12, 26.13 and 26.14).

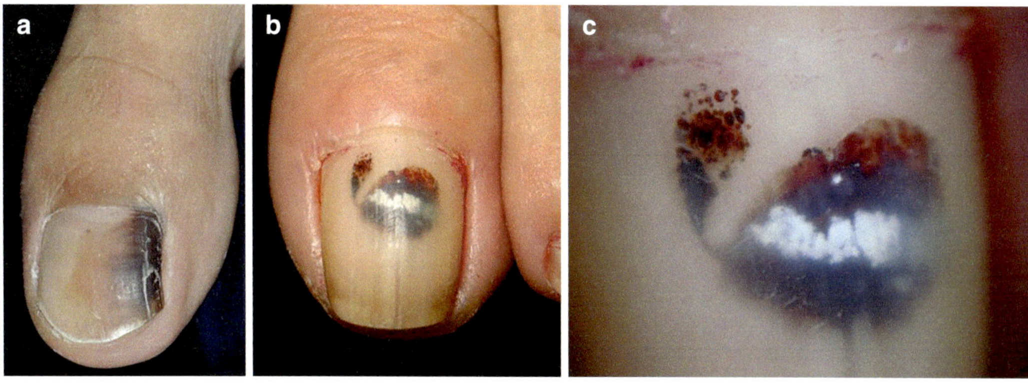

Fig. 26.6 (**a**) Longitudinal pigmented stria on the tennis player's hallux, diagnostic of subungual hematoma, mimicking subungual melanoma. (**b**) Subungual hematoma and (**c**) dermoscopy showing subungual hemorrhage, useful to rule out melanocytic lesions. (Courtesy: Prof. Doctor Hamilton Stolf, Faculty of Medical Sciences, Unicamp)

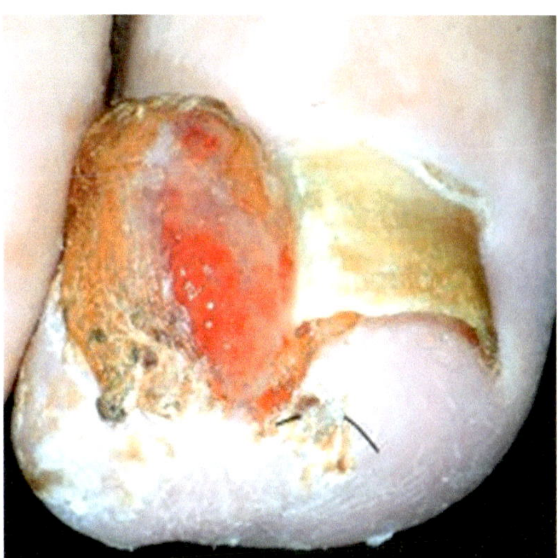

Fig. 26.7 Onychocryptosis and pyogenic granuloma in a soccer player. (Courtesy: Prof. Doctor Hamilton Stolf, Faculty of Medical Sciences, Unicamp)

Table 26.4 Nail changes caused by acute and chronic sports trauma

Onychocryptosis	The ungual plate penetrates the dermis at the lateral nail as a foreign body and causes inflammation, often associated with bacterial infection and purulent secretion, granulation tissue and persistent edema of the lateral nail folds. It is a common and painful condition, regardless of the sport, in young people and adolescents, and it may compromise training and performance. Trauma, ill-fitting shoes, incorrect nail cutting, and nail misalignment are concomitant factors for ingrown toenails (onychocryptosis). Antiseptics, topical antibiotics, and corticosteroids are recommended, as well as straight nail cutting, canthotomy, and partial matricectomy with phenolization or surgical to reduce the width of the nail plate in cases of recurrent grade 2 and 3 ingrown nails

(continued)

Table 26.4 (continued)

Retronychia	Insertion of the nail plate into the proximal nail fold with separation of the nail matrix, followed by inflammation and pain of the proximal nail fold and the formation of a new nail plate under the detached. The "old" nail plate reduces growth and detaches from the nail bed, and a new nail plate forms beneath it often in association with granulation tissue. It is painful and occurs after trauma, mainly in runners or dancers, to the hallux. Dressings and protection and surgical avulsion of the nail are recommended
Onycholysis and dystrophy	Detachment of the nail plate from the distal and/or lateral nail bed (onycholysis), ungual hyperkeratosis, discoloration, and thickening of the nail plate (**dystrophy**) may be a consequence of repeated trauma to the nail and predispose to fungal infection
Fracture or avulsion of the nail plate	Trauma can lead to partial or total fracture of the nail plate or even avulsion. Seen in sports like soccer, running, tennis, basketball, handball, volleyball, ballet, etc. It is recommended to protect the nail bed until the new lamina grows. Depending on the intensity of the trauma and if there is damage to the nail matrix, there is risk of growth of a dystrophic lamina
Golfers nails	Typical linear or punctiform hemorrhage, due to over-pressure gripping of the club

Adapted from: Schneider et al., Mortimer et al. [20, 24]

Table 26.5 Infectious dermatoses seen in athletes and practitioners of sports activities, agents, clinical manifestations, and treatment

Dermatoses and agent	Clinical presentation	Treatment
Folliculitis, furunculosis (*Staphylococcus aureus*)	Folliculitis mainly in areas of terminal hair, of greater sweating and occlusion by equipment or clothing (thighs and buttocks in cyclists), or in athletes who perform regular shaving, thus facilitating penetration of the agent Furunculosis is deeper and painful and leaves depressed scars and abscesses *S. aureus methicillin-resistant* (MRSA) can be transferred to other athletes who may develop active lesions or become asymptomatic carriers of MSRA, harboring the bacteria in their nostrils	Topical antiseptics and antibiotics, oral antibiotics as well as eradication of *S. aureus* from the nostrils with local mupirocin may be necessary Prevention with soaps with antibacterial agents, moisturizing the skin and ventilated cool clothes Avoid humidity and use drying agents such as boric water
Impetigo (*Streptococcus* sp.)	Impetigo, with exudative erosions and crusts Can be transferred between athletes in sports activities with direct skin contact (wrestling, judo) Can be cause of erysipela and cellulitis	Antibacterial agents, moisturizing the skin and ventilated cool clothes Avoid humidity and drying agents
Keratolysis plantare sulcatum (*Kytococcus sedentarius*)	Prolonged occlusion of footwear in athletes with hyperhidrosis, degradation of the keratin of the thicker stratum corneum in the weight-bearing areas of the feet causing small whitish, crater-like depressions that may coalesce to form annular lesions. Asymptomatic, with a bad odor	Treatment includes reduction of hyperhidrosis (aluminum salts), topical antibacterials (benzoyl peroxide, erythromycin or clindamycin) and keratolytics (urea or salicylic acid)
Dermatophytes (*Trichophyton rubrum* and *T. mentagrophytes*)	Erythema, desquamation, active edges, itching Tinea pedis and tinea cruris are more common Interdigital tinea with maceration, erythema, desquamation Moccasin type, with mild erythema and desquamation in the plantar region and lateral skin of the feet Sharing equipment or facilities without protection (showers without slippers)	Avoid occlusion and sweating of the feet Foot drying Antifungal creams such as imidazole or topical terbinafine Oral antifungal for up to 4 weeks
Onychomycosis (same agents as *Tinea pedis*)	Whitish or yellowish nails, generally from the free edge to the proximal region, opaque, thick, up to detachment and hyperkeratosis Differential diagnosis with chronic trauma or inflammatory nail disease such as psoriasis Direct mycological examination is recommended	Topical with solution or enamel for distal and isolated forms Prolonged oral antifungal therapy, more than four months, such as itraconazole and terbinafine

(continued)

Table 26.5 (continued)

Dermatoses and agent	Clinical presentation	Treatment
Tinea gladiatorum (*T. tonsurans*)	Exposed areas of the skin due to infection by direct contact between athletes. Epidemics of dermatophytosis have been described in several judo, wrestling and sumo wrestling teams, with studies confirming interathlete infection	Topical and oral antifungals 2–4 weeks
Herpes simplex virus (HSV) *Herpes gladiatorum*	Vesicles grouped on erythematous base, progress to pustules, erosions and crusts, resolves in 10–14 days It occurs 3–7 days after infection, by contact with active lesion of another athlete	Topical and oral antiviral for 5 days if primoinfection or very intense episode
Human papilloma virus (HPV)	Firm, skin-colored keratotic papules and black dots that correspond to the thrombosed dermal vessel. They may be asymptomatic, but when located in weight-bearing areas of the body, they cause pain when walking or engaging in sports activities, especially plantar warts	Treatment with curettage and topical application of salicylic acid or 5-fluorouracil under occlusion, trichloroacetic acid, nitric acid, cryotherapy, shaving, and electrocoagulation
Molluscum contagiosum	Smooth, shiny, skin-colored or pinkish, asymptomatic, whitish papule of 1–5 mm. More frequent in areas of eczema. Observed in atopic young people and swimmers	Curettage or application of a caustic liquid in each lesion may resolve, but recurrence is frequent
Larva migrans (larva de *Ancylostoma* sp.)	Linear, erythematous, shape-changing, and very itchy papular lesions. Usually on the feet and buttocks. Seen in practitioners of sand sports such as beach tennis and sand football	Thiabendazole creams 50 mg/g, 2–3 times a day until improvement of symptoms, oral ivermectin single dose. Oral albendazole 3 days
Tungiasis (*Tunga penetrans*)	Blackened, pruritic papules of 1–5 mm, usually on the feet Seen in practitioners of sports in the sand	Manual flea extraction
Pediculosis (*Pediculus capitis*)	Presence of nits and lice in the hair, intense itching, and excoriations in the nuchal region Seen in practitioners of sports with close contact as in wrestling or in frequenters of athletes' quarters	Shampoo of permetrine 5%, leave to act and repeat after 7 days
Scabies (*Sarcoptes scabiei*)	Papular, erythematous lesions, some excoriated, presence of tunnels of millimeters in length, located in the axillary folds, breasts, abdomen, buttocks, thighs, wrists, to disseminate. Pruritus. By body-to-body contact or sharing of clothes and equipment	Permethrin lotion 5% topical use on the whole body, wash after 24 h. Repeat for 3 days. Important to treat contacts, change body, bed and bath clothes during treatment

Adapted from: Nowicka et al., Likness and Emer et al. [2, 25, 26]

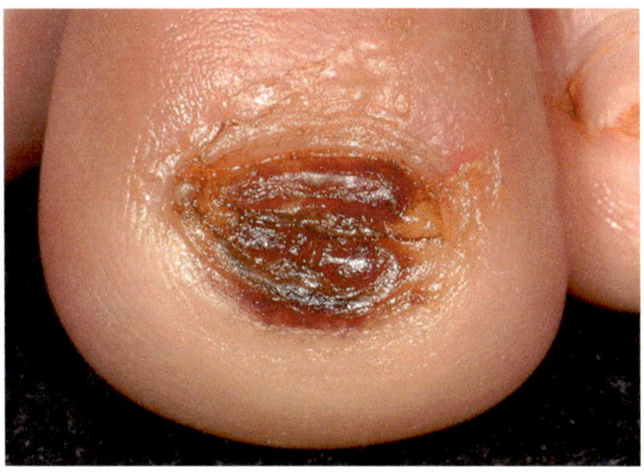

Fig. 26.8 Subungual hematoma and absence of the nail plate after spontaneous avulsion of the second toe in a tennis player. (Courtesy: Prof. Doctor Hamilton Stolf, Faculty of Medical Sciences, Unicamp)

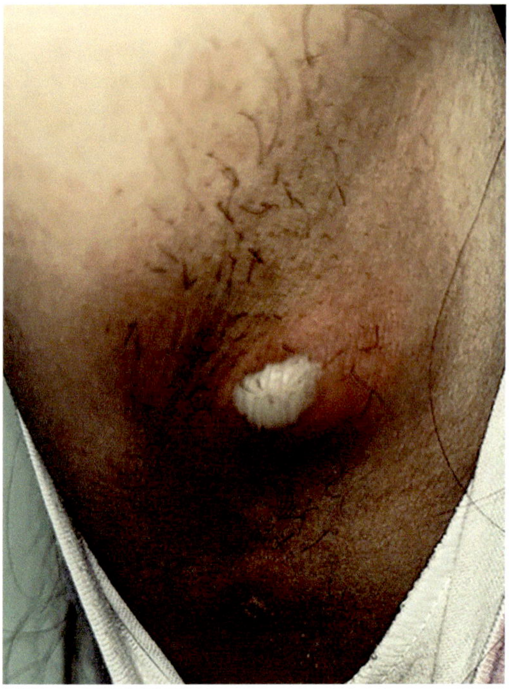

Fig. 26.9 Abscess. (Courtesy: Prof. Dr. Renata Magalhães, Faculty of Medical Sciences, Unicamp)

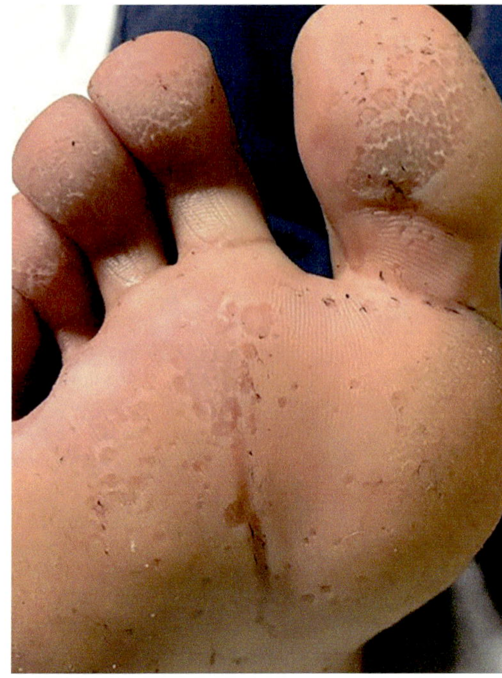

Fig. 26.10 Plantar lesions with rounded depressions accompanied by hyperhidrosis and odor. Keratolysis plantar. (Courtesy: Dr. Elisa Sicamilli, Faculty of Medical Sciences, Unicamp)

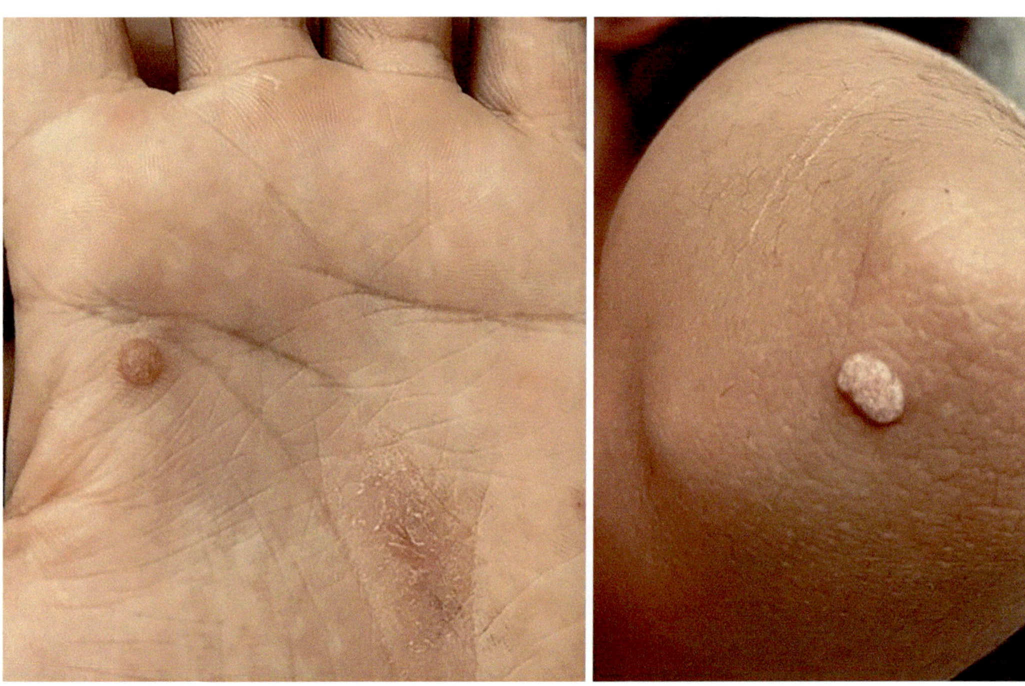

Fig. 26.11 Keratotic papules, diagnosis of viral wart. (Courtesy: Prof. Dr. Renata Magalhães, Faculty of Medical Sciences, Unicamp)

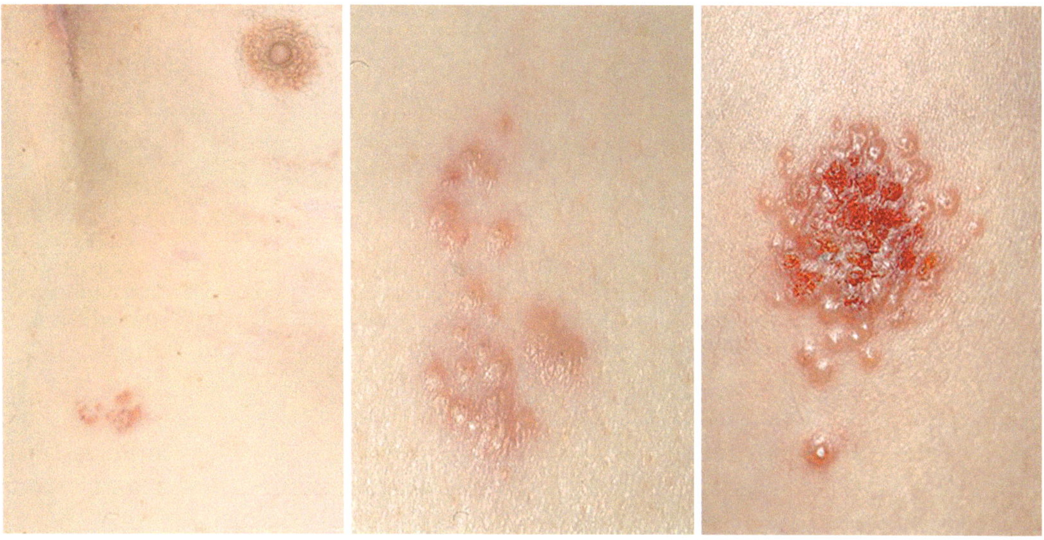

Fig. 26.12 Vesicles on erythematous base on trunk, diagnosis of herpes simplex. (Courtesy: Prof. Doctor Hamilton Stolf, Faculty of Medical Sciences, Unicamp)

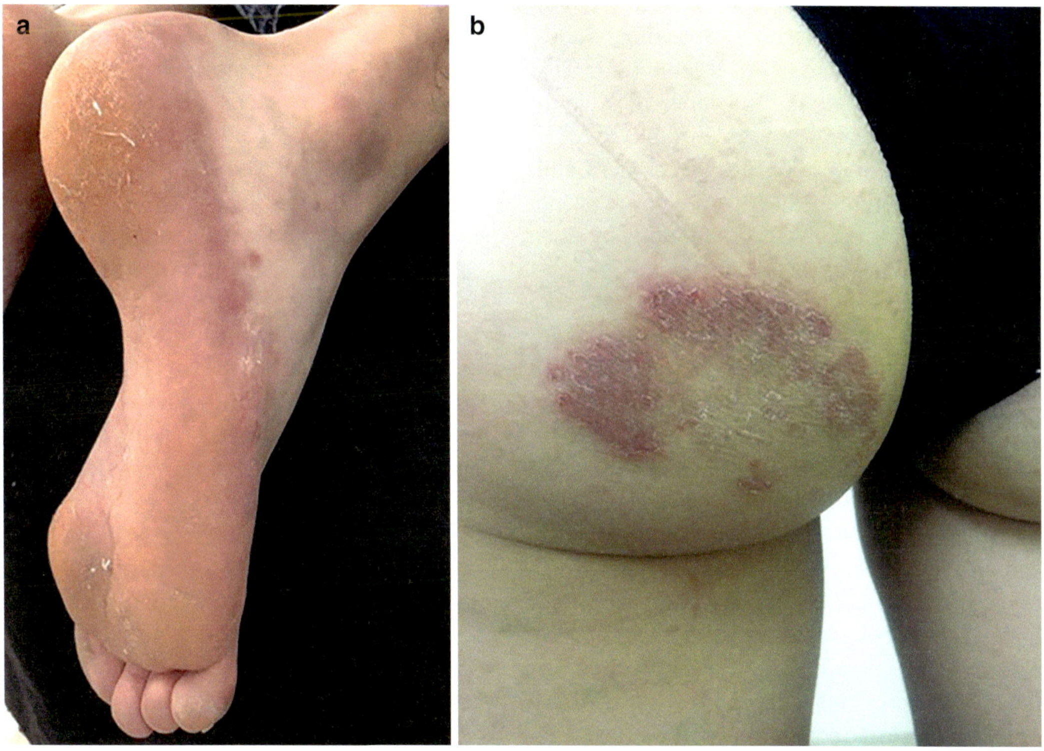

Fig. 26.13 (**a**) Erythema and desquamation on the sole of the foot, mycological examination showing hyphae of dermatophytes, diagnosis of *tinea pedis*. (**b**) Dermatophytosis of the body. (Courtesy: Prof. Doctor Hamilton Stolf, and Prof. Dr. Renata Magalhães, Faculty of Medical Sciences, Unicamp)

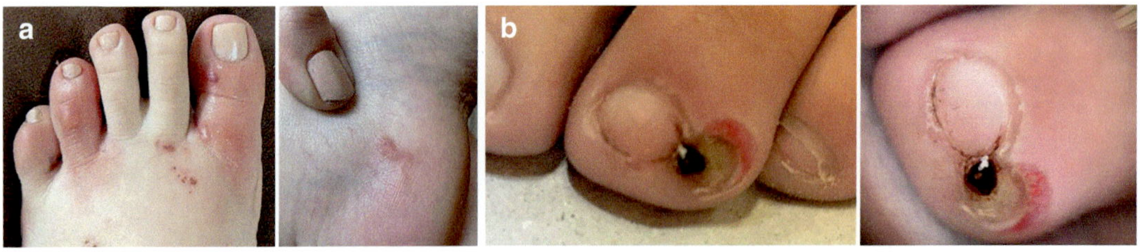

Fig. 26.14 (**a**) Erythematous, papular, linear, pruritic lesions on the dorsum of the fingers and on the medial side of the heel, diagnostic of larva migrans in a beach tennis player. Courtesy: Dr. Elisa Sicamilli, Faculty of Medical Sciences, Unicamp. (**b**) Pigmented papule on the toe, Tunga penetrans, and a dermoscopy image. (Courtesy: Prof. Dr. Hamilton Stolf, Faculty of Medical Sciences, Unicamp)

26.6 Infectious Disorders

Skin infections occur in several sports, either by the transfer of pathogens between athletes through direct contact (wrestling, judo) or by fomites (sharing equipment or facilities) or because activities modify the skin environment, disrupt the skin protective barrier, and/or alter the skin microbiome favoring skin infections (sweating, occlusion, friction, erosions and blisters) [25]. The bacterial, fungal and viral infections most commonly seen in athletes are listed in Table 26.5.

Because of high exposure (swimmers and athletes competing on mats), athletes are prone to a higher risk for mycotic infections by dermatophytes. With close contact during competition, especially wrestlers and judoists, infections by the anthropophilic *Trichophyton tonsurans* are most important (*tinea gladiatorum*) and highly contagious and often cause small epidemics, especially if the primary source of infection is not promptly recognized. The environment of the athletes and asymptomatic carriers may be sources of further spread. Tinea pedis with its clinical manifestations seems to be often underdiagnosed and insufficiently treated. Environmental contamination by fungal spores may be responsible for the significantly higher level of mycotic infections of the feet in children and adolescents active in sports. There is a higher risk of spread of the infection to the toenails. More rarely infections by zoophilic or geophilic dermatophytes are seen in athletes. Education and environmental decontamination are essential for all dermatophytoses associated with sports [25, 27].

About the risk of transmission during sports activity, there are specific recommendations for each type of infection [25, 27].

- Bacterial infections: Avoid contact with other athletes for at least 72 h after starting treatment, but also if there are exudative lesions or if new lesions still appear.
- Herpes infection: Avoid until all lesions are dry and crusted, if you have new lesions or systemic symptoms after 72 h from antiviral start, or wait 120 h from antiviral start.
- Molluscum: Start activity immediately after removal of lesions.
- Infection by dermatophyte fungi: Avoid contacts within 72 h of the start of treatment in the case of skin lesions and 14 days if scalp.
- Pediculosis: Avoid contacts up to 24 h since the beginning of the treatment, provided there are no signs of the agent.
- Scabies: Avoid contacts until at least 24 h from the beginning of treatment or until there are no clinical signs of infestation.

26.6.1 American Tegumentary Leishmaniasis

It can occur in practitioners of sports in forests, such as running, mountain-bike and tree climbing. It is a noncontagious, chronic infectious dis-

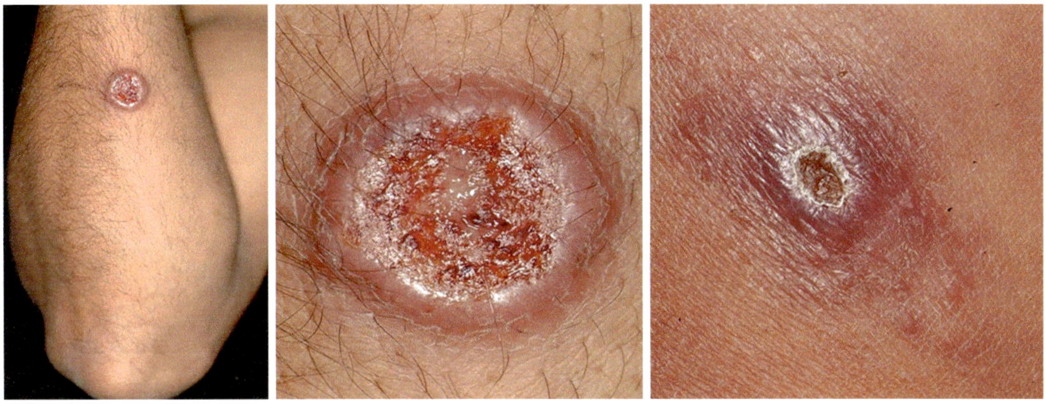

Fig. 26.15 Ulcer with a framed edge, diagnosis of American tegumentary leishmaniasis. (Courtesy: Prof. Doctor Hamilton Stolf, Faculty of Medical Sciences, Unicamp)

ease caused by different species of protozoa of the genus Leishmania that affects the skin and mucosal and naso-buccopharyngeal tissue. It is endemic in 88 countries on five continents, with a worldwide prevalence estimated at 12 million individuals and an incidence of about 600,000 new cases per year. In leishmaniasis in the Americas, several species of sand flies have been reported as vectors of the parasite, whose natural breeding sites include forest areas, tree trunks, and peridomiciliary regions [28–30].

Leishmaniasis infection remains inapparent or asymptomatic in individuals presenting immune resistance. When it evolves into disease, it can present a broad spectrum of clinical manifestations in the skin and/or naso-buccopharyngeal mucosa [29].

The localized form of ATL deserves special attention because it represents the highest percentage of cases (95%) and its great importance in the clinical–immunological unfolding of the disease; the earlier its diagnosis and treatment, the lower the chance of observing more severe forms [29, 30].

The cutaneous form begins after an incubation period of 3–8 weeks, when a papule, nodule or induration appears at the site of the bite. It evolves into an ulcer in its central portion, which gradually increases during the first 3–4 months. The ulcer is characterized by having circular contours, violaceous raised edges and infiltrated, with a coarse granular background, erythematous in color, rarely painful, and with varied diameter. Lesions may occur in several evolutive phases, eventually with satellitosis (flattened and infiltrated papules next to the primary lesion). The lesion may evolve to spontaneous healing or give rise to vegetating and verrucous plaques and nodules [29]. It makes differential diagnosis with several infectious diseases known by the acronym PLECT (Paracoccidioidomycosis, Leishmaniasis, Sporotrichosis, and Tuberculosis) [30].

Confirmation of the diagnosis by demonstrating the agent is important, by smear, culture, pathological examination, or RT-PCR [28, 30].

Treatment is effective, and the first choice drug is pentavalent antimonial (*N*-methyl glucamine) intravenously, at a dose of 15–25 mg of SbV/kg/day (SbV = pure antimony), in 25% glucose serum, infused daily for 6 h, for 20 days. The cycle can be repeated if there is no resolution. Amphotericin B can be used as a second choice [30, 31] (Figs. 26.15 and 26.16).

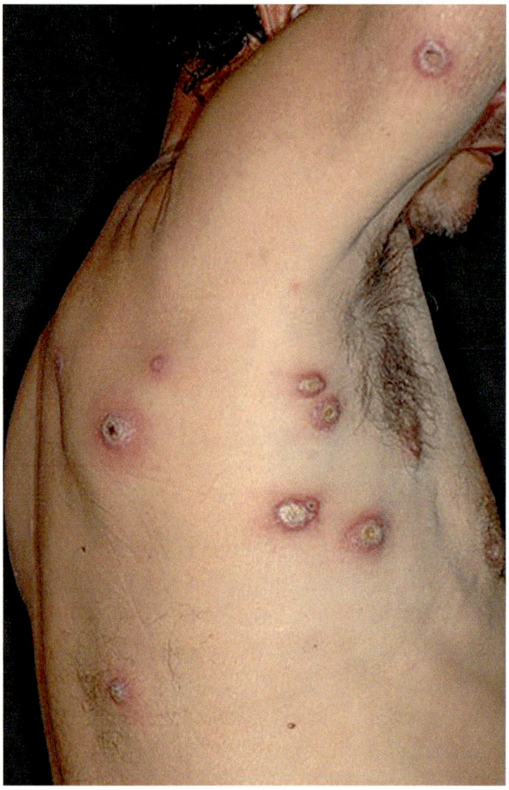

Fig. 26.16 American cutaneous leishmaniasis, disseminated form. (Courtesy: Prof. Doctor Hamilton Stolf, Faculty of Medical Sciences, Unicamp)

26.7 Common Dermatoses Peculiar in Athletes

26.7.1 Acne Mechanica (Sports-Induced Acne)

The most common sports associated with this condition are those that use body protections or head gear, such as American football and hockey, equestrian riders, wrestlers (knee) [5, 32].

Mechanical acne is a papulopustular eruption that simulates acne vulgaris, but is mainly caused by a combination of pressure, occlusion, friction, and/or heat. Stress on the skin appears to be the key element rather than inflammation and hyperkeratinization of the pilosebaceous unit. It is located on the chin, jaw, forehead, neck, or shoulders. It can have association with hormonal or fungal causes. Prevention is recommended, such as wearing moisture-absorbing clothing or clean clothes absorbent cotton shirts under any sports equipment and frequent cleansing of the skin after physical activity. Treatment is similar to other forms of acne with topical or systemic antibiotics, benzoyl peroxide, azelaic acid and topical and systemic retinoids, salicylic acid, and glycolic, trichloroacetic, or resorcinol acid peels. Hair removal, lasers, and microneedle may be indicated. Acne keloidalis nuchae has been described in football players in the occipital region [2].

26.7.2 Rosacea

Rosacea is a chronic inflammatory disease predominantly affecting the centrofacial region (cheeks, chin, nose, and forehead) and the eyes, characterized by recurrent episodes of flushing, persistent erythema, inflammatory papules/pustules, and telangiectasia (Fig. 26.17). Phymatous changes are infrequent, occurring primarily at the nose (rhinophyma). More than half of patients with rosacea have ocular features including dryness, foreign body sensation, photophobia, conjunctivitis, and blepharitis. It is more frequent in northern European descent It can affect athletes who play sports in cold or hot environments and can be exacerbated by extremes of temperature and heat [33]. It is recommended to avoid extreme temperatures, topical and oral metronidazole, topical ivermectin, oral doxycycline, or minocycline, and new biologic agents have been studied. Also, lasers can be used [33].

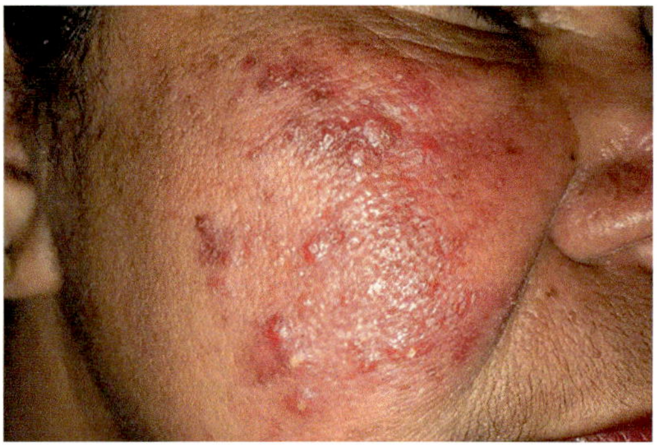

Fig. 26.17 Rosacea. (Courtesy: Prof. Dr. Renata Magalhães, Faculty of Medical Sciences, Unicamp)

26.7.3 Alterations by Food Supplements

Athletes and practitioners of physical activity often supplement proteins, vitamins, and anabolic steroids to improve their performance, causing cutaneous manifestations related to their use [34].

Little is found in the literature about whey protein supplementation and dermatoses. However, studies have related milk protein intake to postprandial insulin and basal insulin growth factor (IGF1) elevation. In addition, when stimulated with whey protein-derived amino acids, enteroendocrine K cells secrete glucose-dependent insulinotropic peptide and stimulate insulin secretion by pancreatic beta cells. Increased insulin and IGF1 activate the phosphatidylinositol 3-kinase pathway, reduce the nuclear amount of the FoxO1 transcriptional factor, and lead to androgen receptor activation, comedogenesis, increased sebaceous lipogenesis, and follicular inflammation, which clinically manifests as acne [34].

The supraphysiological supplementation of anabolic–androgenic steroids (AAS) is better studied. A study conducted in Germany found that 13.5% of gym-goers use AAS substances, and in the USA, among amateur bodybuilders, 80% of men and 40% of women use these substances [35].

Acne is the main side effect reported (Fig. 26.18). The lesions are distributed over the face, shoulders, and chest, do not respond to conventional therapy, and may persist for months after discontinuation of use. There are androgen receptors in sebocytes and follicular keratinocytes. Studies show that AAS increase the size of the sebaceous gland and sebum production, change sebum quality by increasing the percentage of cholesterol and free fatty acids, and promote abnormal follicular keratinization, leading to the formation of comedo. The *Cutibacterium acnes* population is increased while using AAS. Progression to acne fulminans is reported [35, 36] (Fig. 26.18).

Atrophic striae (striae distensae) is related to the anabolic effect of AAS, due to muscle hyper-

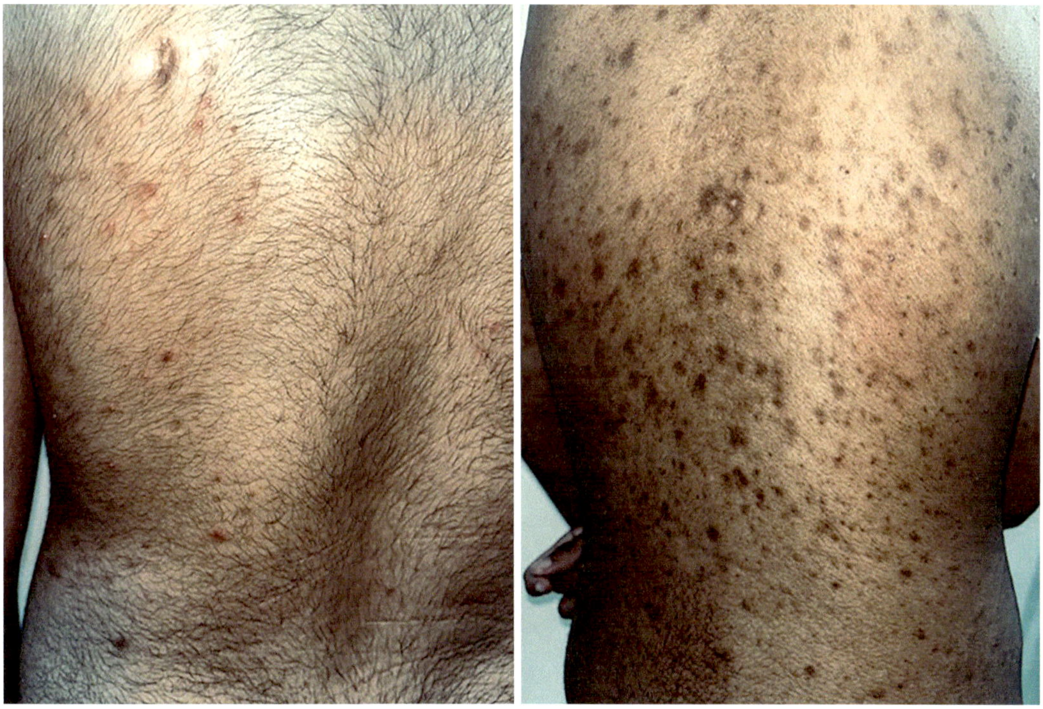

Fig. 26.18 Steroid-induced acne. (Courtesy: Prof. Dr. Renata Magalhães, Faculty of Medical Sciences, Unicamp)

trophy with consequent skin distension and reduction of skin elasticity. The most common sites are neck, chest, shoulders, and upper limbs. Linear keloids have already been described and result from decreased degradation and increased synthesis of type 1 collagen [36].

AAS affect the skin appendages. **Hirsutism** and development or worsening of androgenetic **alopecia** in women or men are described. Other dermatoses are also more frequent in AAS users, such as **gingival hyperplasia, skin infections, rosacea, epidermal cysts, angiolipoma, seborrheic dermatitis, and oiliness** of the skin and hair. It is postulated that oilier skin may lead to increased colonization by Malassezia furfur and increased prevalence of pityriasis versicolor [36].

Patanè et al. [37] performed a systematic review of the side effects of nandrolone decanoate, a drug with a potent anabolic and mild androgenic effect because it is inactivated by 5 alpha-reductase. In this review, the most common skin effects were pruritus, acne, and hyperchromic spots.

Wollina et al. [38] describe a number of cases of side effects of topical or injectable AAS use, such as hirsutism, stretch marks, acne, seborrheic dermatitis, and gynecomastia.

Besides the dermatoses already mentioned, we can mention less prevalent diseases already reported. Cocca and Viviano reported a case of **Stevens–Johnson syndrome** associated with the injectable use of drostanolone propionate, stanozolol, and methenolone enanthate. Pai et al. reported the case of a *Mycobacterium fortuitum* infection in an immunocompetent adult at the site of an anabolic steroid injection (the substance used was not cited). In older reports, exacerbation of psoriasis and induction of acute hereditary coproporphyria are also described [36].

The main therapeutic measure is the suspension of AAS use. The dermatoses described can be treated according to their usual drugs and the authors emphasize the importance of hepatic evaluation before prescribing systemic medications such as antibiotics, isotretinoin, or antiandrogens [35].

26.8 Allergic Conditions

26.8.1 Reactions to Insect Bites

They appear as erythematous and edematous, pruritic papules, and plaques on exposed areas, sometimes with a central vesicle. In some cases, there may be strophilic, i.e., dissemination of similar lesions by sensitization, associated with pruritus. They should be conducted with local cleaning care, topical corticoids if very intense, since they are self-limited. Topical or injectable promethazine should be avoided for its phototoxic potential.

26.8.2 Contact Dermatitis

Eczema is characterized by erythematous lesions, with vesicles in the **acute phase**, desquamation in the **subacute** phase, and lichenification in the **chronic** phase, associated with pruritus. It may be triggered by primary irritation or by sensitization, i.e., participation of acquired immunity after repeated contact with the allergenic substance. Repeated contact with sports equipment (clothing or devices), associated with heat and sweating, may increase the release of allergens from the equipment to the athlete's skin and induce sensitization [39–41].

Immediate reactions with urticaria or angioedema may occur, mainly related to equipment with latex (rubber suits, elastic bandages) [39].

Most cases of allergic contact dermatitis (ACD) are due to chemicals (nickel, rubber chemicals, resins, fragrances, condoms, etc.) and do not occur on first exposure, and it may take several hours or days after contact before lesions appear [39, 42, 43].

Acute lesions may resolve in a few days after removal of the causative allergen, and topical or systemic corticosteroids and antihistamines may be used depending on the intensity of symptoms [39]. Recurrent conditions require investigation through patch testing to identify the agent and arrange for removal or substitution of the substance. In many cases, it is very important to do patch testing in addition to the standard battery with fragments of the equipment or products to which the athlete was exposed [39].

The main agents of allergic contact dermatitis in athletes are as follows

- Chromium of natural leather, rubber chemicals (thiuram, carbamates, mercapto and thiourea derivatives, paraphenylenediamine (PPD), and other compounds) or glues (*p*-butyl phenol-formaldehyde resin). Footwear can be a frequent cause of ACD with lesions that are located on the soles and/or dorsum of the feet and interdigital spaces.
- Thiourea derivatives in rubber are the main allergens of neoprene and diving suits, goggles, and other equipment.
- Black rubber derivatives have been reported as allergens on bicycle handlebars in cycling and swimming fins. Contact dermatitis may resolve leaving long-lasting achromia, simulating vitiligo.
- Acetophenone azine was identified in shin splints causing injuries to pretibial face soccer players [44].
- Colophonium is used in chalk dust to improve the grip of gymnasts' hands.
- Epoxy resin, is used in tennis rackets and as varnish in billiard cues.
- Nickel is found in many gym equipment and can induce eczema of the hands and other locations such as shoulders, arms, and neck in weight lifters.
- Topical medications, anti-inflammatory drugs, antibiotics, and antiseptics or cosmetics can cause dermatitis through direct application to the skin, exposure to contaminated clothing, or contact with a colleague's treated skin [44].

26.8.3 Urticaria

Urticaria is characterized by erythematous, edematous, migratory, and pruritic lesions that occur due to degranulation of mast cells in the dermis and release of histamine and other inflammatory mediators, causing vasodilation of vessels in the upper dermis and causing edema in the dermis. When it affects deep dermis and subcutaneous tissue, angioedema occurs, with an increase of volume in eyelids and lips or other places less commonly. It may be acute, lasting up to 6 weeks, or chronic, lasting longer, continuous, or intermittent. Most often there is a trigger such as an infectious agent or medication, less commonly food or environmental antigens. There are hives of physical causes, triggered by contact with water, cold, vibration, and exercise. These cases may appear during certain physical activity and may be limiting for the athlete [45].

The condition should improve with exercise cessation within hours, and high-dose antihistamines may be necessary to control symptoms or prevent a risk situation [45].

Urticaria is classified into varieties depending on the stimulus (cholinergic, cold, solar, pressure, and aquagenic), and many patients may have a combination. These patients present with itching, burning, tingling, heat, or irritation that precedes the appearance of numerous small (1–4 mm in diameter) pruritic papules with large surrounding eruptions. The papules may occur anywhere on the body and disappear within hours or after removal of the trigger [45].

Cholinergic urticaria is one of the physical hives caused by the stimulation of perspiration, although some consider it secondary to the elevation of the athlete's body temperature [46]. Treatment includes rapid cooling, systemic antihistamines or leukotriene antagonists or corticosteroids, immunotherapy with anti-immunoglobulin E (omalizumab), danazol or, in severe cases, the use of cyclosporine, mycophenolate mofetil, or methotrexate. Patients with cholinergic urticaria should avoid precipitating factors, including exercise and any activity that causes sweating, such as elevated room temperature, hot food, sauna baths, immersion in hot water, and emotional stress [46].

A severe form of activity-exacerbated hives is **exercise-induced anaphylaxis** (EIA), which commonly occurs in atopic or food allergy patients who are also well-conditioned athletes. It develops briefly after exercise with cutaneous pruritus, erythema, and urticaria and then progresses to include angioedema, respiratory distress, gastrointestinal symptoms (nausea, diarrhea, vomiting), and possible vascular collapse. Several mechanisms have been suggested, including histamine- and complement-mediated pathways. In a large retrospective study of EIA cases, 78% of participants noted that running induced their injuries [2, 47, 48].

Individuals reduced their attacks by avoiding exercise in extremely hot or cold weather (44%), avoiding ingestion of certain foods before exercise (37%), and restricting exercise during allergy season (36%) or humid weather (33%). Athletes should learn to avoid the use of certain medications (aspirin and non-drug anti-inflammatory drugs) and foods (wheat, vegetables and shellfish) that could potentiate an attack [2, 49].

Cold urticaria is a type of physical urticaria that results from allergic response to cold, leading to pruritic erythematous lesions with or without angioedema within minutes after exposure to cold environments, activities in cold water, ingestion of cold food, and even contact with cold objects. It is classified into primary or essential (>90%); secondary or acquired, associated with cryoglobulinemia or paroxysmal hemoglobinuria; rarer are delayed cold-induced hives, which occurs 9–18 h after exposure to cold and a familiar cold urticaria in which patients develop an urticarial rash, fever, arthralgia, and conjunctivitis within a few hours. They may have systemic symptoms including fatigue, headache, dyspnea, and tachycardia, rarely anaphylaxis [50].

Cold urticaria affects men and women equally with most patients presenting in young adulthood. It can be diagnosed by the ice cube test (an ice cube is applied to the skin for about 10–20 min, the test is positive if a papule appears in that time). However, approximately 20% of patients have a negative ice cube challenge test.

They may be prophylactically treated with antihistamine medications and may have epinephrine autoinjector in case of anaphylaxis [2, 20].

26.8.4 Anaphylaxis

According to World Allergy Organization Anaphylaxis Guidance 2020, anaphylaxis is highly likely when either of the following two criteria is met [51]:

1. Acute onset of illness (minutes to several hours) with simultaneous involvement of skin, mucous membranes, or both (e.g., generalized urticaria, pruritus or flushing, swollen lips lingual–void);
   And at least one of the following:
   (a) Respiratory compromise (dyspnea, wheezing-bronchospasm, stridor, reduced PEF, hypoxemia).
   (b) Reduced PA or associated symptoms of target organ dysfunction (hypotonia, syncope, incontinence).
   (c) Severe gastrointestinal symptoms (severe colicky abdominal pain, repetitive vomiting).
2. Acute onset of hypotension or bronchospasm or laryngeal involvement following exposure to a highly probable allergen for that patient (minutes to several hours), even in the absence of typical skin symptoms [52].

Anaphylaxis is an acute, life-threatening condition that can occur in the physician's everyday life (Fig. 26.19). Exercise-induced anaphylaxis (EIAn) is characterized by a condition that occurs during physical exercise, with typical symptoms and signs, without other possible triggers. The typical picture includes sudden fatigue, heat, flushing, generalized urticaria, and pruritus. In severe cases, acute angioedema, upper airway obstruction, and shock are observed. These symptoms may occur at any time during exercise and occasionally after. Awareness of this condition is necessary to properly educate patients, reduce the risks, and improve their quality of life [2, 53].

If patients with allergies do not have an identifiable trigger (e.g., food, pollen, alcohol or temperature) that can be avoided, they are strongly recommended to exercise under supervision and to warm up beforehand. If initial symptoms of anaphylaxis appear, it is recommended to stop immediately. Generalized pruritus and the increase in symptoms by exercise favor the diagnosis [2, 53, 54].

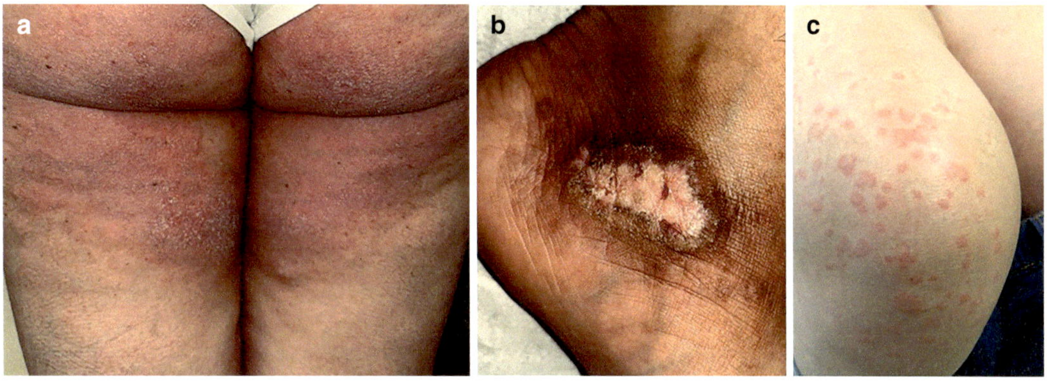

Fig. 26.19 (**a**) Erythematous, scaly, pruritic lesions, diagnosis of subacute contact eczema. (**b**) Lichenified plaque on the medial malleolus, diagnosis of chronic contact eczema. (**c**) Erythematous and edematous lesions, migratory, typical of urticaria. (Courtesy: Prof. Dr. Renata Magalhães, Faculty of Medical Sciences, Unicamp)

Important differential diagnoses are cholinergic urticaria, systemic mastocytosis, hypertryptasemia, cold-induced anaphylaxis, exercise-associated reflux, cardiovascular events, exercise-induced bronchoconstriction, hypoglycemia, neoplastic disorder, postural orthostatic tachycardia syndrome, and exercise exacerbation of primary food allergy.

Treatment is based on rest and rapid infusion of 0.9% sodium chloride, and even epinephrine may be required in severe cases. For patients with frequent and severe symptoms, antihistamines may be useful before activity or continuously. The prognosis is favorable, but there are reports of fatal cases, due to comorbidity or underdiagnosis. Recognition of early signs of anaphylaxis, potential triggers, and modification of exercise habits may control the risk. Intramuscular epinephrine injection for may be recommended for people at high risk or with intense symptoms [52, 54, 55].

26.9 Disorders of Environmental Causes (Light, Sun, Hives, Cold)

Several environmental factors may lead to dermatological manifestations when engaging in high-altitude activity in the mountains. At higher outdoor altitude there is more exposure to cold, as air temperature decreases by approximately 2 °C for every increase in 310 m (1000 ft), as well as low humidity, high wind speed, and excessive exposure to ultraviolet (UV) light [20, 56].

26.9.1 Cold

Playing winter sports with inadequate protection or in very extreme conditions (mountain trekking, ice skating) or water sports in cold water can induce cold-related dermatoses, as shown in Table 26.6.

There are four overlapping phases in the pathogenesis of freezing

- Pre-freezing, tissue decreases in temperature causing vasoconstriction and ischemia, which manifests as hyperesthesia and paresthesia.
- During the freeze-thaw cycle, ice crystals form in the extracellular medium slower or intracellular medium faster, causing cell membrane lysis and apoptosis.
- Vascular stasis, in which vessel oscillations between constriction and dilatation result in leakage and coagulation.
- Late ischemia, which initiates a cellular cascade and increases inflammation by the release of thromboxane A2, prostaglandin F2-alpha, bradykinin, and histamine, causing destruction of the microcirculation, which also leads to cell death [20, 57, 58].

Table 26.6 Injuries caused by cold, clinical manifestations and prognosis

Type of injury	Clinical feature and mechanism	Prognosis
Frostbite	Freezing injury, intraepidermal icicles facilitate cellular damage and death; erythema, vesicles, and eschar	Reversible damage to surgical intervention
Frostnip	Non-freezing injury associated with severe vasoconstriction—icicle formation on skin's surface causing temporary pallor	No long consequences
Trench-foot	Non-freezing injury to feet, from erythema to edema, bullae and gangrene—paresthesias and numbness	Worse prognosis
Chilblains (perniosis)	Non-freeing injury characterized by painful or pruritic erythematous papules—painful or pruritic erythematous papules	Resolves over weeks
Cold panniculitis	Non-freezing injury of tender erythematous areas of induration	Resolves over weeks
Raynaud's phenomena	Vasoconstrictive disorder—skin discoloration ranging from white to blue (cyanosis) to red (rewarming)	Long-term-disease, prevention can avoid future crisis, common in patients with lupus or other rheumatic conditions
Cold urticaria	Physical urticaria triggered by cold-erythematous pruritic papules or plaques	Antihistamine or rarely epinephrine if anaphylaxis

Adapted from: Schneider et al. [20]

It is important to estimate the severity in order to think about treatment and exercise interruption. There are two classification schemes to describe the severity of frostbite: The four classic grades based on acute physical findings after warm-up and the simpler field classification are as follows:

- First- or second-degree freezing: superficial, leaving no or minimal expected tissue loss;
- Third- and fourth-degree freezing: deep, with loss of tissue [20, 58, 59].

Treatment is rapid rewarming in all patients, and prognosis depends on tissue demarcation after 3–4 weeks of healing. Adequate protection from cold is recommended, with proper clothing and equipment, planning of activities, avoidance of smoking, and other factors that induce vasoconstriction. Vasoconstriction phenomena can benefit from calcium channel blockers, sildenafil and platelet antiaggregant and anticoagulants in extreme cases. Also, surgical debridement may be necessary in cases of necrosis [59, 60].

26.9.2 Heat

Heat exposure occurs primarily from heat treatment for sports injuries and can induce various acute and chronic lesions (Table 26.7).

26.9.3 Water

It can be seen in swimmers, surfers and divers. **Water** exposure in susceptible individuals, mainly women, can induce skin damage by several mechanisms, such as loss of the lipid mantle causing xerosis and eczema, besides barrier breakdown, humidity, and maceration, facilitating infections [5]. Several skin alterations are caused in athletes by prolonged contact with water, mainly in susceptible people or with previous dermatoses, as shown in Table 26.8.

26.9.4 Accidents with Marine Animals

It can be seen in water marathoners, surfers, and divers. Accidents involving aquatic invertebrate animals (especially marine animals) reach their peak during the summer due to the higher number of humans in the water, lack of information, and care for these animals. Bathers constitute more than 90% of the victims, and the incidence of this type of accident is 0.1%, or 1 in 1000, in emergency units. Among the victims, approximately 50% are swimmers who step on sea urchins and present traumatic accidents, 25% are swimmers who have contact with cnidarians (Portuguese jellyfish and caravels), and 25% are fishermen injured by poisonous fish such as catfish and rays. Water sports athletes are exposed to these accidents as well (Table 26.9).

Wounds may be stinger-like punctures with spines or rare spines (mandis, stingray, sea urchins, scorpionfish, and toadfish), hives-like eruptions (jellyfish, Portuguese men-of-war, corals, and anemones) or eczema (marine and freewater sponges, marine warms, sea cucumbers) and lacerations with cyanosis or pallor (catfish, marine, or freshwater stingrays) or pain (sharks, morays, piranhas) (Fig. 26.20).

Table 26.7 Injuries caused by heat

Dermatological condition	Treatment
Burns Erythema, blisters, local pain	Wound care, cleaning, debridement if deeper burns, silver sulfadiazine, and other topical healing compounds, plus monitoring for infection and analgesia
Erythema *ab igne* Erythematous or brownish, reticulated patches in areas of chronic heat contact	Avoid contact with hot surfaces such as compresses or physiotherapy equipment, moistening, photoprotection, monitoring for the risk of developing carcinomas in the region
Miliaria Erythematous vesicles and superficial, asymptomatic or slightly pruritic micropapules due to sweat accumulation in eccrine ducts, folds, or dorsum	Cool environment, cold compresses, and topical corticosteroid creams if very intense and long-lasting
Heat urticaria	Transitory, self-limited, antihistamines

Adapted from: Schneider et al., Dissemond et al. [20, 23]

Treatment depends on the agent's accident [61]

- Immersion in hot water for 30–90 min (50 °C), extraction of spicules and fragments, anesthetic infiltration, tetanus prophylaxis, and imaging exam if does not improve.
- Washing the site or compresses with saltwater ice, apply vinegar (acetic acid), analgesia. Do not use fresh water.
- Extensive washing and exploration for removal of fragments.
- Antibiotic therapy and tetanus prophylaxis should always be employed.

26.9.5 Lightning Accidents

It may affect practitioners of extreme sports, mountaineering, climbing, and runners. Lightning is the second leading cause of storm-related deaths, affecting up to 400 people annually in the United States, most commonly men (>80%) between the ages of 20 and 45, with mortality estimated at 10% of cases. Lightning can have

Table 26.8 Dermatoses caused by exposition to water during exercising

Dermatoses	Clinic manifestation	Recommendations
"Water sports hands" or aquagenic acrokeratoderma	Papules on the palms and soles, keratotic and hypopigmented after submersion in water. Symptoms include a burning pain, hyperhidrosis, but disappear as the skin dries	Skin drying
Dry skin of swimmers	Dry skin, especially in winter, due to prolonged immersion and reduction of the lipid mantle	Moisturizing
Green hair	More frequent in children and men with light skin and hair. Due to copper present in algaecides and pipes or chlorine used in water treatment	Treatment is with hydrogen peroxide 2–3% for 30 min

Adapted from: Basler et al. [5]

Table 26.9 Accidents caused by marine animals, agents, clinical manifestations, and treatment

Agents	Clinical manifestation	Treatment
Sponges	Eczematous reaction at the site of contact, with erythema, edema, vesicles and blisters, itching, and pain, resolving in 2 weeks. May be accompanied by polymorphous erythema after a few days	Spike extraction with tape, topical corticoid, antihistamine
Jellyfish (Cnidarians)	Animals with tentacles and with nematocysts. Pain, papuloerythematous rash and linear urticarial plaques, sometimes vesicles, blisters, and superficial necrosis. Rarely pulmonary edema and death	Compress saltwater frost for 10 min, acetic acid (vinegar), remove remaining tentacles
Linuche unguiculata (*cypromedusae planulae larvae*) Swimmer's itch	Papuloerythematous, pruritic eruption in the region covered by the bathing costume, during or after exposure to seawater Seen in the Caribbean Sea, Mexico, Florida, Brazil. Trapping of larvae that release nematocysts. Rarely, fever nausea, vomiting, diarrhea, headache, more in children	Antihistamines, topical corticosteroids Resolution in 1 or 2 weeks
Sea urchin, cucumber, and starfish	Accidents by penetration of thorns, with erythema, edema, and papules, vesicles, and even superficial necrosis. Some species have venom with hypotensive, cardio and neurotoxic and hemolytic action. Risk of bacterial infection and tetanus	Immediate removal of the spicules with forceps and local anesthesia, diluted ammonia may help dissolve residuals. Tetanus prophylaxis and antibiotic therapy
Corals	Cuts, eczematous and irritative reactions, foreign body reactions	Removal of foreign bodies, cleaning and topical corticosteroids if necessary

Adapted from: Haddad et al. [61]

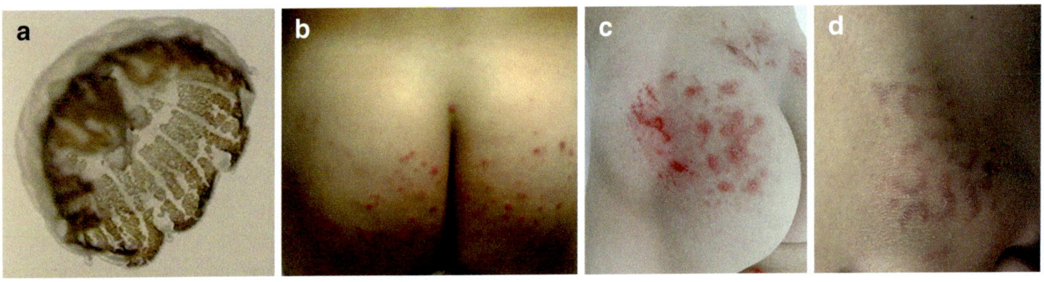

Fig. 26.20 (**a**) *Linuche unguiculata*. Courtesy: Fábio Lang da Silveira. (**b**, **c**) Seabather's eruption, by *Linuche unguiculata*. Courtesy: Prof. Dr. Vidal Haddad Junior, Botucatu School of Medicine, Sao Paulo, Brazil, and André Luiz Rossetto, Universidade do Vale do Itajaí, Santa Catarina, Brazil. (**d**) Coral dermatosis, Dr. Elisa Secamilli. Faculty of Medical Sciences, Unicamp

positive or negative charge and direct or alternating current. A single lightning strike contains 30,000–110,000 A. However, the energy is only applied for a few milliseconds creating little opportunity for transfer to the body [20, 62].

There are several types of injury mechanisms: direct, by contact (when lightning strikes an adjacent object that touches the patient), lateral splash (when the current bounces off a nearby object), and current ground (when lightning travels along the ground and strikes the patient) [20, 62].

The amperage that the patient receives determines the severity of the injury. A low amperage injury can lead to paresthesia, while a high amperage injury can cause ventricular fibrillation or cardiac arrest [20, 62].

After a lightning strike, an initial assessment of cardiac and respiratory function is paramount, followed by the initiation of cardiopulmonary resuscitation while awaiting emergency medical service.

The dermatological manifestations are as follows

- **Lichtenberg's figure**, pathognomonic finding, an erythematous lesion in a fern pattern, known as a lightning tree burn or fringe. It is considered a physical manifestation of lightning and not a true burn. It usually appears within an hour of the lightning strike and resolves within 24–48 h.
- **Linear burns**, from sweat vaporized during the current causing a partial thickness burn (flashover).
- **Punctiform burns**, at the site of the lightning strike exit causing a circular. Larger full-thickness burns, when a patient is in contact with an object that has been struck by lightning or by clothing melting secondary to lightning [63–65].

It is recommended to prevent these kind of accidents: examine weather pattern and storm signs such as clouds, increased wind, thunder. Signs of impending lightning include blue haze around objects (known as St. Elmo's fire), static electricity on the skin or hair, smell of ozone, or a popping sound nearby. In the city, the recommendation is to seek shelter indoors. Outdoors should avoid being in high-risk areas such as on summits, tall objects, or in isolated areas such as trees. Isolation should be attempted by getting up from the ground by sitting on a backpack (after removing any metal), wrapped dry rope or a foam sleeping pad. Groups should spread out to avoid mass casualties.

Treatment is routine burn care, with cleansing, healing, dressing, and debridement if necessary [20, 62].

26.9.6 Ultraviolet Light

Solar radiation is composed of three components: approximately 50% visible light, 40% infrared light and 9% ultraviolet radiation. Ultraviolet radiation (UV) is the cause of damage when discussing solar dermatological exposures [66].

There are three types of UVR light classified by the wavelengths they emit: UVA (320–400 nm), UVB (280–315 nm), and UVC (200–290 nm). The most important types of UVR in relation to exposures are UVA and UVB, since UVC is filtered by the ozone layer. Only about 5% of UVB reaches the Earth's surface, and it damages the DNA of the keratinocyte. UVB exposure causes pyrimidine dimers of cyclobutane and pyrimidone, pyrimidone photoproducts, which leads to errors in DNA repair creating the potential for oncogenesis [20, 66].

Outdoor sports in areas of high ultraviolet (UV) radiation (beaches, sea, mountains, spots, snow) for a long time, without protection, can induce acute lesions such as **sunburn from erythema to blisters, and chronic ones such as spots, aging, and skin cancer**.

26.9.6.1 Phototoxic and Photoallergic Reactions

Phototoxic and photoallergic reactions may occur in athletes with phototypesetting and vitiligo or exposed to plants containing phototoxic chemicals (fig trees, *Ruta graveolens*) during outdoor activities or under treatment with topical or systemic photosensitizing drugs (tetracyclines, quinolones, amiodarone, phenothiazines, psoralens). Photoallergic reactions are of an eczematous pattern, with erythema, vesiculation, desquamation and pruritus, in exposed areas or widespread, in people sensitized by drugs such as piroxicam and other NSAIDs, fenofibrate, quinolones, thiazides, cyclins). Treatment consists of adequate photoprotection, antihistamines, and topical or systemic corticosteroids in severe cases [20].

26.9.6.2 Prolonged Exposure Dermatosis

Prolonged exposure dermatosis is a phenomenon recently described by Totten et al. (2015). An observational study of 74 participants in a ski class in Wyoming showed that 26% of the participants had similar lesions, described as pale edematous papules and erythematous plaques with erosions and crusts, on the face in 90% of the cases. The lesions occurred after approximately 8 days of exposure and resolved within 10 days. The affected individuals had no history of polymorphous eruption to light [67].

26.9.6.3 Actinic Prurigo

It is a pruritic eruption induced by sunlight and at higher altitudes that may occur in all races, although it is particularly common in Native Americans. It often develops in childhood with good resolution, but in some cases may persist into adulthood. These are intensely pruritic papules, sometimes with vesicles and crusts that appear on sun-exposed areas, particularly on the face, neck, and limbs. It is thought to be possibly a persistent variant of polymorphous eruption to light. Photoprotection is recommended in the prevention of outbreaks, and treatment is with topical corticosteroids, topical tacrolimus, narrow-band UVB, and PUVA in an attempt to desensitize, chloroquine, and oral thalidomide [20].

26.9.6.4 Seborrheic Dermatitis

Seborrheic dermatitis is a mild chronic inflammatory skin condition affecting areas of the skin with more sebaceous glands. Increased sebum production and the presence of the yeast *Malassezia furfur play* a role in the pathogenesis. Adult seborrheic dermatitis is considered the most common type of eczema affecting 2–5% of the population, it occurs by the fourth to seventh decade of life, and there is a higher incidence in men. Erythematous lesions and yellowish fatty scales are observed on the scalp, in the creases of the face, eyebrows, sternum and upper back, or in the axillary and inguinal folds. UV radiation may aggravate seborrheic dermatitis. A study in the 1990s examined the prevalence of seborrheic dermatitis in mountain guides in Austria, Switzerland, and Germany and found that 16.3% had seborrheic dermatitis and attributed it to UV-induced immunosuppression due to their chronic occupational exposure or difficulty with hygiene or alterations by topical products [20].

26.10 Skin Cancer

Skin cancer is the most common type of cancer in the United States with approximately two million new diagnoses each year. Sunburn from UV exposure tends to be the precursor to all skin cancers. Environmental factors can increase the amount of UVR including higher altitudes such as clear skies and reflective surfaces such as snow, sand, and water. Daily UV radiation increases by 32% (UVB increases by 17–22% and UVA by 11%) for every 1000 m above sea level during winter [68].

Athletes performing regular outdoor activities under high sun exposure (cycling, marathon, tennis, sailing) who are chronically exposed to UV light have an increased risk of skin cancer.

Athletes show little knowledge about the increased risk of skin cancer and consequently use inadequate protective measures. Competition organizers in many outdoor sports also demonstrate ignorance of this risk, as they continue to perform these activities in hours with high UV index. In addition to avoiding times of day with higher UV light (11–16 h) and favoring shaded areas, athletes should choose appropriate clothing and regularly apply waterproof sunscreens composed primarily of toasty filters. A single application of a sunscreen screen, particularly in water sports or in situations with intense perspiration, is inadequate, as some of the creams will be removed with water/perspiration and many filters lose their UV protection efficacy after some time of irradiation [20, 69].

The most important risk factors include Fitzpatrick phototypes I–III, cumulative or intermittent exposure to ultraviolet (UV) radiation, immunosuppression, and smoking, among others [70]. Exposure to UV radiation constitutes the most relevant causal factor, identifying two patterns of sun exposure: one occupational, related more to chronic exposure; and the other recreational, related more to sporadic intense exposures and history of sunburn [71, 72].

The main types of cutaneous neoplasms are **basal cell carcinoma (BCC), squamous cell carcinoma (SCC), and melanoma**.

- BCC is an epithelial tumor characterized by clusters of basaloid cells of slow growth, rarely evolving to metastases, but with great potential for local destruction. It is mainly associated with intermittent sun exposure throughout life (Fig. 26.21).

- SCC is the second most common type of skin cancer, associated with chronic cumulative sun exposure. It is formed by an atypical proliferation of keratinocytes and is related to a higher risk of cartilage and bone infiltration and metastasization (Fig. 26.22).
- Melanoma is a malignant neoplasm of melanocytes with a higher risk of metastasis and mortality (Fig. 26.23).

In addition to skin tumors, the preneoplastic lesions, such as actinic keratosis, are also related to this chronic exposure and present risk for progression over the years to SCC.

Exposure to UV radiation is known to be the most important modifiable risk factor for the development of skin tumors, and outdoor sports have increased this exposure time [73]. Consequently, the increased incidence of skin cancer has also been attributed to changes in lifestyle, with many populations receiving intermittent sun exposure due to the increasing popularity of outdoor recreation and leisure activities. Several studies address sun protection habits in athletes, sun protection practices, attitudes, and knowledge on the subject among them [74].

A Spanish observational study conducted among paralympic sailors showed that the majority (76.8%) reported a history of sunburn in child-

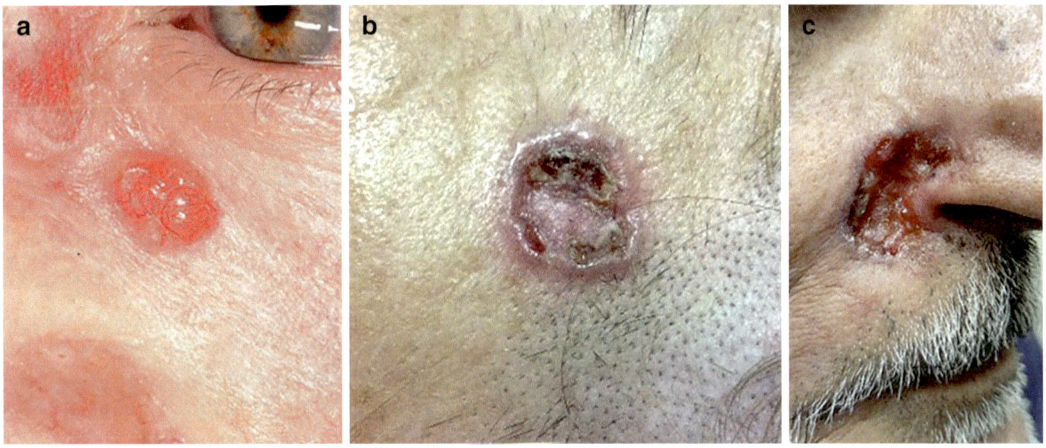

Fig. 26.21 (**a**) Smooth, shiny erythematous papule, diagnostic of basal cell carcinoma. Courtesy: Prof. Doctor Hamilton Stolf, Faculty of Medical Sciences, Unicamp. (**b**, **c**) Ulcerated tumor in a sun-exposed area, diagnostic of infiltrative basal cell carcinoma. (Courtesy: Dr. Thaís Helena Buffo, Faculty of Medical Sciences, Unicamp)

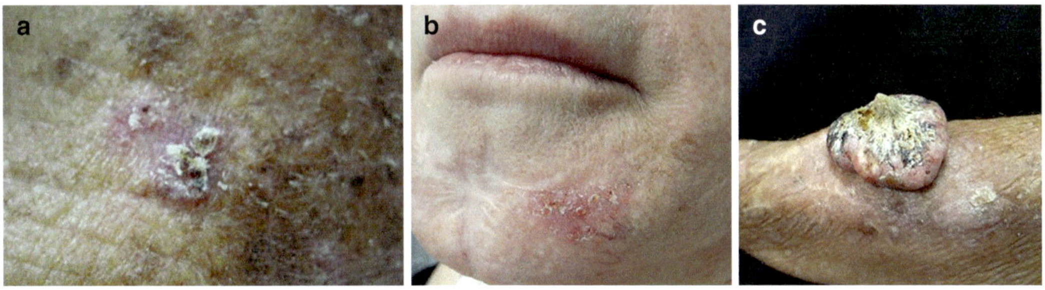

Fig. 26.22 (**a**) Keratotic papules on the forearms, diagnostic of actinic keratoses on a field of cancerization. (**b**) Erythematous and mildly keratotic plaque, diagnostic of carcinoma in situ or Bowen disease. (**c**) Tumor with a keratotic center in a sun-exposed area, diagnostic of invasive squamous cell carcinoma. (Courtesy: Dr. Thaís Helena Buffo, Faculty of Medical Sciences, Unicamp)

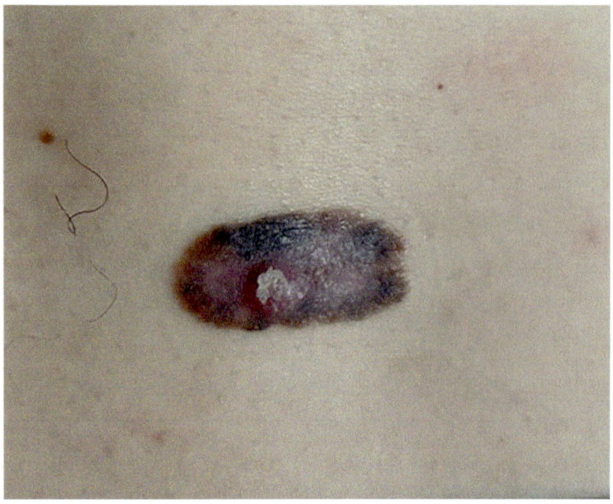

Fig. 26.23 Pigmented lesion, with various colors and irregular outline in the lumbar region, diagnostic of superficial extensive melanoma. (Courtesy: Dr. Thaís Helena Buffo, Faculty of Medical Sciences, Unicamp)

hood, one of the risk factors for skin cancer, including melanoma. They also reported that, despite using sunscreen, sunglasses, and hats, they were not in the habit of reapplying the sunscreen and avoiding the sun at peak risk times [75].

Another Spanish study, among kitesurfers, an aquatic sport whose practitioner is exposed not only to direct sunlight, but also to the reflection of the water surface, aggravating the impact of solar radiation on the skin. Among the 72 athletes, 69.4% were Fitzpatrick phototypes I and II, practiced the activity for more than 10 years for an average of almost 14 h per week with episodes of sunburn [76].

One of the factors that increase overexposure to UV radiation is the performance of outdoor sports. These athletes perform long training and competition sessions outdoors and, in addition, sweating due to physical exertion can facilitate sun damage by having a magnifying effect of UV radiation on the skin and, therefore, increase the risk of sunburn and skin cancer. Training in the central hours of the day, altitude in the case of mountain runners, the absence of shade, and the type of sports clothing they wear for each training session are other factors that increase the risk [77].

Elite athletes in water sports often make inadequate use of photoprotection measures and suffer frequent episodes of sunburn. This puts them at high risk of skin damage. Continuous contact with fast-moving water makes sunscreen lotions come off more easily or irritate the eyes, making their use difficult [76].

It is estimated that up to 80% of skin cancer cases can be prevented by reducing sun exposure and using protective measures, such as sunscreen, hats, sunglasses and long-sleeved shirts, when activities are performed outdoors on sunny days [78, 79].

A specific group of patients with higher risk of developing skin cancer due to the use of immunosuppressive therapies are transplanted patients. As in the general population, they can also be exposed to the sun during sports and leisure activities, with an increased risk of sunburn. In addition, the tumors may behave more aggressively in these patients. Risk factors that need to be assessed in this population are time to transplant, duration, and intensity of immunosuppressive therapy, personal and family history of cancer, history of sun exposure, and episodes of sunburn since childhood [80].

Sun protection behaviors and attitudes are extremely important to reduce the effects caused. The use of photoprotectors, appropriate clothing, hats, and sunglasses should be encouraged. Awareness-raising campaigns on the risk of excessive sun exposure directed specifically to this target audience, especially regarding the increased risk of developing skin cancer, are needed in order to improve their protection habits and reduce sunburn rates associated with the practice of sports.

26.11 Photoprotection

Photoprotection should be used by all sports practitioners regardless of phototype and location.

- Sunscreen application should be regardless of the UV index (UVI), as prolonged exposure at lower levels can still result in high exposure and sunburn and increase the cumulative risk of aging and cancer.
- Avoid exposure at midday (10 a.m.–2 p.m.).

- There are clothes that provide broad spectrum UV protection and protection against visible light. Athletes should take advantage of sport-specific clothing advantages, such as surfing vests.
- Protective hats or caps, adapted to the sport, are essential, and sunglasses, when possible.
- Sunscreen should have at least SPF 30. SPF is a measure of UVB protection (SPF 30 means it would take 30 times longer for erythema to develop vs unprotected skin), but sunscreen should be broad spectrum to include balanced UVA protection.
- Higher SPFs, (50–100), are beneficial for snow sports and water sports such as surfing or sailing. Organic physical filter is also recommended for skin prone to spots and cancer and for people with photosensitivity.
- It should be applied in sufficient quantity (approximately 2 mg/cm^2) at least 30 min before exposure and should be reapplied every 2 h, especially in water sports.
- Secondary performance attributes are important: sunscreens that are easy to spread, non-greasy, non-sticky, suitable for use on wet skin, non-irritating to eyes, sweat resistant, and do not cause loss of grip are best suited for athletes.
- Routine self-examination of the skin and consultation at least once a year.
- Avoid photosensitizing agents.
- Oral supplementation with antioxidants (polypodium leucotomos, nicotinamide) should be considered, but does not replace sunscreen application and physical measures.
- Use of personalized indicators such as UV detection stickers or apps to track UV exposure could increase appropriate sunscreen use.
- Campaigns.
- Uniform/clothing policies to ensure skin coverage and eye photoprotection at clubs and competitions.
- Visual and verbal alert to remind athletes to wear and reapply sunscreen during training or competition.
- Sunscreens should be readily available in accessible places, such as changing rooms and side of pitch.
- It is important that those involved in sports (coaches, trainers etc.) encourage athletes to protect themselves from the sun, for example.
- Use of elite athletes as role models.
- Organizers can send advance reminders to sporting event participants to bring sunscreen and protective clothing (e.g., text message, email).
- Sunscreen advertising can be used to inform users, participants or viewers how to properly apply sunscreen [81].

References

1. Schwarzenberger K. The essentials of the complete skin examination. Med Clin N Am. 1998;82(5):981–99.
2. Emer J, Sivek R, Marciniak B. Sports dermatology: part 1 of 2 traumatic or mechanical injuries, inflammatory conditions, and exacerbations of pre-existing conditions. J Clin Aesthet Dermatol. 2015;8(4):31–43.
3. Levine N. Dermatologic aspects of sports medicine. J Am Acad Dermatol. 1980;3(4):415–24.
4. Mailler-Savage EA, Adams BB. Skin manifestations of running. J Am Acad Dermatol. 2006;55(2):290–301.
5. Basler RS. Skin injuries in sports medicine. J Am Acad Dermatol. 1989;21(6):1257–62.
6. Herring KM, Richie DH Jr. Friction blisters and sock fiber composition. A double-blind study. J Am Podiatr Med Assoc. 1990;80(2):63–71.
7. Brennan FH Jr. Managing blisters in competitive athletes. Curr Sports Med Rep. 2002;1(6):319–22.
8. Singh D, Bentley G, Trevino SG. Callosities, corns, and calluses. BMJ. 1996;312(7043):1403–6.
9. Dickens R, Adams BB, Mutasim DF. Sports-related pads. Int J Dermatol. 2002;41(5):291–3.
10. Hame SL, Melone CP Jr. Boxer's knuckle. Traumatic disruption of the extensor hood. Hand Clin. 2000;16(3):375–80.
11. Cohen PR, Eliezri YD, Silvers DN. Athlete's nodules: sports-related connective tissue nevi of the collagen type (collagenomas). Cutis. 1992;50(2):131–5.
12. Redbord KP, Adams BB. Piezogenic pedal papules in a marathon runner. Clin J Sport Med. 2006;16(1):81–3.
13. Pharis DB, Teller C, Wolf JE Jr. Cutaneous manifestations of sports participation. J Am Acad Dermatol. 1997;36(3 Pt 1):448–59.
14. André R, Laffitte E. Piezogenic pedal papules. Presse Med. 2019;48(1 Pt 1):88.
15. Koehn GG. Skin injuries in sports medicine. J Am Acad Dermatol. 1991;24(1):152.
16. Tlougan BE, Mancini AJ, Mandell JA, Cohen DE, Sanchez MR. Skin conditions in figure skaters, ice-hockey players and speed skaters: part II—cold-

induced, infectious and inflammatory dermatoses. Sports Med. 2011;41(11):967–84.
17. Fragola LA Jr, Watson PE. Common groin eruptions: diagnosis and treatment. Postgrad Med. 1981;69(5):159–63.
18. Janniger CK, Schwartz RA, Szepietowski JC, Reich A. Intertrigo and common secondary skin infections. Am Fam Physician. 2005;72(5):833–8.
19. Mistiaen P, Poot E, Hickox S, Jochems C, Wagner C. Preventing and treating intertrigo in the large skin folds of adults: a literature overview. Dermatol Nurs. 2004;16(1):43–6.
20. Schneider S, Levandowski CB, Manly C, Dellavalle R, Dunnick CA. Wilderness dermatology: mountain exposures. Dermatol Online J. 2017;23(11):13030.
21. Wilkinson DS. Black heel a minor hazard of sport. Cutis. 1977;20(3):393–6.
22. Ayres S Jr, Mihan R. Calcaneal petechiae. Arch Dermatol. 1972;106(2):262.
23. Dissemond J, Grabbe S. Eritema ab igne. Intern Med J. 2008;38:675.
24. Mortimer PS, Dawber RP. Trauma to the nail unit including occupational sports injuries. Dermatol Clin. 1985;3(3):415–20.
25. Nowicka D, Bagłaj-Oleszczuk M, Maj J. Infectious diseases of the skin in contact sports. Adv Clin Exp Med. 2020;29(12):1491–5.
26. Likness LP. Common dermatologic infections in athletes and return-to-play guidelines. J Am Osteopath Assoc. 2011;111(6):373–9.
27. Zinder SM, Basler RS, Foley J, Scarlata C, Vasily DB. National athletic trainers' association position statement: skin diseases. J Athl Train. 2010;45(4):411–28.
28. Barbosa JF, de Figueiredo SM, Monteiro FM, Rocha-Silva F, Gaciele-Melo C, Coelho SS, et al. New approaches on Leishmaniasis treatment and prevention: a review of recent patents. Recent Pat Endocr Metab Immune Drug Discov. 2015;9(2):90–102.
29. Sabzevari S, Mohebali M, Hashemi SA. Mucosal and mucocutaneous leishmaniasis in Iran from 1968 to 2018: a narrative review of clinical features, treatments, and outcomes. Int J Dermatol. 2020;59(5):606–12.
30. Manual de vigilância da leishmaniose tegumentar. Brasil. 2017. https://bvsms.saude.gov.br/bvs/publicacoes/manual_vigilancia_leishmaniose_tegumentar_americana_2edicao.pdf.
31. Mokni M. Cutaneous leishmaniasis. Ann Dermatol Venereol. 2019;146(3):232–46.
32. Kang YC, Choi EH, Hwang SM, Lee WS, Lee SH, Ahn SK. Acne mechanica due to an orthopedic crutch. Cutis. 1999;64(2):97–8.
33. van Zuuren EJ, Arents BWM, van der Linden MMD, Vermeulen S, Fedorowicz Z, Tan J. Rosacea: new concepts in classification and treatment. Am J Clin Dermatol. 2021;22(4):457–65.
34. Melnik BC. Evidence for acne-promoting effects of milk and other insulinotropic dairy products. Nestle Nutr Workshop Ser Pediatr Program. 2011;67:131–45.
35. Melnik B, Jansen T, Grabbe S. Abuse of anabolic-androgenic steroids and bodybuilding acne: an underestimated health problem. J Dtsch Dermatol Ges. 2007;5(2):110–7.
36. Walker J, Adams B. Cutaneous manifestations of anabolic-androgenic steroid use in athletes. Int J Dermatol. 2009;48(10):1044–8.
37. Patanè FG, Liberto A, Maria Maglitto AN, Malandrino P, Esposito M, Amico F, et al. Nandrolone decanoate: use, abuse and side effects. Medicina (Kaunas). 2020;56(11):606.
38. Wollina U, Pabst F, Schönlebe J, Abdel-Naser MB, Konrad H, Gruner M, et al. Side-effects of topical androgenic and anabolic substances and steroids. A short review. Acta Dermatovenerol Alp Pannonica Adriat. 2007;16(3):117–22.
39. Fisher AA. Sports-related allergic dermatitis. Cutis. 1992;50(2):95–7.
40. Ventura MT, Dagnello M, Matino MG, Di Corato R, Giuliano G, Tursi A. Contact dermatitis in students practicing sports: incidence of rubber sensitisation. Br J Sports Med. 2001;35(2):100–2.
41. Kockentiet B, Adams BB. Contact dermatitis in athletes. J Am Acad Dermatol. 2007;56(6):1048–55.
42. Marzario B, Burrows D, Skotnicki S. Contact dermatitis to personal sporting equipment in youth. J Cutan Med Surg. 2016;20(4):323–6.
43. Corazza M, Schenetti C, Schettini N, Catani M, Cavazzini A, Borghi A. Contact dermatitis due to boxing gloves. Dermatitis. 2021;32(6):e107–e8.
44. Raison-Peyron N, Sasseville D. Acetophenone azine. Dermatitis. 2021;32(1):5–9.
45. Antia C, Baquerizo K, Korman A, Bernstein JA, Alikhan A. Urticaria: a comprehensive review: epidemiology, diagnosis, and work-up. J Am Acad Dermatol. 2018;79(4):599–614.
46. Fukunaga A, Washio K, Hatakeyama M, Oda Y, Ogura K, Horikawa T, et al. Cholinergic urticaria: epidemiology, physiopathology, new categorization, and management. Clin Auton Res. 2018;28(1):103–13.
47. Hough DO, Dec KL. Exercise-induced asthma and anaphylaxis. Sports Med. 1994;18(3):162–72.
48. Shadick NA, Liang MH, Partridge AJ, Bingham IC, Wright E, Fossel AH, et al. The natural history of exercise-induced anaphylaxis: survey results from a 10-year follow-up study. J Allergy Clin Immunol. 1999;104(1):123–7.
49. Carlsen KH, Anderson SD, Bjermer L, Bonini S, Brusasco V, Canonica W, et al. Exercise-induced asthma, respiratory and allergic disorders in elite athletes: epidemiology, mechanisms and diagnosis: part I of the report from the Joint Task Force of the European Respiratory Society (ERS) and the European Academy of Allergy and Clinical Immunology (EAACI) in cooperation with GA2LEN. Allergy. 2008;63(4):387–403.
50. Hochstadter EF, Ben-Shoshan M. Cold-induced urticaria: challenges in diagnosis and management. BMJ Case Rep. 2013;2013:bcr2013010441.
51. Cardona V, Ansotegui IJ, Ebisawa M, El-Gamal Y, Fernandez Rivas M, Fineman S, et al. World allergy

organization anaphylaxis guidance 2020. World Allergy Organ J. 2020;13(10):100472.
52. Shaker MS, Wallace DV, Golden DBK, Oppenheimer J, Bernstein JA, Campbell RL, et al. Anaphylaxis-a 2020 practice parameter update, systematic review, and Grading of Recommendations, Assessment, Development and Evaluation (GRADE) analysis. J Allergy Clin Immunol. 2020;145(4):1082–123.
53. Nolte K, Van Rensburg CJ. Exercise-induced anaphylaxis. Curr Allergy Clin Immunol. 2010;23:78–80.
54. Namiki H. Exercise-induced anaphylaxis in an elderly patient. BMJ Case Rep. 2017;2017:bcr-2017-222297.
55. Hoffman M, Murphy M, Koester MC, Norcross EC, Johnson ST. Use of lifesaving medications by athletic trainers. J Athl Train. 2022;57(7):613–20.
56. Bergeron MF, Bahr R, Bärtsch P, Bourdon L, Calbet JA, Carlsen KH, et al. International Olympic Committee consensus statement on thermoregulatory and altitude challenges for high-level athletes. Br J Sports Med. 2012;46(11):770–9.
57. Monseau AJ, Reed ZM, Langley KJ, Onks C. Sunburn, thermal, and chemical injuries to the skin. Prim Care. 2015;42(4):591–605.
58. Sallis R, Chassay CM. Recognizing and treating common cold-induced injury in outdoor sports. Med Sci Sports Exerc. 1999;31(10):1367–73.
59. McIntosh SE, Campbell A, Weber D, Dow J, Joy E, Grissom CK. Mountaineering medical events and trauma on Denali, 1992–2011. High Alt Med Biol. 2012;13(4):275–80.
60. Murphy JV, Banwell PE, Roberts AH, McGrouther DA. Frostbite: pathogenesis and treatment. J Trauma. 2000;48(1):171–8.
61. Haddad V Jr. Environmental dermatology: skin manifestations of injuries caused by invertebrate aquatic animals. An Bras Dermatol. 2013;88(4):496–506.
62. Davis C, Engeln A, Johnson EL, McIntosh SE, Zafren K, Islas AA, et al. Wilderness Medical Society practice guidelines for the prevention and treatment of lightning injuries: 2014 update. Wilderness Environ Med. 2014;25(4 Suppl):S86–95.
63. Mahajan AL, Rajan R, Regan PJ. Lichtenberg figures: cutaneous manifestation of phone electrocution from lightning. J Plast Reconstr Aesthet Surg. 2008;61(1):111–3.
64. Nagesh IV, Bhatia P, Mohan S, Lamba NS, Sen S. A bolt from the blue: lightning injuries. Med J Armed Forces India. 2015;71(Suppl 1):S134–7.
65. Mutter E, Langley A. Cutaneous Lichtenberg figures from lightning strike. CMAJ. 2019;191(9):E260.
66. Baron ED, Suggs AK. Introduction to photobiology. Dermatol Clin. 2014;32(3):255–66.
67. Totten JE, Brock DM, Schimelpfenig TD, Hopkin JL, Colven RM. Prolonged exposure dermatosis: reporting high incidence of an undiagnosed facial dermatosis on a winter wilderness expedition. Wilderness Environ Med. 2015;26(4):525–30.
68. Lichte V, Dennenmoser B, Dietz K, Häfner HM, Schlagenhauff B, Garbe C, et al. Professional risk for skin cancer development in male mountain guides—a cross-sectional study. J Eur Acad Dermatol Venereol. 2010;24(7):797–804.
69. Moyer VA. Behavioral counseling to prevent skin cancer: U.S. Preventive Services Task Force recommendation statement. Ann Intern Med. 2012;157(1):59–65.
70. Estimativa 2020: incidência de câncer no Brasil Rio de Janeiro. 2019. https://www.inca.gov.br/sites/ufu.sti.inca.local/files/media/document/estimativa-2020-incidencia-de-cancer-no-brasil.pdf.
71. Hoban PR, Ramachandran S, Strange RC. Environment, phenotype and genetics: risk factors associated with BCC of the skin. Expert Rev Anticancer Ther. 2002;2(5):570–9.
72. Carroll RP, Ramsay HM, Fryer AA, Hawley CM, Nicol DL, Harden PN. Incidence and prediction of nonmelanoma skin cancer post-renal transplantation: a prospective study in Queensland, Australia. Am J Kidney Dis. 2003;41(3):676–83.
73. Fernandez-Ruiz J, Montero-Vilchez T, Buendia-Eisman A, Arias-Santiago S. Knowledge, behaviour and attitudes related to sun exposure in sportspeople: a systematic review. Int J Environ Res Public Health. 2022;19(16):10175.
74. Bakos RM, Wagner MB, Sul UFRG, Bakos L, et al. Queimaduras e hábitos solares em um grupo de atletas brasileiros. Rev Bras Med Esporte. 2022;12: 275–8.
75. Gutiérrez-Manzanedo JV, De Castro-Maqueda G, Caraballo Vidal I, González-Montesinos JL, Vaz Pardal C, Rivas Ruiz F, et al. Sun-related behaviors, attitudes and knowledge among paralympic sailors. Disabil Health J. 2021;14(3):101095.
76. de Castro MG, Gutiérrez-Manzanedo JV, González-Montesinos JL, Vaz Pardal C, Rivas Ruiz F, de Troya MM. Sun exposure and photoprotection: habits, knowledge and attitudes among elite Kitesurfers. J Cancer Educ. 2022;37(3):517–23.
77. García-Malinis AJ, Gracia-Cazaña T, Zazo M, Aguilera J, Rivas-Ruiz F, de Troya MM, et al. Sun protection behaviors and knowledge in mountain marathon runners and risk factors for sunburn. Actas Dermo-Sifiliográficas (English Edition). 2021;112(2):159–66.
78. Stanton WR, Janda M, Baade PD, Anderson P. Primary prevention of skin cancer: a review of sun protection in Australia and internationally. Health Promot Int. 2004;19(3):369–78.
79. van der Pols JC, Williams GM, Pandeya N, Logan V, Green AC. Prolonged prevention of squamous cell carcinoma of the skin by regular sunscreen use. Cancer Epidemiol Biomark Prev. 2006;15(12): 2546–8.
80. Navarrete-De Gálvez M, Ruiz Sánchez JM, Navarrete-De Gálvez E, Aguilera J, Rivas-Ruiz F, de Troya-Martín M, et al. Sun exposure and protection habits in transplant athletes: an international survey. Photodermatol Photoimmunol Photomed. 2022;38(4):365–72.
81. Gilaberte Y, Trullàs C, Granger C, de Troya-Martín M. Photoprotection in outdoor sports: a review of the literature and recommendations to reduce risk among athletes. Dermatol Ther (Heidelb). 2022;12(2):329–43.

Dehydration and Hyponatremia

27

William O. Roberts

27.1 Introduction

Finding a balance between over and underhydration is essential for athlete safety; inadequate fluid intake during activity results in dehydration. Too much fluid during physical activity can lead to exertional hyponatremia. Humans can tolerate fluid loss during physical activity and do well when fluids are replaced during and between bouts of exercise. Maintaining hydration improves athlete performance and heat tolerance. Dehydration is relatively rare in supported activities but contributes to a common cause of collapse and death from exertional heat stroke in unsupported activities like hiking in the Grand Canyon [1].

Balancing sweat losses with fluid intake is key to staying appropriately hydrated during training and competition. People with usual sweat rates do not need to take in fluid for training or competitions lasting less than an hour and can usually replace the fluid losses with normal drinking and meals [2]. The best strategy for safe hydration during exercise is to drink when thirsty or to calculate fluid replacement for the environment and replace fluids based on the calculated sweat rate [2]. Individual sweating rates vary on hot and cold days, so there is no single fluid replacement volume that works safely during physical activity for an individual on both hot and cold days [2]. The microenvironment at the skin level is tropical, so an overdressed athlete in cold conditions will have a sweating rate closer to hot conditions and require more fluid replacement than an appropriately dressed athlete. Drinking a small amount of fluid 20–30 min before exercise helps an athlete start with a "full" tank, but it is important to remember that humans do not store water like some other mammals. After exercise, an athlete should eat and drink until back to baseline body weight and urinating normally [2]. Urine color is usually pale yellow, like lemonade, when a person is well hydrated [2].

Exercise-associated hyponatremia (EAH) is defined as low serum sodium (<135 mmol/L) within 24 h of activity. It occurs on a continuum of ingesting too much fluid with inappropriate antidiuretic hormone (AVP) release during physical activity (most common) to high sweat sodium losses combined with hypotonic fluid ingestion during physical activity (rare) [1, 3]. EAH has been reported in endurance competitions like marathons, ultramarathons, triathlons, canoe races, and long-distance swimming and also in American football, rugby, hiking, military exercises, police training, tennis, fraternity hazing, Bikram yoga, and lawn bowling [1, 4–7]. Symptomatic EAH is rare but is associated with at least 14 athlete-related deaths since 1981 [1]. EAH is most seen in

W. O. Roberts (✉)
Department of Family Medicine and Community Health, University of Minnesota Medical School, Minneapolis, MN, USA
e-mail: robert037@umn.edu

S. Rocha Piedade et al. (eds.), *Sideline Management in Sports*,
https://doi.org/10.1007/978-3-031-33867-0_27

endurance activities that last 4 or more hours, but four deaths in high school and college football players emphasize the need for prudent fluid replacement in all athletes [1, 8–10].

Although some cases of EAH may be due to pure water intoxication from the overconsumption of hypotonic fluids, non-osmotic AVP secretion is a key factor contributing to most athlete-related symptomatic cases [1]. AVP secretion is stimulated by factors commonly associated with exercise, including nausea or vomiting; interleukin-6 release; plasma volume contraction; hypoglycemia; and elevated body temperature [1]. Body water will flow across cell membranes to equalize solute concentrations on either side of the membrane (sodium–potassium balance), causing cells to swell; within the cranium, this fluid transfer can increase intracranial pressure and potentially lead to a fatal outcome. Drinking to thirst or weight-based fluid replacement strategies are safest for athletes, and knowing athlete sweating characteristics like sweat rate improves hydration outcomes [1, 2].

27.2 Clinical Presentation and Differential Diagnosis

The differential diagnoses for athletes' non-trauma-related collapse include cardiac arrest, anaphylaxis, exertional heat stroke, heat exhaustion, EAH, hypoglycemia, usually from insulin shock, and exercise-associated postural hypotension. In the first minutes following the collapse, evaluation may include breathing status, airway compromise (bronchospasm and angioedema), CNS status (AVPU), rectal temperature, serum sodium (Na^+), and blood glucose. Exertional heat stroke and heat exhaustion share many signs and symptoms of dehydration and EAH, confounding the true diagnosis. The rectal temperature and keen attention to the clinical situation are often necessary to make the correct diagnosis.

Table 27.1 Signs and symptoms that may be present at various stages in the evolution of EAH are not specific or sensitive and are easily confused with dehydration or heat illness

Early	Severe	Late
Lightheaded Dizzy Nausea Middle Headache	Progressive headache Vomiting "Puffy" Muscle cramps Feeling of "impending doom" Dyspnea Confusion	Ashen appearance Prolonged seizure Obtundation

A progressively worsening headache should raise suspicion in a setting with high hypotonic or isotonic fluid intake. Blood pressure, heart rate, and respiratory rate are usually in the normal range, even in severe and late cases

27.3 Key History and Physical Examination Pearls and Findings

Athletes with dehydration often present with fatigue, decreased performance, nausea, headache, apathy, irritability, and thirst. The hallmarks of EAH include a finish time of >4 h, high fluid intake above sweat losses, no weight loss or weight gain, or hot and humid conditions [1]. The presenting signs and symptoms of EAH are not specific and may include malaise, nausea, fatigue, confusion, mild or progressively increasing headache, seizures, coma, or death (see Table 27.1) [1].

27.4 Indications and Benefits of Additional Testing

Point-of-care Na^+ analysis will prove the diagnosis and is sometimes available at large endurance events [1].

27.5 Incidence, Prevalence, and Predisposing Risk Factors

Symptomatic EAH is exceedingly rare, and at the Twin Cities Marathon, we have documented 1.6 per 100,000 finishers (unpublished data—WOR). The mean serum Na^+ for symptomatic and fatal cases is 121 mmol/L, with a range of 109–131 mmol/L [1]. Risk factors include overdrinking water, sports drinks, and other hypotonic beverages; weight gain during exercise; exercise duration >4 h; event inexperience; inadequate training; slow running or performance pace; high or low body mass index; and readily available fluids. (Note: in general, sports drinks are hypotonic to plasma and their Na^+ content is in the 10–38 mmol/L range) [1].

27.6 Sideline Management and Suggestions

EAH can present well after the fluid ingestion "event" at home, in the car, on the airplane, or at the hotel [1]. It is essential not to assume dehydration is the cause of an athlete's collapse. If EAH is suspected, restrict fluids until the athlete is urinating [1]. Treatment of symptomatic EAH is rapid intravenous administration of 2–5% NaCl in 100 mL aliquots until symptoms improve [1]; usually in an emergency room before doing any brain imaging that may delay diagnosis and treatment [1]. In some large events with point-of-care laboratory devices, hypertonic saline administration may be done on site before transferring the patient to an emergency facility [1]. Athletes presenting with mild symptoms associated with EAH can be treated with either an IV bolus of hypertonic saline or oral hypertonic saline fluids [1]. Giving a large volume of intravenous fluid in the training room, even normal saline, without measuring serum electrolytes, can lead to near-fatal or even fatal hyponatremia [11].

27.7 Suggested Prevention Measures

Education of athletes (and entourage), coaches, and staff regarding the benefits and risks of fluid replacement is essential to reducing the risk of dehydration and EAH. Teach "drink to thirst" and "sweat loss" fluid replacement strategies [3, 11]. Daily weight measurements to estimate day-to-day fluid status and sweating rates are helpful for individualized fluid replacement plans [2]. Careful fluid replacement and early recognition of EAH have reduced the deaths in marathons and other endurance events.

Take Home Messages

- Dehydration is not always the cause of athlete collapse.
- Overhydrating can lead to fatal and non-fatal hyponatremia.
- Know what you are treating before giving large volumes of oral or intravenous fluid.
- Teach drink to thirst or weight-based fluid replacement.

References

1. Hew-Butler T, Rosner MH, Fowkes-Godek S, Dugas JP, Hoffman MD, Lewis DP, Maughan RJ, Miller KC, Montain SJ, Rehrer NJ, Roberts WO, Rogers IR, Siegel AJ, Stuempfle KJ, Winger JM, Verbalis JG. Statement of the 3rd international exercise-associated hyponatremia consensus development conference, Carlsbad, California, 2015. Clin J Sport Med. 2015;25(4):303–20.
2. McDermott B, Anderson S, Armstrong L, Casa D, Cheuvront S, Cooper L, Kenney WL, O'Connor FA, Roberts WO. National Athletic Trainers' Association position statement: fluid replacement for the physically active. J Athl Train. 2017;52(9):877–95.
3. Lewis D, Blow A, Tye J, Hew-Butler T. Considering exercise-associated hyponatraemia as a continuum. BMJ Case Rep. 2018;2018:bcr2017222916.

4. Changstrom B, Brill J, Hecht S. Severe exercise-associated hyponatremia in a collegiate American football player. Curr Sports Med Rep. 2017;16(5):343–5.
5. Dimeff RJ. Seizure disorder in a professional American football player. Curr Sports Med Rep. 2006;5(4):173–6.
6. Jones BL, O'Hara JP, Till K, King RF. Dehydration and hyponatremia in professional rugby union players: a cohort study observing English premiership rugby union players during match play, field, and gym training in cool environmental conditions. J Strength Cond Res. 2015;29(1):107–15.
7. Nolte HW, Hew-Butler T, Noakes TD, Duvenage CS. Exercise-associated hyponatremic encephalopathy and exertional heatstroke in a soldier: high rates of fluid intake during exercise caused rather than prevented a fatal outcome. Phys Sportsmed. 2015;43(1):93–8.
8. Eichner ER. Deaths in athletes: news on hyponatremia, nuances in sickle cell trait. Curr Sports Med Rep. 2015;14(5):349–50.
9. Eichner ER. Hyponatremia associated with exercise versus sickling caused by exercise. Curr Sports Med Rep. 2019;18(9):312–3.
10. Eichner ER. Three uncommon or underrated threats to football players and others: pearls and pitfalls for diagnosis and prevention. Curr Sports Med Rep. 2015;14(4):270–1.
11. Herfel R, Stone CK, Koury SI, Blake JJ. Iatrogenic acute hyponatremia in a college athlete. Southern Medical Association 91st Annual Assembly. 1997; Charlotte, North Carolina.

Orthopedic Oncologic Conditions (Differential Diagnosis)

28

Marcelo Tadeu Caiero, Evandro Tito Oliveira, and Jorge Henrique Narciso

28.1 Introduction

Bone and soft tissue tumors comprehend a large number of diseases that can affect all ages. They are not common in the general population, but they may be kept in mind in differential diagnosis of orthopedics condition in juvenile and young adults.

Sports medicine doctors must suspect a musculoskeletal tumor in the athlete, know basic initial screening exams, and refer the patient to orthopedics oncologist as soon as possible to make the correct diagnosis and initiate proper treatment.

The tumors that most affect bone are metastasis. A patient aged 45 years old or older with bone lesion is highly suspected of metastasis from carcinoma. The carcinoma tumors that most often affect bone are as follows: breast, prostate, lungs, kidney, and thyroid. Therefore, metastatic bone tumors are very rare in athlete considering their low age.

Soft tissue sarcomas are rare, representing only 1% of all cancer cases in the United States. Besides that, soft tissue sarcomas are three times more prevalent than bone sarcomas. Some soft tissue sarcomas have predilection to younger patients such as synovial sarcoma, epithelioid sarcoma, and alveolar soft tissue sarcoma.

The more common primary bone sarcomas are osteosarcoma, Ewing tumor, and chondrosarcoma. The former two affect children and adolescents; chondrosarcoma affects adults. Table 28.1 presents the clinical and radiological findings of some musculoskeletal tumors.

M. T. Caiero (✉) · E. T. Oliveira · J. H. Narciso
Instituto de Ortopedia e Traumatologia de São Paulo—IOT/USP, São Paulo, Brazil

S. Rocha Piedade et al. (eds.), *Sideline Management in Sports*,
https://doi.org/10.1007/978-3-031-33867-0_28

Table 28.1 Main features of musculoskeletal tumors

Tumor (main location)	Clinical findings	Radiology
Lipomas and lipomatous tumor	Small or larger growing mass, non-painful	MRI: Homogeneous high signal in T1 and low signal in T2; no gadolinium enhanced
Pigmented villonodular synovitis (knee joint) Tenosynovial giant cell tumor (hand and feet)	Recurrent joint swelling and pain episodes; nodular/ focal form, mechanical symptoms	MRI: Synovial-based mass from nodular proliferation and joint effusion
Synovial chondromatosis	Reduced joint movement, pain, swelling, popping, and catching of the joint	MRI: Cartilaginous nodules, hypointense in T1, and hyperintense in T2 CT scan: Mineralization patterns
Synovial sarcoma	Little or no symptoms, may mimetics a meniscal cyst	MRI: Low signal in T1, heterogeneous high signal in T2, periferic enhancement with gadolinium
Unicameral bone cyst (metaphysis of long bones, proximal femur, and proximal humerus)	Usually painless, but a pathologic fracture in up to two-thirds of patients	X-ray: Lytic metaphyseal lesion, cortical thinning, well defined, no periosteal reaction
Aneurysmal bone cysts (metaphysis and epiphysis of long bones, proximal humerus, distal femur, and proximal tibia)	Pain, discomfort, and radiculopathy	X-ray: Well-defined, lucent multiloculated eccentric lesions at the metaphysis;
Fibrous dysplasia	Isolated (monostotic) or affect multiple bones (polyostotic), causing significant deformity and functional disability	X-ray: Lytic bone lesion at the metaphysis and/or diaphysis with the classic ground glass appearance; shepherd's crook deformity
Nonossifying fibroma (lower limbs)	Usually asymptomatic unless there is a pathologic fracture	X-ray: Lucent, well-defined lesion with lobulated margins and sclerotic rim, occasionally causing a cortical defect
Osteochondroma The most common bone tumor (metaphysis of long bones)	Asymptomatic and found incidentally	Projections with a narrow and elongated base (pedunculated) or lesions with a continuous aspect and enlarged base (sessile)
Enchondroma (small bones of the hands and feet)	Diagnosed accidentally	X-ray: Centric lesion with uniform calcifications MRI: Low signal on T1-weighted sequences and high signal on T2
Osteoblastoma (posterior elements of the spine, metaphysis of long bones)	Pain is the most common symptom and neurological signs (spine)	CT: Exuberant reactive sclerosis surrounding a lytic center (nidus), generally >2 cm MRI: Variable adjacent edema signal and enhancement in the marrow and peripheral soft tissues
Chondroblastoma (epiphysis of immature long bones)	Insidious pain, swelling, and stiffness involving joints, and infectious arthritis is a differential diagnosis	X-ray: Small (<5 cm), epiphyseal radiolucent lesion with well-defined borders, accompanied by a sclerotic border
Osteoid osteoma (lower extremity and spine)	Pain is severe, occurs at rest and night, and alleviates with NSAIDs or aspirin	X-ray: Lucent area surrounded by reactive osseous sclerosis, resulting in a characteristic radiograph image referred to as a nidus CT scan is often necessary to show the nidus
Osteosarcoma (the most common primary bone cancer in adolescents and young adults) (knee and metaphysis of long bones)	Pain and swelling, confused with a history of previous sports trauma or growing pains; 50% around knee	X-ray: Ill-defined radiodense metaphyseal lesion; codman triangle and sunburst appearance are also common
Ewing sarcoma (diaphysis of lower limbs, pelvis)	Swelling, pain, fever, weight loss and fatigue associated with the rapid growth of the mass and increased pain	X-ray: Permeative, ill-defined, lytic lesion within the diaphysis or metadiaphysis of long bones; reactive bone formation such as periosteal reaction (onion skinning or Codman triangle) is frequent

Table 28.1 (continued)

Tumor (main location)	Clinical findings	Radiology
Chondrosarcoma of bone	Long-standing history of pain, mild swelling and progressive difficulty in practicing sports or daily activities	*Grade 1*: Punctate calcifications and popcorn appearance, cortical integrity, endosteal scalloping *Grade 2*: More aggressive pattern, cortical breakage, soft tissue invasion. Grade 3: Even more bone destruction, large soft tissue mass and no calcification
Giant cell tumor of bone (distal femur, proximal tibia, distal radius)	Pain, swelling, and stiffness involving joints; 50% around the knee	Radiolucent lesion in the metaepiphyseal area with no sclerosis or periosteal reaction; in more aggressive cases there is cortical destruction and soft tissue invasion
Bone metastasis (the most common bone cancer)	*Bone pain, broken bones, urinary and or bowel incontinence, weakness in the legs or arms, hypercalcemia*	Depends on primary tumor: Prostate: Blastic lesion Mama: Blastic and lytic lesion Lung, kidney, thyroid: Lytic lesion
Multiple myeloma (the most common primary malignancy of bone)	Bone pain or a pathologic fracture, hypercalcemia, renal insufficiency, and anemia	Multiple "punched-out" lytic lesions; salt and pepper lesions in skull

28.2 When Should a Musculoskeletal Tumor Be Suspected?

The presence of a soft tissue mass should be evaluated with MRI. It is important that the physician be aware of some features of musculoskeletal tumors. Tumors that are superficial, between skin and deep fascia may be malignant. Some malignant soft tissue tumors have a low growth rate. One third of musculoskeletal sarcomas are superficial. Synovial sarcoma, for example, has low growth and little if no symptoms.

Pain in knee location in children and adolescents should be carefully evaluated because 50% of osteosarcomas arise in this region, in the distal femur, proximal tibia, and proximal fibula.

Most musculoskeletal tumors present pain with activity, but some occur at rest, and pain at rest should raise suspicion of a tumor. Osteoid osteoma is a benign bone tumor that presents classically with night pain.

Bone tumors can show symptoms only after local trauma, such as fall on the knee.

In the vertebral column, some tumors that affect posterior elements such as osteoid osteoma and aneurysmal bone cyst may cause antalgic scoliosis.

28.3 What Exams Are Important in Evaluation?

Plain radiographs remain the initial image exam. It is very important to initial evaluation of bone tumors. Plain radiographs show some characteristics of the tumor that can differentiate between benignant and malignant lesions and combined to clinical features and common sites of involvement can lead to correct diagnosis (Table 28.1); can also identify the matrix type, like chondral, fibrous, cystic, or bone form lesions. In some cases, plain radiographs are always necessary to make the correct diagnosis. Benign lesions are well limited, without periosteal reaction, cortical destruction, and soft tissue invasion. Malignant counterparts are ill-limited, can present onion skin reaction, usually destruct bone cortical and spread to soft. Bone tumors have radiograph features that can be used to identify precisely the type of tumor in some cases. For example, giant cell tumor of bone affects epiphysis and metaphysis of long bones with closed physis. If we consider that most GCTB occur in patients between 20 and 40 years of age, we can have a high suspicion that the patient has GCTB with only plain radiography.

CT scan is used to identify pulmonary metastasis in sarcomas, which is much more common to spread to the lungs. Carcinoma lesions show metastatic potential to lungs, liver, and bone. CT scan is superior in demonstrating osteoid osteoma than MRI. A bone scan with Tc99m is used to evaluate if the tumor has osteoblastic activity. It can be used to show metachronous lesions in osteosarcoma and Ewing sarcoma. It can show bone metastasis from carcinomas such as breast and prostate carcinomas. Ultrasound is less used in soft tissue tumors because MRI can show much more information. It serves to evaluate soft tissue mass and should be complemented with MRI. The US guides soft tissue biopsies and can help determine intraoperative location of deep-seated tumors.

MRI is the best image exam for soft tissue evaluation. MRI can evaluate medullary extension of a bone lesion and tumor spread to soft tissues in case of bone tumors. It is of utmost importance in preoperative planning because it shows which muscles must be resected, the proximity with neurovascular structures, subcutaneous invasion, and the need of soft coverage after resection. Contrasted MRI with gadolinium can differentiate a bone cyst from a well-hydrated bone lesion. MRI sequences such as T1, T2, and others permit that the radiologist predict histologic type of tumor in some cases. Soft tissue tumors of homogeneous high signal in T1 and low signal after fat suppression sequences highly suggest lipomas and atypical lipomatous tumors and make biopsy unnecessary.

28.4 Biopsy

Biopsy is the last exam to be asked for the patient, after all image exams have been realized. That is because biopsy should be done in the local area of better tumor representativeness. Besides, biopsy can alter tumor image if it is done first. When a musculoskeletal tumor hypothesis is made, sports medicine doctors must refer the case to a musculoskeletal tumor center. Biopsy should be done by the surgeon that will treat the patient. There are basically 3 types of biopsy: percutaneous, incisional, and excisional. Soft tissue percutaneous biopsy can be executed with core needle or TRUCUT, and bone biopsy can be done with trephine or JAMSHIDI. Incisional biopsy is done with a little access to remove tumor samples and is indicated in cases of tumor proximity to neurovascular structures. In excisional biopsy, the tumor is removed and sent to pathological analysis and is done when the tumor is benign. Biopsy should be done in longitudinal direction in members in the same incision that will be used to remove the tumor because the biopsy scar must be resected along with the mass to decrease the risk ok relapse. Biopsy can be done with CT scan or US aid to improve accuracy.

28.5 Most Often Musculoskeletal Tumors Seen in Athletes

28.5.1 Lipomas and Lipomatous Tumors

Lipomas are the most common tumors observed by orthopedic surgeons. They can be classified as superficial or deep in relation to the deep fascia. The so-called atypical lipomatous tumor is a borderline premalignant lesion. There is a slight male-to-female predominance, most commonly present in middle-aged adults. Truncal locations are more common than the extremities, and the proximal extremity is more common than the distal extremity. Superficial lipomas present as a small growing mass, <5 cm, non-painful, just below the skin. Deep lipomas are usually larger, >10 cm inside muscle, and may not be palpable. Pain can occur if the tumor encroaches adjacent nerves.

MRI shows a high signal intensity in T1 and low signal intensity on T2-weighted imaging. MRI cannot distinguish lipoma from atypical lipomatous tumor [1]. It can only be observed when lipoma is located in a subcutaneous location and smaller than 5 cm. In this case, some patients complain of cosmesis and request excision. Larger-size lesions and lesions that continue to grow can be resected too. Lipomas inside muscle should be resected especially in the lower limb because there is a possibility of atypical lipoma. Marginal resection is sufficient to treat both lipomas and atypical lipomas. Recurrence

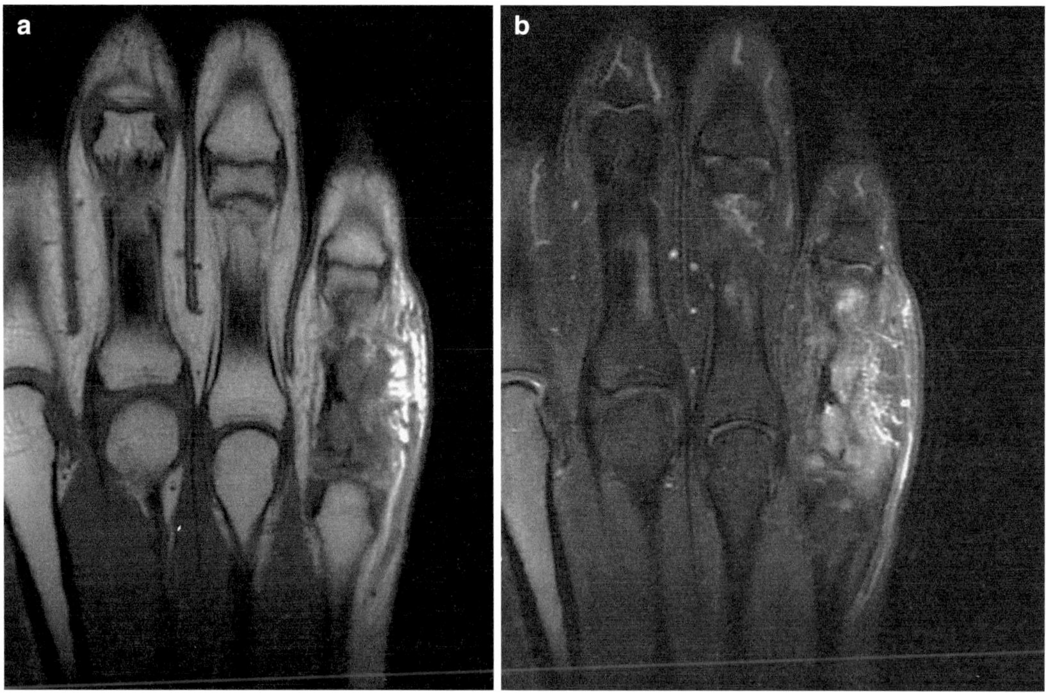

Fig. 28.1 Tenosynovial giant cell tumor of the tendon sheath in the fifth finger. MRI sequences on T1 (**a**) and T2 (**b**) weighted images

rate is minimal. Malignant degeneration of lipoma to liposarcoma is extremely rare. Atypical lipomatous tumor, instead, can dedifferentiate to high-grade malignant liposarcoma.

Lipoma arborescens is most common in the knee, and it is a fat infiltration of synovial tissue of a joint. It almost always occurs with another joint condition. Treatment includes arthroscopic or open synovectomy of the joint if symptomatic.

28.5.2 Pigmented Villonodular Synovitis and Tenosynovial Giant Cell Tumor

Pigmented villonodular synovitis and tenosynovial giant cell tumor of the tendon sheath represent parts of the same disease spectrum; thus, they were grouped as a sole entity named tenosynovial giant cell tumor (TGCT).

TGCT is a proliferative disease of the synovium. It may be focal or diffuse. Clinically, it presents with pain and swelling. Deposition of hemosiderin gives its typical appearance macroscopically and radiographically. In late stages, it may cause articular destruction.

Its incidence is slightly higher in female individuals, peak incidence between 30 and 50 years of age. Any joint can be affected, but the knee is the most common.

The progression is insidious with recurrent episodes of joint swelling and pain. Nodular/focal form presents mechanical symptoms. In late stages, degenerative articular disease is found. Eventually, there is a palpable soft tissue mass. Malignant forms are extremely rare. Joint aspiration can be useful in diagnosis and alleviating the symptoms. The appearance of the aspirated fluid is classically hemorrhagic.

Plain radiography is usually normal. In late stages, articular erosion and severe arthritis are seen. MRI is the gold standard for the diagnosis, showing a synovial-based mass from nodular proliferation and joint effusion (Fig. 28.1a, b). Deposition of hemosiderin gives the classical aspect of low-intensity signal on all sequences (Fig. 28.2a, b). The gross appearance is that of a

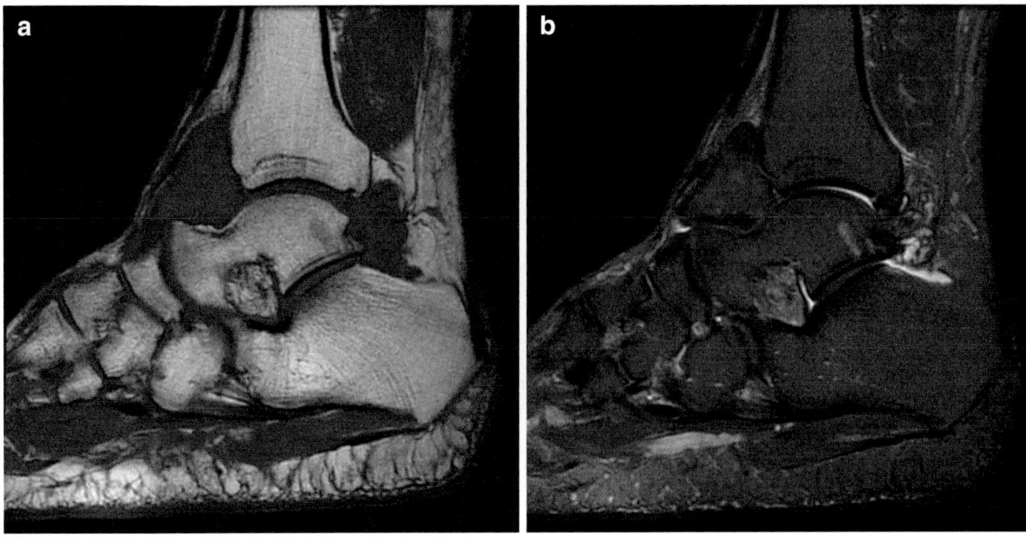

Fig. 28.2 Pigmented villonodular synovitis on T1 (**a**) and T2 (**b**) weighted MRI. Low signal is typically noted on both sequences

brown nodular proliferative synovium highly vascularized.

Surgical management is the mainstay of treatment and open procedure is the benchmark, due to its lower recurrence rates compared to arthroscopic resection. Overall recurrence is up to 30%, and external beam radiation may be used as an adjuvant.

28.5.3 Synovial Chondromatosis

Synovial chondromatosis corresponds to a metaplastic (rather than a true neoplastic) process that affects synovial joints. Synovial cells produce cartilaginous loose bodies into the joint cavity and symptoms occur due to mechanical damage and inflammatory response.

It is a rare condition that affects mostly males between the ages of 30 and 50 years. The most affected joint is the knee, followed by the hip, shoulder, elbow, and ankle. Symptoms include reduced ROM (range of movement), pain, swelling, popping, and catching of the joint. Although considered a benign entity, malignant transformation has been reported.

It may not be visible on plain radiography until calcification of the loose bodies has occurred. The calcification pattern is typically denser in the periphery. As the disease progresses, radiographic findings of osteoarthritis/degenerative joint disorder overlap those of the synovial chondromatosis. Differential diagnoses include myositis ossificans, synovial sarcoma, and synovial chondrosarcoma.

On MRI, they appear as cartilaginous nodules, i.e., hypointense on T1 and hyperintense on T2 (Fig. 28.3a, b). Calcifications are seen as signal voids. The mineralization pattern is best seen on CT images.

Histologically, synovial chondromatosis is characterized by well-circumscribed nodules of hyaline cartilage with clusters of chondrocytes.

Surgery is the primary and best treatment for synovial chondromatosis, which includes removal of the loose bodies and synovectomy of the joint (open or arthroscopically). Recurrence rates are higher for the arthroscopically procedure. With regard to the hip, arthroscopic procedure may be preferred, as the open approach may require dislocation of the femoral head, thus increasing the risk of osteonecrosis.

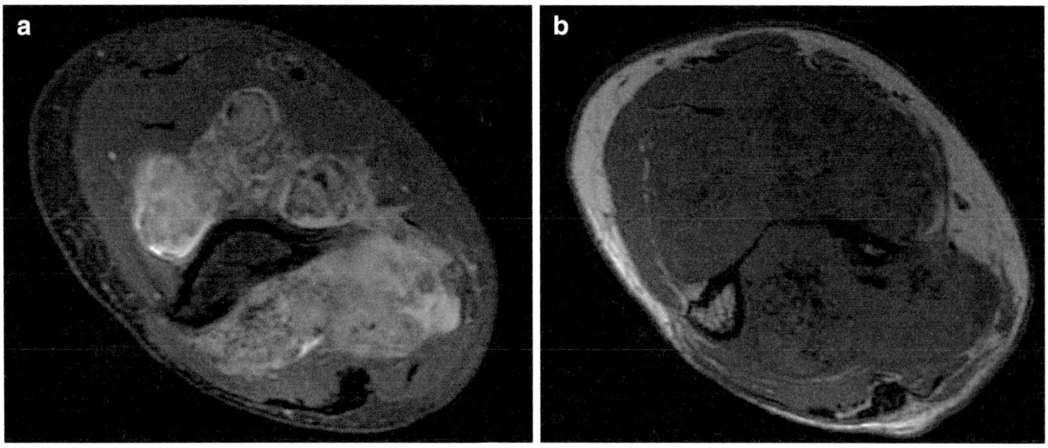

Fig. 28.3 Synovial chondromatosis on T2 (**a**) and T1 (**b**)weighted sequences. The signal intensity is similar to normal cartilage

28.5.4 Synovial Sarcoma

Synovial sarcoma often arises near joints but rarely is intra-articular. Its name is derivated from microscopic resemblance to mature synovial cells but the cellular origin of synovial sarcoma is unknown. This proximity with articulations, specially knee, ankle, and hip and low-growing features can lead to misdiagnosis, when tumor is diagnosed to parameniscal cyst or synovial cyst. It is a high-grade malignant neoplasm with variable biological behavior. Some tumors show rapid growth, but others have low-growing mass, with little or no symptoms. Even little tumors can develop pulmonary metastasis. Synovial sarcoma affects young adults and can show linfonodal spread that should be evaluated. MRI with gadolinium is the best exam to evaluate this tumor (Fig. 28.4a, b). Biopsy is mandatory. Synovial sarcoma is a soft tissue sarcoma that is more chemosensitive and is often used with radiotherapy. Surgical resection with wide margins complemented with radiotherapy is the keystone of treatment.

28.5.5 Unicameral Bone Cyst

Unicameral or simple bone cysts are the most common lesions found in the immature skeleton. It is more seen in the proximal humerus and proximal femur, typically occurring in the first two decades of life. In adults, they are found in less usual locations, such as calcaneus and ilium. The lesions are usually painless but may evolve to pathologic fracture up to two-thirds of patients. Lesions large enough or in weight bearing areas may have an increased risk for pathologic fracture and present with pain. Simple plain radiography is usually diagnostic: a radiolucent unicameral cystic centric lesion at the metaphysis of the bone. The cortex may be thinned but not distorted nor disrupted (Fig. 28.5). No soft tissue extension is seen. Periosteal reaction is not seen, unless a pathologic fracture has occurred. Simple bone cysts are classified as active or latent according to its distance to the physis: active lesions are found up to 1 cm of the physis, whereas farther lesions are considered latent. As the bone grows, the lesion may seem to move toward the diaphysis. It may heal spontaneously with skeletal maturity or after a pathologic fracture. In some cases, surgical treatment is required due to impending risk of fracture. The lesion can be observed when there is a low concern for pathologic fracture, but some restriction from sports and activities is recommended.

28.5.6 Aneurysmal Bone Cyst

Aneurysmal bone cysts (ABC) are metaphyseal and epiphyseal lesions of long bones (commonly proximal humerus, distal femur, and proximal tibia). It is more frequently seen during the second decade of life with a slightly female predomi-

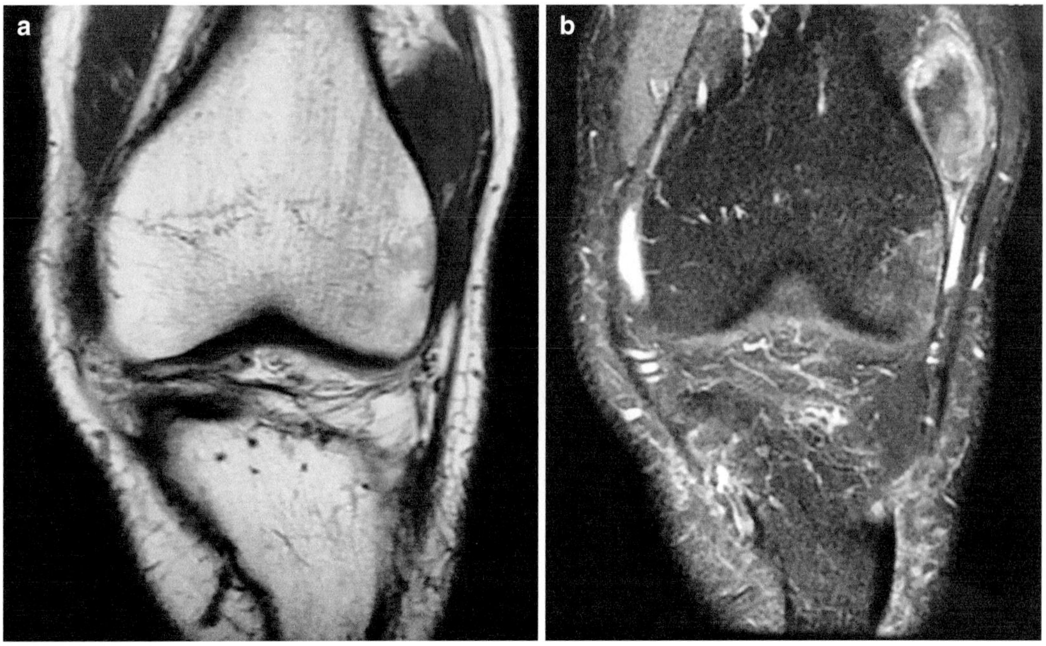

Fig. 28.4 Synovial sarcoma. Coronal T1 (**a**) and coronal fat-suppressed T1 with gadolinium (**b**) enhanced images. Note low T1 signal and heterogeneous image after gadolinium. The lesion has a high signal at the periphery and low signal in the center showing a necrotic central area

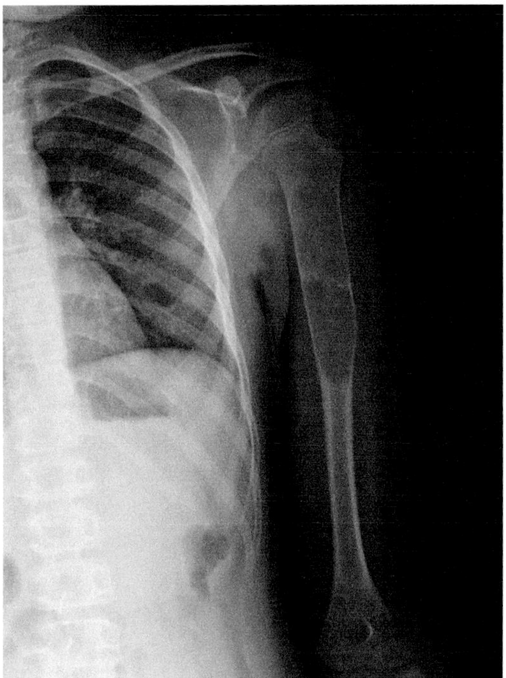

Fig. 28.5 UBC in the proximal humerus. Note that the distance from the physis in this simple radiography indicates an older and less active lesion

nance. Spinal lesions are uncommon, generally located in the posterior elements of the vertebrae and may cause radiculopathy, vertebral collapse, scoliosis, and neurologic deficits. Aneurysmal bone cysts may be seen secondary to another bone lesion in approximately 30% of cases. On plain radiographs, ABCs are seen as lucent eccentric lesions at the metaphysis (Fig. 28.6). The width of the cyst may surpass that of the metaphysis, but no cortical discontinuity is found. The cyst is multiloculated, containing multiple fluid-filled chambers separated by bone septa. Soft tissue mass expanding from the bone lesion may be also seen. The management consists of surgical treatment with recurrence rates as high as 31%. Pathologic fracture may occur and restriction from sports is recommended until the surgical management.

28.5.7 Fibrous Dysplasia

Fibrous dysplasia (FD) is an entity characterized by replacement of cancellous and marrow bone with abnormal fibrous tissue. It may be

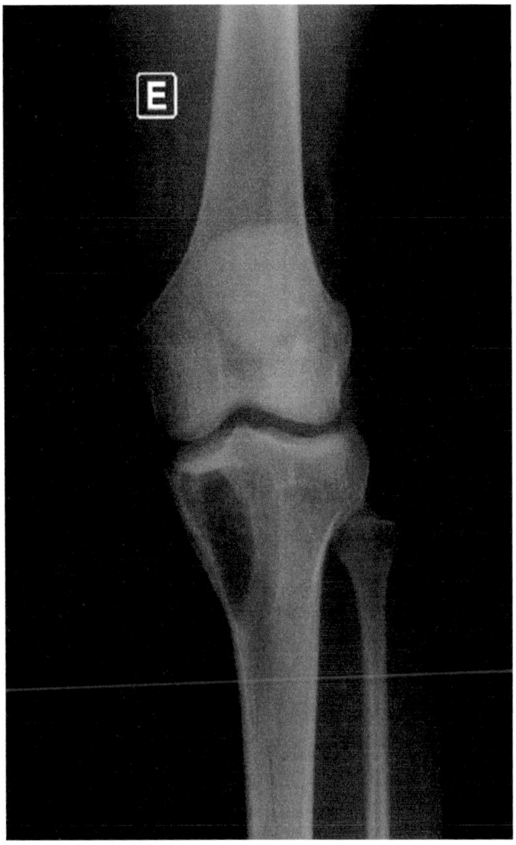

Fig. 28.6 ABC in a 16-year-old patient. An epiphyseal lytic lesion can be observed in the medial tibial plateau

isolated (monostotic) or affect multiple bones (polyostotic), causing significant deformity and functional disability. FD is also associated with McCune Albright syndrome (polyostotic FD, café au lait spots, and precocious puberty) and Mazabraud syndrome (polyostotic FD and soft tissue myxomas). This lesion is usually found incidentally on plain radiography but pain, swelling, and stress fractures may also occur. Most affected bones include the femur, the tibia, the pelvis, foot, and craniofacial bones. Varus deformity of the proximal femur is frequent and described as "shepherd's crook deformity." Plain radiography shows a lytic bone lesion at the metaphysis and/or diaphysis with the classic ground glass appearance (Fig. 28.7). The management is usually conservative, unless there is a high risk for a pathologic fracture. Surgical indications include persistent pain, significant

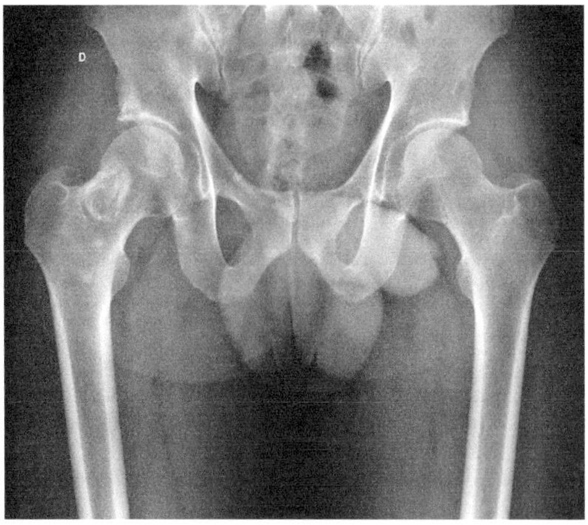

Fig. 28.7 Fibrous dysplasia in the right femoral neck

bone deformity, fracture, and nonunion. Diphosphonates can be used as a treatment for polyostotic disease.

28.5.8 Nonossifying Fibroma

Nonossifying fibroma is a benign fibrous lesion found eccentrically in the metaphysis of skeletally immature patients and occasionally in young adults. They are most commonly seen in the distal femur, proximal tibia, distal tibia, and proximal fibula. 80% occur in individuals younger than 20 years. Lesions found in older individuals are often regressing. They are usually asymptomatic unless there is a pathologic fracture. Pain without fracture must be considered a red flag to a more aggressive process. On plain radiography, NOF presents as a lucent well-defined lesion with lobulated margins and sclerotic rim, longer and larger than wider, occasionally causing a cortical defect between 1 and 3 cm in diameter (Fig. 28.8a, b). Secondary aneurysmal bone cysts can develop within a NOF. Management usually consists of serial radiographs as most of these lesions regress as the individual grows older and reaches skeletal maturity. The surgical treatment is reserved to the lesions with impending risk of pathologic fracture or those that have already fractured.

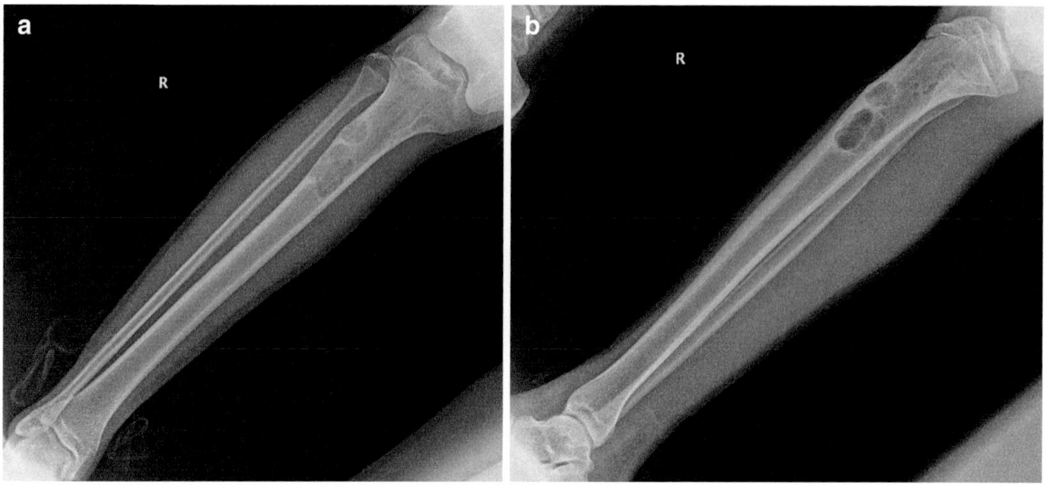

Fig. 28.8 Nonossifying fibroma of the proximal tibia. Image of an eccentrical lytic lesion in the immature skeleton on AP (**a**) and lateral X-ray (**b**) views

28.5.9 Osteochondroma

Osteochondroma consists of an exophytic lesion covered by a cartilaginous layer, which projects from the surface of the bone, and is considered the most common benign bone tumor affecting commonly metaphyseal region of proximal humerus, distal femur, and proximal tibia (physis of accentuated growth) in males around 18 years of age.

The lesions are typically asymptomatic and found incidentally. The lesions increase in size during the first decade of life and symptoms (due to friction of musculotendinous and compression of vascular structures) are related to the size and location of the lesion. Because they are associated with the growth process, these lesions generally stop their growth after skeletal maturity.

Osteochondromas can present on radiographs in two main forms: projections with a narrow and elongated base (pedunculated) or lesions with a continuous aspect and enlarged base (sessile) (Fig. 28.9a). The lesion continuing bone marrow with the host bone is essential for the diagnosis, visualized in MRI (Fig. 28.9b) or CT.

Excision of the lesion is curative although incomplete resections can lead to recurrences. Many surgeons prefer to wait until puberty for the surgery in less symptomatic osteochondromas.

28.5.10 Enchondroma

Enchondroma is a benign hyaline cartilage tumor, common in the small bones of the hands and feet. When affecting the metaphysis of long bones, especially the distal femur and proximal humerus the lesions are typically intramedullary. Usually is diagnosed accidentally, in the investigation of a painful condition in the shoulder or knee, in patients around the third-fourth decades of life, asymptomatic in the majority cases.

A solitary enchondroma can be described as a centric lesion, usually <3 cm, with uniform calcifications (Fig. 28.10a). MRI presents a low signal on T1-weighted sequences and high signal on T2 (Fig. 28.10b, c). When occurs the small bones of the hands and feet, the lesions can be more aggressive, with cortical expansion and rupture. Ollier disease and Maffucci syndrome are nonhereditary forms of multiple enchondromatosis, with multiple soft tissue hemangiomas in Maffucci disease.

Malignant transformation of single lesions is rare, around 1%. The majority will not require any intervention. Tumors with cortical expansion, pain, and pathologic fractures can be treated with intralesional resection and grafting.

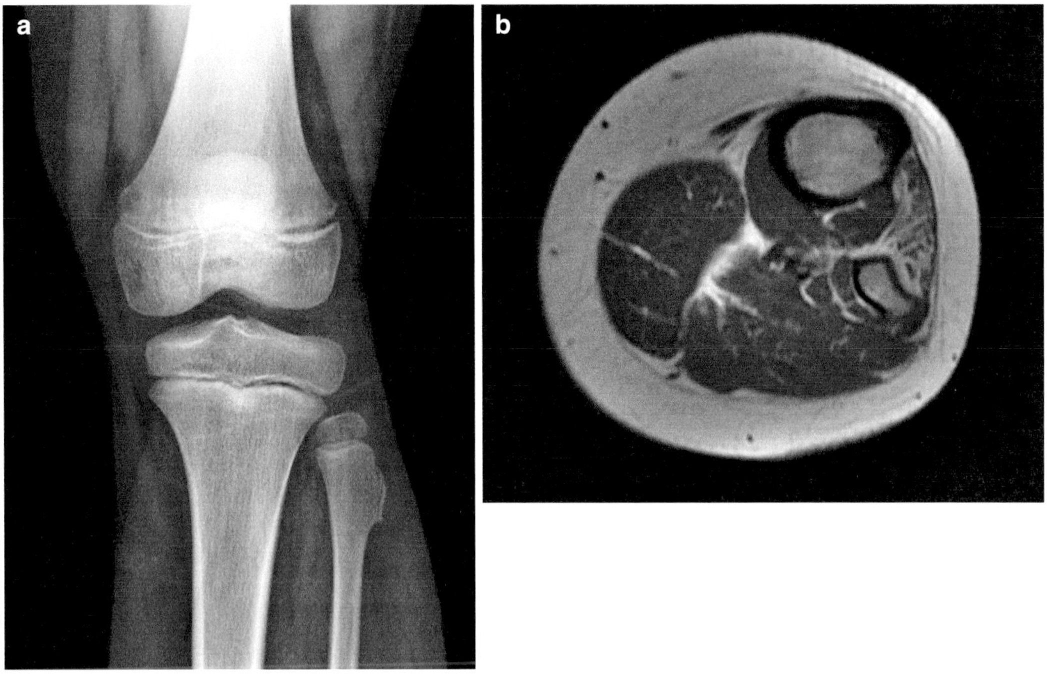

Fig. 28.9 (**a**) X-ray shows pedunculated osteochondroma in the proximal fibula's lateral aspect, inducing fibular nerve compression and foot dorsiflexion deficit. On MRI (**b**), the continuous bone marrow of the lesion can be observed

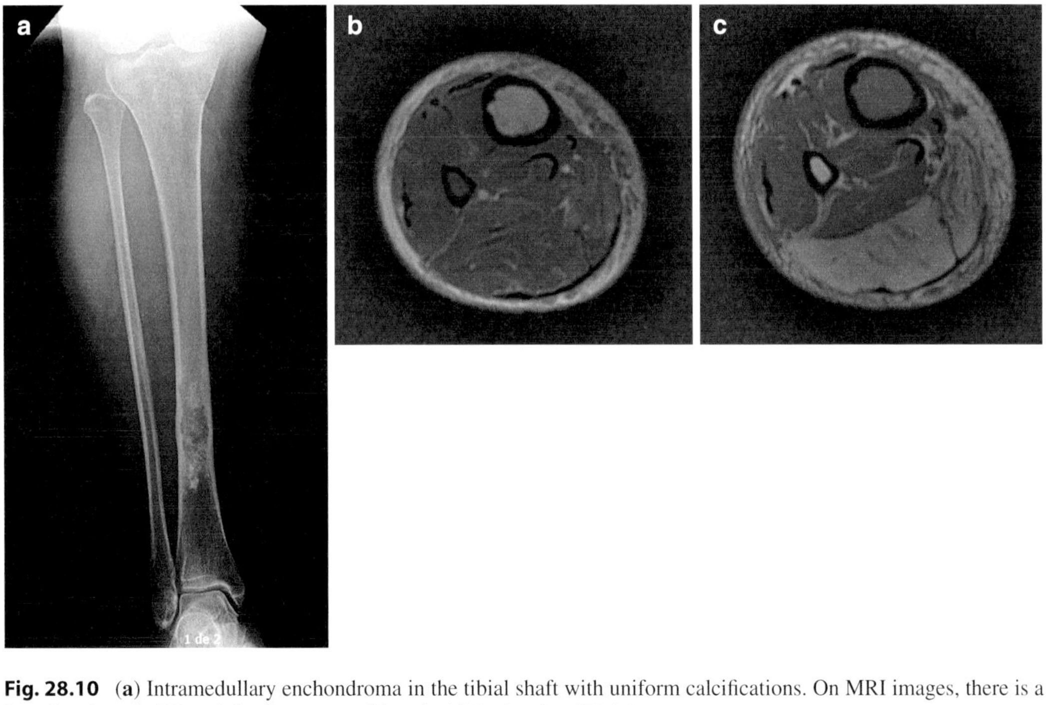

Fig. 28.10 (**a**) Intramedullary enchondroma in the tibial shaft with uniform calcifications. On MRI images, there is a low signal on the T2-weighted sequence (**b**) and a high signal on T1 (**c**)

28.5.11 Osteoblastoma

Osteoblastoma consists of a locally aggressive bone tumor, generally >2 cm, with a very similar morphology with osteoid osteoma affecting commonly the spine, in particular the posterior elements, in males around the second and third decades of life.

Pain is the most common symptom and neurological signs can occur in spinal lesions. On CT, osteoblastomas present as an exuberant reactive sclerosis surrounding a lytic center (nidus) (Fig. 28.11). MRI demonstrates a variable adjacent edema signal and enhancement in the marrow and peripheral soft tissues.

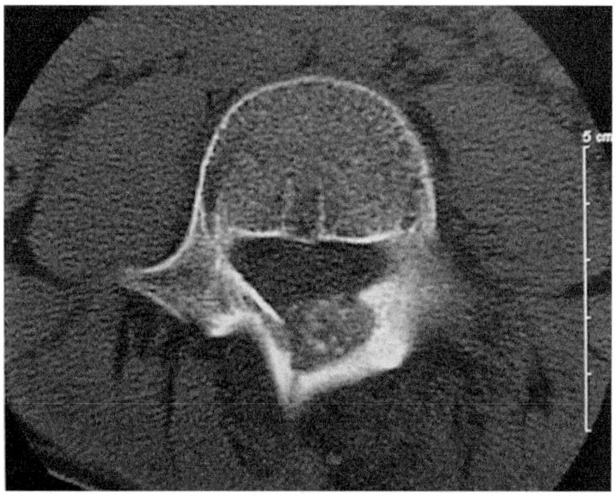

Fig. 28.11 Osteoblastoma of left laminae of the vertebra

Recurrences are uncommon and less invasive techniques including CT-guided drill excision, image-guided percutaneous radiofrequency, cryoablation, high-intensity focused ultrasound, and laser photocoagulation can be used. In some cases, near to the spinal cord, with a potential risk of injury, the open surgical resection of the lesions will be necessary.

28.5.12 Chondroblastoma

Chondroblastoma (epiphyseal chondroblastoma or Codman's tumor) is a relatively uncommon benign cartilaginous tumor that characteristically affects the epiphysis of immature long bones. More common in males, this lesion usually manifests unifocally in the femur.

Symptoms such as insidious pain, swelling, stiffness involving a joint, often the knee, are common, making pyoathritis a great differential diagnosis.

Despite the benign nature of the lesion, chondroblastoma is a locally destructive tumor, described as a small (<5 cm), radiolucent lesion with well-defined borders, accompanied by a sclerotic border (Fig. 28.12a–c).

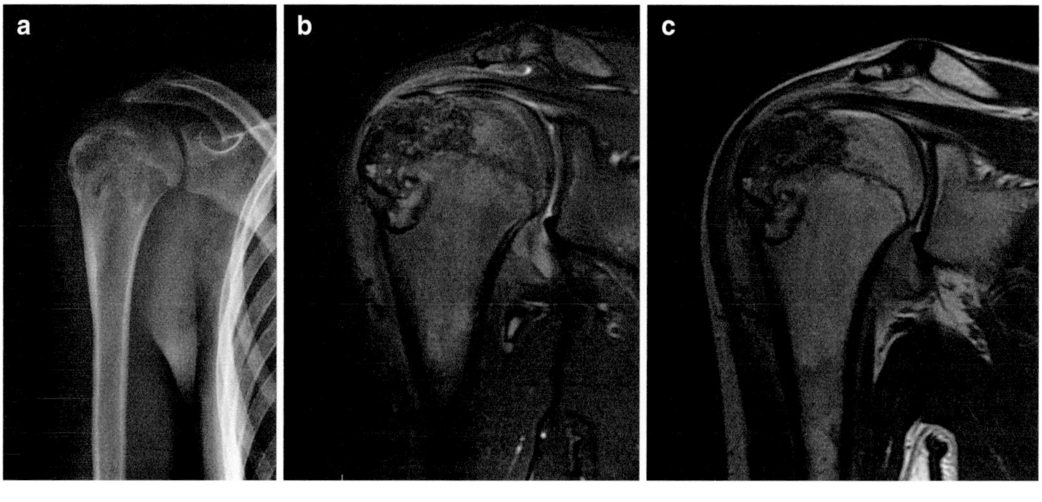

Fig. 28.12 Chondroblastoma in the proximal humerus of a 12-year-old male child. On radiography (**a**), is possible to observe a destructive aspect of the lesion, that extends to the metaphysis. MRI (**b** and **c**) demonstrate the condral matrix of the lesion

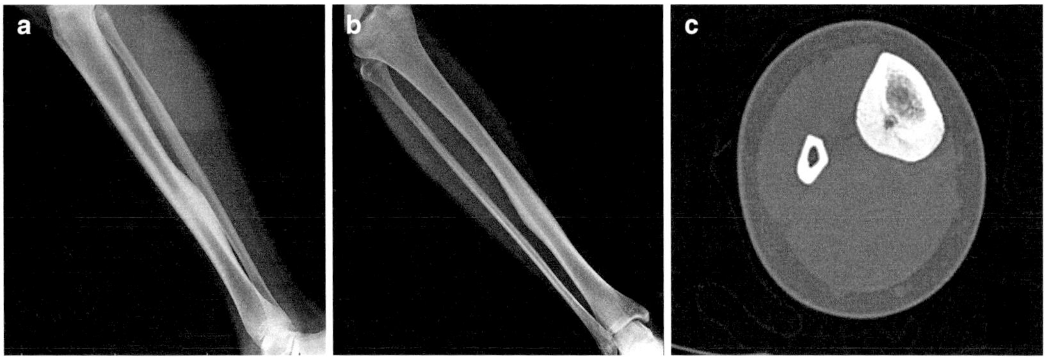

Fig. 28.13 Osteoid osteoma in the tibial shaft with an exuberant osteogenic reaction (**a** and **b**). On CT (**c**), the nidus (lytic center lesion) is surrounded by gross sclerosis

Due to this locally aggressive nature and the discomfort in joints affected, surgical treatment of chondroblastoma with extended intralesional curettage and grafting is indicated. Local recurrence is low, but significant when compared to other benign cartilaginous tumors.

28.5.13 Osteoid Osteoma

Osteoid osteoma is a benign bone-forming tumor usually less than 1.5 cm in diameter and has a peak incidence in the second decade of life. Males are more commonly affected with the range male-to-female ratio 3:1. Fifty percent of these tumors occur in the long bones of the lower extremities. In the spine, it affects the posterior elements of the vertebrae. Pain is severe and occurs at rest and at night. Pain is alleviated with use of NSAIDs or aspirin. Plain radiographs show a Lucent area surrounded by reactive osseous sclerosis (Fig. 28.13a, b), resulting in a characteristic radiograph image referred to as a nidus [2]. CT scan is often necessary to show the nidus because X-ray may not show the nidus because of the sclerotic rim (Fig. 28.13c). MRI can demonstrate osseous and soft tissue edema and is inferior to CT to show the nidus. Nuclear imaging with technetium Tc-99 m is very sensitive for detection of osteoid osteoma [3]. Osteoid osteoma must be distinguished from a cortical stress fracture in young athletes.

Chronic NSAID administration may manage patients with mild symptoms, and some of these lesions have been reported to resolve over time [4]. Surgical treatment of osteoid osteoma consists of nidus resection or, more frequently, CT-guided radioablation of the nidus.

28.5.14 Osteosarcoma

Osteosarcoma is the most common primary bone cancer and most often arises in adolescents and young adults. It has a predilection to long bone metaphyseal portions, such as distal femur, proximal tibia, and proximal humerus. Fifty percent of osteosarcoma cases arise near the knee joint. This is important because knee symptoms are very frequent in the young athletic population, so osteosarcoma may be kept in sports medicine doctor's mind. Diagnosis can be confused with history of pain related to previous trauma in sports practice or growing pains [5]. More than 90% of osteosarcomas are high grade, with rapid development and early metastatic potential to lungs. Patients with clinically detectable metastasis, with axial tumors and early relapse despite treatment have a poorer prognosis.

Pain and swelling are the most common complaints. Pain initially worsens with physical activity but soon is noted even with rest. Plain radiography, MRI of the entire bone affected, whole body scan, and chest CT scan are used for initial evaluation. After these exams, biopsy is made to confirm diagnosis. Plain radiography shows an ill-defined radiodense metaphyseal

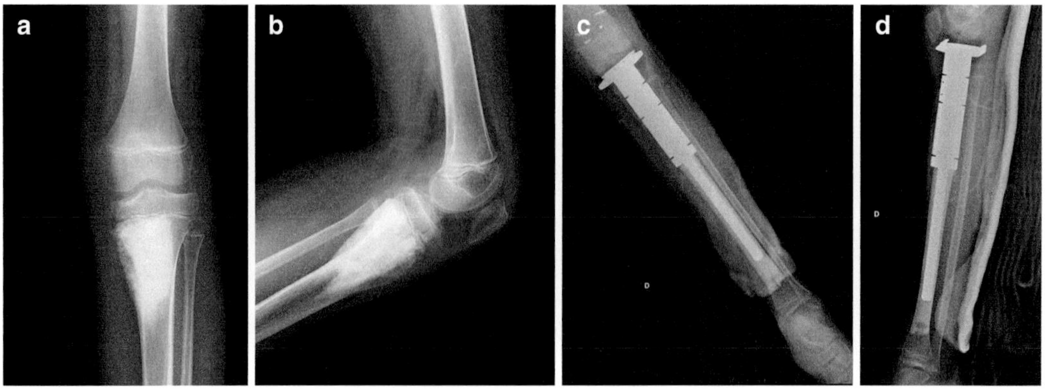

Fig. 28.14 Osteosarcoma of proximal tibia in an adolescent. X-ray (**a** and **b**) of the lesion shows an ill-defined osteoblastic lesion in proximal tibial metaphysis with sunburst appearance. (**c** and **d**) Resection of the tumor with wide margins and reconstruction with proximal partial tibial endoprosthesis. This type of prosthesis permits spare distal femur physis and less leg length discrepancy

lesion (Fig. 28.14a, b). Codman triangle and sunburst appearances are also common.

The treatment of osteosarcoma is based in pre-op multiagent chemotherapy, surgery, and post-op chemotherapy that can be modified based on the study of specimen response. With this treatment and wide surgical margins, 70% of the patients can expect long-term relapse-free survival. Tumor-free margins are of utmost importance to avoid recurrence and improve survival. Multiple studies have shown no statistical difference between patients treated with amputation versus limb salvage [6]. Even in cases with pathological fracture, limb salvage surgery is advocated when local control can be achieved [7]. It is often difficult to choose between limb sparing or amputation and the patient and family must participate in decision-making. The most important factor is local control. There are several reconstruction options available. That includes modular megaprosthesis (Fig. 28.14c, d), allografts alone, or allograft-prosthetic composites. Rotationplasty can be used in selected cases. With the advent of modern prosthesis, amputation may be a good choice.

28.5.15 Ewing Sarcoma

Ewing sarcoma is a small, round-cell sarcoma with varying neuroectodermal differentiation and high-grade malignancy with a strong propensity for metastasis. This tumor is characterized by a translocation between 11 and 22 chromosomes and has a slight male predominance. It is the second most common primary malignancy of bone in children and adolescents and much more common in Caucasians than in Africans. The lower extremity is the most common osseous site, followed by pelvis, chest wall, and upper extremity.

Swelling, pain, fever, weight loss, and fatigue may be present. There is a rapid growth of the mass and increased pain, and Ewing sarcoma differs from osteosarcoma because the former frequently causes systemic compromise. Another important differential diagnosis is with osteomyelitis because of fever and rapid onset of symptoms. Physical examination shows a mass or asymmetric fullness of the affected extremity. Regional lymphadenopathy may be present, but is rare. Metastasis to lungs almost always be present by hematogenous spread. The second most frequent site of metastasis is bone.

Laboratory evaluation is used to determine the health status and prognosis. It includes complete blood cell count, erythrocyte sedimentation rate, C-reactive protein, metabolic panel, and lactate dehydrogenase (LDH). An elevated lactate dehydrogenase at the time of diagnosis is associated with an increased risk of recurrence and decreased survival [8].

In the plain radiographs, Ewing sarcoma shows a permeative, ill-defined, lytic lesion

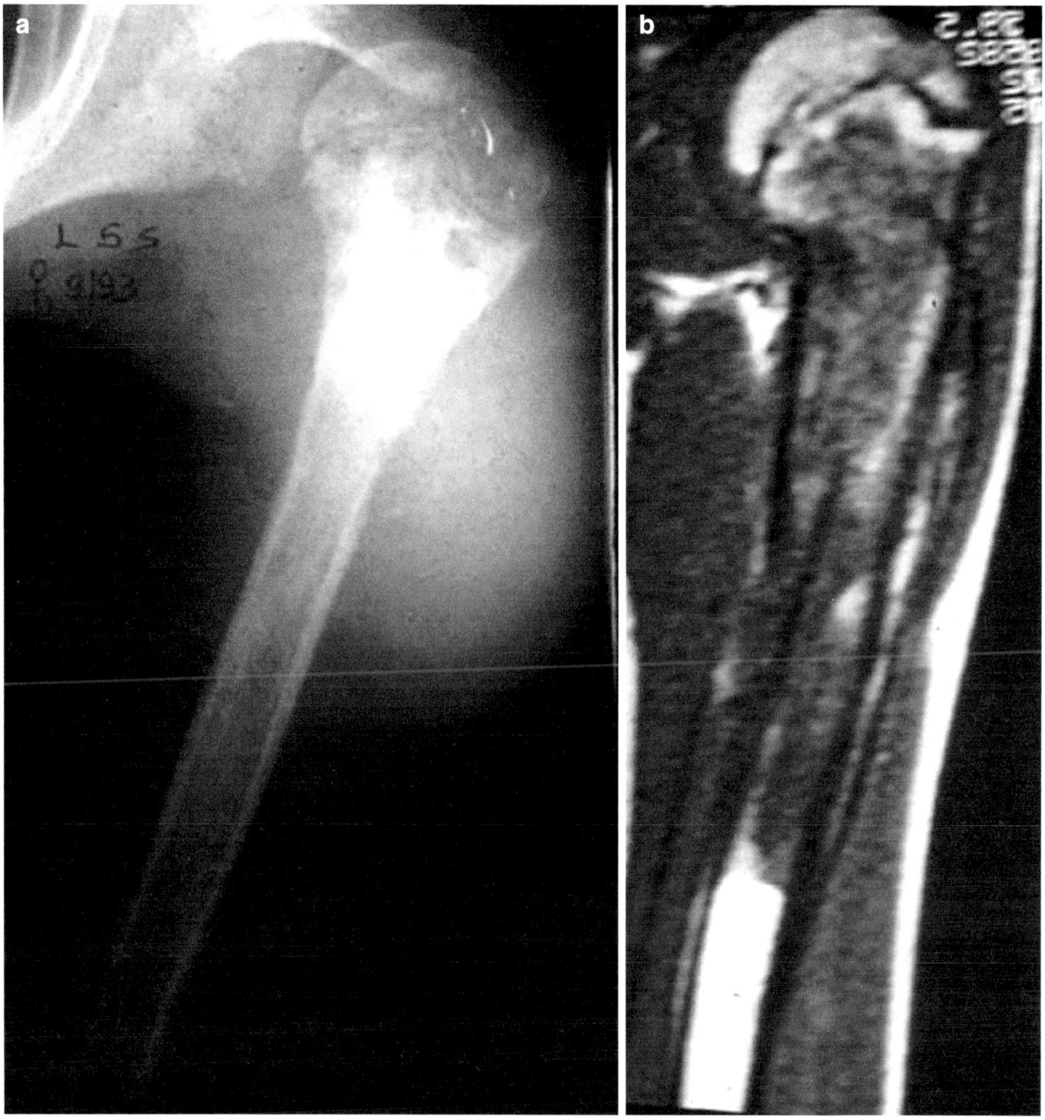

Fig. 28.15 Ewing sarcoma of the proximal humerus. (**a**) X-ray shows an ill-defined lytic metadiaphyseal lesion. (**b**) MRI shows cortical breakage and soft tissue invasion. Medullary spread is clearly demonstrated in MRI

within the diaphysis or metadiaphysis of long bones (Fig. 28.15a). Reactive bone formation such as periosteal reaction (onion skinning or Codman triangle) is frequent. MRI shows the extent of medullary involvement (Fig. 28.15b), presence of skip metastasis, soft tissue invasion, and involvement of major neurovascular structures. CT of the chest is used to search for lung metastasis. Technetium bone scan is used as a sensitive test for bone metastasis. PET/CT is useful in assigning stage for Ewing sarcoma [9].

The 5-year overall survival rate is 76% in children younger than 15 years. Metastatic disease remains the strongest indicator of poor prognosis. Other indicators of poor prognosis are pelvic lesions, great tumor volume, and elevated LDH.

Treatment of Ewing sarcoma includes induction chemotherapy, surgery with wide margins, reconstruction of bone defect, and post-op chemotherapy. Chemotherapy generally includes vincristine, doxorubicin, and cyclophosphamide alternating with ifosfamide and etoposide [10].

Almost 74% of Ewing sarcoma underwent limb salvage versus amputation from 1988 to 2007 [11]. Limb salvage was associated with improved survival, good functional outcomes, and patient satisfaction. Options of reconstruction include megaprosthesis, allografts, and vascularized fibula augmentation.

28.6 Chondrosarcoma of Bone

Chondrosarcoma is a malignant primary bone tumor that affects adults and older individuals. It differs in many aspects with osteosarcoma and Ewing sarcoma, which affects children and adolescents. There are many subtypes of chondrosarcoma, varying from indolent low-grade to high-grade fulminant cancer. Classifying this tumor is often difficult because needle biopsy is often inaccurate to show the correct diagnosis. Chondrosarcoma is resistant to chemotherapy and radiotherapy; therefore, the treatment is almost always surgical. Unless of high grade, chondrosarcoma tends to present with a long-standing history of pain, mild swelling, and progressive difficulty to practice sports or daily activities [12].

Chondrosarcoma affects the axial and proximal appendicular skeleton most often, and most axial cartilage neoplasms behave more aggressively than appendicular tumors. Grade 1 chondrosarcoma is slow-growing, insidious, and mild pain and may be confused with other orthopedics diseases, such as low back pain, sciatica, and rotator cuff disorders. A soft tissue mass is uncommon because the tumor remains for a long time inside the bone. Actually, low-grade chondrosarcoma of the extremities has been reclassified to low-grade cartilage neoplasm. In such cases, the risk of metastasis is lower than 1%. When axial chondrosarcoma is included, the metastatic rate increases to 8% [13]. Low-grade chondrosarcoma can dedifferentiate from a high-grade neoplasm. This may happen after a long lag period. Increased tumor size and pain increase may raise suspicion to a malignant dedifferentiation. Grade 2 chondrosarcomas may present similarly to their grade 1 counterparts. Tumors with more myxoid components tend to grow faster. Grade 3 chondrosarcoma and dedifferentiated chondrosarcoma usually present with a very aggressive course. A soft tissue mass is common and the tumor can destroy cortical bone and invade neurovascular structures and adjacent muscles. Secondary chondrosarcomas arise from a benign cartilage tumor, such as enchondroma, periosteal chondromas, and synovial chondromatosis [14]. Other types of chondrosarcoma are juxtacortical chondrosarcoma, mesenchymal chondrosarcoma, clear cell chondrosarcoma, and extraskeletal myxoid chondrosarcoma.

Plain radiographs are very important to determine tumor grade; they show the rate between tumor growth and bone ability to react and preserve its structure. MRI is the second-line study and is often used to follow up. CT scan is superior to MRI in showing cortical integrity, basically endosteal scalloping which is useful to differentiate between enchondroma and low-grade chondrosarcoma. Deeper scallops are a hallmark of more active tumors. As the lesion ages, the intramedullary lesion progressively calcifies and shows a typical aspect of punctate calcifications and popcorn appearance. Biopsy unfortunately cannot differ from enchondroma to grade 1 chondrosarcoma. Grade 2 chondrosarcoma demonstrates a more aggressive pattern, breaks the cortex, destroys bone, and invades surrounding soft tissue (Fig. 28.16a). Grade 3 chondrosarcoma shows even more bone destruction, large soft tissue mass, and no calcification.

The treatment of chondrosarcoma depends on the tumor grade. Grade 1 chondrosarcoma of the appendicular skeleton is managed with intralesional curettage use of adjuvants such as phenol and liquid nitrogen [15], and the defect is filled with cement such as PMMA. Protecting long bones from iatrogenic fractures is advisable using plates to bypass the lesion. Grade 2 chondrosarcoma is managed with marginal or wide resection [16] (Fig. 28.16b) and bone reconstruction with an endoprosthesis. Grade 3 chondrosarcoma is managed with wide resection and bone reconstruction if possible. Although this tumor is generally radioresistant and chemoresistant,

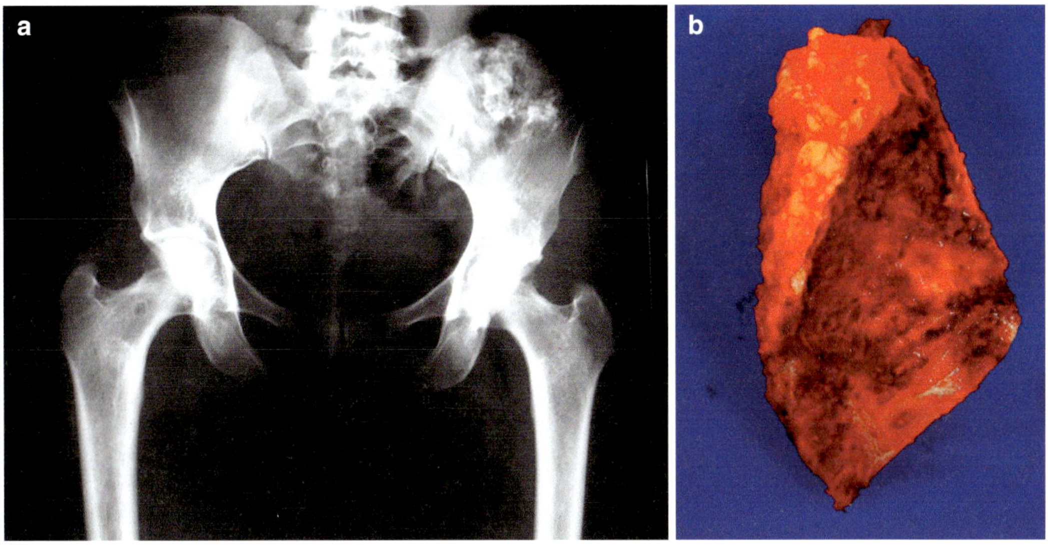

Fig. 28.16 X-ray shows type II chondrosarcoma of the left iliac wing (**a**). (**b**) specimen resected. No reconstruction was needed

chemotherapy may be used in mesenchymal and dedifferentiated chondrosarcoma.

28.7 Giant Cell Tumor of Bone

GCTB was previously considered a benign locally aggressive tumor, but now is considered an intermediate neoplasm. It affects young adult patients between 20 and 40 years of age. It has the predilection to metaphysis and epiphysis of long bones such as distal femur, proximal tibia, and distal radius; 50% of GCTB arise near the knee joint [17]. GTTB affects the vertebral body in the vertebral column and can present with radicular symptoms. Pain and joint effusion are common due to epiphyseal involvement. The symptoms are pain that often begins insidiously that increases over time. Approximately 20% of patients will have pathologic fracture [18]. CGTB has a capacity to develop lung metastasis in 2–9% of the cases [19].

The X-ray GCTB shows a radiolucent lesion in the metaepiphyseal area with no sclerosis or periosteal reaction (Fig. 28.17a, b). In more aggressive cases, there is cortical destruction and soft tissue invasion. MRI is effective to demonstrate cortical destruction and the spread to soft tissue. T1-weighted MRI demonstrates low to intermediate signal homogeneous, and T2 sequences show heterogeneity. Gadolinium-enhanced images confirm a solid lesion. CT is used to access pulmonary status.

Bone destruction seen in GCTB is mediated by multinucleated osteoclast-like giant cells and receptor activator of nuclear kappa-b (RANK) ligand pathway plays an essential role in osteoclastogenesis.

The surgical treatment of GCTB varies from curettage with adjuvant in cases with no cortical destruction to en bloc resection and bone reconstruction with megaprosthesis in more aggressive cases. Simple curettage can result in high local recurrence rate of 25–65%. More recently, denosumab, a human monoclonal antibody that can inhibit RANKL, has been used with success in challenging cases such as pelvic and vertebral severe compromise.

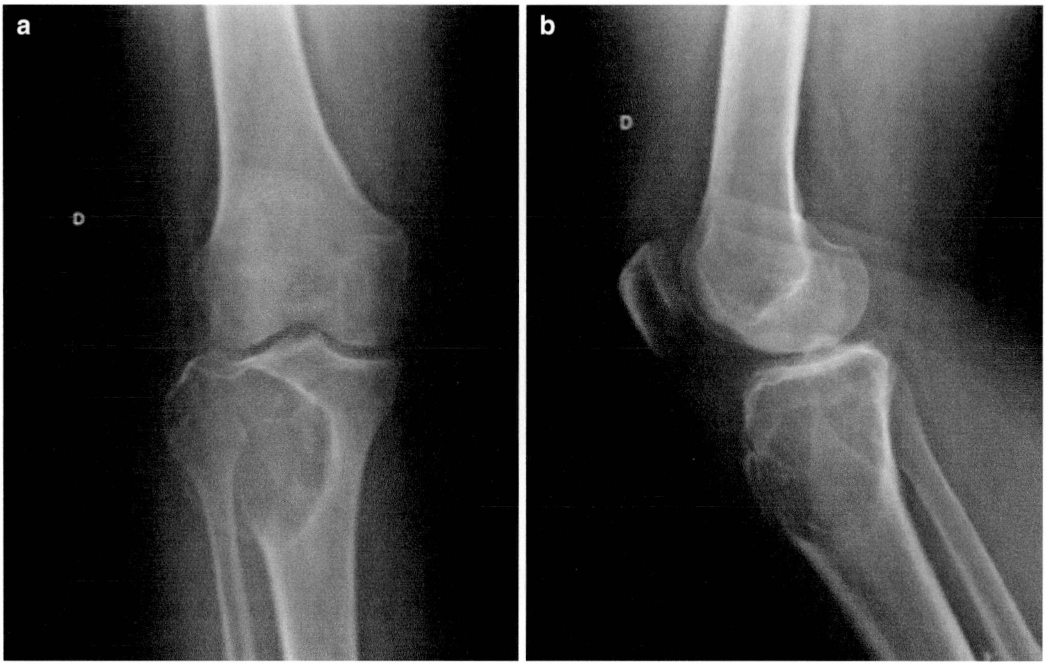

Fig. 28.17 Giant cell tumor of bone (**a** and **b**). X-rays show a lytic metaepiphyseal lesion in the proximal tibia. The lateral cortical bone is thinned and destructed

28.8 Bone Metastasis

Bone metastasis refers to a secondary bone implant following a primary neoplasm whose origin may be or not known. It means that some patients receive cancer diagnosis after a pathologic fracture has occurred or following suggestive incidental findings during a radiologic investigation of vague complaints (such as pain or mild trauma).

Metastases are the most common malignancy of the bone, corresponding to up to 90% of all bone tumors. Those of known origin is usually derived from the breast, prostate, or lung (Fig. 28.18), while those of unknown origin are often from the kidney, lung, or thyroid.

Prognostic and treatment rationale depends on the primary malignance stage and histologic degree. The number and site of metastases in the bone are also considered when choosing the optimal treatment. The presence of mechanical pain (that limits daily activities), high-risk sites (lower limbs, especially proximal femur), purely or predominantly osteolytic lesions, and size of the lesion (greater than two-thirds of the bone diameter) indicate restrictions to weight bearing in the affected limb, as well as prophylactic surgical fixation of the bone. If the patient has no mechanical pain nor the metastasis is in a high-risk site, no restriction to sports and activities is recommended.

Treatment options for bone metastasis include surgery, radiation therapy, and chemotherapy. Impending pathologic fractures must be treated surgically—unless the risks of the procedure and the patient's clinical conditions are prohibitive. Depending on the primary malignancy, good response to radiation therapy is expected and can be considered as the first line of treatment. Bone metastasis can also respond to chemotherapy, but usually it is not considered adequate as a single modality treatment.

It must be kept in mind that metastatic disease generally has a poor prognosis itself. A pathologic fracture worsens this clinical scenario and must be avoided by precisely indicating weight-bearing restrictions and prophylactic fixation whenever needed.

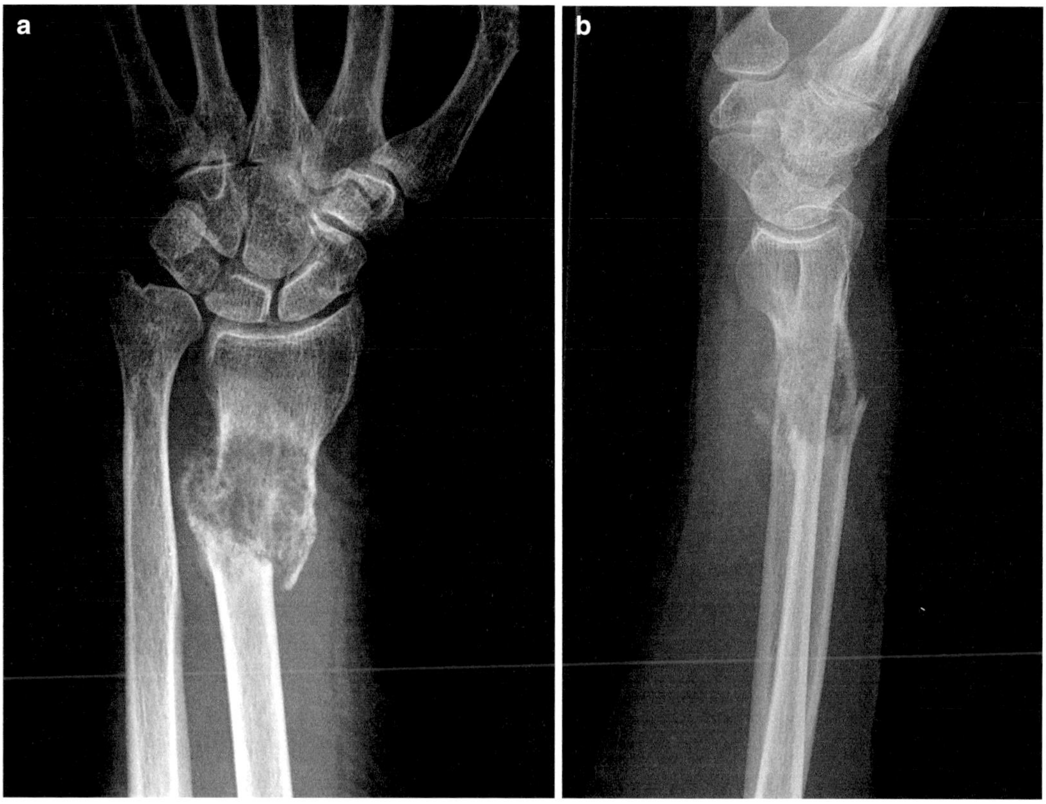

Fig. 28.18 Lung cancer metastasis to bone. Purely lytic lesion. Pathologic fracture of the distal diaphysis of the radio can be observed at the AP (**a**) and lateral (**b**) X-ray views

28.9 Multiple Myeloma

Myeloma is the most common primary malignancy of bone and can be described as a neoplastic proliferation of plasma cells that most commonly affects African descent males >40 years and results in multiple skeletal lesions (with bone pain or a pathologic fracture), hypercalcemia, renal insufficiency, and anemia.

Painful bony symptoms are one of the most common symptoms and multiple "punched-out" lytic lesions can be observed at the diagnosis. In an orthopedic scenario, the presence of M globulin spike in serum protein electrophoresis associated with classic lesions is sufficient, but the diagnostic criteria include monoclonal plasma cells ≥10% on bone marrow biopsy and ≥ 1 of the CRAB (hypercalcemia, renal insufficiency, anemia, bone lesions) features of end-organ damage (Fig. 28.19).

This disease takes multiple forms that vary in treatment and prognosis. The solitary plasmacytoma is a plasma cell tumor occurring in a single skeletal location and lacking appropriate criteria for diagnosis of multiple myeloma.

Treatment is usually based on chemotherapy, with radiotherapy used in adjuvance for pain control. Surgical management is indicated for associated fractures or prophylactic fixation in lesions with a high Mirel's score (≥8 points).

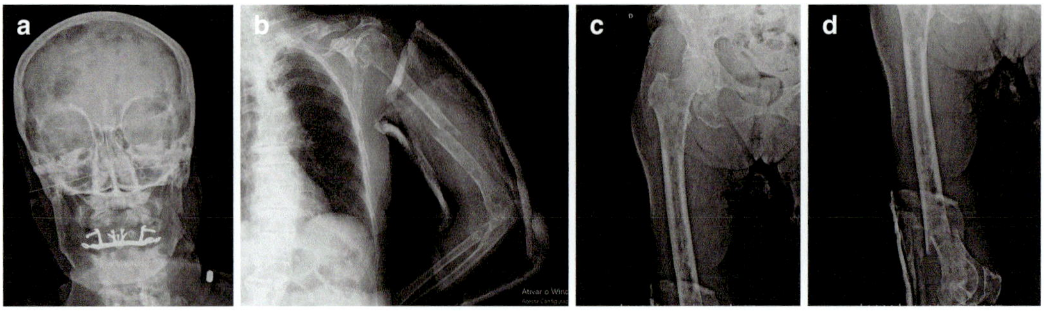

Fig. 28.19 Radiographs of a patient with multiple myeloma. Note the multiple "punched-out" lytic lesions in the skull (**a**), humerus (**b**), and femur (**c**) with pathological fractures of the distal femur (**d**) and humeral diaphysis (**b**)

Take Home Messages

- Always keep in mind musculoskeletal tumors as a differential diagnosis.
- Suspect of soft tissue nodules that occur in different sites or with no clear explanation, such as perimeniscal cysts with no meniscus disease.
- Suspect of fractures that occur with very low energy of trauma: it could be an osteosarcoma,
- Rapid referral to orthopedic oncologist is of utmost importance to give the best treatment and best chance to resume sports activities.

References

1. Toirkens J, De Schepper AM, Vanhoenacker F, et al. A comparison between histopathology and findings on magnetic resonance imaging of subcutaneous lipomatous soft-tissue tumors. Insights Imaging. 2011;2(5):599–607.
2. Jaffe H. Osteoid osteoma: a benign osteoblastic tumor composed of osteoid and atypical bone. Arch Surg. 1935;31:709–28.
3. Bilchik T, Heyman S, Siegel A, Alavi A. Osteoid osteoma: the role of radionuclide bone imaging, conventional radiography and computed tomography in its management. J Nucl Med. 1992;33(2):269–71.
4. Kneisl JS, Simon MA. Medical management compared with operative treatment for osteoid-osteoma. J Bone Joint Surg Am. 1992;74(2):179–85.
5. Meyers PA, Gorlick R. Osteosarcoma. Pediatr Clin N Am. 1997;44(4):973–89.
6. Rougraff BT, Simon MA, Kneisl JS, Greenberg DB, Mankin HJ. Limb salvage compared with amputation for osteosarcoma of the distal end of the femur: a long-term oncological, functional, and quality-of-life study. J Bone Joint Surg Am. 1994;76(5):649–56.
7. Ferguson PC, McLaughlin CE, Griffin AM, Bell RS, Deheshi BM, Wunder JS. Clinical and functional outcomes of patients with a pathologic fracture in high grade osteosarcoma. J Surg Oncol. 2010;102(2):120–4.
8. Li S, Yang Q, Wang H, et al. Prognostic significance of serum lactate dehydrogenase levels in Ewing's sarcoma: a meta-analysis. Mol Clin Oncol. 2016;5(6):832–8.
9. Treglia G, Salsano M, Stefanelli A, et al. Diagnostic accuracy of 18F-FDG-PET and PET/CT in patients with Ewing sarcoma family tumours: a systematic review and a meta-analysis. Skelet Radiol. 2012;41(3):249–56.
10. Grier HE, Krailo MD, Tarbell NJ, et al. Addition of ifosfamide and etoposide to standard chemotherapy for Ewing's sarcoma and primitive neuroectodermal tumor of bone. N Engl J Med. 2003;348(8):694–701.
11. Schrager J, Patzer RE, Mink PJ, Ward KC, Goodman M. Survival outcomes of pediatric osteosarcoma and Ewing's sarcoma: a comparison of surgery type within the SEER database, 1988-2007. J Registry Manag. 2011;38(3):153–61.
12. Marco RA, Gitelis S, Brebach GT, Healey JH. Cartilage tumors: evaluation and treatment. J Am Acad Orthop Surg. 2000;8:292–304.
13. Andreou D, Gilg MM, Gosheger G, et al. Metastatic potential of grade I chondrosarcoma of bone: results of a multi-institutional study. Ann Surg Oncol. 2016;23(1):120–5.
14. Unni KK, Inwards C. Dahlin's bone tumors: general aspects and data on 10,165 cases. 6th ed. Philadelphia: PA, Lippincott-Raven; 2012.
15. DiGiorgio L, Touloupakis G, Vitullo F, Sodano L, Mastantuono M, Villani C. Intralesional curettage with phenol and cement as adjuvants for low-grade intramedullary chondrosarcoma of the long bones. Acta Orthop Belg. 2011;77:666–9.

16. De Camargo OP, Baptista AM, Atanasio MJ, Waisberg DR. Chondrosarcoma of bone: lessons from 46 operated cases in a single institution. Clin Orthop Relat Res. 2010;468:2969–75.
17. Errani C, Ruggieri P, Asenzio MA, et al. Giant cell tumor of the extremity: a review of 349 cases from a single institution. Cancer Treat Rev. 2010;36(1):1–7.
18. Salunke AA, Chen Y, Chen X, et al. Does pathological fracture affect the rate of local recurrence in patients with a giant cell tumour of bone?: a meta-analysis. Bone Joint J. 2015;97-B(11):1566–71.
19. Niu X, Zhang Q, Hao L, Ding Y, Li Y, Xu H, et al. Giant cell tumor of the extremity: retrospective analysis of 621 Chinese patients from one institution. J Bone Joint Surg Am. 2012;94(5):461–7.

Rheumatologic Issues

29

Sérgio Rocha Piedade, Zoraida Sachetto, Guilherme Grisi Mouraria, and Daniel Miranda Ferreira

29.1 Introduction

A rheumatological disease comprises an autoimmune dysfunction that triggers an inflammatory process affecting muscles, tendons, ligaments, joints, and synovial tissue, consequently causing tissue degeneration—a connective tissue disorder [1–3]. It encompasses different diseases and may involve several anatomical sites such as the spine, hip, knee, shoulder, elbow, hand, ankle, and foot joints [2, 4] Moreover, rheumatological diseases can also present systematic manifestations on the skin, oral ulcers, serositis, eyes, heart, and disorders in hematological and neurological systems, presenting an underlying clinical sign of the disease.

Many times, the passion for sports may produce "heroes or even demigods" on earth, people that in our minds will not be touched by any clinical disease, except by traumatic events, because they seem to be genetically, physically, and mentally well-protected from that. Unfortunately, it is not true; athletes are not free from diseases such as rheumatological disorders.

Although journals, TV shows, and social media have already reported stories of famous athletes diagnosed with a rheumatological disease, as well as the repercussions to their athletic career to go forward practicing sports and competing, literature has not yet given close attention to the occurrence of rheumatic disease in the athletic population. This fact could influence some sports medicine physicians and orthopedists not to include rheumatic disease in differential diagnoses for musculoskeletal complaints [1, 5–10]. Understanding that rheumatic disease may mimic musculoskeletal complaints commonly associated with traumatic events or mechanical joint overload is essential to call the attention of sports medicine physicians and orthopedists to these diseases as a possible differential diagnosis in athletes or regular sports practitioners.

Clinically, the disease may alter from a period of more important clinical manifestations to the remission of the symptoms [11, 12]. The main complaints of musculoskeletal disorders are persistent pain and discomfort associated with joint swelling or effusion and muscle weakness resulting in a progressive decline in sports performance due to the active inflammatory process of the disease [13]. In this context, the early diagnosis of a rheumatological disease could allow better control of the inflammatory process and the fast

S. R. Piedade (✉) · Z. Sachetto · G. G. Mouraria
Exercise and Sports Medicine, Department of Orthopedics, Rheumatology, and Traumatology, University of Campinas—UNICAMP, Campinas, SP, Brazil
e-mail: piedade@unicamp.br; zoraida@unicamp.br; mouraria@unicamp.br

D. M. Ferreira
Department of Radiology, University of Campinas—UNICAMP, Campinas, SP, Brazil

Department of Radiology, São Leopoldo Mandic Faculty of Medicine, Campinas, SP, Brazil

S. Rocha Piedade et al. (eds.), *Sideline Management in Sports*,
https://doi.org/10.1007/978-3-031-33867-0_29

evolution of rheumatological disorders and injuries, which could be vital for the athlete's career in sports [8–10, 12, 13].

Therefore, the sports medicine physician should be aware of that when assessing an athlete's musculoskeletal persistent complaints, mainly even if training re-adaptation and physiotherapy approach had no benefits to remission of the symptoms. Therefore, we should think out of the box and remember that rheumatological diseases also affect athletes!

Rheumatological diseases have a large spectrum of clinical presentations; therefore, the knowledge and familiarity with these clinical features are essential for the physician to establish the correct diagnosis and start adequate treatment soon [4, 5, 11].

This chapter explores and discusses the different rheumatological diseases, their main clinical features, laboratory tests, and radiological signs involved in the diagnosis, mimicking differential diagnosis, the importance of early diagnosis in the treatment, and drug medication implication in sports performance—doping.

29.2 The Diagnosis of Rheumatological Disorders

29.2.1 When Should We Suspect a Rheumatological Disease?

In sports practice, the diagnosis of rheumatological disease is not always considered because the leading reported complaints and injuries in the low back, neck, hip, groin, knee, and ankle are commonly related to a traumatic event, overtraining, or even psychological distress [9, 12]. However, the physician should be aware of that because these clinical complaints *could overlap and mimic underlying symptoms of a rheumatological disorder.*

In this context, the physician should pay close attention to the athlete's reports of joint pain, swelling, warmth, redness, no sports trauma history, and no remission even after a customized training program, according to the athlete's complaints or a rest period [6, 9]. Moreover, it is essential to be aware of systematic signs such as anorexia, weight loss, and fever that could signify features related to some rheumatological diseases such as systemic lupus erythematosus, rheumatoid arthritis, vasculitis, and polymyalgia [2–4, 14–17].

Therefore, careful anamnesis and physical assessment remain the primary tools to identify the symptoms related to rheumatological disorders helping to identify possible diagnoses. Next, lab exams will be required to confirm which rheumatological disease is affecting the athlete.

29.2.2 Main Clinical Signs of Rheumatological Disorders

In general, the clinical features of rheumatological diseases show the response of soft tissues and joints to the autoimmune and inflammatory processes that will chronically affect different organs and systems of the human body, such as musculoskeletal symptoms of arthralgia, myalgia, fever, warmth, and redness [2, 5]. *Moreover, there are systemic manifestations of the disease that may be presented by weight loss, dry skin, skin rashes, dry eyes, and so on* [12, 18].

The onset of joint symptoms combined with the clinical joint involvement features may indicate some specific rheumatic disease. Therefore, monoarticular arthritis of large joints of lower limbs is commonly related to reactive arthritis, while rheumatoid arthritis initially affects small joints of the hands symmetrically [2, 9, 12].

29.2.3 Laboratory Exams

In clinical practice, once the clinical suspicion of rheumatological disease has been raised, some blood tests should be requested, such as rheumatoid factor (RF); anti-citrullinated protein autoantibodies (ACAPA); erythrocyte sedimentation rate (ESR); and C-reactive protein (CPR) [3, 15, 19].

The laboratory exams should be complemented by other exams such as monosodic urate (MSU) and ANA: antinuclear antibody (ANA). In addition, tissue samples and joint liquid are also done to investigate and exclude other causes, such as infection, and confirm the diagnosis [15, 20].

29.3 Radiological Exams

Radiological exams include X-ray, ultrasound (US), magnetic resonance (MR), and computed tomography (CT). However, in the initial stages of the disease, the radiological exams will not add factual information because they could show no evidence of joint degeneration and slight soft tissue edema or synovitis. With the progression and more activity of the inflammatory process of the disease, the radiological changes in the soft tissue and joint will be more significant [21–24].

29.4 Rheumatological Diseases

29.4.1 Rheumatoid Arthritis

Rheumatoid arthritis is an inflammatory polyarthritis resulting from a systemic autoimmune disease that can also affect several organs [25]. The initial and most prevalent reported clinical signs are symmetric inflammation of small joints of the hands and feet. Early morning joint pain is a typical complaint and is one of the diagnostic criteria. The appearance of rheumatoid nodules can be present in 20% of patients. Although the rheumatoid blood factor is present in 80% of cases, it cannot be considered a pathognomonic finding for this disease. Soft tissue swelling, joint effusion, synovial hyperemia, and hyperplasia are the early radiographic findings (Fig. 29.1). According to the American Academy of Rheumatology, the diagnosis of Rheumatoid arthritis is considered positive in the presence of four clinical signs for at least 6 weeks or three clinical signs and a positive rheumatoid factor [26]. The clinical signs are as follows:

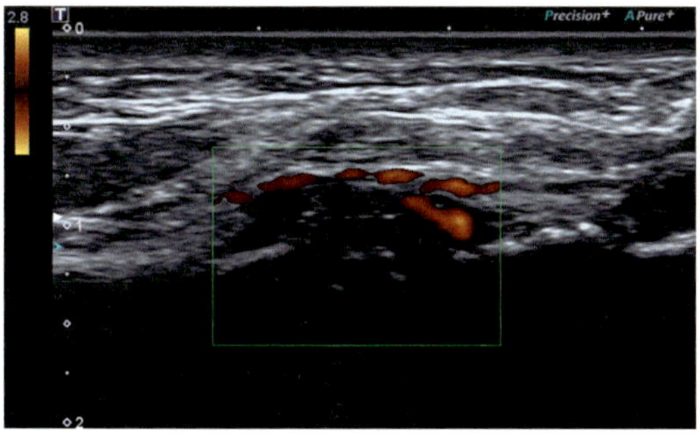

Fig. 29.1 Ultrasound with Doppler of the metacarpophalangeal joint (MCP) with synovial proliferation and inflammation

- Edema in 3 or more joints,
- Edema in both hands,
- Symmetric joints swelling,
- Bone erosions on hand on radiographic exams,
- Rheumatoid nodules,
- Morning stiffness for at least 1 h.

29.4.2 Ankylosing Spondylitis

Ankylosing spondylitis is a chronic inflammatory disease involving the axial or peripheral skeleton and touches young men between 30–40 years of age [7]. The main complaints reported are pain and progressive loss of mobility of the spine and sacroiliac joint, fingers, enthesitis, and eyes (anterior uveitis). The sacroiliac joint is one of the first to be affected by this disease. In clinical practice, the pain may improve with physical activity but worsens at awakening (inactivity during sleeping).

The radiological assessment of the spine and pelvis may show the joint structural changes—so-called ankylosing spondylitis, and diagnose and classify the disease. Sacroiliitis and Romanus lesions is usually the first radiological manifestation finding in inflammatory spondyloarthropathies (Fig. 29.2). However, even when the radiograph shows no joint changes, the diagnosis can also be confirmed by pain in the axial skeleton, with joint alterations on MRI or positive HLA-27 test. However, it is essential to remember that this test cannot be used isolated to confirm the diagnosis of ankylosing spondylitis because, despite the fact that 90% of the patients have a positive HLA-B27, only 10% of individuals will develop the disease [27].

29.5 Gout Arthritis

This painful inflammatory arthritis is caused by crystals formed in the joints because of the high serum dosage of uric acid (hyperuricemia), triggering an inflammatory cascade mediated by

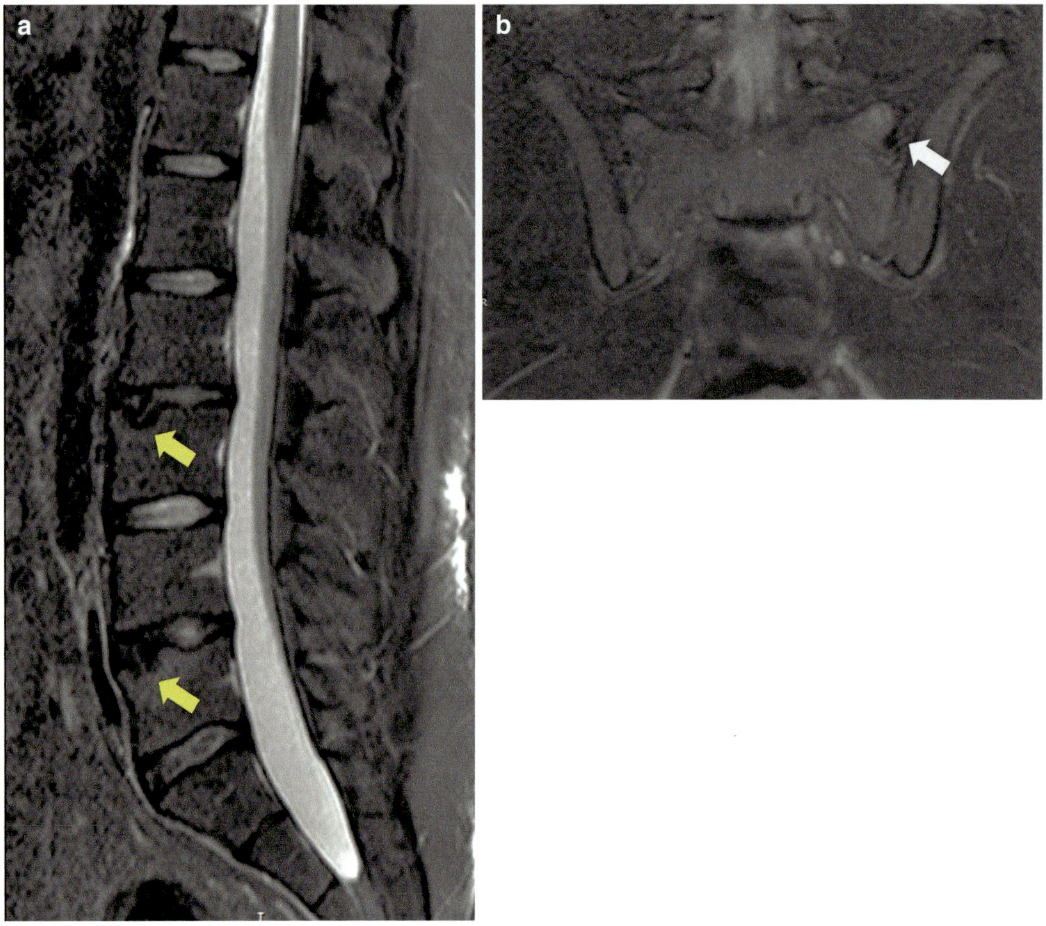

Fig. 29.2 (**a**) Irregularity and erosion involving the anterosuperior edges of the L3 and L5 vertebral endplates (Romanus lesion). (**b**) Marrow edema across the superior sacral margin of the left sacroiliac joint, reflecting initial sacroiliitis

macrophage action against the crystals on the joint surface. The most common clinical features are edema and hyperemia, mainly in the foot and ankle, but it may also progress to the upper limb joints. Gout tophus may be present in more severe cases or in those with inadequate treatment [15]. Initially, the radiographs show only soft tissue edema (Fig. 29.3), while bone destruction will occur in more advanced cases [16]. The presence of monosodium urate crystals in the synovial fluid analyzed under microscopy can make the diagnosis [28]. However, not all patients with hyperuricemia will develop arthritis.

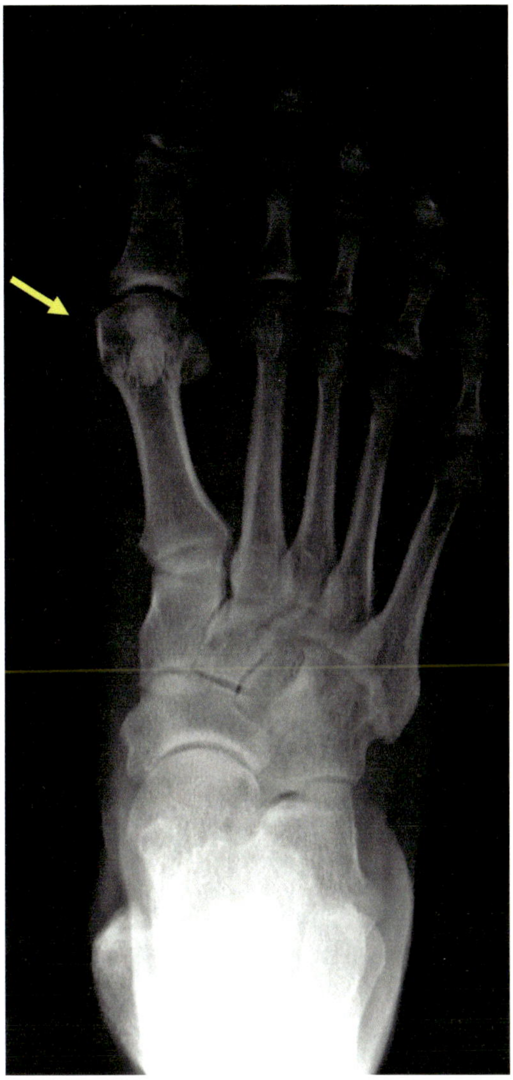

Fig. 29.3 Periarticular soft tissue swelling around the first metatarsophalangeal joint

29.6 Systemic Lupus Erythematosus

This chronic autoimmune disease results from the immunological system's action against tissues, such as skin, joints, blood vessels, kidneys, lungs, and brain, causing generalized inflammation and damage to them [14]. The disease can be classified as systemic, cutaneous, drug-induced, and neonatal. The most common clinical features are fatigue, weight loss, fever, rash, hair loss, and arthritis [14]. 85% of patients will present arthritis, more commonly, in the interphalangeal and metacarpophalangeal joints of the hands, followed by the knee and wrist. The chronic use of corticosteroid drugs for treating underlying clinical conditions can predispose the onset of osteoporosis and osteonecrosis.

29.7 Fibromyalgia

This syndrome is characterized by diffuse pain, fatigue, and changes in the sleep/wake cycle. The complaint of diffuse pain without a known cause for 3 months clinically confirms the diagnosis [29]. Moreover, the association with psychiatric disorders such as depression and anxiety are common. Although laboratory tests help diagnose, it is essential to assess the thyroid function (TSH), level of C-reactive protein, and blood count test for other diseases.

29.8 Behcet's Disease

It is a rare disorder that leads a blood vessel inflammation (vasculitis) affecting the whole body, mainly the mucosa, lungs, and central nervous system [30]. The primary manifestation is the presence of oral and genital ulcers and uveitis. In the most severe clinical presentations, it can progress to aneurysms in the central nervous system [30].

Arthritis can occur intermittently in 40–60% of cases, usually manifested as an oligoarticular of large joints such as the knee and ankle. The diagnosis is made by assessing the various symptoms of *Behcet's disease and excluding other pathologies* [31].

29.9 Polymyalgia Rheumatica

It is an inflammatory disorder more prevalent in individuals over 50 years of age. It is clinically manifested by severe muscle pain and joint stiffness, particularly in the bilateral shoulder, upper arms, elbows, neck, hips, and knees [17]. General clinical signs and symptoms include fatigue, mild fever, loss of appetite, and feeling of not being well. In the acute phase, there was an increase in CPR level. The ultrasound evaluation may show a joint and subacromial effusion resulting from the inflammatory response of the macrophage action on the synovial membrane [32]. The signs of polymyalgia rheumatic may start quickly and worsens in the morning.

29.10 Sarcoidosis

This disease is systemic granulomatosis that may affect any part of the human body, but mostly the lungs and lymph nodes, the skin, eyes, muscles, and tendons [33]. The diagnosis is made by the clinical symptoms and histopathology [33]. In the acute form, the patient may present edema and arthralgia, especially in the ankles, while in the chronic phase, it may progress to deformities [34].

29.11 Sjogren's Syndrome

It is a chronic autoimmune disease that could be primary or secondary to another condition, such as rheumatoid arthritis, affecting the entire body. The lymphocytic invasion of exocrine glands causes its dysfunction, clinically manifested by extensive dryness of the eyes and mouth. Musculoskeletal system disorder occurs in up to 70% of patients, and fatigue is a prevalent symptom and joint pain, especially in the knees and small joints of the hands and wrists [35].

29.11.1 Differential Diagnosis in Monoarthritis

In a clinical diagnosis of acute monoarthritis, the sports medicine physician should consider the possibility of joint infection and perform a careful investigation before ruling out this diagnosis [9]. In clinical practice, the pain, swelling, hyperemia, and increased joint temperature characterize the arthritis inflammatory process, which can manifest as polyarticular, oligo, or monoarticular. Polyarticular presentation is commonly seen in inflammatory or autoimmune diseases, while acute monoarthritis may result from infection, deposits of crystals, or even an autoimmune/inflammatory disease [15, 20].

As in the general population, the diagnosis of monoarthritis in athletes is based on their clinical history, reported complaints, and physical evaluation. For example, if an athlete complains of acute knee pain and temporary discomfort that resolves spontaneously, it might be diagnosed as monoarthritis secondary to crystal-induced arthritis [20]. On the other hand, the presence of a red joint may indicate an infectious process or crystal-induced arthritis [19]. However, the sports medicine physician should be aware that a fever does not necessarily confirm the joint infection diagnosis because it could also result from crystal-induced arthritis leading to misdiagnosis. In this context, the synovial fluid analysis is the main laboratory test to confirm the diagnosis [28]. Table 29.1 compares the findings of the synovial liquid analysis of different etiologies of monoarthritis and the normal synovial fluid.

Table 29.1 Main clinical findings, laboratory tests, and radiology of different rheumatological diseases

Rheumatological disease	Diagnosis		
	Main clinical findings	Laboratory tests	Radiology
Rheumatoid arthritis	Polyarthritis, ocular (scleritis, uveitis, keratitis), interstitial lung disease, rheumatoid nodule, systemic vasculitis, pericarditis, pleuritis	RF, ACPA Elevated ESR, CRP: Nonspecific	X-ray: Symmetrical abnormalities, periarticular osteopenia, narrowing of the joint spaces and marginal degradation, swelling of the soft tissues and synovial cysts and nodules MR: Synovitis, bone erosion and bone marrow edema
Ankylosing spondylitis	Inflammatory back pain and progressive spinal rigidity, arthritis (hips, shoulders, peripheral joints and finger/toes)	HLA-B27	X-ray/MR: Sacroiliitis, syndesmophytes, erosions RM: Bone marrow edema, Romanus lesions
Gout	Arthritis (mono, oligo or polyarticular)	Hyperuricemia (uric acid level above 7 mg/dl) MSU in synovial fluid (negative birefringence) Elevated ESR, CRP: Nonspecific	US/CT/MR: MSU crystal deposition US: Double contour sign, tophus, aggregates and erosion MR: Tophus, synovitis, bone marrow edema, bone erosion X-ray: Bone erosion—Chronic cases
Systemic lupus erythematosus	Polyarthritis, photosensitivity, malar rash, oral or nasal ulcers, serositis, glomerulonephritis, hematological and central nervous system manifestations	ANA Antibodies: Anti-dsDNA, anti-smith, antiphospholipid antibodies Hypocomplementemia, direct Coombs test, proteinuria, red blood cell casts, leukopenia, lymphopenia, thrombocytopenia Elevated ESR, CRP: Nonspecific	–
Polymyalgia rheumatica	Proximal (shoulder/hip girdle) pain and stiffness, peripheral arthritis	Elevated ESR, CRP: Nonspecific	–
Inflammatory MISOISTIS	Dermatomyositis—Proximal weakness of arms and legs, dysphagia, Gottron papules, periorbital edema (heliotrope), erythema of the anterior upper chest (V-sign) or posterior neck (Shaw sign), interstitial lung disease Polymyositis—proximal weakness of arms and legs, dysphagia	Creatine phosphokinase elevated Elevated ESR, CRP: Nonspecific	–
Sjogren's syndrome	Dry eye, soreness, arthritis, peripheral nervous system (sensitivomotor and autonomic), nonspecific and/or usual interstitial pneumonia	Autoantibodies: Anti-Ro (SSA), anti-La (SSB) RF, ANA Elevated ESR, CRP: Nonspecific	–

(continued)

Table 29.1 (continued)

Rheumatological disease	Diagnosis		
	Main clinical findings	Laboratory tests	Radiology
Behcet's disease	Oral and genital ulcers, pseudofolliculitis, nodosum erythema, uveitis, central nervous system (parenchymal and non-parenchymal), thrombophlebitis, colitis	There is no specific diagnostic test	–
Inflammatory EYE disease (non-infectious uveitis)	Anterior, intermediates, posterior or pan uveitis	Elevated ESR, CRP: Nonspecific	–
Sarcoidosis	Lymphadenopathy, nodosum erythema, uveitis, arthritis, hepatic and splenic nodules	Hypercalcemia, hypercalciuria Elevated ESR, CRP: Nonspecific	Torax CT: Hilar and mediastinal nodes, lung interstitial disease
Fibromyalgia	Muscle and joint stiffness, insomnia, fatigue, mood disorders, cognitive dysfunction, anxiety, depression	–	–

RF rheumatoid factor, *ACPA* anti-citrullinated protein autoantibodies, *ESR* erythrocyte sedimentation rate, *CRP* C-reactive protein, *MR* magnetic resonance, *CT* computed tomography, s*MSU* monosodic urate, *ANA* antinuclear antibody

29.12 The Importance of Early Diagnosis

The early diagnosis of a rheumatological disorder allows control and minimizes the inflammatory process and deleterious effects on the musculoskeletal system—especially on the joints and surrounding soft tissues [8, 9, 12]. Therefore, the orthopedists' and sports physicians' knowledge of these diseases plays a crucial role in identifying underlying symptoms and clinical features of the rheumatological disease, requesting a rheumatological assessment, and starting the treatment soon [1, 6, 9, 10]. Table 29.1 presents the main clinical findings, laboratory tests, and radiology of different rheumatological diseases.

29.13 Treatment

The activity of the inflammatory process is approached and treated by the rheumatologist. Non-steroids, steroids, analgesics, and physiotherapy are the main strategies for treating the disease. According to the level of clinical complaints and the progression of the joint degeneration, different strategies such as a period of immobilization for pain relief, using orthoses, and surgical intervention in cases of severe joint degeneration could be necessary [1, 6, 18].

29.13.1 Rheumatological Drugs and Athlete's Doping

Some drugs were banned in world sports, while others were prohibited only during competition seasons. Although some substances used to treat rheumatological diseases can be considered doping by the World Anti-Doping Agency (WADA), others, especially potent analgesics, **are allowed as long as the athlete proves that there is no other medication or substance as an alternative for treating their disease**.

WADA consider that the "in-competition" period begins before midnight (11:59 pm) the day before a competition in which the athlete is scheduled to participate, with the possibility of AMA-WADA approval for a different period for a particular sport. The "in-competition" period finishes at the end of the competition, only after the completion of the sample collection process. Prohibited at "all times" means that the substance or method is prohibited "in-competition" and "out-of-competition" as defined in the World Anti-Doping Code.

Any pharmacological substance that is not on any of the subsequent sections of the prohibited list and without current approval by any governmental health regulatory authority for human therapeutic use, for example: drugs in pre-clinical or clinical development or discontinued, synthetic drugs (designer drugs), and substances approved for veterinary use only are banned "at all times." The WADA's complete list of drugs can be found on the website: https://www.wada-ama.org/.

29.13.1.1 Prognosis of Rheumatological Athlete's Career

The sports career of a rheumatoid athlete is strictly linked to controlling the activity of the inflammatory process of this autoimmune and chronic disease, reinforcing the importance of early diagnosis. It will allow starting the treatment to mitigate and slow down the harmful effects of rheumatological disease on the musculoskeletal system.

At the same time, it is essential to consider that the level of inflammatory activity of the disease could be more or less intense, and therefore, each patient has a range of particular clinical features for the same rheumatological disease.

Therefore, athletes diagnosed with a rheumatological disease need a systematic follow-up with a rheumatologist, sports medicine physician, physiotherapist, and under some circumstances, an orthopedic surgeon's assessment, especially when the musculoskeletal system has a more severe injury.

Take Home Messages

- Be aware of an athlete's musculoskeletal persistent complaints, mainly even if training re-adaptation and physiotherapy approaches had no benefits to remission of the symptoms.
- The lack of a mechanism of trauma or injury may suggest an underlying disease.
- Think out of the box and remember that rheumatological diseases also affect athletes!
- The early diagnosis of a rheumatological disorder allows to control and minimizes the inflammatory process and deleterious effects on the musculoskeletal system—especially on the joints and surrounding soft tissues.

References

1. Metsios GS, Kitas GD. Physical activity, exercise and rheumatoid arthritis: effectiveness, mechanisms and implementation. Best Pract Res Clin Rheumatol. 2018;32:669–82. https://doi.org/10.1016/j.berh.2019.03.013.
2. McInnes IB, Schett G. The pathogenesis of rheumatoid arthritis. N Engl J Med. 2011;365:2205–19. https://doi.org/10.1056/NEJMra1004965.
3. Scott DL, Wolfe F, Huizinga TWJ. Rheumatoid arthritis. Lancet (London, England). 2010;376:1094–108. https://doi.org/10.1016/S0140-6736(10)60826-4.
4. Gutiérrez-González LA. Rheumatologic emergencies. Clin Rheumatol. 2015;34:2011–9. https://doi.org/10.1007/s10067-015-2994-y.
5. Pan JC, Bressler DN. Fatigue in rheumatologic diseases. Phys Med Rehabil Clin N Am. 2009;20:373–87. https://doi.org/10.1016/j.pmr.2008.12.008.
6. Proschek D, Rehart S. Sport and rheumatoid arthritis. Z Rheumatol. 2014;73:434–8. https://doi.org/10.1007/s00393-013-1341-4.
7. Raychaudhuri SP, Deodhar A. The classification and diagnostic criteria of ankylosing spondylitis. J Autoimmun. 2014;48–49:128–33. https://doi.org/10.1016/J.JAUT.2014.01.015.
8. Jennings F, Lambert E, Fredericson M. Rheumatic diseases presenting as sports-related injuries. Sports Med. 2008;38:917–30. https://doi.org/10.2165/00007256-200838110-00003.
9. Flemming DJ, Bernard SA. Arthritis mimicking sports-related injuries. Clin Sports Med. 2013;32:577–97. https://doi.org/10.1016/j.csm.2013.03.003.

10. Harvey J, Tanner S. Low back pain in young athletes. A practical approach. Sports Med. 1991;12:394–406. https://doi.org/10.2165/00007256-199112060-00005.
11. Narváez JA, Narváez J, De Lama E, De Albert M. MR imaging of early rheumatoid arthritis. Radiogr a Rev Publ Radiol Soc North Am Inc. 2010;30:143–5. https://doi.org/10.1148/rg.301095089.
12. Littlejohn EA, Monrad SU. Early diagnosis and treatment of rheumatoid arthritis. Prim Care. 2018;45:237–55. https://doi.org/10.1016/j.pop.2018.02.010.
13. Rubin DA. MR and ultrasound of the hands and wrists in rheumatoid arthritis. Part II. Added clinical value. Skelet Radiol. 2019;48:837–57. https://doi.org/10.1007/s00256-019-03180-6.
14. Aringer M, Costenbader K, Daikh D, Brinks R, Mosca M, Ramsey-Goldman R, et al. 2019 European league against rheumatism/American College of Rheumatology classification criteria for systemic lupus erythematosus. Ann Rheum Dis. 2019;78:1151–9. https://doi.org/10.1136/annrheumdis-2018-214819.
15. Dalbeth N, Merriman TR, Stamp LK. Gout. Lancet (London, England) 2016;388:2039–2052. https://doi.org/10.1016/S0140-6736(16)00346-9.
16. Neogi T, Jansen TLTA, Dalbeth N, Fransen J, Schumacher HR, Berendsen D, et al. 2015 Gout classification criteria: an American College of Rheumatology/European league against rheumatism collaborative initiative. Ann Rheum Dis. 2015;74:1789–98. https://doi.org/10.1136/ANNRHEUMDIS-2015-208237.
17. Camellino D, Giusti A, Girasole G, Bianchi G, Dejaco C. Pathogenesis, diagnosis and Management of Polymyalgia Rheumatica. Drugs Aging. 2019;36:1015–26. https://doi.org/10.1007/s40266-019-00705-5.
18. Sommer OJ, Kladosek A, Weiler V, Czembirek H, Boeck M, Stiskal M. Rheumatoid arthritis: a practical guide to state-of-the-art imaging, image interpretation, and clinical implications. Radiogr a Rev Publ Radiol Soc North Am Inc. 2005;25:381–98. https://doi.org/10.1148/rg.252045111.
19. Birch JTJ, Bhattacharya S. Emerging trends in diagnosis and treatment of rheumatoid arthritis. Prim Care. 2010;37(779–92):vii. https://doi.org/10.1016/j.pop.2010.07.001.
20. Ma L, Cranney A, Holroyd-Leduc JM. Acute monoarthritis: what is the cause of my patient's painful swollen joint? C Can Med Assoc J = J l'Association Medicale Can. 2009;180:59–65. https://doi.org/10.1503/cmaj.080183.
21. Weaver JS, Omar I, Mar W, Kauser AS, Mlady GW, Taljanovic M. Magnetic resonance imaging of rheumatological diseases. Pol J Radiol. 2022;87:e93–112. https://doi.org/10.5114/pjr.2022.113390.
22. Chang EY, Chen KC, Huang BK, Kavanaugh A. Adult inflammatory Arthritis: what the radiologist should know. Radiogr a Rev Publ Radiol Soc North Am Inc. 2016;36:1849–70. https://doi.org/10.1148/rg.2016160011.
23. Taljanovic MS, Melville DM, Gimber LH, Scalcione LR, Miller MD, Kwoh CK, et al. High-resolution US of rheumatologic diseases. Radiogr a Rev Publ Radiol Soc North Am Inc. 2015;35:2026–48. https://doi.org/10.1148/rg.2015140250.
24. Burke CJ, Alizai H, Beltran LS, Regatte RR. MRI of synovitis and joint fluid. J Magn Reson Imaging. 2019;49:1512–27. https://doi.org/10.1002/jmri.26618.
25. Kwoh CK, Anderson LG, Greene JM, Johnson DA, O'Dell JR, Robbins ML, et al. Guidelines for the management of rheumatoid arthritis: 2002 update. Arthritis Rheum. 2002;46:328–46. https://doi.org/10.1002/ART.10148.
26. Aletaha D, Neogi T, Silman AJ, Funovits J, Felson DT, Bingham CO, et al. 2010 rheumatoid arthritis classification criteria: an American College of Rheumatology/European league against rheumatism collaborative initiative. Arthritis Rheum. 2010;62:2569–81. https://doi.org/10.1002/ART.27584.
27. Turina MC, de Winter JJ, Paramarta JE, Gamala M, Yeremenko N, Nabibux MN, et al. Clinical and imaging signs of Spondyloarthritis in first-degree relatives of HLA-B27-positive ankylosing spondylitis patients: the pre-Spondyloarthritis (pre-SpA) cohort study. Arthritis Rheumatol (Hoboken, NJ). 2016;68:2444–55. https://doi.org/10.1002/ART.39766.
28. Pascual E, Jovaní V. Synovial fluid analysis. Best Pract Res Clin Rheumatol. 2005;19:371–86. https://doi.org/10.1016/J.BERH.2005.01.004.
29. Jay GW, Barkin RL. Fibromyalgia. Dis Mon. 2015;61:66–111. https://doi.org/10.1016/J.DISAMONTH.2015.01.002.
30. Akdeniz N, Elmas ÖF, Karadağ AS. Behçet syndrome: a great imitator. Clin Dermatol. 2019;37:227–39. https://doi.org/10.1016/J.CLINDERMATOL.2019.01.001.
31. Alpsoy E, Donmez L, Bacanli A, Apaydin C, Butun B. Review of the chronology of clinical manifestations in 60 patients with Behçet's disease. Dermatology. 2003;207:354–6. https://doi.org/10.1159/000074113.
32. Meliconi R, Pulsatelli L, Uguccioni M, Salvarani C, Macchioni P, Melchiorri C, et al. Leukocyte infiltration in synovial tissue from the shoulder of patients with polymyalgia rheumatica. Quantitative analysis and influence of corticosteroid treatment. Arthritis Rheum. 1996;39:1199–207. https://doi.org/10.1002/ART.1780390719.
33. Govender P, Berman JS. The diagnosis of sarcoidosis. Clin Chest Med. 2015;36:585–602. https://doi.org/10.1016/J.CCM.2015.08.003.
34. Nessrine A, Zahra AF, Taoufik H. Musculoskeletal involvement in sarcoidosis. J Bras Pneumol. 2014;40:175–82. https://doi.org/10.1590/S1806-37132014000200012.
35. Fauchais AL, Ouattara B, Gondran G, Lalloué F, Petit D, Ly K, et al. Articular manifestations in primary Sjögren's syndrome: clinical significance and prognosis of 188 patients. Rheumatology (Oxford). 2010;49:1164–72. https://doi.org/10.1093/RHEUMATOLOGY/KEQ047.

Part IV

Environmental Challenges

HEAT (Hyperthermia or Insolation, Exertional Heat Stroke)

30

David Figueroa, Francisco Figueroa, and Minerva Itriago

30.1 Introduction

Hyperthermia or insolation, exertional heat stroke (HEAT) is a medical emergency defined as life-threatening hyperthermia (core body temperature > 40.5 °C), multiorgan failure, and central nervous system (CNS) dysfunction. It occurs during physical activity in athletes (elite and recreational), military personnel, and people performing the physical activity as part of an occupation (e.g., construction workers), usually, but not always, in hot environments. In fact, HEAT is the third leading cause of death among athletes during physical activity [1].

Gardner and Kark were the first to describe serious heat illness as a spectrum of increasing severity that includes heat exhaustion, heat injury, and heat stroke [2].

Heat exhaustion is a mild to moderate condition associated with physical activity characterized by the inability to maintain cardiac output and blood pressure because of high skin blood flow requirements and/or dehydration that may or may not be associated with marked hyperthermia. Heat injury is a moderate to severe syndrome characterized by organ and tissue injury in the presence of severe hyperthermia. Finally, on the most extreme side of the spectrum is HEAT, which is a life-threatening condition defined by profound CNS dysfunction (e.g., confusion, severe disorientation, combativeness, seizures, and coma), hyperthermia, body organ/tissue damage, and often vigorous exercise [3, 4].

The true incidence of HEAT is unknown because of frequent misdiagnoses (e.g., dehydration or heat exhaustion). Epidemiologic surveys of U.S. high-school football players and army personnel reveal a steady increase in morbidity and mortality from exertional heat stroke during the past decade. Nevertheless, because exertional heat stroke most often affects healthy young persons and its recognition and treatment are usually prompt, mortality rates are low (<5%) [5–7].

30.2 Pathophysiology

The primary pathogenic mechanism of heat stroke involves the transition from a compensable thermoregulatory phase (in which heat loss exceeds heat gain) to a non-compensable phase (in which heat gain is greater than heat loss) when cardiac output is insufficient to cope with the high thermoregulatory needs. Consequently, core body temperature continues to rise, leading to a direct cytotoxic effect and an inflammatory

D. Figueroa · M. Itriago
Clinica Alemana-Universidad del Desarrollo, Santiago, Chile

F. Figueroa (✉)
Clinica Alemana-Universidad del Desarrollo, Santiago, Chile

Hospital Sotero del Rio, Santiago, Chile

S. Rocha Piedade et al. (eds.), *Sideline Management in Sports*,
https://doi.org/10.1007/978-3-031-33867-0_30

response, creating a vicious cycle and eventually causing multiorgan failure [8].

Thermoregulation is controlled by the hypothalamus, with compensatory responses mediated principally in the skin (sweating and vasodilation) and cardiovascular system (increased cardiac output and gut vasoconstriction). During strenuous exercise, especially in hot and humid climates, heat is stored faster than the body can dissipate it. Therefore, it is typical to have body temperatures between 38.9 °C and 40.3 °C during intense exercise in the heat. When the cell is heated beyond its thermal threshold, cell damage occurs, which may lead to organ dysfunction and failure/death. Some individuals may have underlying risk factors that can lead to HEAT (Table 30.1). Extrinsic risk factors also play a large role in the risk for HEAT (Table 30.2) [9, 10].

Table 30.1 Intrinsic risk factors

Lack of heat acclimatization
Current febrile illness
Skin disorders: anhidrosis, sunburn, psoriasis, etc.
Dehydration
Medications/supplements (e.g., diuretics, CNS stimulants, and antidepressants)
Sleep deprivation
Recent alcohol use
Low physical fitness
Overweight/obesity
Cardiovascular disorders (e.g., hypertension and peripheral vascular disease)
Malignant hyperthermia susceptibility

Table 30.2 Extrinsic risk factors

Hot, humid environment (especially wet bulb globe temperature exceeding 28 °C)
Exercise intensity
Inappropriate work-to-rest ratios
Heavy equipment/clothing
Lack of education and awareness among athletes, coaches, and medical staff
Lack of emergency plans to identify and treat EHS
Lack of proper infrastructure (heat acclimatization period, access to fluids, preventive cooling strategies, etc.)

30.3 Diagnosis

The diagnosis of HEAT is largely clinical, based primarily on the triad of hyperthermia, neurologic abnormalities, and recent exposure to physical exertion. Early signs and symptoms include the following: [1] CNS dysfunction (disorientation, irrational behavior, combativeness, convulsions, collapse, and loss of consciousness); [2] rectal temperature > 40.5 °C taken at point of collapse; [3] dizziness and lightheadedness; [4] extreme fatigue not typical for that activity; [5] headache; [6] nausea, vomiting, and diarrhea; [7] tachycardia; [8] tachypnea; [9] hypotension; and [10] ataxia [3].

The disorder has three phases: a hyperthermic–neurologic acute phase, a hematologic–enzymatic phase (peaking 24–48 h after the event), and a late renal–hepatic phase (if clinical symptoms are sustained for 96 h or longer). The most critical is the acute phase since prompt recognition and treatment of heat stroke in the acute phase may be lifesaving [4].

Adequate measurement of core (rectal) temperature is critical in persons who may have heat stroke. Hyperthermia is expected, but reliance on a core body temperature of more than 40.5 °C as a diagnostic yardstick could be misleading, since the temperature may be falsely low if the measurement is delayed or performed inappropriately (e.g., if the temperature is measured orally or from the forehead or the axilla). Nevertheless, extreme hyperthermia during physical exertion does not always indicate heat stroke; many marathon runners finish the race with a high core body temperature but without accompanying changes associated with the clinical picture of heat stroke [5].

Given the brain's extreme sensitivity to hyperthermia, CNS disturbances are inevitable in heat stroke. Early symptoms include behavioral changes, confusion, delirium, dizziness, weakness, agitation, combativeness, slurred speech, nausea, and vomiting. Seizures and sphincter incontinence may occur in severe cases.

Consciousness commonly deteriorates but is usually regained once the temperature falls below the critical level of 40.5 °C [5].

Multiorgan system dysfunction and failure may peak within 24–48 h. If treatment is prompt, clinical signs become milder in most cases and abate within a few days, and most patients recover without lasting effects. Possible complications range from sustained alteration in consciousness to disseminated intravascular coagulation, acute respiratory distress syndrome, and acute renal, cardiac, and hepatic dysfunction and failure. Rhabdomyolysis, although not pathognomonic, is typical of exertional heat stroke. The prognosis worsens when kidney and liver dysfunction are sustained for more than 96 h. Autopsy studies show that end-organ failure after heat stroke is due primarily to heat-induced necrotic and apoptotic cell death accompanying widespread microthrombosis, hemorrhage, and inflammatory injury. Some neurologic sequelae (e.g., cerebellar ataxia, dysarthria, cognitive disorders, and anterograde amnesia) may persist for several weeks to months. One study indicates that the risk of death during the months and years after recovery from heat stroke may be higher than the risk in the general population [11–13].

30.4 Treatment (Fig. 30.1)

HEAT-related death is preventable through immediate recognition of symptoms, core (rectal) temperature assessment, and rapid treatment via cold-water immersion (CWI). The primary objective is the alleviation of hyperthermia; thus, HEAT victims should be aggressively cooled, onsite, if possible, within the "golden half-hour" after collapse/cessation of activity. Morbidity and mortality are more strongly linked to duration, rather than degree, of hyperthermia; hence, the "cool first, transport second" principle. CWI provides the fastest whole-body cooling rate and the lowest morbidity and mortality for HEAT. When body temperature is reduced to <40 °C within 30 min of symptom onset, mortality approaches 0%, and most recover without sequelae. Contrarily, the prognosis worsens if the core body temperature is sustained above the critical threshold of 40.5 °C. In the absence of a specifically defined end-point temperature for safe cessation of cooling, common practice dictates a target temperature below 39 °C (preferably 38.5–38.0 °C) to lessen the risk of clinical deterioration [3].

For exertional heat stroke, a cooling rate faster than 0.10 °C per minute is safe and is desirable for improving the prognosis. CWI can achieve a cooling rate of 0.20–0.35 °C per minute. Under military or desert field conditions where ice is not readily available, a cooling rate of approximately 0.10 °C per minute can be achieved by pouring copious amounts of water over the body and fanning [5].

No pharmacologic agents accelerate cooling. Antipyretic agents such as aspirin and acetaminophen are ineffective in patients with heat stroke since fever and hyperthermia raise the core body temperature through different physiological pathways. Furthermore, antipyretic agents aggravate coagulopathy and liver injury in patients with heat stroke [5].

Prompt recognition and effective cooling will in most cases rapidly reverse heat-induced organ dysfunction. However, cooling may not suffice to obtain a full recovery, and prompt administration of adjuvant treatments may be critical for survival. The standard of care should be immediate intervention with symptomatic support of organ functions and awareness of the possible development of systemic inflammatory response syndrome.

Fig. 30.1 Algorithm for HEAT management

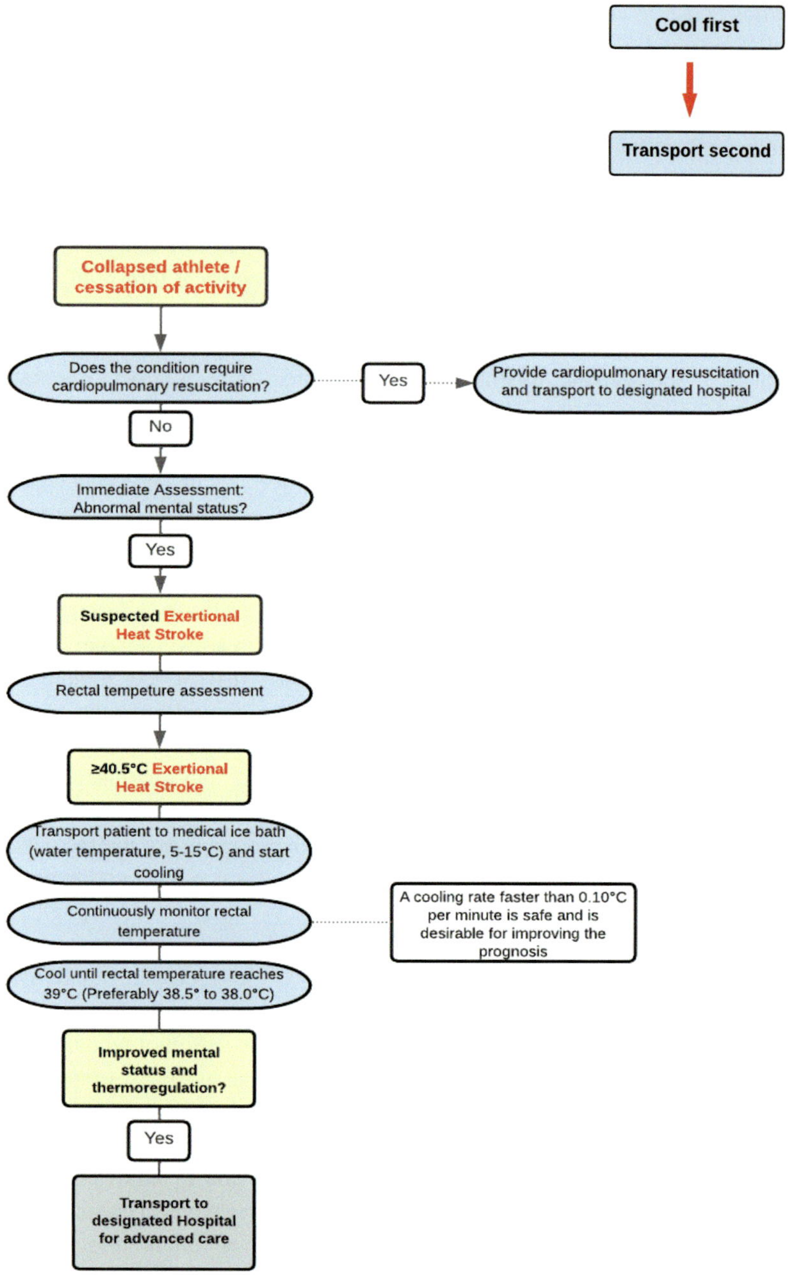

30.5 Return to Play Guidelines

For workers, athletes, or military personnel recovering from exertional heatstroke, there are no comprehensive guidelines for returning to work, play, or duty. Common sense dictates waiting for clinical and laboratory findings to return to normal and cautiously reintroducing exercise.

The American College of Sports Medicine recommends the following: (1) Refrain from exercise for more than 7 days after release from medical care; (2) follow-up in about 1 week for physical examination and repeat laboratory testing or diagnostic imaging of affected organs that may be indicated, based on physician evaluation; (3) when cleared, begin exercise in a cool environment; gradually increase duration, intensity, and heat exposure for 2 weeks to acclimatize; and demonstrate heat tolerance; (4) if return to activity is difficult, consider a laboratory exercise-heat tolerance test about 1 month post-incident; and (5) clear the athlete for full competition if heat tolerance exists after 2–4 weeks of training [1].

Take Home Messages

- HEAT is a medical emergency defined as life-threatening hyperthermia (core body temperature > 40.5 °C), multiorgan failure, and central nervous system (CNS) dysfunction. The diagnosis is largely clinical, based primarily on the triad of hyperthermia, neurologic abnormalities, and recent exposure to physical exertion.
- HEAT-related death is preventable through immediate recognition of symptoms, core (rectal) temperature assessment, and rapid treatment via CWI. The primary objective is the alleviation of hyperthermia; thus, HEAT victims should be aggressively cooled, onsite, if possible, within the "golden half-hour" after collapse/cessation of activity. No pharmacologic agents accelerate cooling.
- When body temperature is reduced to <40 °C within 30 min of symptom onset, mortality approaches 0%, and most recover without sequelae.

References

1. Armstrong LE, Casa DJ, Millard-Stafford M, et al. American College of Sports Medicine position stand. Exertional heat illness during training and competition. Med Sci Sports Exerc. 2007;39:556Y72.
2. Gardner JW, Kark JA. Clinical diagnosis, management, and surveillance of exertional heat illness. In: Pandolf KB, Burr RE, editors. Medical aspect of harsh environments, vol. 1. Washington, DC: Office of the Surgeon General, Department of the Army, United States of America; 2001. p. 231–79. (Textbooks of military medicine;.
3. Navarro CS, Casa DJ, Belval LN, Nye NS. Exertional heat stroke. Curr Sports Med Rep. 2017;16(5):304–5.
4. Laitano O, Leon LR, Roberts WO, Sawka MN. Controversies in exertional heat stroke diagnosis, prevention, and treatment. J Appl Physiol (1985). 2019;127(5):1338–48.
5. Epstein Y, Yanovich R. Heatstroke. N Engl J Med. 2019;380(25):2449–59.
6. Kerr ZY, Marshall SW, Comstock RD, Casa DJ. Implementing exertional heat ill- ness prevention strategies in US high school football. Med Sci Sports Exerc. 2014;46:124–30.
7. Armed Forces Health Surveillance Branch. Update: heat illness, active com- ponent, U.S. Armed Forces, 2017. MSMR. 2018;25:6–12.
8. Leon LR, Bouchama A. Heat stroke. Compr Physiol. 2015;5:611–47.
9. Bouchama A, Knochel JP. Heat stroke. N Engl J Med. 2002;346(1978–88):25.
10. Epstein Y, Roberts WO. The pathophysiology of heat stroke: an integrative view of the final common pathway. Scand J Med Sci Sports. 2011;21:742–8.
11. Roberts GT, Ghebeh H, Chishti MA, et al. Microvascular injury, thrombosis, inflammation, and apoptosis in the pathogenesis of heatstroke: a study in baboon model. Arterioscler Thromb Vasc Biol. 2008;28:1130–6.
12. Lim CL. Heat sepsis precedes heat toxicity in the pathophysiology of heat stroke-a new paradigm on an ancient disease. Antioxidants (Basel). 2018;7(11):149.
13. Wallace RF, Kriebel D, Punnett L, Wegman DH, Amoroso PJ. Prior heat illness hospitalization and risk of early death. Environ Res. 2007;104:290–5.

Cold (Hypothermia) 31

Ryan H. Barnes and Robert A. Magnussen

31.1 Background

Exposure to cold weather and the elements is common for athletes, particularly those who participate in winter, water, wind, or high-altitude sports. Cold-related injuries are secondary to a disruption between the body's natural heat production and heat dissipation [1], as 90% of body heat is lost through the skin [2]. Eventually, the imbalance leads to progressively severe cold-related injuries [3]. In order to protect athletes from cold-related injuries, multiple sports organizations including the International Olympic Committee have released guidelines [4].

Hypothermia is defined as a core body temperature of less than 35 ° C (95 ° F) [5]; however, clinical features of hypothermia can be evident at higher core body temperatures if the body is unable to generate enough heat to maintain physiologic function. The severity of hypothermia is classified based on core body temperature (Table 31.1). Finally, frostbite occurs when tis-

Table 31.1 Severity of hypothermia

Grade/Severity	Definition
MILD	**33° C to 37° C** (91.4° F to 98.6° F)
MODERATE	**29° C to 33° C** (84.2° F to91.4° F)
SEVERE	**< 29° C** (< 84.2° F)

R. H. Barnes · R. A. Magnussen (✉)
Department of Orthopaedics, OSU Sports Medicine Research Institute, The Ohio State University, Columbus, OH, USA

S. Rocha Piedade et al. (eds.), *Sideline Management in Sports*,
https://doi.org/10.1007/978-3-031-33867-0_31

sues freeze. This problem most commonly occurs in exposed areas of the body and the extremities.

Few studies discuss the incidence of cold-related injuries in sports; however, the incidence in cross-country skiing has been reported as high as 20% [6]. Mortality from hypothermia has been quoted as being as high as 17%, with a 1.8% increase in mortality with each 1 °C core body temperature drop [7]. Despite being less frequent than hyperthermia, hypothermia is associated with higher mortality rates, more frequent need for hospital admission, longer hospital stays, and higher total health care costs than hyperthermia [8].

Physiologically, the body counterbalances heat loss by inducing peripheral vasoconstriction, which warms the central organs [9]. In severe cases, this decrease in peripheral blood flow can contribute to frostbite. Shivering occurs as a way to increase muscle activation and metabolism and elevate core body temperature.

Risk factors for cold injury include the environment and weather conditions: rain, wind, temperature, and altitude [1]. It is important to be mindful of changes in weather throughout the event and ensure that the athletes and the coaching staff have proper attire for all weather conditions. It is also important to be mindful of the athletes at increased risk of developing hypothermia. Athletes with lower BMI have higher rates of hypothermia, as fat can act as natural insulation. The age of the athletes can also be important, as younger athletes (less than 12 years old) or older athletes (greater than 60 years old) have more difficulty with natural thermoregulation. Medications can also place athletes more at risk, including central nervous system depressants and phenothiazines [7]. Medical comorbidities such as hypoglycemia, hypothyroidism, peripheral neuropathy, and hypothyroidism can also predispose athletes to cold-related injury.

Fact Box 31.1

- Hypothermia is defined as a core body temperature less than 35 ° C (95 ° F), with varying severities dependent upon core body temperatures.
- Peripheral vasoconstriction occurs in order to shunt blood flow to central organs and decrease heat loss to the environment via the skin.
- Shivering is a natural protective reaction to being cold in order to increase muscle activation and core body temperature.

31.2 Clinical Presentation and Differential Diagnosis

The signs and symptoms of hypothermia are variable depending upon the severity. Those athletes with mild cases of hypothermia will present with shivering [1]. Typically, these athletes will have stable vital signs but could have mild hypertension. They may complain of fatigue, difficulty with fine motor skills, and some mild confusion or altered mental status. Once the severity has progressed to moderate hypothermia, the vitals become more unstable. At this point, the body is unable to maintain continuous shivering and can present with more signs of maximal peripheral vasoconstriction with cool and pale extremities. Finally, with severe hypothermia, there is a progression of altered mental status, slurred speech, gross motor skill impairment, and potentially comatose.

Fact Box 31.2

- Presentation of hypothermia will vary based on severity, but athletes often complain of uncontrollable shivering or in severe cases may demonstrate altered mental status.
- Athletes may complain of trouble with motor skills associated with their sport that they can normally perform with no difficulty.

31.3 Physical Examination

It is important to evaluate patients in a protected, warm environment. The athlete should have all wet or damp clothes removed and be provided with dry, warm clothes prior to completing evaluation. The athlete should have a thorough neurological examination performed, including orientation and motor testing. The skin should be examined to ensure that there are no signs of frostbite. In athletes with frostbite, the appearance of the tissues depends upon the severity of the frostbite and whether it is superficial or deep [1]. In superficial frostbite, the tissues will appear erythematous, mottled, and stiff, and patients may complain of numbness (Fig. 31.1). In deep frostbite, patients will complain of dense numbness, and the tissue will appear firm and may have vesicles.

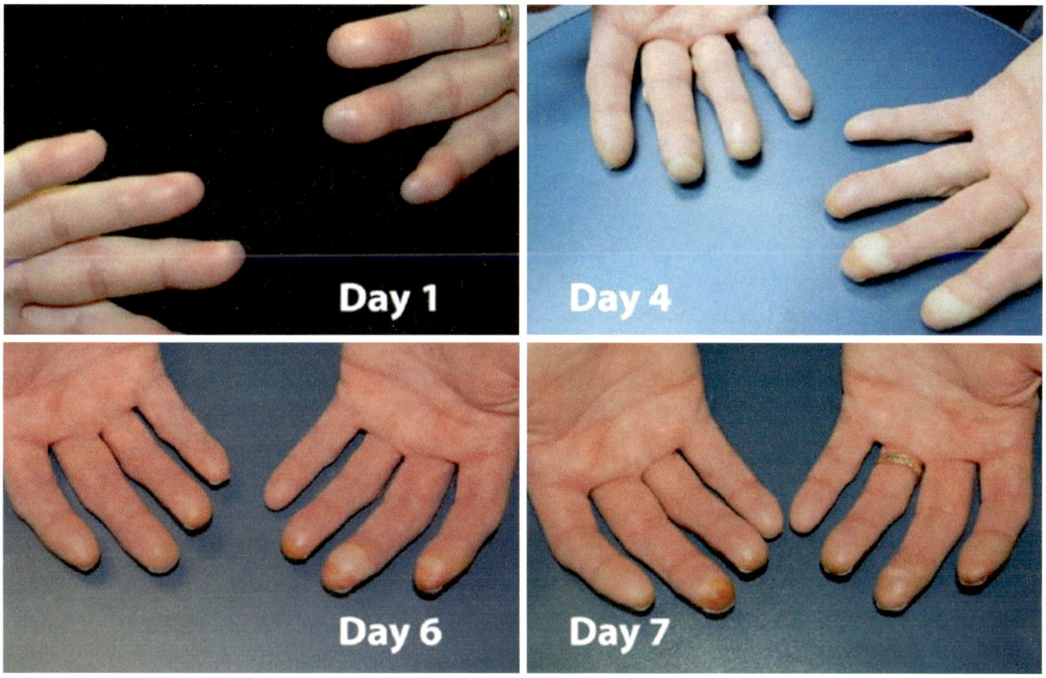

Fig. 31.1 Progression of second-degree frostbite injury, treated with rewarming in a warm water bath, pain medications, and dry bandages [6]

31.4 Additional Testing/Imaging

The only true way to diagnose and stratify the severity of the hypothermia is to assess core body temperature with a rectal thermometer. No additional testing or imaging is required as this is a clinical diagnosis.

31.5 Sideline Management Guidelines

The best management for hypothermia is prevention and taking steps to avoid placing athletes in positions that could leave them more susceptible to their environment. For athletes who are exposed to the elements, it is important to dress athletes appropriately. For winter sports, wearing layers is important. The outer layer should provide warmth and be relatively water- and wind-resistant. The middle layers should provide the most warmth. The inner layers should be relatively lightweight and aid in wicking away moisture from the body.

The main emphasis of treatment is to decrease heat loss and restore the natural homeostasis of heat loss and heat production. If an athlete is identified as being at risk for hypothermia, they should be moved into a protected environment that is warmed and their clothing should be removed if it is wet or damp (Fig. 31.2). Athletes should be properly hydrated. It is also important for providers to consider treating other associated medical comorbidities, which could be contributing to the hypothermia.

Rewarming can occur through both passive and active methods [1]. Passive rewarming is the main management for sidelines and occurs through more gradual methods such as insulated clothing or blankets. If symptoms progress, active rewarming may be required, potentially including warmed intravenous fluids. Active rewarming includes warming the trunk, in order to avoid after-drop, which is caused by the return of cold blood from the extremities if the extremities were preferentially heated, leading to an even further drop in core temperature.

In treatments of frostbite, prior treatments listed still apply. In addition, the area should be rewarmed in a warm water bath from 40 ° C to 42 ° C (104 ° F to 107.6 ° F) for up to 30 min [1]. During the rewarming period, vasoconstrictors should be avoided in order to avoid further reduced blood flow to the extremity. Although rewarming the body is critical, it is also important to be mindful that skin burns can occur in hot water.

Return to play will be variable based on the severity of the hypothermia. In mild cases, once symptoms have resolved with treatments, the athlete can return to play. However, in moderate-to-severe cases, the athlete should not be allowed to return to play in the same game. Once the athlete is stabilized and asymptomatic, return to play can be considered.

Fact Box 31.3

- Removing the athlete from the environment into a protected, warm space is crucial
- Remove all wet clothes and place warm, dry clothes or blankets
- In severe cases, athletes will need to be transported to emergency departments for more invasive treatment methods

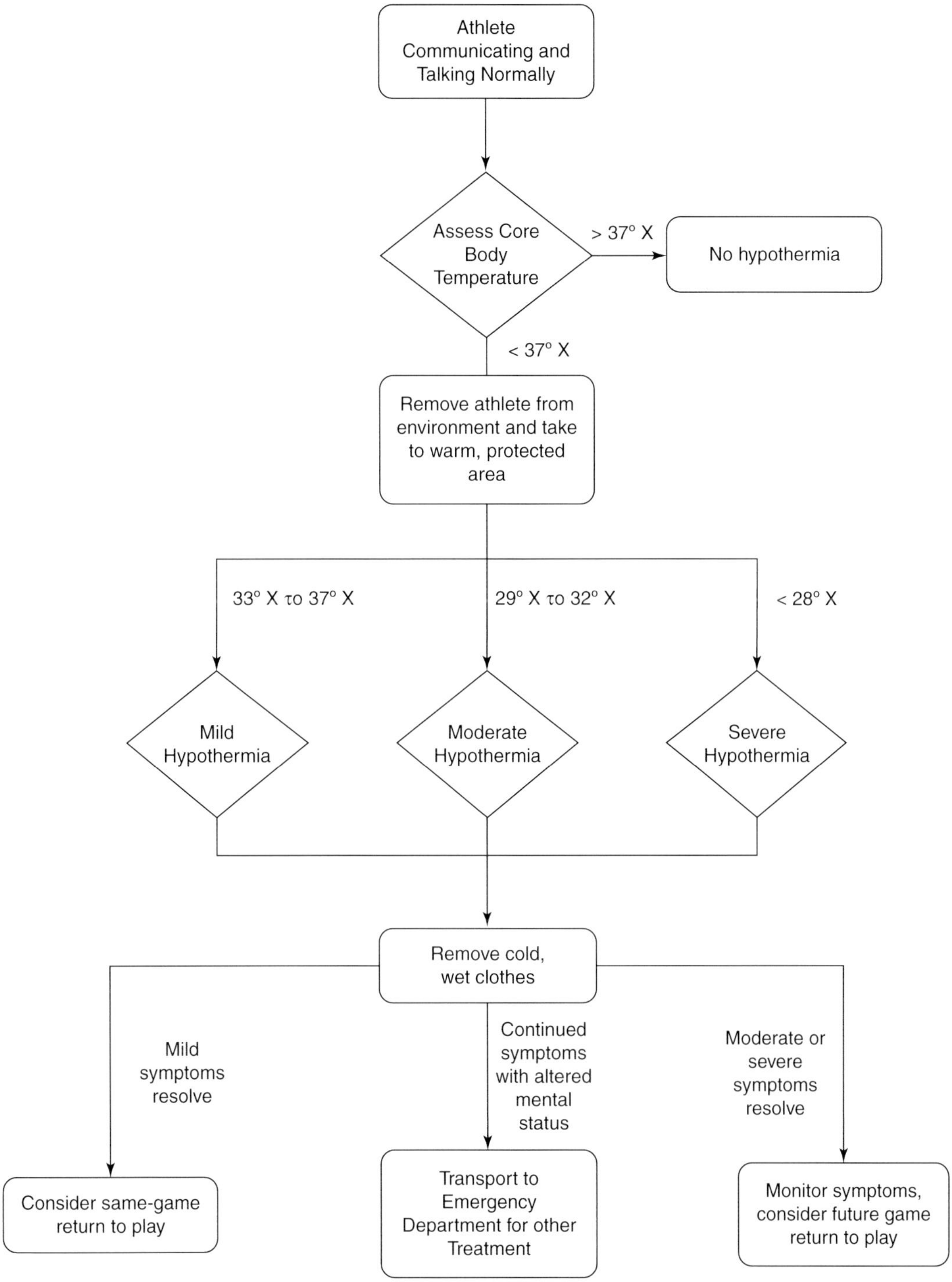

Fig. 31.2 Treatment algorithm

31.6 Suggested Prevention Measures

Prevention is the key to avoid hypothermia. It is important to educate athletes and coaches about the signs and symptoms of hypothermia, so they can readily recognize early signs and symptoms to prevent progression [10]. Having proper attire and recognizing weather conditions are of the utmost importance. In cases of early recognition, it is important to move the athlete to a warm environment. New wearable technologies are being produced that can alert athletes when signs of hypothermia are detected [11].

Take Home Messages

- Prevention is the best treatment for cold-related injuries.
- Core body temperature should be measured with a rectal thermometer.
- Signs and symptoms can range from shivering and difficulties with motor control to altered mental status and frostbite in severe cases.
- Sideline treatment should include moving the athlete to a warm, protected environment, removing wet clothing, and replacing it with dry, insulated clothing.

References

1. Noonan B, Bancroft RW, Dines JS, Bedi A. Heat- and cold-induced injuries in athletes: evaluation and management. J Am Acad Orthop Surg. 2012;20(12):744–54.
2. McDonald A, Stubbs R, Lartey P, Kokot S. Environmental injuries: hyperthermia and hypothermia. MacEwan University Student eJournal. 2020;4(1)
3. Castellani JW, Young AJ. Health and performance challenges during sports training and competition in cold weather. Br J Sports Med. 2012;46(11):788–91.
4. Bergeron MF, Bahr R, Bartsch P, et al. International Olympic Committee consensus statement on thermoregulatory and altitude challenges for high-level athletes. Br J Sports Med. 2012;46(11):770–9.
5. Ulrich AS, Rathlev NK. Hypothermia and localized cold injuries. Emerg Med Clin North Am. 2004;22(2):281–98.
6. Fudge J. Exercise in the cold: preventing and managing hypothermia and frostbite injury. Sports Health. 2016;8(2):133–9.
7. DeFranco MJ, Baker CL, DaSilva JJ, Piasecki DP, Bach BR. Environmental issues for team physicians. Am J Sports Med. 2008;36(11):2226–37.
8. Noe RS, Jin JO, Wolkin AF. Exposure to natural cold and heat: hypothermia and hyperthermia Medicare claims, United States, 2004-2005. Am J Public Health. 2012;102(4):e11–8.
9. McMahon JA, Howe A. Cold weather issues in sideline and event management. Curr Sports Med Rep. 2012;11(3):135–41.
10. Castellani JW, Young AJ, Ducharme MB, et al. American College of Sports Medicine position stand: prevention of cold injuries during exercise. Med Sci Sports Exerc. 2006;38(11):2012–29.
11. Shakeel CS, Hassan U, Ilyas F, Zariwala MM, Ilyas SM, Khan SJ. A prelude to wearable technology for the measurement and restoration of core body temperature and heart rate in athletes suffering from hypothermia. Proc Inst Mech Eng H. 2022;236(1):56–64.

Sports and Altitude

32

Marcello Motta, Gregory Ornon, and Jacques Menetrey

32.1 Introduction

Altitude training or training in hypoxia has the primary aim to increase blood oxygen-carrying capacity and muscular adaptations in order to strengthen performance at sea level, but also in altitude. Since the 1968 Mexico City Olympics, training in altitude has been commonly used by elite athletes in many sports, but also for the acclimatization of mountaineers or trailers. This training strategy is nowadays also used by recreational athletes. At first, only endurance sports were involved, then collective team sports start using hypoxic exposure in their training planning. Hypoxic training was first performed in natural high-altitude areas (hypobaric hypoxia), including places such as Kenya, France, Switzerland, or United States. A variety of artificial altitude environment equipments (normobaric hypoxia), such as altitude centers or hypoxic tents, have been developed since 1990. Although substantial differences exist between these modalities of hypoxic training, both have interesting characteristics which can be used to enhance performance. To date, several forms of hypoxic training and/or altitude strategies exist: traditional "live high-train high," contemporary "live high-train low," or "live low-train high" approaches.

M. Motta
Department of Medical and Surgical Specialties, Radiological Sciences, and Public Health, University of Brescia, Brescia, Italy

G. Ornon
Centre de Médecine du Sport et de l'Exercice (CMSE), Swiss Olympic Medical Center, Hirslanden Clinique La Colline Geneva, Geneva, Switzerland
e-mail: Gregory.ornon@hirslanden.ch

J. Menetrey (✉)
Centre de Médecine du Sport et de l'Exercice (CMSE), Swiss Olympic Medical Center, Hirslanden Clinique La Colline Geneva, Geneva, Switzerland

Orthopaedic Surgery Service, University Hospital of Geneva, Geneva, Switzerland
e-mail: Jacques.Menetrey@hirslanden.ch

32.2 Physiologic Response to Altitude

Regarding human physiology, at high altitude, low atmospheric oxygen concentration and low barometric pressure represent the most important environmental factors. Increased ultraviolet radiation and extreme temperature (cold and hot) constitute other factors that need to be considered. The human body reacts in several different ways in order to adapt to these changes. Hypoxia is the main key factor for all the physiologic changes that occur with altitude: it is defined as combinations of barometric pressure (PB) and an inspired fraction of oxygen (FiO_2) that result in an inspired partial pressure of oxygen (PiO_2) lower than a normoxic value of 150 mmHg [1] (Fig. 32.1). The absolute change in oxygen avail-

S. Rocha Piedade et al. (eds.), *Sideline Management in Sports*,
https://doi.org/10.1007/978-3-031-33867-0_32

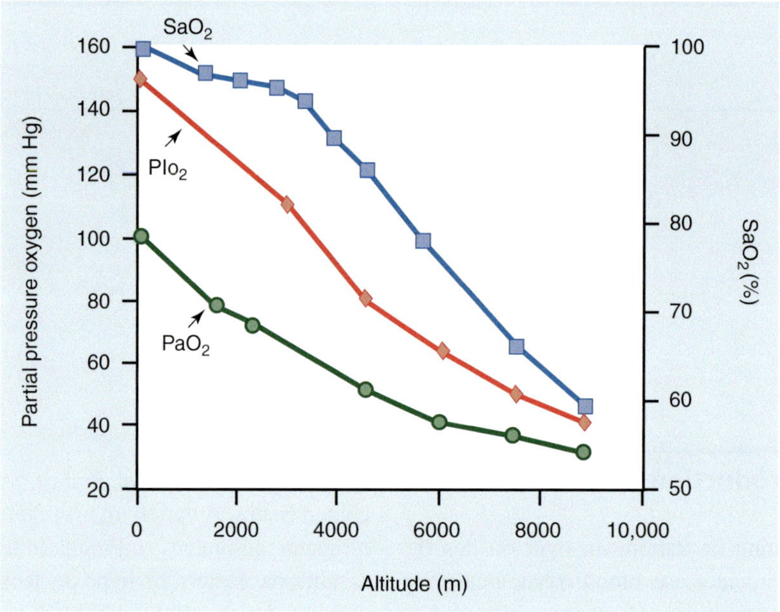

Fig. 32.1 Increasing altitude leads to a decreasing inspired PO_2 (PIO_2), arterial PO_2 (PaO_2), and arterial oxygen saturation (SaO_2). An important note: the difference between PIO_2 and PaO_2 narrows at high altitude because of increased ventilation and that SaO_2 is well maintained while awake until over 3000 m

ability imposed by a given ascent can be calculated easily. Since oxygen represents 21% of normal air, the partial pressure of oxygen (PO_2) at sea level is (21% of 760 mmHg) or 160 mmHg. Once inspired, the air becomes saturated with water vapour (partial pressure 47 mmHg) so that the total gas pressure is reduced to 713 mmHg and PO_2 falls to (21% of 713 mmHg) or 150 mmHg. In the alveoli, the oxygen is diluted further by approximately 50 mmHg, due primarily to the presence of carbon dioxide, resulting in a local PO_2 (P_AO_2) of around 100 mmHg: at equilibrium with the plasma, arterial PO_2 (PaO_2) is, therefore, usually also around 100 mmHg. At an atmospheric pressure of 560 mmHg, which corresponds to an altitude of around 2300 m (7600 ft) or just higher than Mexico City, P_AO_2 can be estimated to be around 60 mmHg (21% of [560–47]—50 mmHg). At altitude of 3500 m (11,000 ft), where atmospheric pressure is 500 mmHg, P_AO_2 will be around (21% of [500–47]—50 mmHg) because it has always to be taken in consideration to the partial pressure water vapour and the oxygen dilution in the alveoli; in the Himalayas and Andes where there are settlement as high as 5000 m (17,500 ft), atmospheric pressure is only 390 mmHg and calculated P_AO_2 is around 25 mmHg. Hypoxic conditions present with increasing altitude (reduction in PB, also referred to as "hypobaric hypoxia" [HH]) or in low-oxygen environments by reducing the oxygen portion in ambient air (reduction in FiO_2, called "normobaric hypoxia" [NH]) [2]. Exposure to hypoxia leads to a decrease in PiO_2 and a subsequent reduction in arterial oxygen pressure (PaO_2) and arterial oxygen saturation ($SaO_{2,3}$). This oxygen deficiency in the blood and muscles is also called "hypoxemia". The human body reacts to hypoxia with hematological and non-hematological adaptations, which in addition have the potential to improve athletic performance.

32.2.1 Acute Exposure

There is strong evidence that the primary regulator of hypoxia-mediated cellular adaptations is hypoxia-inducible factor 1 (HIF-1) [2], a transcription factor that regulates oxygen homeostasis [4]. HIF-1 is responsible for enhanced oxygen transport capacity and/−or improved oxygen extraction/−utilization at the cellular level [5]. The most important physiological adaptation leading to enhanced aerobic performance is a hypoxia-induced increase in erythropoiesis [6, 7].Under hypoxia, erythropoiesis is mainly triggered by an enhanced stimulation of the EPO hormone in the kidneys [8]. After arrival at altitude, EPO increases within hours and peaks after 1–2 days of hypoxic exposure, before it declines toward baseline [8, 9].

32.2.1.1 Haematological Effects

The increased EPO levels lead to an enhanced production of red blood cells (RBC) in the bone marrow, resulting in an elevated Hb mass and thus an improved oxygen transport capacity of the blood, which in turn should enhance exercise performance [10–12]. Not only Hb mass is involved; in fact, soon after ascending to high altitude (HA), plasma volume (PV) begins to decrease, causing hematocrit (Hct) and hemoglobin concentration (Hb) to increase. Arrival at altitude coincides with a rapid fall in plasma volume. Over several days, people experience a fall by up to 20% in their plasma volume because water is excreted as urine or instead shifts into either the interstitium or cells. This results in rapid increase in the concentration of circulating haemoglobin and subsequent rises in Oxygen delivery (DO_2) and arterial oxygen content (CaO_2). Although this process can persist for several weeks, over a prolonged stay at altitude, plasma volume slowly returns to normal. Although the plasma concentration of erythropoietin tends to fall over the course of 3 weeks at altitude, red cell production remains raised for up to 8 months in those new to altitude and can result in 50% increase in red cell mass. This hemoconcentration increases arterial oxygen carrying capacity, thereby satisfying muscle oxygen requirements.

32.2.1.2 Ventilatory Effects

The first reaction of human body to low oxygen concentration (hypoxia) in altitude is an increase in ventilatory response triggered by carotid body receptors [13]. All these changes play an important role in the acclimatization process. Decreased alveolar CO_2, hypocapnia, and respiratory alkalosis, which has an inhibitory effect on the central respiratory center, are effects caused by hypoxic ventilatory response. This inhibitory effect limits further increase in ventilation.

32.2.1.3 Cardiovascular Effects

At altitude, a sympathetic response is elicited to maintain oxygen perfusion to the tissues in the face of hypoxaemia. Hypoxia influences directly the release of catecholamine in the adrenal medulla. For this reason, athletes at altitude show higher epinephrine levels compared with those at sea-level. The increased release of catecholamine has several effects: increased heart rate, cardiac output, and blood pressure due to increment in sympathetic activity.

32.2.1.4 Skeletal Muscle Effects

Hypoxia leads to specific changes in gene transcription, muscle metabolism, and muscle buffering capacity. Upregulation of GLUT-4 transporter mRNA has been found in skeletal muscle following 6 weeks of altitude training, which facilitates a longer-lasting uptake of glucose during exercise. There is also an upregulation of angiogenin, higher production of IL-8 and VEGF that promotes formation of new capillaries and improves muscle blood flow. Another adaptive response is an upregulation of monocarboxylate transporters which handle lactate and carbonic anhydrase enzymes which influence hydrogen and bicarbonate ion transport. This is the reason for an increase in lactate exchange and removal and, consequently, a slower pH decrease within "glycolytic" exercise and an improvement in muscle buffer capacity [14].

32.2.1.5 Other System Effects

The response of the renal system, at early stage of acclimatization, consists in excreting bicarbonate and conserving hydrogen ions (altitude-induced diuresis) [15]. There is also an increase in parathyroid hormone level that led to higher plasma calcium and phosphate levels. From the neuropsychologic point, there is a decreased synthesis of neurotransmitters, cerebral vasodilatation, mood changes, and reduced cognitive function.

The better performance results are apparently the consequence of haematological and peripheral adaptations, and not mandatory associated with an increment in VO^2max in elite athletes.

32.2.2 Chronic Exposure

Chronic exposure has the major effect of haemoglobin concentration increase as a haematologic adaptation to high altitude; this has been reported for over a century among highlanders (typically residents at altitude >4000 m) after at least 2 weeks. This phenomenon is due to higher erythropoietin production by the kidneys [13]. Other effects of chronic exposure to high altitude, on various system, comprehend: increased lung capillary blood volume and lung diffusion capacity, right ventricular hypertrophy, decreased systolic/diastolic blood pressure, increased plasma triglyceride level, hyperuricemia, albuminuria, reduced renal plasma flow, glomerular hypertrophy, cerebral hypoxia, decreased sleep quality, and increased mood disorder [13, 16, 17].

32.3 Side Effects

32.3.1 High Altitude Illness

The term altitude illness refers to a series of conditions related to an increased altitude. The main cause of these conditions is the low ambient oxygen (hypoxia) that is brought about by the low atmospheric pressure at altitude. During athletic competitions such as mountain races, athletes may experience very rapid ascent, with high risk of high-altitude illness (HAI). Risk factors HAI include previous episodes of high altitude illness, a faster rate of ascent, poor hydration, increased intensity of physical activity, and individual variability [18, 19]. A progressive ascent to altitude is the main key of prevention for all acute high altitude illnesses (AHAIs). The guidelines recommendations predict that above 2500 m, altitude should be increased at a rate of 600 to 1200 m per 24-h period [19]. Athlete's residing altitude and the altitude to which the athlete plans to ascend are factors related to the duration of an effective acclimatization. With acute mountain sickness (AMS) one should not progress in the ascent until resolution of symptoms and should consider descent if medical management does not resolve symptoms. HAI can progress in some case to high altitude cerebral edema (HACE) or high altitude pulmonary edema (HAPE); in these situations, immediately descending to a lower altitude is required. Inside HAI spectrum, there is also the Chronic mountain sickness (CMS), an uncommon condition among highlanders, directly related to altitude of residence, that is characterized by extreme polycythemia, pulmonary hypertension, severe right ventricular hypertrophy, low systemic blood pressure, hypoventilation, and chronic arterial oxygen desaturation [13].

32.3.2 Ultraviolet Radiation

Deleterious effects of ultraviolet (UV) radiation are experienced sometimes by high altitude athletes. Every altitude increase of 1000 m is accompanied by UV-A and UV-B exposure increase around 10% to 20% [19]. Skin cancer, seborrheic dermatitis, and cataract formation are related to greater UV exposure [20, 21]. Athletes should wear sunglasses with UV protection, adequate clothing, and sunscreen with a sun protection factor of at least 30; in fact, snow leads to increase in UV exposure risk by providing a reflective surface.

32.3.3 Sleep Hygiene

At high altitude, athletes often accuse insomnia, frequent awakening, and restless sleep [22–24]. Some athletes may experience sensation of suffocation or apnea and relieved by wakening and several deep breaths, resulting in restless sleep. The reason behind all of these problems is due to hyperventilation secondary to high altitude that is associated with hypoxia, subsequent hypocapnia, and decreased respiratory drive, which is followed by apnea and resumption of the cycle [23, 24].

32.3.4 Nutrition

A correct nutrition is an important aspect to take care about for athletes at high altitude. First of all, because chronic high altitude exposure leads to significant weight loss, caused primarily due to loss of fat-free mass, with negative effects on physical performance [25]. Factors possibly contributing to this weight loss are decreased physical activity, hypoxia, irregular sleep pattern, cold exposure, and nutritional imbalance related to protein metabolism [25, 26]. There is also a tendency for hypohydration at high altitude. Adequate fluid intake is essential to avoid underperformance due to hypohydration particularly in warm climates. Because of strong demand for erythropoiesis, athletes should increase dietary and supplemental iron before traveling to high altitude [19]. Certainly, the most important micronutrient at altitude is iron. An appreciation of baseline iron status and appropriate supplementation are fundamental nutritional interventions that facilitate the Hbmass responses at altitude. There is a dose–response relationship between the amount of iron supplemented and Hbmass gains at altitude; the most effective iron supplementation is represented by a single 200 mg dose of elemental iron taken in the evening to potentially minimize the iron and exercise-induced increases in hepcidin. Athlete's nutritional strategy, at high altitude, should include adequate caloric intake. In fact, inadequate caloric intake may lead to significant weight loss for athletes staying at high altitude for more than 3 weeks. Glycogen storage deficit could be prevented with a diet strategy that consists of about 60% carbohydrates, 25% fat, and 15% protein [26].

32.4 Altitude Training

Altitude training has turned up recently as a way to obtain an advantage over other athletes. It involves breathing in a reduced percentage of oxygen, hypoxia, in either simulated or natural environment, with the primary aim to improve the athletic performance. To date, the optimal altitude for this kind of training remains unknown; nevertheless, the majority of research studies have been performed at moderate altitudes, normally between 2000 and 3000 m. At these heights, a safe erythropoietin response has been noticed with minimal side effects [27].The altitude training consists of 3 possible basic models: live high, train high (LHTH); live high, train low (LHTL); and live low, train high (LLTH) [12]. In some places, training at altitude is not always feasible, so simulated altitudes are often used. The simulation for altitude training (normobaric hypoxia) occurs through tent, hypobaric chamber, or altitude simulation room. The optimal altitude is very hard to find; altitude training has to take in account both the physiological altitude stress and the recovery of the athletes in order to minimize the stress and make the recovery faster.

32.4.1 Live High, Train High

Live High Train High (LHTH) refers to athletes living and training at natural altitude for a period of time (usually 2–4 weeks). LHTH duration is between 2 and 4 weeks, because the increase in red cell mass that starts after 12 days reaches a plateau after 24 days. LHTH is often used because of a general consensus among athletes that it strengthens and enhances endurance performance [28]. The reason is a dose-response relationship with the level of hypoxia resulting in increased blood red cell mass. However, there is concern that altitudes higher than 3000 m could lead to loss in intensity of exercise and sequent muscle wasting, excess ventilatory work, and higher probability to develop acute mountain sickness [29]. All of these side effects, causing stress and tension in the athletes, can overcome the positive erythropoietic benefits [27]. In LHTH, the athletes first face the acclimatization phase that lasts around 7–10 days. During this first phase, high intensity exercises are not suggested. Then primary training period is used to increment the energy and duration of training. The final phase lasts 2–5 days: the intensity and volume of training are progressively decreased, in order to recover from the altitude-induced fatigue. Even if altitude training permits acclimatization, athletes mostly are not able to train at the same intensity as compared with sea level [30]. Coming back then to sea level, three phases are usually observed by athletes. A first positive phase for some athletes, during 2–4 days, followed by a phase of reduction in the athletic performance. Most of athletes are able to reach their peak performance 15–20 days after return to sea level. In the literature there are not so many well-controlled studies on LHTH, but the effect of LHTH is well known: hypoxic exposure leads to an increase in haemoglobin mass (Hbmass) [31, 32],as shown in a study by Siebenmann et al. [33] who reported an increase of 5% in Hb mass after 4 week at 3450 m of altitude. The most important controlled studies about LHTH are: the study of Rodriguez et al. [34] that considered two groups of swimmers, showed an increase in aerobic performance (400-m freestyle) in LHTH group (who lived and trained permanently for 4 weeks at 2320 m) more than the control group (4.7% vs. 1.6%); the study of Bonne et al. [32] that examined two groups of elite swimmers, reported an Hbmass increase (by 6.2%) and improved aerobic performance in the LHTH group (who lived and trained 3 to 4 weeks between 2000 and 3000 m) much more than sea-level control group; similarly, Mellerowicz et al. [35] registered, in a group of trained athletes who performed 4 week at 2000 m, an higher improvement in VO^2max and aerobic performance than a SL group.

32.4.2 Live Low, Train High

LLTH consists in an altitude training program where athletes live in a natural environment (normobaric normoxic) and train in short intervals (5–180 min) at simulated normobaric hypoxia or hypobaric hypoxia [30]. Normobaric hypoxia can be obtained through nitrogen dilution, oxygen filtration, or inspiration of hypoxic gas. LLTH program can be helpful for athletes in the resting state (intermittent hypoxic exposure; IHE) or during training sessions (intermittent hypoxic training; IHT). Intermittent hypoxic training (IHT) combines episodes of hypoxia, interspersed with episodes of normoxia, hypoxia of lesser severity, hypercapnia, or hyperoxia. The IHT schemes used in experiments vary greatly in the duration of the cycle, the number of hypoxic episodes, and the number of days of training. Technically, hypoxia can be achieved by breathing gas hypoxic mixtures (GHM) through special equipment (hypoxicators, rebreathers), based on the principle of return breathing. (Fig. 32.2) Within the LLTH model, there are further subdivisions into different types: continuous training, resistance training, interval training, repeated sprint training, and passive exposure at rest [36, 37]. In all of these different methods, the lack of oxygen leads to adaptive processes in the body and mostly in the muscles [38]. In the last years, a new method of LLTH, the repeated-sprint training in hypoxia (RSH), has gained a lot of popularity [39]. This method consists of repetitive short maximal intensity exercises (<30 s) with short incomplete recoveries. In normoxia, a larger maximal repeated sprinting performance enhancement and fatigue resistance have been registered, without any effect on the erythropoietic pathway. The efficacy of RSH is based on

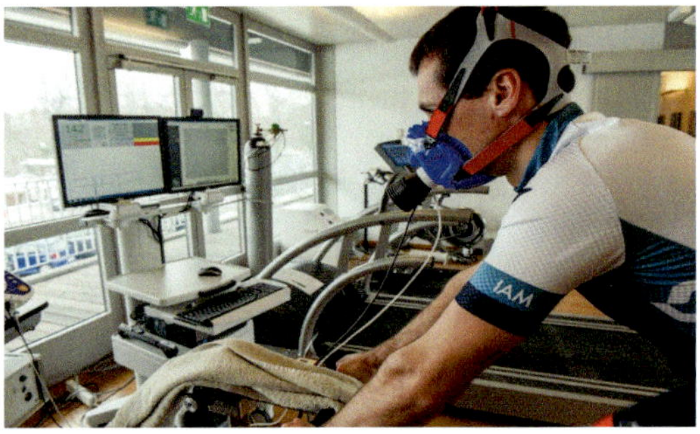

Fig. 32.2 Intermittent Hypoxia Training (HIT) with Altitrainer (Switzerland) of a cycling athlete; AltiTrainer enables subjecting individuals to physical exercise in conditions of hypoxia, hyperoxia, and hypercapnia

specific skeletal muscle tissue changes mediated by an oxygen-sensing pathway [40](i.e. hypoxic-inducible factors) likely to be fiber-type specific, which ends in an improved exercise tolerance through a greater buffering capacity, lactic acid tolerance, and/or O_2 extraction in the working muscle. These adaptations are very important for some intermittent sports such as soccer, rugby, Australian football, and ice hockey. The appropriate training conditions (frequency, duration, intensity of exercise, and altitude of training,) are still under debate. The physical and psychological state of subject, sport event altitude, performance level, and support of nutrition are certainly related to the positive effect of this method.

32.4.3 Live High, Train Low

LHTL represents an altitude training program in which athletes rest and live at moderate altitude (2000 to 3000 m; hypobaric hypoxia) or use simulated altitude (normobaric hypoxia) while train at lower altitude or sea level. The Living High Training Low (LHTL) strategy has the advantage of altitude acclimatization, without training intensities' reduction that are one of the main limitations of the LHTH program. With LHTL, athletes can improve exercise performance at altitude and sea level, have the physiological benefits of altitude, and at the same time keep the volume and intensity of training at a lower altitude [30]. The hypoxic erythropoietic effect of altitude appears when the athlete has spent approximately 300–400 h of living at a minimum altitude of 2000 m for more than 14–16 h per day for at least 19–20 days [41]. The altitude response in training is individualized, and not everyone experiences the same changes and improvements [42]. Some studies register a reduction of altitude potential physiological response, especially in athletes with high red cell volume (elite endurance athletes) [38]. A meta-analysis showed that hypobaric hypoxia LHTL represents the best chance for improving endurance performance in elite and sub-elite athletes [43]. In another study, significant differences in the responses to LHTL were registered between hypobaric hypoxia groups and normobaric hypoxia groups [44], with an higher performance improvement and increased hematological changes in the hypobaric hypoxia group 3 weeks after LHTL. Similar results were encountered in a study by Bedleman et al. [45], where hypobaric hypoxia exposure was compared to normobaric hypoxia in cyclists, with conclusion that normobaric hypoxia may not induce the same hypoxic stimulus and training benefit as hypobaric hypoxia exposure. For resting and sleeping, the athlete can select between natural and utilize artificial altitude to reduce the fatigue and stress of traveling to and from training sites. For this reason, there has been a development of hypoxic facilities such as hypoxic tents and hypobaric chambers for improving the opportunity for hypoxic altitude training, especially when it is geographically challenging. With hypoxic/nitrogen house, altitudes around 2500 m can be simulated through reduction of oxygen percentage from 21% to 15% by diluting it with nitrogen. Also with hypoxic tents, very easy to use and portable, the simulation of altitude can reach 4000 m. In addition, barometric steel chambers are available, but these are really expensive and limited in availability. At least 10–12 h per 24 h have to be passed in a low oxygen environment, with beneficial effect observed after at least 4 weeks of training twice a week; the maintenance of these positive effects is registered to be around a period of 3 weeks. The optimal altitude for athletes is related to the specific sport, current residing altitude, and altitude of the event [28]. As previously reported, Hypobaric hypoxia LHTL represents the best method for improving performance in elite and sub-elite athletes, especially in endurance athletes.

32.5 Athlete's Monitoring During Altitude Training

To enhance the possible benefits of altitude training, an effective monitoring system that assesses fitness and fatigue responses to training of athletes is fundamental. This is very important given that the additional stress imposed by the hypoxic environment may lead to an increased risk of maladaptation, illness, or overtraining [46, 47]. Detailed longitudinal monitoring of an athlete's physical responses to training is required: [1] in the lead-up period to assure an optimal physical condition to maximize the advantage of altitude training; [2] at altitude to lower the risk of maladaptation and overtraining; and [3] post-altitude, as training quality may be higher as a result of adaptations conferred from altitude, and optimal loads during this period are critical. Simultaneously, monitoring of internal and external training loads is mandatory in the assessment of individual response to hypoxia. The external training load is an objective measure of athlete's work in training (e.g. running speed, distance completed, total elevation gain). Alternatively, the internal workload estimates the biological stress imposed by the training session and is normally defined by the disturbance in homeostasis of physiological and metabolic processes [48].

32.5.1 Blood Monitoring

RBC parameters are commonly used to study and also to monitor the effect of high-altitude training in athletes. RBC parameters are usually expressed as concentration rather than total amount. However, relative parameters are affected by changes in blood volume (BV) and could therefore lead to misinterpretation and incorrect conclusions. Absolute parameters are not affected by changes in BV and should be preferred to confront high altitude athletes with sea level athletes and to estimate the effect of altitude training. The determination of Hbmass has become increasingly important in recent years, mostly to assess the efficiency of training interventions [49, 50], especially altitude training methods and the impact of iron supplementation. Monitoring the Hbmass response to altitude is possible through various methods; the most used one is carbon monoxide rebreathing [51]. Nowadays, it is one of the most widely used methods for determining the Hbmass, given that is minimally invasive, not harmful, and enables quantification of the total Hbmass independent of plasma volume. Furthermore, the method allows for reliable Hbmass determinations from capillary blood samples. A strong relationship was reported between changes in Hbmass, VO^2max, and endurance performance observed with altitude training [52], facilitating an increase in Hbmass during altitude exposure; this increase contributes towards a positive performance outcome following altitude training [10]. Adequate iron stores are necessary to withstand increases in erythropoiesis and Hbmass with chronic altitude exposure [53]. In non-supplemented, iron-deficient runners, red cell volume remained unchanged in contrast with their non-iron-deficient counterparts. As such, monitoring an athlete's full iron profile about 4–6 weeks prior to altitude exposure is critical [54]. Iron supplementation prior to altitude exposure is important to normalize iron stores and promote adaptation upon arrival to altitude. In order to maximize the Hbmass response at altitude, daily supplementation with ~100 to 200 mg of elemental iron may be required [54].

32.5.2 Blood Oxygen Saturation Monitoring

Information about athlete's hematological response to altitude may be revealed by measurement of peripheral oxygen saturation (SpO_2) at rest [55]. The rise in levels of erythropoietin is proportional to the degree of hypoxia and decline in SpO_2. Athletes with a higher saturation value or faster increase in SpO_2 during altitude exposure may need to extend the length of an exposure, increase exposure to a higher altitude, or complete more high-intensity exercise at altitude to get higher desaturation [55]. Athlete's ability to maintain SpO_2 has been strongly linked to the maintenance of both VO^2max and performance at altitude [56]. VO^2max is generally accepted as the single best measure of the functional limit of the combined respiratory and circulatory systems to deliver oxygen to active muscles and the ability of the muscles to use oxygen and is reproducible. Moreover, VO^2max is the most often studied and well-described effect of altitude exposure on exercise performance and is more or less independent of exercise protocol. At altitude, VO^2max is mainly affected by the reduction of air pressure that leads to reduced partial pressure of oxygen and consequently reduced oxygen flux at every step along the oxygen cascade. Consequently, VO^2max is reduced at altitude and this reduction is directly related to increased relative training intensity for the same absolute work load. At altitude, the decreased PO_2 and resultant hypoxemia lower maximal oxygen uptake (VO^2max) by approximately 6–7% per 1000 m increase at altitude from sea level to 3000 m [57], and that there is a substantial individual difference in the reduction of VO^2max with increasing altitude. This reduction was highly correlated with the decrease in SpO_2, and of course, with the increase in relative training intensity for the same absolute running speed. According to Ferretti et al. [58], the decrease in SpO_2 accounts for about 86% of the decrease in VO^2max, and the reduction of 1% in SpO_2 below 92–93% causes a decrease of ~1% of VO^2max. Hence, the main mechanism for the hypoxia-induced decrease in VO^2max at low and moderate altitude is the decrease in SpO 2max. Maximal heart rate tended to decrease by about 2 beats per 1000 m increasing altitude. Submaximal values showed as expected that VO^2 for the same absolute speed is the same independent of altitude. SpO_2 reduced curvilinearly as did heart rate increase to compensate for the reduced oxygen content of the arterial blood. With living for 2–3 weeks LHTH acclimatization, the initial deficit in VO^2max can be reduced by about 1/3, whereas this deficit has been shown to be reduced by about 50–70% with the LHTL approach. This altered O_2 intake is the principal factor limiting aerobic performance at altitude compared to sea level. The decrease in endurance exercise performance is lower in normobaric hypoxia, due to reductions in the inspired fraction of oxygen (FIO_2) than equivalent reductions in hypobaric hypoxia [59], since the intensity of the normobaric hypoxia stimulus may be lower. In either case, maximal cardiac output declines since both maximal stroke volume and heart rate are lower during hypoxia, whether due to decreased barometric pressure or FIO_2. Elite athletes may be more susceptible to this situation than lesser trained individuals due to the fact that elite athletes have exercise-induced arterial hypoxemia, even at sea level [60]. Even among elite athletes frequently exposed to altitude, some are more negatively affected than others during exercise in hypoxia [60]. Pre-screening of an athlete's desaturation response during maximal exercise, as well as the hypoxic ventilatory response, could provide information that may foresee their response to altitude, which could be used to make modifications to training at altitude (e.g. lengthened recoveries, more sessions at lower altitude) necessary to maintain exercise intensity. In addition, maximal heart rate (HRmax) declines at altitude; this decrease was reported already at low altitude (<1000 M) and is less in normobaric than in hypobaric hypoxia [61].

32.5.3 Overreaching and Overtraining at Altitude

A well-managed period of intensified altitude training can be used to increase performance level in elite endurance athletes [62]; however, this may have at the same time negative consequences for performance. While altitude training can lead to improvements in athletes performance, it can also increase the level of fatigue state given the higher intensity of exercise, and therefore render athletes more susceptible to undesirable outcomes [63]. Monitoring of objective measures such as body mass, resting heart rate, urinary specific gravity, blood/serum urea and creatine kinase concentration, and heart rate variability has been suggested to establish the level of fatigue during altitude training, but subjective measures may be more responsive to training-induced changes in athlete [64]. The use of questionnaires that includes items pertaining fatigue, health, and sleep quality (among other factors) is a simple and also reliable method of monitoring athlete wellness, and this strategy can be recommended over measures that require an extended period of monitoring with frequent data collection. A very good method to assess the perceived exertion is the Borg Scale [65]: it is a simple method of rating perceived exertion (RPE) to gauge an athlete's level of intensity in training and competition. Perceived exertion is an individual's rating of exercise intensity, formed by assessing their body's physical signs such as heart rate, breathing rate, and perspiration/sweating. There are several RPE scales, but the most common are the 15-point scale [6–20] and the 11-point scale (0–10), with 0 being a resting state and 10 being a maximum effort. Borg's RPE scale was not intended simply for athletics. Among other things, it can be quite useful in terms of occupational health and safety for workers performing physical labor. However, it has become most popular in the fields of sports science and sports medicine and is often used to help put together training regimens. In its simplest terms, it provides a measure of how hard it feels that the body is working based on the physical sensations that the subject experiences, including increased heart rate, increased respiration or breathing rate, increased sweating, and muscle fatigue. The symptom of exertion is unique to an individual and can be used as a subjective estimate of the work intensity undertaken across a variety of populations. The intensity of work is important because of the risks of musculoskeletal injuries and disorders arising from a mismatch between the worker's capability and the physical demands of their job. Finally, it is important to underline that altitude training has to be scheduled very well and it's not advisable to start it really near a major event because it's necessary to test the athlete's response to altitude.

32.6 Specificity for Altitude in the Athletes

32.6.1 Responders vs. Non-responders

The concept of responders and non-responders started with the study by Levine et al. [66], in which athletes were exposed to 4 weeks of living at 2500 m and training according to various protocols at either 2500–3000 or 1250 m. Authors registered, at the end of the period, a wide variability in their response and result and so they divided athletes into a "responder" and a "non-responders" group. Responders were the ones who had their EPO increased twice that of non-responders and concomitantly showed an increase in erythrocyte volume and VO^2max. Their running economy, buffer or anaerobic capacity, as well as the measured oxidative enzymes remained essentially unchanged. Non-responders included natives to high altitude as well as sojourners. What they did share was a lower level of EPO, iron concentration, erythroid cell lines, and red cell survival time soon after return to sea level—which may lead to rapid destruction of HIF-1α, compromising the ability of short duration hypoxia to increase red cell mass.

32.6.2 Team Sports

Over the last two decades, team sports have faced a tremendous increase in the time of play and energy demands during matches. So there is a never-ending research of innovative ways to improve match outcomes, and altitude training (~2000–3000 m) [67] has emerged as a popular solution. The physical (total distance covered, high-speed running or sprinting) and physiological (cardiovascular load, blood lactate concentration) demands of major team (football, rugby or Australian football) and racket sports (tennis and squash) have considerably increased in recent years due to new tactical approaches that have been adopted by many teams, thereby increasing the importance of endurance capacity. Team sports share the common feature of intermittent, high-intensity, exercise patterns with continuously changing pace and also face high variability of game characteristics between sports, between playing positions, and playing styles within the same sport and even from one match to the next [68]. This creates a diversity of physiological challenges and performance needs across team-sport players. While elite team-sport players do not exhibit the specific physical/physiological capacities of elite endurance and sprint athletes, they generally possess an efficient combination of 'aerobic' and 'anaerobic' potential. Although aerobic metabolism dominates the energy delivery during most team sports, decisive actions (e.g. sprints, jumps, and tackles) are covered by means of anaerobic metabolism [69]. As a result, the demands of team sports lend themselves towards a potential gain from adaptations to hypoxia from aerobically (maximal oxygen uptake (VO^2max)), economy and Phosphocreatine resynthesis) and anaerobically (muscle buffer capacity) derived mechanisms. However, because the extent to which a player may benefit from different altitude training methods may differ according to both their general and specific training focus (more aerobic vs. anaerobic type of adaptations), no uniform recommendations can be made across all team sports. Altitude training may have greater benefits for players involved in covering large distances (>100 m/min) with high-intensity repeated efforts (i.e. 'invasion' sports), as Australian football players do, compared with volleyball players, who run relatively less (distance covered generally). In team sports, where a high Hbmass is not necessarily a pre-requisite in all positions, players are generally characterized by a low to moderate Hbmass (or VO^2max values usually ranging from 55 to 65 mL/min/kg) [70] in comparison with endurance athletes [71], whose performance is largely related to aerobic capacity. Artificial altitude models (LHTL) may be more convenient for the team-sport players with the possibility of remaining in one training venue, while individualizing the 'altitude dose' and training contents in line with their characteristics and field positioning.

32.6.3 Endurance Sports

Elite endurance athletes have been using altitude training for decades in order to improve both their altitude and sea level performance [72, 73]. Both with live high–train high (LHTH) or live high–train low (LHTL), the physiological rationale for altitude training is that the decreased barometric and partial pressure of oxygen lead to lowered oxygen availability causing the signaling of hypoxia-inducible factor-1α (HIF-1α), which then causes an increased erythropoietic response and increased hemoglobin mass (Hbmass). Incorporation of altitude exposure into elite endurance athletes' training schedules is becoming more common in order to induce short- and long-term physiological adaptations that may enhance performance [74–76]. Due to the effects of acclimatization to altitude on performance and to the fact that optimal performance is achieved after acclimatization to the altitude where the competition takes place, live high and train high is very likely the optimal concept [77]. Altitude training is typically included in the annual training plan as 2–4-week camps at low to moderate altitudes. Acclimatization to altitude is necessary for optimal performance at altitude. Current recommendations suggest that ~ 14 days of acclimatization at the same altitude as the competition is sufficient at moderate to high altitudes (i.e. 2000–4500 m) [74]. However, since the time required for acclimatization is likely to be altitude-dependent, less time may be sufficient to acclimatize to lower altitudes. Whether altitude training is employed to improve subsequent sea-level performance or to prepare for competition at altitude, a main aim is to maximize the positive physiological adaptations. Careful monitoring of individual responses to training loads (TLs) and acclimatization is essential for optimizing these adaptations and for reducing the risk of adverse effects, such as over-training, illness, and/or dehydration. Given the combined stress of hypoxia and potential increases in TLs, individual monitoring is especially important during altitude training camps where large inter-individual differences in responses to hypoxia may manifest [60] that repeated altitude exposures over time could be an adequate strategy for an elite athlete to maximally benefit from altitude training. This approach allows repeating the stimulus for Hbmass increases and non-hematological training adaptations, while decreasing the negative effects of altitude ascents due to faster acclimatization via 'hypoxic memory', which together result in minimal chances of 'non-responding. The systematic altitude training approach of several of the top well-funded American endurance running groups (e.g.

Bowerman Track Club, Nike Oregon Project) and British Athletics' endurance running program comprehend three to six altitude camps per year [78]. The capacity to train at a higher altitude level, achieved through repeated exposures, could be an important contributor to an overall altitude-induced improvement. Performing regular natural altitude training camps has been recommended as part of a season-long training program for swimmers. Endurance athletes may utilize a combination of LHTH, LHTL, and IHT models to ensure peak fitness at the time of main competition. Millet [75] proposes a triphasic training cycle for endurance athletes involving each training model at various time points. In the preparation phase, two or three Living High Training High sojourns at 2200–2500 m are recommended as "base training", while in pre-competition training, similar training at lower altitudes of 1800–2000 m may facilitate more intense interval training. During the competitive phase, athletes benefit from a combination of Intermittent Hypoxic Training and Living High—Training Low training.

32.7 Conclusion

We conclude that there is sufficient evidence to suggest that all methods of altitude training can benefit athletic performance in some way; however, to gain improvement in sea-level performance for the top elite athletes, a Live High-Train Low method is recommended. Nevertheless, performance enhancement for athletes as a result of altitude training is not always guaranteed. Indeed, some athletes may be unable to handle the extra stress that accompanies hypoxia, especially when they may be already working close to their physical limits. In such cases, maladaptation and detraining may occur and the athlete's performance may decrease rather than increase. Through rigorous preparation, adequate training and recovery, and thorough planning, altitude training can be successful. Maintaining detailed longitudinal data on individual athletes including subjective and objective measures of stress and performance will allow the early detection of problems and increase the chances of a positive altitude training block. However, questions still remain to be answered including what is the most effective hypoxic dosage, what is the best way to monitor adaptation during hypoxia, and discovering the best way to delineate responders from non-responders.

References

1. Conkin J, Wessel JH. Critique of the equivalent air altitude model. Aviat Space Environ Med. 2008;79(10):975–82.
2. Favier FB, Britto FA, Freyssenet DG, Bigard XA, Benoit H. HIF-1-driven skeletal muscle adaptations to chronic hypoxia: molecular insights into muscle physiology. Cell Mol Life Sci. 2015;72(24):4681–96.
3. Hamlin MJ, Draper N, Hellemans J. Real and simulated altitude training and performance. In: Hamlin M, editor. Current issues in sports and exercise medicine. InTech; 2013. http://www.intechopen.com/books/current-issues-in-sports-and-exercise-medicine/real-and-simulated-altitude-training-and-performance.
4. Semenza GL. HIF-1: mediator of physiological and pathophysiological responses to hypoxia. J Appl Physiol. 2000;88(4):1474–80.
5. Lindholm ME, Rundqvist H. Skeletal muscle hypoxia-inducible factor-1 and exercise: skeletal muscle hypoxia-inducible factor-1 and exercise. Exp Physiol. 2016;101(1):28–32.
6. Chapman RF, Stray-Gundersen J, Levine BD. Individual variation in response to altitude training. J Appl Physiol. 1998;85(4):1448–56.
7. Wehrlin JP, Zuest P, Hallén J, Marti B. Live high-train low for 24 days increases hemoglobin mass and red cell volume in elite endurance athletes. J Appl Physiol. 2006;100(6):1938–45.
8. Jelkmann W. Regulation of erythropoietin production: erythropoietin production. J Physiol. 2011;589(6):1251–8.
9. Robach P, Fulla Y, Westerterp KR, Richalet JP. Comparative response of EPO and soluble transferrin receptor at high altitude. Med Sci Sports Exerc. 2004;36(9):1493–8.
10. Levine BD, Stray-Gundersen J. Point: positive effects of intermittent hypoxia (live high:train low) on exercise performance are mediated primarily by augmented red cell volume. J Appl Physiol. 2005;99(5):2053–5.
11. Stray-Gundersen J, Chapman RF, Levine BD. "Living high-training low" altitude training improves sea level performance in male and female elite runners. J Appl Physiol. 2001;91(3):1113–20.

12. Wilber RL, Stray-Gundersen J, Levine BD. Effect of hypoxic 'dose' on physiological responses and sea-level performance. Med Sci Sports Exerc. 2007;39(9):1590–9.
13. Whayne TF. Cardiovascular medicine at high altitude. Angiology. 2014;65(6):459–72.
14. Feriche B, Schoenfeld BJ, Bonitch-Gongora J, de la Fuente B, Almeida F, Argüelles J, et al. Altitude-induced effects on muscular metabolic stress and hypertrophy-related factors after a resistance training session. Eur J Sport Sci. 2020;20(8):1083–92.
15. Goldfarb-Rumyantzev AS, Alper SL. Short-term responses of the kidney to high altitude in mountain climbers. Nephrol Dial Transplant. 2014;29(3):497–506.
16. Penaloza D, Arias-Stella J. The heart and pulmonary circulation at high altitudes: healthy highlanders and Chronic Mountain sickness. Circulation. 2007;115(9):1132–46.
17. Zhang G, Zhou SM, Yuan C, Tian HJ, Li P, Gao YQ. The effects of short-term and long-term exposure to a high altitude hypoxic environment on neurobehavioral function. High Alt Med Biol. 2013;14(4):338–41.
18. Fulco CS, Beidleman BA, Muza SR. Effectiveness of Preacclimatization strategies for high-altitude exposure. Exerc Sport Sci Rev. 2013;41(1):55–63.
19. Koehle MS, Cheng I, Sporer B. Canadian academy of sport and exercise medicine position statement: athletes at high altitude. Clin J Sport Med. 2014;24(2):120–7.
20. Cheng I, Kiss A, Lilge L. An observational study of personal ultraviolet dosimetry and acute diffuse reflectance skin changes at extreme altitude. Wilderness Environ Med. 2013;24(4):390–6.
21. Rigel EG, Lebwohl MG, Rigel AC, Rigel DS. Ultraviolet radiation in alpine skiing: magnitude of exposure and importance of regular protection. Arch Dermatol. 2003;139(1):60–2.
22. Bloch KE, Buenzli JC, Latshang TD, Ulrich S. Sleep at high altitude: guesses and facts. J Appl Physiol. 2015;119(12):1466–80.
23. Tseng CH, Lin FC, Chao HS, Tsai HC, Shiao GM, Chang SC. Impact of rapid ascent to high altitude on sleep. Sleep Breath. 2015;19(3):819–26.
24. Weil JV. Sleep at high altitude. High Alt Med Biol. 2004;5(2):180–9.
25. Wing-Gaia SL. Nutritional strategies for the preservation of fat free mass at high altitude. Nutrients. 2014;6(2):665–81.
26. Kechijian D. Optimizing nutrition for performance at altitude: a literature review. J Spec Oper Med. 2011;11(2):12.
27. Saunders PU, Pyne DB, Gore CJ. Endurance training at altitude. High Alt Med Biol. 2009;10(2):135–48.
28. Girard O, Amann M, Aughey R, Billaut F, Bishop DJ, Bourdon P, et al. Position statement—altitude training for improving team-sport players' performance: current knowledge and unresolved issues. Br J Sports Med. 2013;47(Suppl 1):i8–16.
29. Levine BD, Stray-Gundersen J, Mehta RD. Effect of altitude on football performance: football at altitude. Scand J Med Sci Sports. 2008;18:76–84.
30. Wilber RL. Application of altitude/hypoxic training by elite athletes. Med Sci Sports Exerc. 2007;39(9):1610–24.
31. Wachsmuth NB, Völzke C, Prommer N, Schmidt-Trucksäss A, Frese F, Spahl O, et al. The effects of classic altitude training on hemoglobin mass in swimmers. Eur J Appl Physiol. 2013;113(5):1199–211.
32. Bonne TC, Lundby C, Jørgensen S, Johansen L, Mrgan M, Bech SR, et al. "Live High–Train High" increases hemoglobin mass in Olympic swimmers. Eur J Appl Physiol. 2014;114(7):1439–49.
33. Siebenmann C, Cathomen A, Hug M, Keiser S, Lundby AK, Hilty MP, et al. Hemoglobin mass and intravascular volume kinetics during and after exposure to 3,454-m altitude. J Appl Physiol. 2015;119(10):1194–201.
34. Rodríguez FA, Iglesias X, Feriche B, Calderón-Soto C, Chaverri D, Wachsmuth NB, et al. Altitude training in elite swimmers for sea level performance (altitude project). Med Sci Sports Exerc. 2015;47(9):1965–78.
35. Mellerowicz H, Meller W, Wowerier J, Zerdick J, Ketusinh O, Kral B, et al. Comparative studies on the effect of high altitude training on permanent performance at lower altitudes. Schweiz Z Sportmed. 1971;Suppl:5–17.
36. McLean BD, Gore CJ, Kemp J. Application of 'live low-train high' for enhancing normoxic exercise performance in team sport athletes. Sports Med. 2014;44(9):1275–87.
37. Millet GP, Faiss R, Brocherie F, Girard O. Hypoxic training and team sports: a challenge to traditional methods? Br J Sports Med. 2013;47(Suppl 1):i6–7.
38. Lundby C, Millet GP, Calbet JA, Bärtsch P, Subudhi AW. Does 'altitude training' increase exercise performance in elite athletes? Br J Sports Med. 2012;46(11):792–5.
39. Millet G, Girard O, Beard A, Brocherie F. Repeated sprint training in hypoxia—an innovative method. Dtsch Z Für Sportmed. 2019;2019(5):115–22.
40. Vogt M, Puntschart A, Geiser J, Zuleger C, Billeter R, Hoppeler H. Molecular adaptations in human skeletal muscle to endurance training under simulated hypoxic conditions. J Appl Physiol. 2001;91(1):173–82.
41. Wilbur RL. Live high + train low: thinking in terms of an optimal hypoxic dose. Int J Sports Physiol Perform. 2007;2(3):223–38.
42. Chapman RF, Karlsen T, Resaland GK, Ge RL, Harber MP, Witkowski S, et al. Defining the "dose" of altitude training: how high to live for optimal sea level performance enhancement. J Appl Physiol. 2014;116(6):595–603.

43. Bonetti DL, Hopkins WG. Sea-level exercise performance following adaptation to hypoxia: a meta-analysis. Sports Med. 2009;39(2):107–27.
44. Saugy JJ, Schmitt L, Cejuela R, Faiss R, Hauser A, Wehrlin JP, et al. Comparison of "Live High-Train Low" in Normobaric versus Hypobaric Hypoxia. PLoS One. 2014;9(12):e114418.
45. Beidleman BA, Fulco CS, Staab JE, Andrew SP, Muza SR. Cycling performance decrement is greater in hypobaric versus normobaric hypoxia. Extreme Physiol Med. 2014;3(1):8.
46. Bailey DM, Davies B. Physiological implications of altitude training for endurance performance at sea level: a review. Br J Sports Med. 1997;31(3):183–90.
47. Saw A, Halson S, Mujika I. Monitoring athletes during training camps: observations and translatable strategies from elite road cyclists and swimmers. Sports. 2018;6(3):63.
48. Mujika I. Quantification of training and competition loads in endurance sports: methods and applications. Int J Sports Physiol Perform. 2017;12(s2):S2-9–S2-17.
49. Gore C, Hahn A, Burge C, Telford R. VO_2 max and Haemoglobin mass of trained athletes during high intensity training. Int J Sports Med. 1997;28(06):477–82.
50. Schmidt W, Prommer N. Effects of various training modalities on blood volume: Total hemoglobin mass and altitude training. Scand J Med Sci Sports. 2008;18:57–69.
51. Gore CJ, Sharpe K, Garvican-Lewis LA, Saunders PU, Humberstone CE, Robertson EY, et al. Altitude training and haemoglobin mass from the optimised carbon monoxide rebreathing method determined by a meta-analysis. Br J Sports Med. 2013;47(Suppl 1):i31–9.
52. Saunders PU, Garvican-Lewis LA, Schmidt WF, Gore CJ. Relationship between changes in haemoglobin mass and maximal oxygen uptake after hypoxic exposure. Br J Sports Med. 2013;47(Suppl 1):i26–30.
53. Govus AD, Garvican-Lewis LA, Abbiss CR, Peeling P, Gore CJ. Pre-altitude serum ferritin levels and daily oral iron supplement dose mediate iron parameter and hemoglobin mass responses to altitude exposure. PLoS One. 2015;10(8):e0135120.
54. Stellingwerff T, Peeling P, Garvican-Lewis LA, Hall R, Koivisto AE, Heikura IA, et al. Nutrition and altitude: strategies to enhance adaptation, improve performance and maintain health: a narrative review. Sports Med. 2019;49(S2):169–84.
55. Płoszczyca K, Langfort J, Czuba M. The effects of altitude training on Erythropoietic response and hematological variables in adult athletes: a narrative review. Front Physiol. 2018;9:375.
56. Chapman RF, Stager JM, Tanner DA, Stray-Gundersen J, Levine BD. Impairment of 3000-m run time at altitude is influenced by arterial oxyhemoglobin saturation. Med Sci Sports Exerc. 2011;43(9):1649–56.
57. Wehrlin JP, Hallén J. Linear decrease in.VO2max and performance with increasing altitude in endurance athletes. Eur J Appl Physiol. 2006;96(4):404–12.
58. Ferretti G, Moia C, Thomet JM, Kayser B. The decrease of maximal oxygen consumption during hypoxia in man: a mirror image of the oxygen equilibrium curve. J Physiol. 1997;498(1):231–7.
59. Saugy JJ, Rupp T, Faiss R, Lamon A, Bourdillon N, Millet GP. Cycling time trial is more altered in hypobaric than Normobaric hypoxia. Med Sci Sports Exerc. 2016;48(4):680–8.
60. Chapman RF. The individual response to training and competition at altitude. Br J Sports Med. 2013;47(Suppl 1):i40–4.
61. Mourot L, Millet GP. Is maximal heart rate decrease similar between Normobaric versus hypobaric hypoxia in trained and untrained subjects? High Alt Med Biol. 2019;20(1):94–8.
62. Sharma AP, Saunders PU, Garvican-Lewis LA, Clark B, Welvaert M, Gore CJ, et al. Improved performance in National-Level Runners with Increased Training Load at 1600 and 1800 m. Int J Sports Physiol Perform. 2019;14(3):286–95.
63. Schmitt L, Willis SJ, Coulmy N, Millet GP. Effects of different training intensity distributions between elite cross-country skiers and Nordic-combined athletes during live high-train low. Front Physiol. 2018;9:932.
64. Saw AE, Main LC, Gastin PB. Monitoring the athlete training response: subjective self-reported measures trump commonly used objective measures: a systematic review. Br J Sports Med. 2016;50(5):281–91.
65. Borg GAV. Psychophysical bases of perceived exertion. Med Sci Sports Exerc. 1982;14(5):377–81.
66. Levine BD, Stray-Gundersen J. "Living high-training low": effect of moderate-altitude acclimatization with low-altitude training on performance. J Appl Physiol. 1997;83(1):102–12.
67. Bärtsch P, Saltin B, Dvorak J. Consensus statement on playing football at different altitude: consensus statement on playing football at different altitude. Scand J Med Sci Sports. 2008;18:96–9.
68. Bradley PS, Carling C, Archer D, Roberts J, Dodds A, Di Mascio M, et al. The effect of playing formation on high-intensity running and technical profiles in English FA premier league soccer matches. J Sports Sci. 2011;29(8):821–30.
69. Faude O, Koch T, Meyer T. Straight sprinting is the most frequent action in goal situations in professional football. J Sports Sci. 2012;30(7):625–31.
70. Wachsmuth N, Kley M, Spielvogel H, Aughey RJ, Gore CJ, Bourdon PC, et al. Changes in blood gas transport of altitude native soccer players near sea-level and sea-level native soccer players at altitude (ISA3600). Br J Sports Med. 2013;47(Suppl 1):i93–9.
71. Heinicke K, Wolfarth B, Winchenbach P, Biermann B, Schmid A, Huber G, et al. Blood volume and hemo-

globin mass in elite athletes of different disciplines. Int J Sports Med. 2001;22(7):504–12.
72. Daniels J, Oldridge N. The effects of alternate exposure to altitude and sea level on world-class middle-distance runners. Med Sci Sports. 1970;2(3):107–12.
73. Tønnessen E, Sylta Ø, Haugen TA, Hem E, Svendsen IS, Seiler S. The road to gold: training and peaking characteristics in the year prior to a gold medal endurance performance. PLoS One. 2014;9(7):e101796.
74. Burtscher M, Niedermeier M, Burtscher J, Pesta D, Suchy J, Strasser B. Preparation for endurance competitions at altitude: physiological, psychological, dietary and coaching aspects. A narrative review. Front Physiol. 2018;9:1504.
75. Millet GP, Roels B, Schmitt L, Woorons X, Richalet JP. Combining hypoxic methods for peak performance. Sports Med. 2010;40(1):1–25.
76. Mujika I, Sharma AP, Stellingwerff T. Contemporary periodization of altitude training for elite endurance athletes: a narrative review. Sports Med. 2019;49(11):1651–69.
77. Chapman RF, Laymon AS, Levine BD. Timing of arrival and pre-acclimatization strategies for the endurance athlete competing at moderate to high altitudes. High Alt Med Biol. 2013;14(4):319–24.
78. Turner G, Fudge BW, Pringle JSM, Maxwell NS, Richardson AJ. Altitude training in endurance running: perceptions of elite athletes and support staff. J Sports Sci. 2019;37(2):163–72.

Lightning 33

Tori A. Edmiston, Luke Zabawa,
and Mark R. Hutchinson

Abbreviations

ABC	Airway, breathing, circulation
ABCDE	Airway, breathing, circulation, deformities, exposure
ACLS	Advanced cardiovascular life support
AED	Automated external defibrillator
AVPU	Alert, verbal, pain, unresponsive
BLS	Basic life support
CBC	Complete blood count
CK	Creatine kinase
CMP	Comprehensive metabolic profile
CNS	Central nervous system
CPR	Cardiopulmonary resuscitation
CT	Computed tomography
CTA	Computed tomography angiography
EKG	Electrocardiogram
EMG	Electromyography
FIFA	Federal International Football Association
GCS	Glascow coma scale
IEA	Interscholastic Equestrian Association
IOC	International Olympic Committee
IV	Intravenous
LOC	Loss of consciousness
MLB	Major League Baseball
MRI	Magnetic resonance imaging
NCAA	National Collegiate Athletic Association
NOAA	National Oceanic and Atmospheric Administration
NSSL	National Severe Storms Laboratory
PGA	Professional Golfers' Association
UA	Urinalysis
USOPC	United States Olympic and Paralympic Committee
USSF	United States Soccer Federation

T. A. Edmiston · L. Zabawa · M. R. Hutchinson (✉)
University of Illinois, Chicago, IL, USA

Orthopedic Surgery Resident, University of Illinois, Chicago, IL, USA

Department of Orthopaedics and Sports Medicine, University of Illinois, Chicago, IL, USA
e-mail: mhutch@uic.edu

Fact Box

- Lightning is the most consistent and significant weather hazard that may affect intercollegiate athletics [1].
- National Severe Storms Laboratory (NSSL) estimates that within the US, 100 fatalities and 400–500 injuries requiring medical treatment occur from lightning strikes every year [1].
- Approximately 10% of people who are struck by lightning are killed, the remaining 90% exhibit various degrees of disability.
- The National Weather Service. [2, 3] reported data from 2010 and 2011, with

S. Rocha Piedade et al. (eds.), *Sideline Management in Sports*,
https://doi.org/10.1007/978-3-031-33867-0_33

48% and 62% of lightning fatalities attributed to sport and recreation, respectively.
- High risk groups and risk factors: outdoor activities, mountain climbers/hikers, swimmers, field athletes (javelin, shot-put), golfers, bicyclists.
- Three quarters of all lightning casualties occur between May and September, nearly four fifths occur between 10:00 AM and 7:00 PM, which coincides with the hours for most athletic or recreational activities.
- Preventative measures: education, implementation of lightning safety policy including avoidance of sheltering under trees and avoiding open fields and spaces, designating safe locations for shelter, monitoring local weather forecasts with a designated weather watcher, establish a chain of command.

33.1 Introduction

Lightning is the most consistent and significant weather hazard that may affect intercollegiate athletics [1]. Within the United States, the National Severe Storms Laboratory (NSSL) estimates that 100 fatalities and 400–500 injuries requiring medical treatment occur from lightning strikes every year [1]. While the probability of being struck by lightning continues to be extremely low, the risks are significantly higher in areas where the storm is in close proximity and proper safety precautions are not followed or clear guidelines are not outlined and implemented [1]. A lightning strike can result in fatal cardiac arrest at the time of injury or in the subsequent days following resuscitation on the day of injury due to irreversible ischemic brain injury, etc. [4]

Lightning is a widespread danger to the physically active population, in part because of the prevalence of afternoon to early evening thunderstorms from late spring to early fall and a societal trend toward outdoor physical activities during those times [5–8]. Certain areas of the United States have greater thunderstorm activity than others. The areas with the most lightning activity are Florida, the Gulf States, the Mississippi and Ohio River Valleys, the front range of the Southern Rocky Mountains, and parts of the Southwest [9].

Many athletic events occur outdoors, and these activities may rely on coaches, officials, athletic trainers, team physicians, and athletic administrators to make safety decisions for continued play. It is therefore essential that everyone involved understand the dangers of lightning, have a safety plan in place, and abide by the safety plan once thunder or lightning is heard/seen. The assistance of weather watchers, real-time weather forecasts, and commercial weather warning devices/services may be of use as tools to aid in monitoring and notification of threatening weather situations, decision making regarding stoppage of play, evacuation, and return to play [10].

33.2 Basic Lightning Facts

Lightning is a giant spark of electricity in the atmosphere between clouds, the air, or the ground [11].

Lightning can occur between opposite charges within the thunderstorm cloud (intra-cloud lightning) or between opposite charges in the cloud and on the ground (cloud-to-ground lightning) [11].

Lightning is one of the oldest observed natural phenomena on earth [11].

Lightning actually causes thunder. Energy from a lightning channel heats the air to approximately 50,000 °F. This in turn causes the air to explode outward with a huge amount of pressure. This pressure decreases rapidly with increasing distance, and within approximately ten yards, becomes small enough to be perceived to the human ear as the sound we call thunder [11].

Thunder can be heard up to 25 miles from the lightning discharge. The frequency of the sound changes with distance [11]. The initial thunder you hear produces a tearing sound since the thunder contains the highest frequencies. Subsequently, you hear a sharp click or loud crack to a low-frequency rumbling [11].

As light travels through air much faster than sound does (~ one million times), we can use thunder to estimate the distance to lightning. Counting the number of seconds from the time the flash is observed to the sound heard and dividing by 5 (sound travels at ~1/fifth of mile/s and 1/third of km/s) gives an estimate of the number of miles (dividing by 3 for an estimate of kilometers) to the flash [11].

Most of the lightning flashes produced by storms start inside the cloud. If the flash strikes the ground, a channel develops downward toward the surface. When the channel approaches ~100 yards of the surface, objects on the surface (trees, bushes, and buildings) send up sparks to meet it. If these sparks connect with the downward channel, a large electrical current surges quickly down the channel to the object that produced the sparks. This explains why skyscrapers and tall objects are more likely to be struck by lightning.

33.3 Clinical Presentation

History: Lightning injuries are typically obvious if they occur in an athletic setting with witnesses present. However, lightning injuries can be difficult to diagnose if the person presents without a witness is unable to provide details of the injury or is found dead in a field or mountain side. Typically, the victim can provide basic details of the injury, but it is common for the person to have some degree of anterograde amnesia or confusion. Keen assessment of the victim's ability to relate the details of the event should be observed as they may be able to provide basic details of the event or participate in a reasonably coherent social conversation. Conversely, they may repeat the same question multiple times or may not remember the events as time progresses from onset. More severe symptoms such as not recognizing a family member or coach are not present and should be observed carefully as they may be signs of intended secondary gain [12].

Physical presentation after lightning injury is varied and can range from mild disorientation with no immediate signs to cardiac arrest (only direct cause of death) and anoxic brain injury. Conscious athletes often report muscle aches, dysesthesias, headaches, weakness, or other neurologic/musculoskeletal problems [13].

33.4 Injury Types

Classically, there are five mechanisms for lightning to conduct through and injure the body. A sixth modality was observed recently and described.

1. *Direct strike:* Occurs when the victim is in the open, away from protection, and directly injured by a cloud-to-ground burst. This is one of the less-frequent sources of injury (3– 5%), as most people generally seek shelter when storms approach. This mechanism would intuitively cause the highest mortality, but surprisingly does not for unknown reasons [14–16].
2. *Contact:* Often associated with indoor strikes or when a victim is within a location considered safe (i.e., when talking on a corded telephone, showering, or doing dishes while indoors). Occurs when an electrical surge passes through wiring, scaffolding, or plumbing and transmits to the victim by direct contact with that object [14, 16].
3. *Sideflash (also known as "splash")*: Occurs in up to 30% of injuries. Commonly seen in outdoor settings, where the victim seeks shelter beneath a tree or within a shelter that has not been grounded. May affect several members of a group if they are clustered together, such as scout groups gathered under a tree during a storm [14–16].
4. *Step voltage (ground potential):* The conductive nature of the earth acts to transport a current from a potentially distant strike to the victim. The voltage difference is increased with a greater separation of contacts. For example, a hiker lying down on the ground will have a greater potential for injury than one who is crouching down with their feet only a few inches apart [14].

5. *Upward streamer:* This injury occurs when the victim acts as a conduit for the positively charged upward streamer from the ground and helps transmit the charge toward the negatively charged stepped leaders coming from the clouds [14, 17].
6. *Barotrauma:* This most recently described mechanism of injury is associated with the sonic blast and pressure differential that accompanies a lightning strike. This mechanism may account for traumatic brain injury, as well as such injuries such as ruptured tympanic membranes [14, 18].

33.5 Lightning Effects by System

Cardiac: Cardiac arrest is the only known cause of death following a lightning strike. Lightning may cause a temporary momentary asystole from which the heart spontaneously recovers. Autonomic nervous system control of cardiac rhythm has been shown to be affected by lightning. At times the initial respiratory arrest may last longer than the cardiac arrest and cause a secondary cardiac arrest due to hypoxia. A more serious brain injury can also cause a prolonged cardiac or respiratory arrest [13].

QTc prolongation is the most common EKG abnormality which tends to resolve over the course of several months and commonly does not require treatment or intervention [13].

Neurologic: The immediate effect of the electrical current of a lightning strike on the central nervous system (CNS) in an alerted level of consciousness (LOC) [14]. In severe cases as mentioned above, damage to the respiratory centers within the brainstem may occur and cause sudden death or substantial anoxic brain injury even if the athlete is resuscitated. Rarely, rapid onset of cerebral edema develops causing brainstem herniation. Contusion and intracranial hemorrhage have also been reported. In unconscious athletes, anoxic brain injury or underlying brain trauma should be suspected.

Athletes who are awake and lucid may experience subsequent disabling neurocognitive deficits similar to those with concussion or blunt brain injury. These symptoms may not be present or apparent until the survivor attempts to return to their previous activities. Typical presentations are the inability to process new information, organize, and multitask [13].

Acute pain/debilitating headaches, numbness, or other dysesthesias may be apparent. Chronic pain syndromes may develop subsequently following a lightning strike injury due to nerve injury, sympathetic nervous system injury, spinal cord injury, or other causes [13].

Initial sympathetic nervous injury may cause vascular spasm; temporary paralysis and mottling of an extremity (keraunoparalysis); transient self-limited hypertension; and late problems with positive tilt test results, vertigo or dizziness, hypertension, and pain syndromes [13].

Mechanical trauma from a fall after a lightning strike may also contribute to the neurologic sequelae found on exam. Rarely, a lightning strike may cause the athlete to fall or be thrown with sufficient force to cause a skull fracture and intracranial hemorrhage. It can be difficult to distinguish if the comatose or semicomatose state is secondary to electrical shock or intracranial hematoma until lateralizing signs develop [13].

Musculocutaneous: Fractures of the skull, ribs, extremities, and spine have been reported but are rare [13]. As stated before, chronic pain syndromes may develop subsequently.

As the electric current passes through tissue, it is converted to heat, which has the potential to damage muscle tissue. Muscle necrosis may cause rhabdomyolysis, compartment syndrome, or renal failure, all of which are very rare [13].

Ocular/Ophthalmic: Nearly every type of eye injury has been reported with lightning injury, including cataracts, macular holes, retinal separation, and iritis. Cataracts may occur early or late after the initial lightning injury [13].

Disruption of autonomic nervous system can cause dilated and/or nonreactive pupils. This short-term reaction to lightning strikes cannot be used to assess brain death.

Cataracts are the most common intraocular lesions caused by lightning. Two types are seen, traumatic cataract (shortly after injury from a concussion, due to multiple tears of the lens capsule) versus cataract characteristic of an injury from either lightning or high voltage current (appears first few days or weeks, anterior subcapsular changes).

Retinal involvement is less frequent, although chorioretinal atrophy, macular holes, macular cysts, papilledema, hemorrhage, and detachment have been noted. Retinal damage should be investigated when assessing vision, even in a developed/developing cataract patient [13].

Lid lesions are varied from partial thickness burn to ulcerated necrotic lesions. Conjunctival chemosis frequently occurs and corneal lesions vary from transitory punctate keratitis to severe interstitial keratitis. Iridocyclitis can be mild and temporary to severe and chronic. Paresis of accommodation may also occur.

Otic: Ear injuries are common following lightning injury and are seen in up to half of patients. Direct electrical injury and blast effects can injure the ears with significant ear damage and hearing loss. Tinnitus and other eighth nerve symptoms, such as dizziness and balance deficiencies, are also common [13].

Temporal bone pathology such as tympanic membrane rupture (>1/2 of more severely injured patients), middle ear and mastoid effusion of blood, total rupture of the Reissner membrane, degeneration of the stria vascularis and organ of Corti, edema of the intracanalicular portion of the facial nerve, herniation of a portion of cerebellum into the internal auditory meatus, and a possible microfracture of the otic capsule are also common [13].

Seldom, unilateral hearing loss is present with audiograms demonstrating typical nerve-type hearing loss [13]. The tympanic membrane is typically intact but significantly inflamed in these athletes. Hearing disability may be temporary or permanent.

Essentially, all lightning strike survivors report chronic tinnitus, which tends to be quite an irritating sequalae.

Dermatologic

Burn types caused by the lightning strike:

- Feathering (Lichtenberg figures, keraunographic markings).
- Linear.
- Punctate—Multiple, closely spaced, discrete, circular, usually full-thickness lesions (due to current passing through dry skin, resembles a cigarette burn).
- Thermal (ignites or melts clothing, usually full thickness.
- Contact—Occurs when metal, such as jewelry, zippers, or belt buckles, contacts the skin during a lightning strike; sporadic full-thickness burn or can actually "tattoo" metal, such as a necklace, into the skin.
- Flash—Superficial burn that results in brown discoloration of the skin.

A pathognomonic cutaneous feature is feathering, which includes linear feather-like superficial skin markings (keraunographic marks) and usually disappear after a few days. Typical cutaneous manifestations consist of erythematous streaks that do not blanch [13].

Linear burns are usually partial-thickness, 1–4 cm wide, that occur on sweat/rain-covered areas of the body, such as beneath the breasts or mid chest, and in the midaxillary line. These burns present minutes to hours after the lightning strike [13].

Full thickness burns rarely result from lightning [13].

Myoglobinuria should be ruled out in these cases.

Some possible findings on physical exam of an athlete with lightning injury:

- Cold, mottled, pulseless extremities.
- Confusion, amnesia, paralysis, and loss of consciousness.
- Temporary hearing loss or tympanic membrane rupture.
- Hypotension.
- Prolonged paresis or paralysis of the extremities.
- Fixed and dilated pupils.
- Lichtenberg figures/Feathering.
- Clothing that is singed, shredded, or blown apart.

Others—*Blunt Injury*: Organ contusions, pulmonary hemorrhage, pneumothorax, and cardiac contusions have been reported but are rare. If the patient has a history of a fall or being thrown a distance, investigate for fractures and blunt injuries. A patient may also have experienced explosive trauma and shrapnel effects if he or she was close to an object that was exploded by lightning [13].

Differential Diagnosis

- Electrical injuries
- Ventricular fibrillation
- Intracranial hemorrhage
- Seizure
- Syncope
- Cardiorespiratory arrest
- Ventricular fibrillation
- CNS injury or stroke
- Autonomic nervous system injury
- Peripheral nervous system injury
- Blunt and explosive trauma
- Musculoskeletal injury
- Acoustic injury
- Barotrauma

33.6 Indications/Benefits of Additional Testing

Laboratory evaluation: routine testing not typically warranted: CBC, CK with isoenzymes, UA, Urine myoglobin level, CMP.

EKG

EMG

Neurophysical battery.

Plain Radiographs.

CT head W/ and W/O contrast, CTA head, MRI head.

33.7 Incidence and Prevalence

Within the United States, the National Severe Storms Laboratory (NSSL) estimates that 100 fatalities and 400–500 injuries requiring medical treatment occur from lightning strikes every year [1]. According to the NWS Storm Data, over the last 30 years (1989–2018), the US has averaged 43 reported lightning fatalities per year [4]. Based on reported and collected data, approximately 10% of people who are struck by lightning are killed. The remaining 90% exhibit various degrees of disability. More recently, in the last 10 years (2009–2018), the US has averaged 27 lightning fatalities [4]. Worldwide, lightning causes an estimated 24,000 deaths and about 240,000 injuries annually [18]. On average, 25 million lightning flashes strike the ground each year in the United States [6, 19].

Data from 2005 indicated that approximately 15% of lightning casualties arose in organized sports, and an additional 25–30% resulted from recreational activities [20]. The National Weather Service [2, 3] reported more recent data from 2010 and 2011, with 48% and 62% of lightning fatalities attributed to sport and recreation.

According to statistics from the National Weather Service, a person living in the United States will have a 1:10,000 chance of being struck by lightning by 80 year of age [21]. However, considering this statistic is for the general population, it can be assumed that a person will have a much higher chance of being struck if they enjoy outdoor activities [14].

33.8 High-Risk Groups/Risk Factors

High-risk groups and risk factors include outdoor activities, mountain climbers/hikers, swimmers, field athletes (javelin, shot-put), golfers, and bicyclists. Three quarters of all lightning casualties occur between May and September, nearly four fifths occur between 10:00 AM and 7:00 PM, which coincides with the hours for most athletic or recreational activities.

33.9 Treatment

Before evaluating an injured athlete, it is important to assess the scene for safety first. If the scene is deemed safe, immediate assessment and treatment of the injured athlete can begin. Otherwise, safe evacuation to a substantial building is indicated prior to assessment and treatment. No place outside is safe when thunderstorms are in the area and rescuers/physicians, athletes, and spectators may be at significant risk. National lightning safety guidelines indicate that significant risk continues for 30 min after the last lightning is seen or thunder is heard [13].

If the athlete is unresponsive, shout for help and activate the emergency response system via call to 911 or the local agency immediately prior to providing any treatment (if only one on the scene). Get an AED or send someone to do so. Initial examination of an athlete on the sideline with observed or suspected lightning injury should include evaluation of airway, breathing, and circulation with intervention being provided if any findings of deficiency are elicited on exam. Basic life support (BLS) or advanced cardiac life support (ALCS) care should be initiated and followed according to treatment algorithm and access to medications/advanced airway (including cardiopulmonary resuscitation and rescue breaths, AED assessment, and shock if indicated as well as medication administration if available and rapid transport to the emergency room). Immobilization should be considered in those who are unresponsive or altered because of risk of blunt trauma from the lightning concussion or from being thrown by involuntary muscle contraction. Others with keraunoparalysis, evidence of head injury/tenderness, or hematomas of the neck or back should alert the rescuer to the possibility of an injury to the spinal cord. In such cases, stabilize the head until the person is secured to a long backboard by emergency medical technicians [13] (Figs. 33.1 and 33.2).

Next, carefully assess level of alertness (AVPU) and orientation. Evaluate for any disabilities followed by exposure/skin exam including wounds and burns. (ABCDE approach). Vital signs should be obtained as soon as completing ABC's and assessing for level of consciousness and alertness. An accurate blood pressure reading is necessary to determine if the athlete is hypertensive and needs immediate transportation and IV fluid hydration. Obtain a heart rate to determine if the patient is tachycardic or bradycardic with rhythm assessment as soon as possible to evaluate for any arrythmias that may progress or become lethal as treatment options are available if identified early. Respiratory rate is important to determine if tachypneic or labored; supplemental oxygen or an advanced airway may be necessary. Temperature is important as hyper or hypothermia may complicate the clinical presentation and needs to be addressed during early management. A full neurologic examination should be completed when the athlete has been stabilized (Fig. 33.3) (Tables 33.1, 33.2 and 33.3).

Perform an electrocardiography (EKG) or telemetry for rate, rhythm, and other abnormality assessment as soon as possible. EKG changes following a lightning strike are typically due to vascular spasm and arrythmia without coronary artery occlusion. Occasionally, there is direct damage to the myocardium. Electrocardiographic evidence for direct myocardial damage includes ST segment elevation, T-wave inversion, and prolongation of the QT interval, typically temporary without serious cardiac complications [13].

Severe burn injuries should include cleansing the wound, followed by treatment with a topical antimicrobial cream containing polymyxin (10,000 U/g), nystatin (4000 U/g), and nitrofurantoin (0.3%) or other burn cream. Tetanus prophylaxis should be updated. Any devitalized skin should be excised, and autogenous, split-thickness skin grafts considered [13].

Use NSAIDS and narcotics for acute pain.

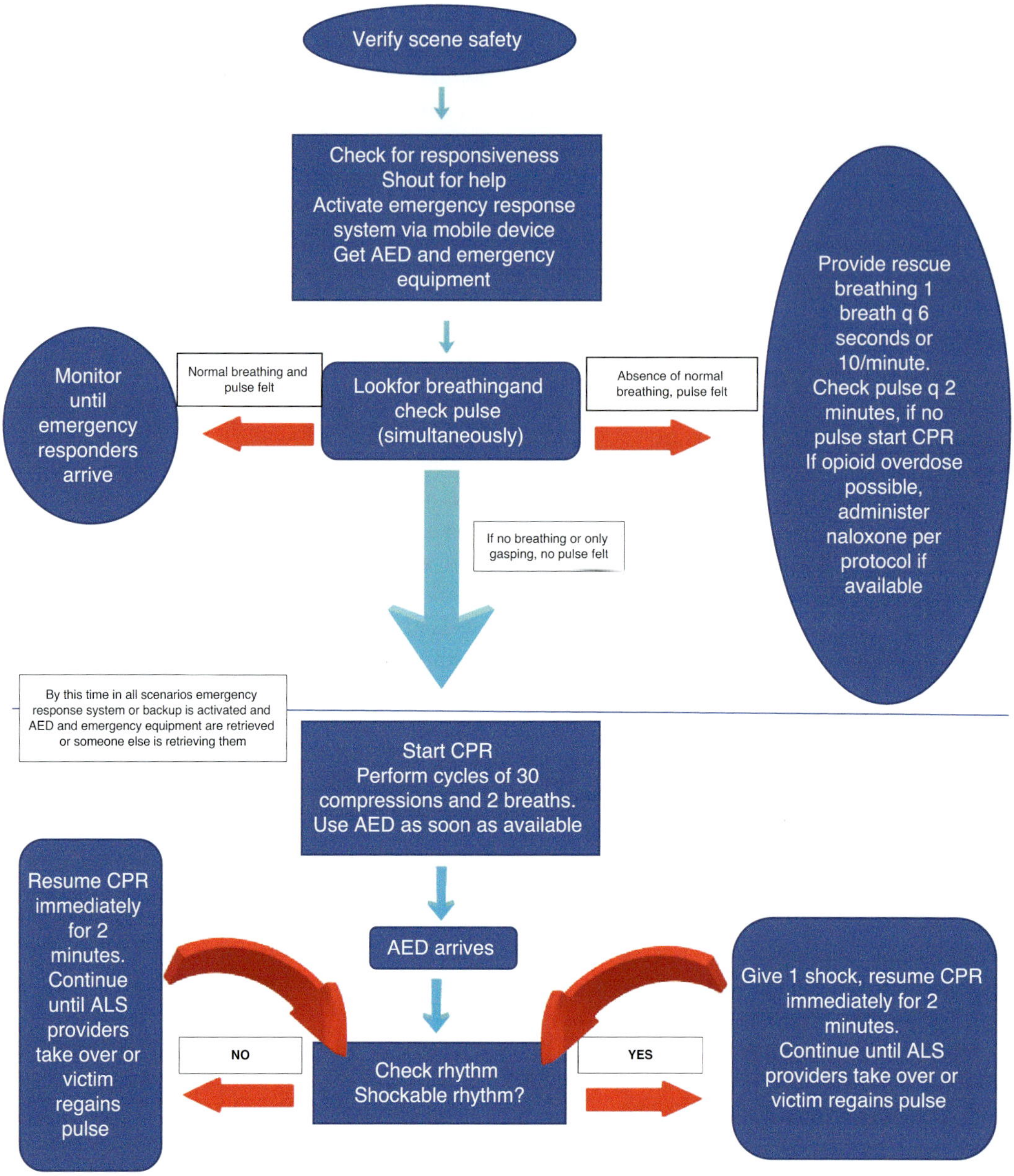

Fig. 33.1 Advanced basic life support

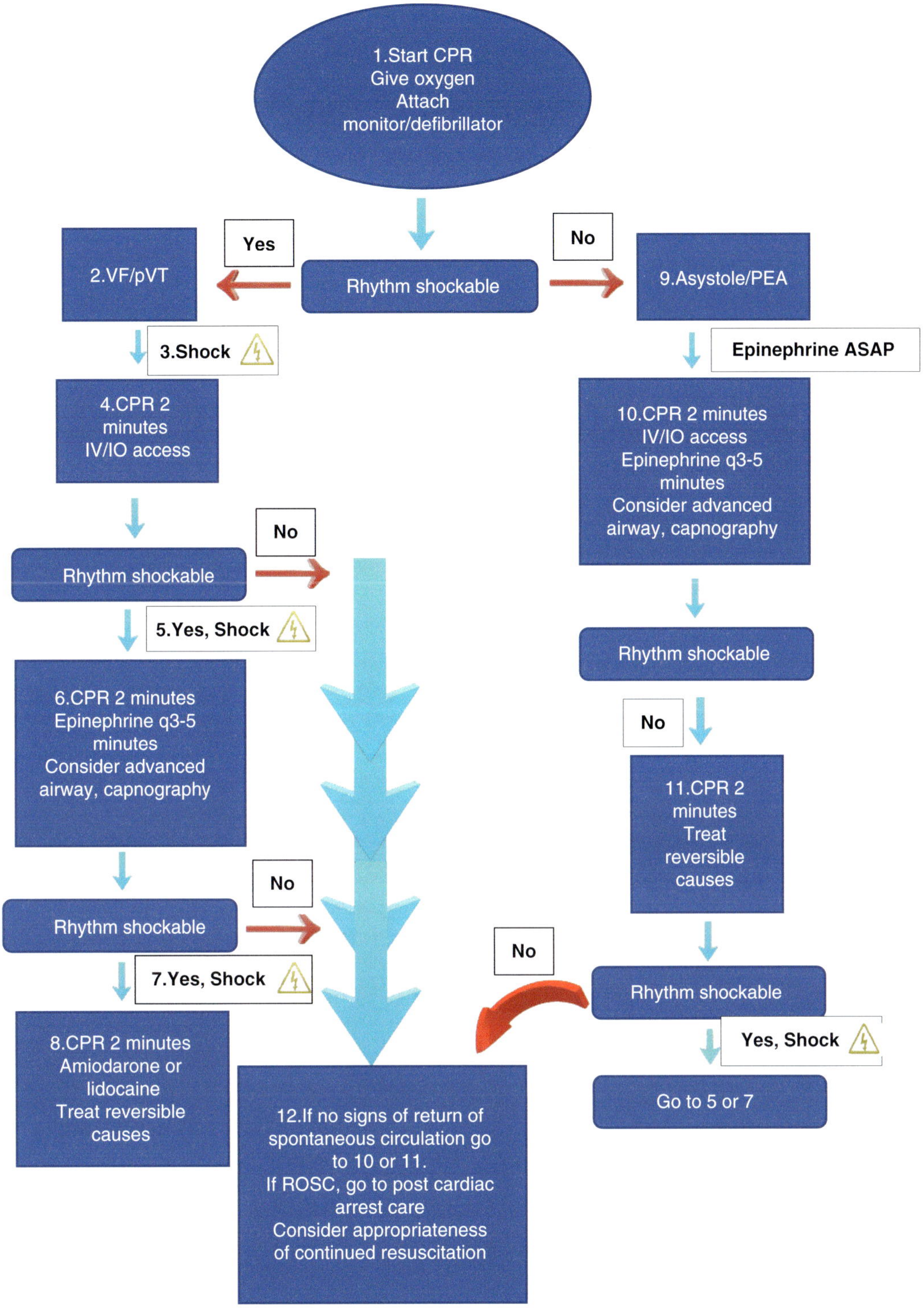

Fig. 33.2 Adult cardiac arrest algorithm

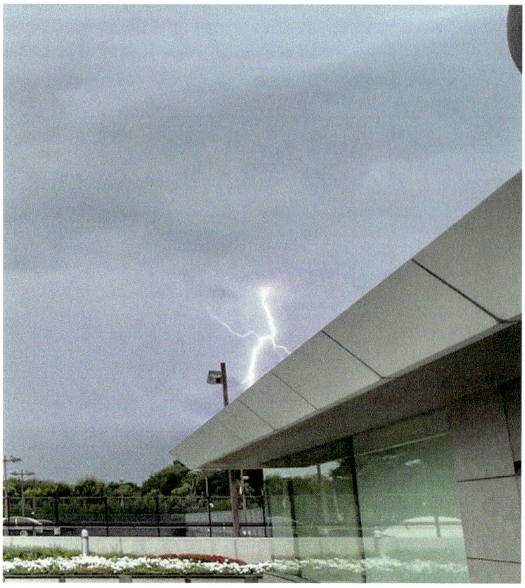

Fig. 33.3 Lightning strikes at sporting events, United States High Performance Center, Tokyo Olympic Games, 2021

Table 33.1 Trauma evaluation (ABCDE approach)

A	Airway
B	Breathing
C	Circulation
D	Deformity
E	Exposure

Table 33.2 Orientation assessment

Person	Able to relate person = 1	Unable to relate person = 0
Place	Able to relate place = 1	Unable to relate person = 0
Time	Able to relate time = 1	Unable to relate time = 0

Commonly reported A&O × 0 to3

Table 33.3 GCS (LOC Assessment). Created by Graham Teasdale and Bryan Jennett in 1974. Clinical scale to assess level of consciousness

	1	2	3	4	5	6
Eye (E)	Does not open eyes	Opens eyes in response to pain	Opens eyes in response to voice	Opens eyes spontaneously	N/A	N/A
Verbal (V)	Makes no sounds	Incomprehensible sounds	Inappropriate words	Confused and disoriented, but able to answer questions	Oriented to time, person and place, converse normally	N/A
Motor (M)	Makes no movements	Abnormal extension (decerebrate posture)	Abnormal flexion (decorticate posture)	Withdrawal to painful stimuli	Moves to localize pain	Obeys commands

Commonly reported as GCS of 3–15

33.10 Prevention

Preventative measures include education and implementation of lightning safety policy including avoidance of sheltering under trees and avoiding open fields and spaces. Additionally, designating safe locations for shelter and monitoring local weather forecasts with a designated weather watcher. It is also important to establish a chain of command (Fig. 33.3).

33.11 Current Recommendations

The *National Athletic Trainers' Association* recommends a proactive approach to lightning safety, including the implementation of a lightning-safety policy that identifies safe locations for shelter from the lightning hazard. Further components of this policy are monitoring local weather forecasts, designating a weather watcher, and establishing a chain of command.

Additionally, a flash-to-bang count of 30 s or more should be used as a minimal determinant of when to suspend activities. Waiting 30 min or longer after the last flash of lightning or sound of thunder is recommended before athletic or recreational activities are resumed [9].

The *National Collegiate Athletic Association* recommendations are as follows: education and prevention are the keys to lightning safety [10].

Prevention should begin long before any athletically related activity, event, or practice by having an institutional lightning safety plan in place. The following steps are recommended by the NCAA and NOAA to mitigate risk of a lightning hazard: (1) Develop a lightning safety plan for each outdoor venue. (2) Designate a person to monitor threatening weather and to notify the chain of command who can make the decision to remove a team, game personnel, television crews, and spectators from an athletics site or event. A lightning safety plan should include prearranged instructions and announcements for participants and spectators, designation of warning and all-clear signals, proper signage, and designation of safer places from the lightning hazard. (3) Monitor local weather reports daily. Be diligently aware of potential thunderstorms that may form during scheduled athletics events or practices and monitor warning signs of developing thunderstorms in the area, such as high winds or darkening skies. Weather information can be found through various means: local television news coverage, online, cable and satellite weather programming, a lightning detection and notification app, or the National Weather Service (NWS) website at www.weather.gov. (4) Be informed of National Weather Service- (NWS) issued thunderstorm watches or warnings and know the difference between a severe thunderstorm watch and a severe thunderstorm warning. A watch indicates that severe thunderstorms are possible in and near the watch area. Stay informed and be ready to act if a severe thunderstorm warning is issued. A warning is issued when severe weather has been reported by spotters or indicated by radar. Warnings indicate imminent danger to life and property. It should be noted that neither watches nor warnings are issued for lightning. A NOAA weather radio is particularly helpful in providing this information. (5) Know where the closest "safer structure or location" is to every outdoor venue and know how long it will take to evacuate everyone to that safer location. A safer structure or location is defined as: (a) Any building normally occupied or frequently used by people, e.g., a building with plumbing and/or electrical wiring that acts to electrically ground the structure. Avoid the shower, plumbing facilities, contact with electrical appliances, and open windows and doorways during a thunderstorm. (b) In the absence of a sturdy, frequently inhabited building, any vehicle with a hard metal roof (neither a convertible, nor a golf cart) with the windows shut provides a measure of safety. *The hard metal frame and roof, not the rubber tires, are what protect occupants by dissipating lightning current around the vehicle and not through the occupants.* It is important not to touch the metal framework of the vehicle. Some athletics events rent school buses to provide safer locations around open courses or fields. (6) Lightning awareness should be heightened at the first flash of lightning, clap of thunder, and/or other signs of an impending storm, such as increasing winds or darkening skies, no matter how far away. These types of activities should be treated as a warning or wake-up call to athletics personnel [15]. Lightning safety experts suggest that if you hear thunder, begin preparation for evacuation. If you see lightning, consider suspending activities and evacuating to designated safer locations. For large-scale events, continuous monitoring of the weather should occur from the time pre-event activities occur and throughout the event. Specific lightning safety guidelines have been developed with the assistance of lightning safety experts. Institutions should design a lightning safety plan that considers local safety needs, local venues (including access to those venues), weather patterns, and storm types [10].

As a minimum, lightning safety experts strongly recommend that by the time the weather monitor observes 30 s between seeing the lightning flash and hearing its associated thunder or by the time the leading edge of the storm is within 6 miles of the venue, all individuals should have left the athletics site and be within a safer structure or location. Individuals just entering the outdoor venue should be directed to the safer location. Use the Flash to Bang method to estimate the distance between your location and the lighting flash. Thunder may be hard to hear if there is an athletics event going on, particularly in stadiums with large crowds. Implement your lightning safety plan accordingly. Ensure a safe and orderly evacuation from the venue with announcements, signage, safety information in programs, and entrances that can also serve as mass exits. Planning should account for the time it takes to move the teams and spectators to their designated safer locations. Lightning can strike from blue sky and in the absence of rain. At least 10% of lightning occurs when there is no rainfall and when blue sky is visible; this is especially prevalent with summer thunderstorms. Lightning can, and does, strike as far as ten (or more) miles away from the rain shaft. If you hear thunder, lightning is close enough to pose an immediate threat. Be aware of local weather patterns and review local weather forecasts before an outdoor practice or event. Avoid using landline telephones, except in emergency situations. People have been killed while using a landline telephone during a thunderstorm. Cellular or cordless phones are safe alternatives to a landline phone, particularly if the person and the antenna are located within a safer structure or location, and if all other precautions are followed. To resume athletics activities, lightning safety experts recommend waiting 30 min after both the last sound of thunder and after the last flash of lightning is at least 6 miles away and moving away from the venue. If lightning is seen without hearing thunder, lightning may be out of range and therefore less likely to be a significant threat. At night, be aware that lightning can be visible at a much greater distance than during the day as clouds are being lit from the inside by lightning. This greater distance may mean that the lightning is no longer a significant threat. At night, use both the sound of thunder and seeing the lightning channel itself to decide on when to reset the 30-min return-to-play clock before resuming outdoor athletics activities [10].

Table 33.4 Flash bang techniq

If thunder is heard	The lightning is..
5 s after a flash	1 mile away
10 s after a flash	2 miles away
15 s after a flash	3 miles away
20 s after a flash	4 miles away
25 s after a flash	5 miles away
30 s after a flash	6 miles away
35 s after a flash	7 miles away
40 s after a flash	8 miles away

The current NCAA policy requires that play be suspended if there is lightning within 8 miles of the stadium. It requires a 30-min delay, but this may vary because the time count will restart if a lightning strike occurs within the 8-mile radius [10] (Table 33.4).

The *PGA tours lightning protocol* is as follows which states officials are constantly monitoring the weather with an on-site meteorologist and state of the art technology. In the event that lightning is detected at a distance from the course that threatens the safety of the individuals at the event, play is immediately suspended and the course is evacuated for safety precautions. The distance from the course, however, is not explicitly documented [22].

USA rugby recommends obtaining a weather forecast before an outdoor event in addition to knowing your local weather patterns. They also advise identifying and staying within traveling range of a proper shelter. Employ the "30–30 Rule" to know when to seek a safer location [23]. The "30–30 Rule" states that when you see lightning, count the time until you hear thunder. If this time is 30 s or less, go immediately to a safer place. If you can't see the lightning, just hearing the thunder means lightning is likely within striking range. After the storm has apparently dissipated or moved on, wait 30 min or more after hearing the last thunder before leaving the safer location [24].

The *United States Soccer Federation (USSF)* position is that if you can hear thunder, you are within reach of lightning and that referees must protect the safety of all participants by stopping game activities quickly, so that participants and spectators may retire to a safer place before the lightning threat becomes significant. Applying the 30–30 rule is recommended and to wait 30 min or more after hearing the last thunder before leaving shelter [25].

USA equestrian and the Interscholastic Equestrian Association (IEA) recommends having a plan and a safe place to take shelter in the event of lightning as it is an important step in risk management. It is recommended that outdoor events be suspended or moved indoors if a storm is less than 6 miles away (including mounting and warm-ups) [26]. In order to determine the distance of a storm in miles, use the Flash-to-Bang Method by counting the number of seconds between seeing lightning and hearing thunder and dividing it by five (lightingsafety.noaa.gov) [2].

The Major League Baseball (MLB) states the home team shall be the sole judge as to whether a game shall not be started because of unsuitable weather conditions or the unfit condition of the playing field, except for the second game of a conventional or split doubleheader. Nothing in this rule is intended to affect a Club's ability to suspend or resume any game pursuant to a policy governing severe weather, significant weather threats, and lightning safety that has been filed with the league office prior to the championship season [27]. It is noted, however, that there is no specific lightning guidance or protocols are outlined as it is up to the home team to determine safety and whether game should be started.

Review of the lightning policy guidelines for *Major League Baseball, Major League Soccer, and the National Football League* reveals minimal, highly variable lightning policy recommendations for either the teams or the spectators, with a great amount of the decision being placed on the umpires and referees [14].

USA open water swimming protocol is as follows, "2019 Plan: The following priority will occur in this order, if the Safety Officer, Meet Referee, Meet Director, or Independent Safety Monitor becomes aware of any situation requiring abandonment (including inclement weather). (1) Radio Communication to Officials and Safety Personnel on Course. (2) All Lifeguards issue a 3 loud short blast whistle command and instruct all swimmers to evacuate the course. (3) Announcer instructs all swimmers, safety personnel, and Officials, to exit the course. If the reason for abandonment is inclement weather, announcer will instruct all athletes, coaches, parents, and meet personnel to go to the shelter, team bus, or vehicles, until inclement weather passes. (4) Everyone will be instructed to go to vehicles, until safe conditions return." [28] Of note, there remains no specific distance regulations or detection methods outlined.

USA tennis notes lightning is a potential severe hazard and life-threatening consequence of an approaching storm near outdoor tennis matches. It is important to be prepared for immediate cessation of all matches or warm-up in the event of lightning. In essence, if lightning is sighted, stop all activity and direct everyone to seek appropriate shelter. A 30–30 rule may be used [29].

USA beach volleyball notes, "The weather must not present any danger of injury to the players." [30] The NCAA beach (sand) volleyball states that the weather must not present any danger of injury to the players. Referees should consult with coaches regarding suspension of play to ensure safety. While play should continue through most rain and wind, lightning represents a very real hazard and should be carefully and conservatively considered. Full procedure listed in NCAA Modifications and Conference Guidelines" [30].

The *USOPC (United States Olympic and Paralympic Committee)* no longer has information regarding lightning safety or severe weather protocols listed on its website. No policy or protocol found [31].

The *IOC (International Olympic Committee)* no longer has information regarding lightning safety or severe weather protocols listed on its website. No policy or protocol found [32].

World Rugby recommends the following, (1) live data: in circumstances, where live data are available from local meteorological services along with advice from an expert, these data should be used to assist in the decision about whether to allow the event/match to commence, continue, or be abandoned. (2) Determination of a chain of command which clearly identifies the person with ultimate responsibility to stop the event, either temporarily or indefinitely, or to evacuate the venue. It should be ensured that this person is familiar with local protocols and is provided with accurate and up to date information. (3) Communication with local weather services or tracking of Weather alerts should be established in advance of any event.

When the lightning strike is within 6 miles of the venue, it is recommended that players are removed from the pitch. Flash bang technique to determine distance when live data direct from local weather services is available. Recommended safe distances from the lightning event is 6 miles.

For events/venues where live data direct from local weather services is not available, the 30/30 rule should be used to ensure participant and spectator safety: (1) *Shelter should be sought when there are 30 s or less between the flash and the associated thunderclap.* (2) *Safe to return to the field of play is considered only after a minimum of 30 min after the final flash of lightning or clap of thunder has been seen/heard.*

The 6-mile recommendation may be altered depending on the topography of the area. For example, to increase this distance in flat open areas such as deserts or decrease it if the storm is located on the other side of a mountain range.

For spectators, individual stadium safety protocols should be followed in the event of a strike risk. For events which are not taking place in a stadium, the same protocols as those for players should be followed [33].

Federal International Football Association (FIFA) no longer has information regarding lightning safety or severe weather protocols listed on its website. No policy or protocol found [34] (Table 33.5).

Table 33.5 Quick reference: lightning protocols/policies by organization

Lightning protocols/policies by organization	
Organization	Policy
National Athletic Trainers' Association	Implementation of a lightning-safety policy that identifies safe locations for shelter from the lightning hazard Monitoring local weather forecasts, designating a weather watcher, and establishing a chain of command Flash-to-bang count of 30 s or more should be used as a minimal determinant of when to suspend activities Waiting 30 min or longer after the last flash of lightning or sound of thunder is recommended before athletic or recreational activities are resumed [9]
National Collegiate Athletic Association	Education and prevention are the keys to lightning safety Prevention: Develop a lightning safety plan for each outdoor venue. 1. Designate a person to monitor threatening weather and to notify the chain of command 2. Monitor local weather reports daily 3. Monitor local weather reports daily 4. Be informed of National Weather Service (NWS) issued thunderstorm watches or warnings and know the difference between a severe thunderstorm watch and a severe thunderstorm warning 5. Know where the closest "safer structure or location" is to every outdoor venue and know how long it will take to evacuate everyone to that safer location 6. Lightning awareness should be heightened at the first flash of lightning, clap of thunder, and/or other signs of an impending storm, such as increasing winds or darkening skies, no matter how far away. These types of activities should be treated as a warning or wake-up call to athletics personnel 7. Use the Flash to Bang method to estimate the distance between your location and the lighting flash 8. To resume athletics activities, lightning safety experts recommend waiting 30 min after both the last sound of thunder and after the last flash of lightning is at least 8 miles away, and moving away from the venue 9. Play be suspended if there is lightning within 8 miles of the stadium. [1, 10]

Table 33.5 (continued)

Lightning protocols/policies by organization	
Organization	Policy
PGA tour	Officials are constantly monitor the weather with an on-site meteorologist and state of the art technology In the event that lightning is detected at a distance from the course that threatens the safety of the individuals at the event, play is immediately suspended and the course is evacuated for safety precautions The distance from the course however is not explicitly documented [22]
USA rugby	Obtain a weather forecast before an outdoor event in addition to knowing your local weather patterns. Identify and stay within traveling range of a proper shelter. Employ the "30–30 Rule" to know when to seek a safer location [23]
United States Soccer Federation (USSF)	If you can hear thunder you are within reach of lightning Referees must protect the safety of all participants by stopping game activities quickly, so that participants and spectators may retire to a safer place before the lightning threat becomes significant Apply the 30–30 rule and wait 30 min or more after hearing the last thunder before leaving shelter [25]
USA equestrian and the Interscholastic Equestrian Association	Having a plan and a safe place to shelter in the event of lightning Outdoor events be suspended or moved indoors if a storm is less than 6 miles away (including mounting and warm-ups) [26] In order to determine the distance of a storm in miles use the Flash-to-Bang Method by counting the number of seconds between seeing lightning and hearing thunder and dividing it by five (lightingsafety.noaa.gov) [2]
MLB	Home team shall be the sole judge as to whether a game shall not be started because of unsuitable weather conditions or the unfit condition of the playing field, except for the second game of a conventional or split doubleheader [27] No specific lightning guidance or protocols are outlined as it is up to the home team to determine safety and whether game should be started
USA open water swimming	"2019 Plan: The following priority will occur in this order, if the Safety Officer, Meet Referee, Meet Director, or Independent Safety Monitor becomes aware of any situation requiring abandonment (including inclement weather) 1. Radio Communication to Officials and Safety Personnel on Course 2. All Lifeguards issue a 3 loud short blast whistle command, and instruct all swimmers to evacuate the course 3. Announcer instructs all swimmers, safety personnel, and Officials, to exit the course. If the reason for abandonment is inclement weather, announcer will instruct all athletes, coaches, parents, and meet personnel to go to the shelter, team bus, or vehicles, until inclement weather passes 4. Everyone will be instructed to go to vehicles, until safe conditions return." [28] No specific distance regulations or detection methods outlined
USA tennis	Lightning is a potential severe hazard and life-threatening consequence of an approaching storm near outdoor tennis matches. Important to be prepared for immediate cessation of all matches or warm-up in the event of lightning If lightning is sighted, stop all activity and direct everyone to seek appropriate shelter A 30–30 rule may be used [29]
USA beach volleyball	"The weather must not present any danger of injury to the players" [30] No specific guidelines noted
The USOPC (United States Olympic and Paralympic Committee)	No longer has information regarding lightning safety or severe weather protocols listed on its website. No policy or protocol found [31]

(continued)

Table 33.5 (continued)

Lightning protocols/policies by organization	
Organization	Policy
IOC (International Olympic Committee)	No longer has information regarding lightning safety or severe weather protocols listed on its website. No policy or protocol found [32]
World Rugby	Live data: in circumstances, where live data is available from local meteorological services along with advice from an expert, this data should be used to assist in the decision about whether to allow the event/match to commence, continue or be abandoned Determination of a chain of command which clearly identifies the person with ultimate responsibility to stop the event, either temporarily or indefinitely or to evacuate the venue is vital. It should be ensured that this person is familiar with local protocols and is provided with accurate and up to date information Communication with local weather services or tracking of Weather alerts should be established in advance of any event When the lightning strike is within 6 miles of the venue, it is recommended that players are removed from the pitch [33] Flash bang technique to determine distance when live data direct from local weather services is available Recommended safe distances from the lightning event is 6 miles For events/venues where live data direct from local weather services is not available, the 30/30 rule should be used to ensure participant and spectator safety: • Shelter should be sought when there are 30 s or less between the flash and the associated thunder clap • Safe to return to the field of play is considered only after a minimum of 30 min after the final flash of lightning or clap of thunder has been seen/heard. The 6 mile recommendation may be altered depending on the topography of the area. For example, to increase this distance in flat open areas such as deserts or decrease it if the storm is located on the other side of a mountain range For spectators, individual stadium safety protocols should be followed in the event of a strike risk. For events which are not taking place in a stadium, the same protocols as those for players should be followed [33]
FIFA	No longer has information regarding lightning safety or severe weather protocols listed on its website. No policy or protocol found [34]

33.12 Future Recommendations

In the future, it would be helpful and beneficial to have universal lightning regulations, policies, and protocols that apply broadly among multiple sports and organizations as well as across nations. Having a universal policy allows for less uncertainty and hesitation. It allows for congruency when participating at multiple locations both internationally and nationally with various clubs/team organizations [34–39]. This chapter has used the United States as an example, but the hope is to internationalize recommendations widely as recommendations and policies vary widely abroad as well. In the United States, it appears that the NCAA has the most comprehensive protocol and has been referenced by multiple other organizations to formulate their protocols and procedures. Having a complete and clear understanding of the protocols and procedures as well as an explicit chain of command in each instance can significantly reduce the chance of harm and injury and allow for more extensive preventative measures, education, and preparation. There have been many examples of missteps/misunderstandings and unclear protocols which could have resulted in significant injury and harm in sport both in the United States and internationally. Widely, the most accepted current protocols revolve around the flash bang technique as well as the 30–30 rule. Ideally, there would be a universal rule or technique for determination of suspension/discontinuation of play in the aim of player, spectators, and staff safety.

Take Home Messages

- Lightning is the most consistent and significant weather hazard that may affect intercollegiate athletics [1]. Within the United States, the National Severe Storms Laboratory (NSSL) estimates that 100 fatalities and 400–500 injuries requiring medical treatment occur from lightning strikes every year [1].
- A lightning strike can result in fatal cardiac arrest at the time of injury or in the subsequent days following resuscitation due to irreversible ischemic brain injury, etc.
- Medical management of the lightning victim continues to primarily be supportive and resuscitative care [14].
- High-Risk Groups/ Risk factors: Outdoor activities, mountain climbers/ hikers, Swimmers, Field athletes (javelin, shot-put), Golfers, Bicyclists.
- Three quarters of all lightning casualties occur between May and September, nearly four fifths occur between 10:00 AM and 7:00 PM, which coincides with the hours for most athletic or recreational activities.
- Action plans and procedures for lightning safety are essential. These plans should include the following:
  - An evacuation plan for players and spectators.
  - A designated person monitoring all weather forecasts and reports.
  - Designated chain of command.
  - Clear notification system to alert athletes, fans/spectators, and staff.
  - A safe shelter.
- Current recommendations by organization are varied and no specific universal lightning protocol for sport exists.
- The NCAA currently appears to have the most comprehensive and specific lightning safety protocol and policy. It has been referenced by multiple organizations across the board.
- Additional research is needed to formulate a universal lightning safety protocol with specific policies in distance and technique for determination of play cessation in the aim of player, staff, and spectator safety.

References

1. NCAA lightning safety guidelines. NCAA; 2001. http://files.leagueathletics.com/Images/Club/14690/NCAALightningGuidelines.pdf.
2. National Weather Service. *Lightning fact page*. 2012. http://www.lightningsafety.noaa.gov/statistics.html.
3. National Weather Service. *Lightning fatalities*. 2012. http://www.nws.noaa.gov/om/hazstats.shtml. Accessed 29 Feb 2012.
4. US Department of Commerce, NOAA. "How Dangerous Is Lightning?" *National Weather Service*, NOAA's National Weather Service. https://www.weather.gov/safety/lightning-odds. Accessed 12 Mar 2019.
5. Lopez RE, Holle RL, Heitkamp TA, Boyson M, Cherington M, Langford K. The underreporting of lightning injuries and deaths in Colorado. Bull Am Meteorol Soc. 1993;74(11):2171–8.
6. Lopez R, Holle R, Heitkamp T. Lightning casualties and property damage in Colorado from 1950 to 1991 based on storm data. Forecast. 1995;10(1):114–26.
7. Bennett B, Holle R, Lopez R. Lightning safety guidelines. In: Klossner D, editor. National Collegiate Athletic Association Sports Medicine Handbook. Overland Park, KS: National Collegiate Athletic Association; 2011; 2012.
8. Uman M. All about lightning. New York, NY: Dover Publications; 1986.
9. Walsh KM, Cooper MA, Holle R, Rakov VA, Roeder WP, Ryan M, National Athletic Trainers' Association. National Athletic Trainers' Association position statement: lightning safety for athletics and recreation. J Athl Train. 2013;48(2):258–70. https://doi.org/10.4085/1062-6050-48.2.25.
10. *2014–15* NCAA sports medicine handbook. NCAA; 2014. http://www.ncaapublications.com/product-downloads/MD15.pdf.
11. "Lightning Basics." *NOAA National Severe Storms Laboratory*. https://www.nssl.noaa.gov/education/svrwx101/lightning/#:~:text=Lightning%20is%20a%20giant%20spark,the%20cloud%20and%20the%20ground.
12. Cooper MA. Lightning injuries clinical presentation: history, physical examination, complications. In: Lightning injuries clinical presentation: history, phys-

ical examination, complications. Medscape; 2021. emedicine.medscape.com/article/770642-clinical.
13. "Lightning Injuries." *Lightning Injuries*. misc.medscape.com/pi/android/medscapeapp/html/A770642-business.html.
14. Thomson EM, Howard TM. Lightning injuries in sports and recreation. Curr Sports Med Reports. 2013;12(2):120–4. https://doi.org/10.1249/JSR.0b013e318287728f.
15. Cooper MA, Holle RL, Andrews C. Distribution of lightning injury mechanisms. In: Proceedings for the 20th international lightning detection conference. Tucson, AZ; 2008. http://www.vaisala.com/Vaisala%20Documents/Scientific%20papers/Distribution_of_lightninginjury_mechanisms.pdf.
16. Cooper MA, Andrews CJ, Holle RL. Lightning injuries. In: Auerbach PS, editor. Wilderness medicine. 5th ed. Philadelphia, PA: CV Mosby; 2007. p. 66–108.
17. Cooper MA. A fifth-mechanism of lightning injury. Acad Emerg Med. 2002;9:172–4.
18. Blumenthal R, Jandrell IR, West NJ. Does a sixth mechanism exist to explain lightning injuries?: investigating a possible new injury mechanism to determine the cause of injuries related to close lightning flashes. Am J Forensic Med Pathol. 2012;33:222–6. (medline)
19. Holle R, Cummins K. Monthly distributions of U.S. NLDN cloud-to-ground lightning. 2010 Paper presented at international lightning detection conference, 21–22 April, Orlando, FL.
20. Holle R, Lopez R, Navarro B. Deaths, injuries, and damages from lightning in the United States in the 1890s in comparison with the 1990s. J Appl Meteorol. 2005;44(10):1563–73.
21. National Oceanic and Atmospheric Administration's National Weather Service Web Site. Silver Spring (MD): National Weather Service. http://weather.gov. [cited 2012 July 30].
22. Tour, Pga. "Frequently Asked Questions." *PGATour*, PGATOUR.COM. https://www.pgatour.com/company/pga-tour-faqs.html. Accessed 2 Feb 2022.
23. *This document represents the USA rugby policy with regard to lightning...* https://cdn1.sportngin.com/attachments/document/0085/8691/usar-lightning-policy.pdf.
24. *Lightning safety facts—National Weather Service.* https://www.weather.gov/media/zhu/ZHU_Training_Page/lightning_stuff/lightning/lightning_facts.pdf.
25. *AYSO thunder/lightning policy—dt5602vnjxv0c. Cloudfront.net.* https://dt5602vnjxv0c.cloudfront.net/portals/14043/docs/ayso%20thunder.pdf.
26. *IEA Weather Guidelines Rev 6.19.15—Rideiea.org.* https://www.rideiea.org/wp-content/uploads/2019/11/H.-IEA-Weather-Guidelines-rev-7.29.15.pdf.
27. *2019 Official Baseball Rules 2019 Official Baseball Rules—Mlb.com.* https://content.mlb.com/documents/2/2/4/305750224/2019_Official_Baseball_Rules_FINAL_.pdf.
28. *Open Water Race Management 101—USA Swimming.* https://www.usaswimming.org/docs/default-source/open-water-resources/open-water-race-management-101.pdf?sfvrsn=7d853f32_6.
29. 2022 Friend of the court, handbook of tennis rules and regulations. USTA. 2022. https://www.usta.com/content/dam/usta/2022-pdfs/2022%20Friend%20at%20Court.pdf.
30. Rule differences: USAV beach, USAV indoors. NCAA Indoors. http://ncva.com/downloads/Referee%20Beach%20Rules%20Comparisons.pdf.
31. "United States Olympic & Paralympic Committee." *Team USA*. https://www.teamusa.org/about-the-usopc.
32. IOC. "IOC—International Olympic Committee." *International Olympic Committee*, IOC, https://olympics.com/ioc. Accessed 11 Aug 2022.
33. Worldrugby.org. "Player Welfare Guidelines." *World Rugby*. https://www.world.rugby/the-game/player-welfare/guidelines/lightning.
34. *FIFA Stadium Safety and Security Regulations.* https://digitalhub.fifa.com/m/682f5864d03a756b/original/xycg4m3h1r1zudk7rnkbpdf.pdf.
35. Holle R. Lightning fatalities in tropical and subtropical regions. 29th Conference on Hurricanes and Tropical Meteorology.

Tables and Figures

36. "Algorithms." *Cpr.heart.org*. https://cpr.heart.org/en/resuscitation-science/cpr-and-ecc-guidelines/algorithms.
37. Staff SI. Lightning strikes at sporting events. *Sports Illustrated*, Sports Illustrated. https://www.si.com/extra-mustard/2013/08/12/lightning-strikes-sporting-events. Accessed 12 Aug 2013.

Others

38. "Lightning Safety." *NCAA.org*. www.ncaa.org/sports/2014/4/9/lightning-safety.aspx.
39. "Lightning Information for Organized Sporting Events." *Centers for Disease Control and Prevention*, Centers for Disease Control and Prevention. https://www.cdc.gov/disasters/lightning/sportingevensts.html. Accessed 7 Jun 2022.

Extraction and Rescue Challenges

34

Omar Farah, Ghassan Farah,
and Mark R. Hutchinson

Fact Box

- When an athlete is injured in a loose foam pit, primary attention should be given to not propagating further damage. Coaches and athletes should avoid aggressive entry to a foam pit that contains an injured athlete. Their entry may cause movement of the foam blocks and subsequent movement of the injured athlete, with potential for further injury to an unstable cervical spine injury.
- As in all cases of environments that introduce challenges to extraction, medical personnel covering an indoor ice event should practice rescue on the ice surface prior to the event to accustom themselves to entrance and exit of the rink and movement along the ice.
- Indeed, such extremes of location and weather can preclude helicopter access. This creates increased pressure on the medical management team managing injuries since they must simultaneously tend to the injury itself while mitigating the environmental conditions that threaten to destabilize the injured athlete.

O. Farah
Columbia Vagelos College of Physicians and Surgeons, New York, NY, USA

G. Farah
Orthopaedic Surgery Resident, University of Illinois-Chicago, Chicago, IL, USA

M. R. Hutchinson (✉)
Department of Orthopaedic, Sports Medicine, University of Illinois-Chicago, Chicago, IL, USA

34.1 Introduction

Sports take place in a spectrum of environments and arenas, some of which may create significant physical and practical barriers to emergency medical care. Whether the sport is played on unusual playing surfaces, on ice, in the water, in environmental extremes or at challenging locations, sport physicians must be able to reach an acutely injured athlete within a reasonable time frame so as not to delay necessary treatment. Further, proper medical care must be tailored to the unique environment, oftentimes requiring the clinician to be cognizant of various impeding and possibly dangerous factors. Meanwhile, the provider must avoid putting themselves at risk while providing necessary urgent care. This chapter provides a review of the rescue and extraction challenges that a covering clinician may face in

S. Rocha Piedade et al. (eds.), *Sideline Management in Sports*,
https://doi.org/10.1007/978-3-031-33867-0_34

unique environments of gymnastics, indoor ice, indoor water, and extreme sports events. The overarching philosophy of being prepared for the unique environment that a specific sport introduces will hopefully assist the reader in applying these concepts to other events and sports.

34.2 Gymnastics: The Unstable Surface Environment

Some sports provide unique access and extraction problems due to the stage that the athletes are performing on, the unique equipment demands of a sport, or the practice surface they train on. Gymnastics is a classic example. Gymnastics is one of the oldest sports, dating back to the age of the Ancient Greeks [1]. Despite being around for more than 2000 years, gymnastics developed into a competitive sport approximately 100 years ago [2]. A sport involving high-flying acrobatics and feats of strength, with notable amounts of upper and lower extremity contortion, flipping, and hard landings, gymnastics is associated with relatively high injury rates and increased risk for catastrophic head and spine injuries [1, 3–5]. Medical coverage of gymnastics competitions may be challenging and requires sufficient knowledge of the sport, the injury epidemiology, and competition-specific obstacles to providing acute medical care to an injured athlete.

More than five million athletes participate in gymnastics in the United States, the majority of participants being female (76%). Approximately 80% of athletes are 18 years or younger, implying a large majority of injured athletes will be pediatric, who present with their own unique challenges [1]. Two major disciplines of gymnastics exist: artistic and rhythmic. Artistic gymnastics, the more common of the two, consists of women's and men's competitions. Women's events include vault, balance beam, uneven parallel bars, and floor exercise. Men's events include floor exercise, pommel horse, still rings, vault, parallel bars, and horizontal bar [2]. Other events include trampoline, tumbling, acrobatic, and group gymnastics [2].

More than 86,000 gymnastics-related injuries are treated each year. Injury risk increases with level of performance, as well as number of training hours [3]. Among collegiate sports, women's artistic gymnastics ranks second only to American football with respect to practice injury rate, and fourth overall when including competition injuries [4]. The absolute risk of injury is significantly higher during practice sessions, accounting for up to 97% of injuries. However, if evaluated in reference to exposure time, the risk of injury during competition is nearly twice as high as during practice sessions [4, 6]. This may be explained by increased fatigue of completing an entire routine versus a single individual skill, decreased protective equipment (foam pits, resi-mats), absence of spotting coaches, and increased intensity and pressure during competitions. While spotting coaches are allowed during competition, they may come with a score deduction, thereby discouraging their use. The most frequently encountered injuries involve the lower extremity, with ankle sprains being the most common injury [3–5]. Vault and floor exercises account for the vast majority of acute injuries [1, 4]. Accordingly, a covering sports medicine physician should pay particular attention to vault and floor exercise events. The clinician should assess the general floor layout as well as access points and should position themselves close to the at-risk skill apparatus and be prepared for acute injuries during dismounts and landings.

As mentioned above, gymnastics consists of various disciplines. A single gymnastics meet may extend over multiple days and include multiple competition activities. It is critical for the covering medical personnel to prepare ahead of time for event coverage. Specific aspects to focus on in preparation for a gymnastics competition include administrative personnel, location and venue of competitions and practice sessions, gymnastics disciplines and levels competing, and number of athletes competing. Many elite competitions are held on a podium, or raised competition surface, in which the competitive equipment and competition is 2–3 feet off the floor of the arena. (Fig. 34.1—*Elevated Podium*) With athletes performing their skills on an elevated sur-

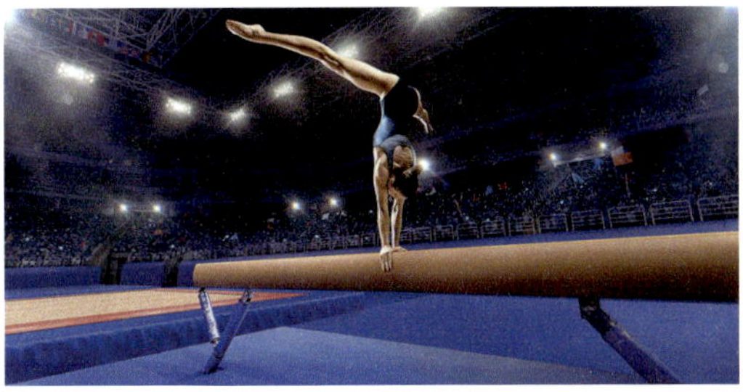

Fig. 34.1 Elevated Podium. Example of a competitive gymnastics stadium. Note the possible challenges to timely access to an injured athlete, including the elevated podiums upon which the events are held. (Source: Adobe Stock)

face, the covering sports medicine clinician needs to account both for the risk of falling off the podium as well as any navigation challenges in getting onto and off the podium in times of emergency. It may take more time to reach an injured athlete. Access and egress pathways for emergency responders, emergency medical services, and extraction equipment need to be considered for each apparatus. The covering physician should also be aware of emergency action plans, including whether emergency medical services (EMS) will be present on-site. It is recommended to practice retrieval of an injured athlete from specific competition surfaces, including pits and trampolines. As mentioned above, a large majority of gymnastic athletes are pediatric, and thus will require appropriately sized medical equipment (e.g., backboards). Finally, a medical staff meeting prior to the event is essential to cover logistics, review the plan, and address any questions or concerns.

During the event, medical staff is responsible for providing timely medical care to the acutely injured athlete. Concussions are the most common head injury sustained by gymnasts, usually secondary to head impact on the mat, floor, or an apparatus [3]. Diagnosis is clinical and treatment is generally similar to other sports; however, special consideration should be given to more conservative return to play recommendations due to the risk of returning these athletes to high-risk apparatus. Symptoms of concussion, including headache, dizziness, abnormal balance, delayed reaction time, and visual disturbance, may incapacitate an athlete performing a high-flying skill, thereby increasing the risk for further, potentially catastrophic, injury [4].

Gymnastic athletes are at particularly high risk of cervical spine injuries secondary to the acrobatic nature of the sport in which they are at height and their bodies are inverted. Mechanisms for cervical spine injury include landing directly on the head, landing on the upper back with a hyperflexed neck, and landing on the chest with a hyperextended neck [4]. Management should adhere to Advanced Trauma Life Support (ATLS) protocols, including stabilization of the cervical spine with assessment of airway, breathing, circulation, and disability. As a large proportion of gymnasts are pediatric, it is critical to ensure availability of appropriately sized equipment, including pediatric-sized backboards.

Practice and competition surfaces can provide an additional challenge for the covering clinician due to access challenges, poor footing, and unstable surfaces when attempting to respond to or extracting an injured athlete. Loose foam pits are in-ground, or above-ground, six to eight foot deep pits of varying length and width filled with loose foam blocks. Loose foam pits are training tools that serve to provide a relatively safe landing environment. Similarly, resi-pits are training-specific, 32-inch deep mats. The mats are soft and located within a large hole in the ground, providing a soft, landing surface. Competitive trampolines stand approximately four feet high and are intentionally springy. (Fig. 34.2—*Pit*, Fig. 34.3—*Trampoline)* The above surfaces are particularly unstable. Merely walking on a loose foam pit, resi-pit, or trampoline may add insult to injury in an athlete with an unstable cervical spine injury. The following is a suggested protocol for management of cervical spine injuries in loose foam pits. It may be extended to other uneven and unstable surfaces. When an athlete is injured in a loose foam pit, primary attention should be given to not propagating further damage. Coaches and athletes should avoid aggressive entry to a foam pit that contains an injured athlete. Their entry may cause movement of the foam blocks and subsequent movement of the injured athlete, with potential for further injury to an unstable cervical

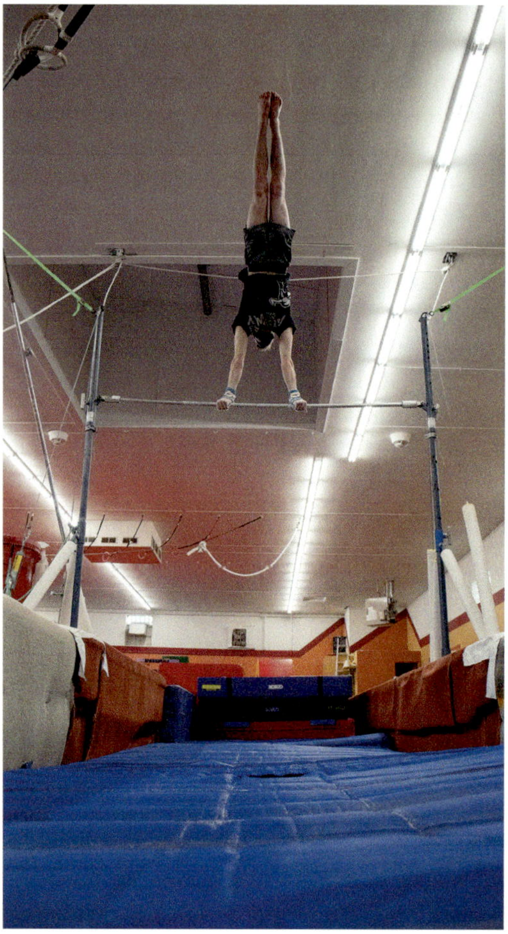

Fig. 34.2 Pit. Gymnast performing aerobic stunt in pit. (Source: Unsplash)

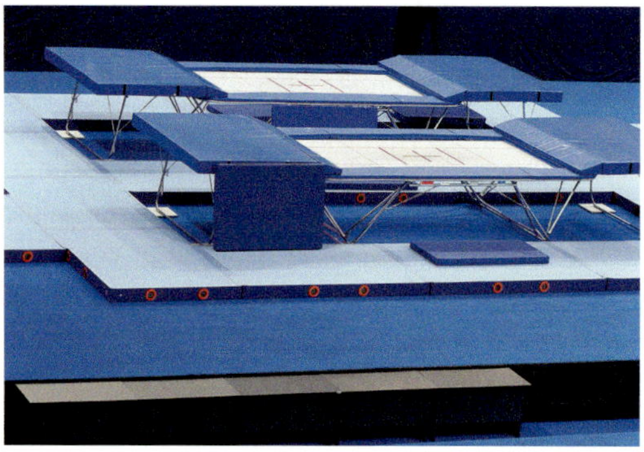

Fig. 34.3 Trampoline. Gymnastics trampolines. Trampolines are elevated from the ground surface and present a challenging, unstable surface for the physician attempting to reach an injured athlete. (Source: Adobe Stock)

spine injury. Nonemergency responders should be instructed to stay out of the pit unless directed to enter by the medical staff. Prior to entering the foam pit, the covering sports physician should assess the environment and attempt to talk to the athlete from outside the pit. Again, it is prudent to avoid entering the pit unless absolutely necessary. If the injury is life-threatening, the pit is entered directly without the use of a mat. Meanwhile, another member of the staff or meet official should contact emergency medical services (EMS). Socks and shoes should be removed prior to entering the pit as they may impede progress through the foam blocks. Four to six individuals are recruited to aid in extraction of the injured athlete from the pit. Slow and steady movements are required while approaching the athlete. Once near the athlete, airway, breathing, and circulation status are assessed as per ATLS protocol. If possible, the C-spine is stabilized manually. Caution should be taken to avoid moving any of the foam blocks from beneath the gymnast, as this may cause the gymnast to sink further into the pit, thereby making extraction more difficult. If available, the athlete may be directly transferred onto a backboard. Otherwise, a mat may be used to transport the athlete outside of the pit. The mat is slid beneath the athlete while having the C-spine stabilized manually. If the injury is deemed to be non-life-threatening and time permits, medical personnel should obtain several mats. Mats are laid onto the foam blocks and used as platforms, allowing the entering person to remain afloat in the pit and minimize any disturbance of the foam blocks. Mats are then placed on either side of the athlete, and one in front of the athlete's head. Using slow and steady movements, the athlete is approached by a crawling maneuver upon the mats. The C-spine is stabilized manually followed by an ATLS primary assessment. Once again, a coordinated effort requiring multiple people will be needed to carefully transfer the athlete onto a mat or backboard (if available) for extraction. Given the complexity of the extraction, pre-competition training and practice of rescue maneuvers from loose foam pits and other uneven surfaces are recommended.

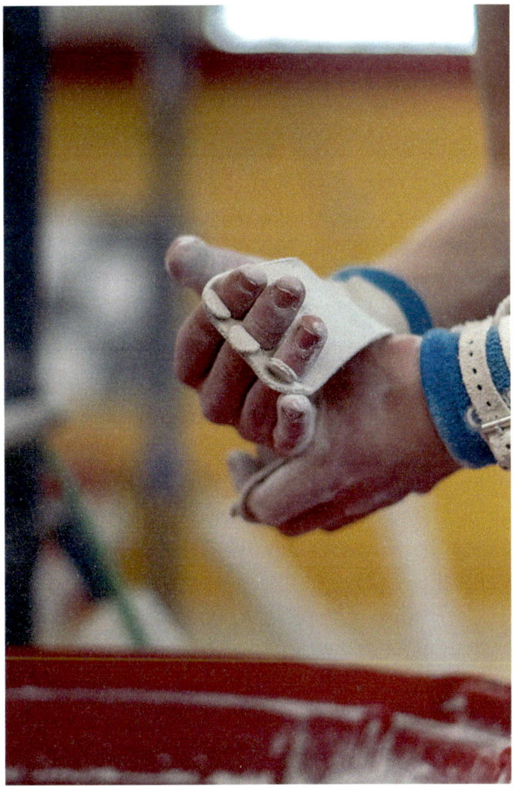

Fig. 34.4 Leather Grips. Leather grips. While commonly worn by gymnasts performing on uneven or horizontal bars, leather grips are associated with "grip lock" injuries, in which the gymnast's body rotates around a locked and static hand, ultimately resulting in a forearm fracture. (Source: Unsplash)

"Grip locks" are injuries unique to gymnastics. Gymnasts often use leather grips to improve performance on uneven or horizontal bars. (Fig. 34.4—*Leather Grips*) Leather grips may occasionally lock in place while the remainder of the gymnast's body continues to revolve around the bar. This causes the forearm to wrap around the bar and ultimately fracture. Extraction of this injured athlete may require multiple people. The athlete will be hanging from the bar, often using the contralateral uninjured extremity to offload the injured side. The athlete should first be supported, relieving weight off the injured extremity. The grip on the injured extremity is gently loosened and released. The injured extremity is stabilized as the athlete is removed from the apparatus.

Gymnastics is a popular sport involving acrobatic and aerial stunts, thereby predisposing athletes to risk for potentially catastrophic injuries. It is also a classic sport that represents the challenges of extraction on an unstable surface or in an environment that introduces unique access problems. The sports medicine clinician covering a gymnastics practice or competition should be well-acquainted with common sports injuries and their management, as well as injuries unique to gymnastics competition. The covering physician should be aware of the unique challenges of caring for an athlete in the gymnastics environment, including the presence of podiums, loose foam pits, resi-pits, and trampolines. Thorough preparation, including a well-thoughtout emergency plan regarding extraction, is critical to providing timely and optimal medical care to any injured athlete.

34.3 Ice Hockey and Skating: The Slippery Surface Environment

The ice environment introduces critical emergency access and extraction challenges for sports such as ice hockey, figure skating, and speed skating. Ice hockey is a team sport in which players traverse an ice-skating rink on knife-like ice skates attempting to shoot a rubberized puck into the opposing team's goal. The goalposts are typically made of steel. Each player, barring the goalie, carries a hockey stick that is made of wood or carbon fiber to guide the puck on the ice and to strike the puck when passing or shooting for goal. Players can move at speeds up to 30 miles per hour, and the rubberized puck can travel at speeds up to 100 miles per hour [7]. Despite players being dressed in protective body gear and helmets, the numerous solid objects that are part of the playing field in addition to the full contact nature of the sport present risk for injury.

Figure skating is a sport in which individuals, pairs of individuals, or groups perform on an ice-skating rink using sharp skates. Historically, the sport objective was limited to athletes tracing figures in the ice. However, with the evolution of the sport, performances have grown to include jumps, spins, throw jumps, lifts, and death spirals, each of which are extremely physically demanding on the athlete [8].

Although injuries are common in all levels of ice hockey play, injury patterns are strikingly different depending on the age group of the athletes. The number of injuries peaks in adolescence, with athletes between the ages of 12 and 17 accounting for 47% of injuries, correlating with the age at which body checking is typically introduced into gameplay [9]. Bodychecking is the act of using one's torso, shoulder, or hips to make contact with the opposing player most recently in possession of the puck [10]. Most injuries among athletes below the age of 18 affect the upper extremities [9]. Compared to athletes below 18 years of age, athletes older than 18 have a significantly higher rate of lacerations [9]. However, throughout all age groups, fractures are the most common type of injury (30%), followed by sprains/strains (24%) and open wounds (21%). Regarding location of injury, head and neck injuries (concussions, cervical spine injuries, facial fractures, etc.) and lower extremity injuries are the most common [11]. Despite the growing ice hockey participation among female athletes, male athletes continue to account for a significant majority of ice hockey players, and as a result, make up 90% of injuries [9, 12]. Due to the aggressive gameplay and presence of high-velocity moving objects during competition, the most common causes of injury in ice hockey are collisions with other players, falls, and being struck by or colliding with a solid object [12]. In singles figure skating, overuse injuries are more common than acute injuries [8]. However, given the incorporation of lifts, jumps, and throws in pair skating, there is a higher incidence of acute injuries in pair skating compared to singles [13]. The majority are of musculoskeletal nature and involve the lower extremities (56.4%), followed by upper extremities (25.4%) and back (14.6%) [14]. Other common injuries include lacerations and head injuries.

Despite significant differences in the gameplay and injury patterns of ice hockey and figure skating, both sports face similar extraction challenges when an athlete suffers an injury on the ice. The walled off skating rink is the first barrier to reaching the injured athlete. Although there will always be a slight delay when getting into the walled-off skate rink, it is critical that the skate rink entry and exit paths be unobstructed and the emergency equipment be located near the access point to the ice surface [13]. The entry, access, and egress routes for EMS support to both the building and playing surface should be well-planned before the event. Once the rescue team enters the rink, the slippery ice surface creates a stability issue as rescuers are attempting to reach the injured athlete, as well as when the athlete is being removed from the rink. To prepare for the slippery ice surface, nonslip shoe covers such as cleats or crampons should be used by medical personnel. (Fig. 34.5—*Nonslip shoe covers*) These should be readily available for anyone assisting the extraction. A scoop-type stretcher is easiest to use on the slippery ice surface and can be used instead of a backboard [13]. It is also recommended that a team of responders with stable footing is present to assist in any need to log-roll an athlete found face down on the ice. The lead clinician should be responsible for maintaining the cervical spine and be the sole person managing the timing of when the torso is rolled. As in all cases of environments that introduce challenges to extraction, medical personnel covering an indoor ice event should practice rescue on the ice surface prior to the event to accustom them-

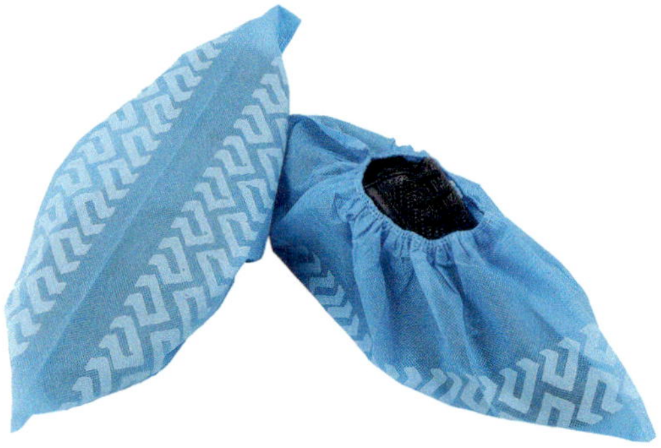

Fig. 34.5 Nonslip Boot Covers. Nonslip boot covers. Ribbed surface along the plantar aspect of the covers allows for increased stability while traversing icy surfaces. (Source: Shutterstock)

selves to the entrance and exit of the rink and movement along the ice.

Once the athlete is reached, costumes in figure skating and protective gear in ice hockey provide another set of barriers for treatment of the injured athlete. Figure skating costumes are expensive and can cost upwards of $1000, thus, the medical team should be mindful of this. Nevertheless, costumes should be cut if deemed necessary for management of the injury. A large towel or blanket can be used to maintain the athlete's modesty. Ice hockey and figure skating skates are typically tied tightly. Thus, the removal of the skates can create undesired traction on the lower leg which can be detrimental in the setting of a lower extremity injury. To avoid this, the laces should be loosened as much as possible prior to skate removal [11, 13].

Helmets provide a unique problem in cervical spine stabilization for injured ice hockey athletes. External stabilization of the helmet does not necessarily ensure that the head inside the helmet is stabilized [15]. Thus, the National Athletic Trainers' Association has established proper cervical spine management guidelines in helmet sports. For athletes in which the helmet is properly applied by the athlete and adequately secures the head, the helmet should not be removed to avoid unnecessary movement of the neck. Instead, the helmet itself should be stabilized [16]. If, however, the helmet is not providing adequate immobilization of the cervical spine, the helmet AND shoulder pads should BOTH be removed to allow for proper immobilization and alignment of the spine [17]. Moreover, helmets and facemasks should be removed urgently if there is any concern regarding airway access. Powered screwdrivers, Trainer's angels, clip scissors, or whatever tool are necessary to remove face masks should be immediately available.

It is also critical for medical personnel covering ice sport events to be prepared for the injury patterns common to these sports. Splints, immobilizers, cervical spine collars, stretchers, backboards, gauze, facemask removal tools, and suture kits should all be readily available to treat and manage fractures and lacerations, the most common injuries in ice hockey and figure skating [8, 13, 18].

Due to the unique nature and environment of sports played on slippery surfaces, injury management faces numerous obstacles that can hinder or delay treatment. Thus, it is imperative that medical professionals covering ice events such as ice hockey and figure skating are prepared to encounter delays during entrance and exit of the ice rink, a slippery ice surface, helmets, and barriers of clothing and costumes. They must also be prepared to confront the various fracture and open wound injuries that are common in these sports.

34.4 Swimming and Diving: The Water Environment

Competitive swimming gained its initial widespread popularity in the nineteenth century [19]. Both open water and pool swimming are included within competitive swimming and each can provide unique environmental access challenges. By total number of participants, indoor competitions are more popular and take place in an indoor swimming pool and can range from 50 to 1500 m in length. Swimming styles include freestyle, backstroke, breaststroke, or butterfly; races can be performed individually or in medley relays with four athletes per team [20].

Another popular indoor water sport is competitive diving, in which athletes jump or fall from a platform or springboard into a pool, performing acrobatics while airborne. While its origins date back to the nineteenth century, competitive diving did not gain its popularity until the early 1900s [21]. Since then, the sport has continued to grow. Currently, competitive diving has multiple events in the Olympics, including jumps from three- and ten-meter-high boards as well as single athlete and synchronized (two athletes jumping and performing simultaneous acrobatics) events.

Similar to other sports, athletes participating in competitive swimming and diving are at risk of developing injuries during practice or competition. In both sports, overuse injuries are significantly more common than acute injuries. The majority of swimming injuries are overuse injuries due to chronic overload [22]. These injuries typically manifest in the shoulders, hips, and knees of swimmers. On the other hand, acute injuries in swimmers typically affect the hands and feet of athletes. Metacarpal and calcaneal fractures are examples of acute injuries that are caused by striking a lane line, another hand of a player, or the wall at the end of a lap. Other less common acute swimmer injuries include shoulder or patellar subluxation, but these typically occur in the setting of chronic injury and repetitive overuse of the joints [22].

Competitive diving injuries have a similar incidence and severity level as swimming injuries [20]. The most commonly reported diving injury is injury to the lumbar spine. The anterior segments of the vertebral bodies are vulnerable to compressive loading. With time, this can lead to overuse injury and lower back pain in divers [23]. Although cervical spine injuries in competitive diving have been studied in depth, the majority of the cervical spine injuries occur in non-organized and noncompetitive diving. Thus, cervical spine injuries are of high incidence in recreational diving activities, specifically due to the lack of experience of individuals performing such dives in the recreational setting. Cervical spine injury in organized diving events is relatively less common [24]. Other diving injuries tend to be localized to the upper extremity and affect the wrists, elbows, and shoulders. Again, most of these injuries are due to chronic overuse. However, acute stress fractures during hard impact with the water can manifest in the setting of repetitive trauma that has weakened the osseous structures of the upper extremities. Such injuries include but are not limited to carpal bone contusions, scaphoid stress fractures, olecranon stress fractures, and midclavicular stress fractures [22].

Since overuse injuries tend to dominate the injury profiles of these sports, the incidence of catastrophic events that would require rescue and extraction in the water environment is thankfully rare; nonetheless, pre-event planning and creation of an emergency plan to address the possibility are critical. For example, if an acute hand or foot fracture occurs during competition, the athlete can independently remove themselves from the pool and seek medical attention; however, in the face of a suspected cervical spine injury, the emergency response plan needs to be initiated. Pre-event planning should include a clear understanding of which responder is trained and certified to enter the water and which provider may need to stay on the pool deck until the athlete can be extracted and brought to them. In-water, lifesaving responders should be prepared to immobilize the head and neck of an athlete who is still in the water. Only those trained in life-saving should actually enter the water. Two functional, manual, in-line stabilization techniques have been described: the hip and shoulder support and the head splint. The hip and shoulder support is used exclusively for a face-up athlete, in which one arm is placed below the athlete's hips and the other is placed below the athlete's shoulders. The athlete should not be lifted in this technique, but rather supported so that movement of the head is minimal and yet the face remains above water. The head splint technique can be used for face-up or face-down athletes and uses the extended arms of the athlete to squeeze the ears and immobilize the head [25]. (Fig. 34.6—*Aquatic C-spine stabilization*) Both of these techniques are only used until a back-

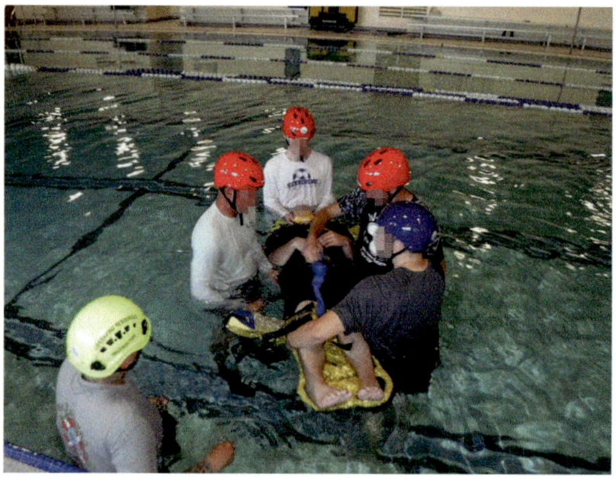

Fig. 34.6 Aquatic C-Spine Stabilization. Example of aquatic C-spine stabilization with use of a backboard. Note the provider at the head maintaining C-spine stability during manipulation and movement of the injured athlete. (Source: Lifesaving Resort)

board is prepared and brought into the water to lift the injured athlete. The backboard should be inserted under the athlete while in the water and should always be operated by at least two medical providers, while a third manually immobilizes the head [23, 26]. Additional swimmers can be used to stabilize the board as the athlete is being transferred to the pool deck. The athlete may then be removed from the water and further assessed and treated appropriately.

Ultimately, the philosophy of water extraction is the same as any challenging environment. Pre-event planning including location of emergency equipment, access for EMS, and a practiced response by a team who understands their individual roles will assure success when extracting an athlete from a water environment. Uniquely, critical members of the team need to be identified in advance regarding who is qualified and trained to enter the water.

34.5 The Extreme Sport Environment

Extreme sports (ES) are a category of sports that involve intense speeds, heights, high levels of physical exertion, specialized gear, and typically contribute to high levels of thrill, energy, and anxiety for the participants and the viewers [27]. While there may exist some controversy regarding the definition of extreme sports, this section refers to sports that are high-risk, performed in extreme environmental conditions, and in which the participant has to accept risk of extreme injury or death [28]. Extreme sports are usually performed in beautiful, remote, hard-to-get-to, and extreme locations, ranging from colossal mountains to raging waters. Examples of extreme sports include skydiving, BASE (buildings, antenna, spans, and earth) jumping, rock and ice climbing, surfing, skiing, and snowboarding [29].

Risk-taking in sport has become more popular each year, and extreme sports are currently at an all-time high in level of participation [30]. This can partly be explained by increase in mass media interest, showing impressive and beautiful views alongside exhilarating sport maneuvers which have struck an appeal with younger audiences [31]. Skydiving is a perfect example of this recent trend in extreme sports. The United States Parachute Association (USPA) has recorded that the 39,412 USPA members aggregated a total of 3.57 million jumps in the year 2021, compared to a mere 10,000 registered members in the 1970s [32]. This trend is similarly seen across BASE jumping, sports climbing, and other extreme sports [31, 33].

Due to their extreme nature, most extreme sports exhibit a considerable risk of severe injury and death. However, there is still significant variability between the injury profiles of each extreme sport. Some extreme sports can have a relatively safer injury profile compared to even traditional sports. For example, sports climbing has a significantly lower injury rate than American football and horse riding [34]. Other extreme sports, such as skydiving, can have moderate injury rates, with severe injuries (requiring visit to an emergency department) summing approximately 50 jumps per 100,000 jumps. BASE jumping exhibits an even riskier injury profile, with up to 300 of 100,000 jumps resulting in severe injury or death [29].

Analyzing all extreme sports jointly, the most common type of injury is a thoracolumbar vertebral fracture (31.5%), followed by severe traumatic brain injury (9.1%), rib fracture (8.7%), pneumothorax (7.8%), and femoral fracture (7.3%) [35]. Although each individual extreme sport has its own unique dangers and distinct injury patterns, the trends in each sport match the overall trend of extreme sports: a majority of injuries are orthopedic in nature [29, 31, 34, 36]. Generally, there exist two cohorts of athletes within extreme sports that exhibit the highest rate of injuries: those that are inexperienced and new to the sport, and those that are experienced experts in the sport. The rate of injury tends to be significantly higher during competitions compared to times of practice and training, likely secondary to the increased pressure to perform well during competitions [31]. Due to the extreme nature of these sports, multiple injuries typically occur simultaneously, with each injury often being of high severity (high Injury Scale and

Severity scores) [37]. In addition to sport-specific injuries, all extreme sports athletes are subject to extreme environmental conditions, including but not limited to exercise-associated hyperthermia, hypothermia, frostbite, shallow water black-out, and high-altitude sicknesses (i.e., cerebral edema, retinal hemorrhage, acute hypoxia) [38].

To achieve the environmental extremes required, athletes must often travel to remote locations that are typically far from civilization, and by extension, far from established medical care. Thus, when an athlete becomes injured during participation within this genre of sport, there exist numerous rescue and extraction challenges for the medical provider team. Most important of these challenges is medical response time. Emergency extraction is typically performed by helicopters that have the ability to reach remote locations [39]. Though helicopters are a rapid mode of transportation, the closest medical center can be hours away from the geographical location of injury, placing a significant time barrier to emergency medical treatment. Professional ES sporting events (e.g., Winter X-Games) typically have private medical coverage that are on-site and prepared for rescue and extraction. However, recreational athletes face the struggles of dealing with local and governmental assistance which may involve significant delays and long response times [31].

In addition to extended times for EMS arrival, athletes injured during ES participation must also endure the extremes of their environment while awaiting rescue and extraction, including turbulent waters, high-altitude mountains, and severely cold temperatures. Indeed, such extremes of location and weather can preclude helicopter access. This creates increased pressure on the medical management team managing injuries since they must simultaneously tend to the injury itself while mitigating the environmental conditions that threaten to destabilize the injured athlete. This is all especially difficult when dealing with multiple injuries simultaneously.

Therefore, when covering ES athletes and events, it is important for medical personnel to be prepared to stabilize the injured athlete amidst these challenges. In sports that have a high incidence of lower extremity orthopedic injuries such as skydiving and BASE jumping, medical personnel should ensure medical kit contents are divided into primary equipment (carried by each jumper) and secondary equipment (available for use, but does not need to be carried by each person). Primary equipment includes an emergency whistle and/or GPS beacon, small roll of tape, multitool, dental floss, and extra water. Secondary equipment includes equipment specific to the common orthopedic injuries in these sports, including SAM splints, femoral traction splints, pelvic binders, and vertical rescue equipment [40, 41].

Sports that involve turbulent waters, such as whitewater rafting and surfing, have a relatively high incidence of vertebral column injuries. Stabilization is an important aspect of management of vertebral column injury, which can be extremely difficult in moving waters. Therefore, medical personnel should be trained in using in-water immobilization techniques which include vice-grip, body-hug, and extended-arm head splint techniques. Using the vice-grip technique, the chin is stabilized with the arm that is resting on the sternum of the athlete, and the back of the head is cupped with the other hand, with this second arm running along the athlete's spine. In the body-hug technique, the rescuer is on the posterior side of the face-up and floating victim, with their arms passing underneath the armpits of the victim and their hands cupping the ears of the victim to stabilize the head. In the extended-arm head splint technique, the arms of the victim are extended above the head of the victim and pressed to the victim's ears providing stabilization of the head [42]. The medical provider must also be prepared for extreme temperatures associated with snow (skiing and snowboarding) and desert sports that can make it difficult to endure the wait of EMS. Thus, warming blankets and extra water should always be packed in case of extreme colds or heats, respectively.

The environmental extremes that are associated with extreme sports create numerous challenges during injury rescue for athletes participating in these sports and require extensive planning and preparation. There have been some systemic efforts to mitigate these challenges, such as implementing rescue teams close to areas that have become popular for BASE jumping/skydiving, or establishing hyperbaric chambers near popular diving locations [31]. However, it is essential for medical professionals covering extreme sport athletes to be prepared to stabilize injured athletes in the setting of long EMS response time, multiple simultaneous orthopedic injuries, and extreme environmental conditions such as strong waters, high altitudes, and extreme temperatures.

Ultimately, sports take place in a spectrum of environments and arenas, some of which may create significant physical and practical barriers to emergency medical care. Whether the sport is played on unusual playing surfaces, on ice, in the water, in environmental extremes or at challenging locations, sport physicians must be able to reach an acutely injured athlete within a reasonable time frame so as not to delay necessary treatment. The key to success is pre-event planning that includes an understanding and respect of the environmental challenges for both access to and egress from the site of an injured athlete, preparation for the unique injury patterns and risks of the individual sport, and development of a knowledgeable, efficient, and well trained response team that has practiced the emergency response to unique environments.

References

1. Hecht SS, Burton MS. Medical coverage of gymnastics competitions. Curr Sports Med Rep. 2009;8(3):113–8. https://doi.org/10.1249/JSR.0b013e3181a61993.
2. USA Gymnastics | USA Gymnastics. https://usagym.org/. Accessed 12 Aug 2022.
3. Desai N, Vance DD, Rosenwasser MP, Ahmad CS. Artistic gymnastics injuries; epidemiology, evaluation, and treatment. J Am Acad Orthop Surg. 2019;27(13):459–67. https://doi.org/10.5435/JAAOS-D-18-00147.
4. Marshall SW, Covassin T, Dick R, Nassar LG, Agel J. Descriptive epidemiology of collegiate Women's gymnastics injuries: National Collegiate Athletic Association Injury Surveillance System, 1988–1989 through 2003–2004. J Athl Train. 2007;42(2):234–40.
5. Kruse DW, Nobe AS, Billimek J. Injury incidence and characteristics for elite, male, artistic USA gymnastics competitions from 2008 to 2018. Br J Sports Med. 2021;55(3):163–8. https://doi.org/10.1136/bjsports-2019-101297.
6. Caine DJ, Nassar L. Gymnastics injuries. Med Sport Sci. 2005;48:18–58. https://doi.org/10.1159/000084282.
7. Flik K, Lyman S, Marx RG. American collegiate Men's ice hockey: an analysis of injuries. Am J Sports Med. 2005;33(2):183–9. https://doi.org/10.1177/0363546504267349.
8. Han JS, Geminiani ET, Micheli LJ. Epidemiology of figure skating injuries: a review of the literature. Sports Health. 2018;10(6):532–7. https://doi.org/10.1177/1941738118774769.
9. Hostetler SG, Xiang H, Smith GA. Characteristics of ice hockey-related injuries treated in US emergency departments, 2001-2002. Pediatrics. 2004;114(6):e661–6. https://doi.org/10.1542/peds.2004-1565.
10. Willer B, Kroetsch B, Darling S, Hutson A, Leddy J. Injury rates in house league, select, and representative youth ice hockey. Med Sci Sports Exerc. 2005;37(10):1658–63. https://doi.org/10.1249/01.mss.0000181839.86170.06.
11. Moslener MD, Wadsworth LT. Ice hockey: a team Physician's perspective. Curr Sports Med Rep. 2010;9(3):134–8. https://doi.org/10.1249/JSR.0b013e3181dfccd9.
12. Ashby K, Cassell E. Injury in snow and ice sports. 2007:24.
13. Lambrinakos-Raymond K, FitzGerald B, Geminiani ET. Sideline coverage of figure skating events. Curr Sports Med Rep. 2019;18(5):166–71. https://doi.org/10.1249/JSR.0000000000000597.
14. Fortin JD, Roberts D. Competitive figure skating injuries. Pain Physician. 2003;6(3):313–8.
15. Mihalik JP, Beard JR, Petschauer MA, Prentice WE, Guskiewicz KM. Effect of ice hockey helmet fit on cervical spine motion during an emergency log roll procedure. Clin J Sport Med. 2008;18(5):394–8. https://doi.org/10.1097/JSM.0b013e31818115e3.
16. Division I intercollegiate ice hockey team coverage. Br J Sports Med. https://bjsm.bmj.com/content/43/13/1000.short?casa_token=_3vkOqMj9P4AAAAA:3gvW5pjBCoiVd8hdNtlU6OzLURpxP7Rgitdg8oA3EywzjH0RGxyJ-CIP9%2D%2DSGgHq3C6Alxp6q74. Accessed 12 Aug 2022.
17. Swartz EE, Boden BP, Courson RW, et al. National Athletic Trainers' association position statement: acute management of the cervical spine–injured athlete. J Athl Train. 2009;44(3):306–31. https://doi.org/10.4085/1062-6050-44.3.306.
18. Anderson GR, Melugin HP, Stuart MJ. Epidemiology of injuries in ice hockey. Sports Health. 2019;11(6):514–9. https://doi.org/10.1177/1941738119849105.
19. Lohn J. Below the surface: the history of competitive swimming. Rowman & Littlefield; 2021.

20. Kerr ZY, Baugh CM, Hibberd EE, Snook EM, Hayden R, Dompier TP. Epidemiology of National Collegiate Athletic Association men's and women's swimming and diving injuries from 2009/2010 to 2013/2014. Br J Sports Med. 2015;49(7):465–71. https://doi.org/10.1136/bjsports-2014-094423.
21. History of Diving. British Swimming. https://www.britishswimming.org/browse-sport/diving/learn-more-about-diving/history-diving/. Accessed 12 Aug 2022.
22. Khodaee M, Edelman GT, Spittler J, et al. Medical Care for Swimmers. Sports Med Open. 2016;2:27. https://doi.org/10.1186/s40798-016-0051-2.
23. Rubin BD. The basics of competitive diving and its injuries. Clin Sports Med. 1999;18(2):293–303. https://doi.org/10.1016/S0278-5919(05)70145-9.
24. Jones NS. Competitive diving principles and injuries. Curr Sports Med Rep. 2017;16(5):351–6. https://doi.org/10.1249/JSR.0000000000000401.
25. SWS_Manual_sample_2.pdf. https://www.redcross.org/content/dam/redcross/atg/PDFs/Take_a_Class/SWS_Manual_sample_2.pdf. Accessed 12 Aug 2022.
26. Werniki P, Fenner P, Szpilman D. Spinal injuries: immobilization and extraction. In: Bierens J, editor. Drowning:Prevention, Rescue and Treatment. Springer-Verlag; 2005. p. 291–5.
27. Kraeutler MJ, Laver L, Mei-Dan O. Extreme Sports. In: Khodaee M, Waterbrook AL, Gammons M, editors. Sports-related fractures, dislocations and trauma: advanced on- and off-field management. Springer International Publishing; 2020. p. 857–64. https://doi.org/10.1007/978-3-030-36790-9_54.
28. Cohen R, Baluch B, Duffy LJ. Defining extreme sport: conceptions and misconceptions. Front Psychol 2018;9. https://www.frontiersin.org/articles/10.3389/fpsyg.2018.01974. Accessed 8 Aug 2022.
29. Laver L, Pengas IP, Mei-Dan O. Injuries in extreme sports. J Orthop Surg Res. 2017;12(1):59. https://doi.org/10.1186/s13018-017-0560-9.
30. Pain MT, Pain MA. Essay: Risk taking in sport. Lancet. 2005;366:S33–4. https://doi.org/10.1016/S0140-6736(05)67838-5.
31. Mei-Dan O, Carmont M. Adventure and extreme sports injuries: epidemiology, Treatment, Rehabilitation and Prevention. Springer Science & Business Media; 2012.
32. USPA > United States Parachute Association. https://uspa.org/. Accessed 8 Aug 2022.
33. Brymer E, Gray T. Dancing with nature: rhythm and harmony in extreme sport participation. J Adventure Educ Outdoor Learn. 2009;9(2):135–49. https://doi.org/10.1080/14729670903116912.
34. Schöffl V, Morrison A, Schwarz U, Schöffl I, Küpper T. Evaluation of injury and fatality risk in rock and ice climbing. Sports Med. 2010;40(8):657–79. https://doi.org/10.2165/11533690-000000000-00000.
35. Gosteli G, Yersin B, Mabire C, Pasquier M, Albrecht R, Carron PN. Retrospective analysis of 616 air-rescue trauma cases related to the practice of extreme sports. Injury. 2016;47(7):1414–20. https://doi.org/10.1016/j.injury.2016.03.025.
36. Soreide K, Ellingsen CL, Knutson V. How dangerous is BASE jumping? An analysis of adverse events in 20,850 jumps from the Kjerag massif, Norway. J Trauma Acute Care Surg. 2007;62(5):1113–7. https://doi.org/10.1097/01.ta.0000239815.73858.88.
37. Greenspan L, McLellan BA, Greig H. Abbreviated injury scale and injury severity score: a scoring chart. J Trauma. 1985;25(1):60–4. https://doi.org/10.1097/00005373-198501000-00010.
38. Trease L, Albert E, Singleman G, Brymer E. What is an extreme sports healthcare provider: an auto-ethnographic study of the development of an extreme sports medicine training program. Int J Environ Res Public Health. 2022;19(14):8286. https://doi.org/10.3390/ijerph19148286.
39. Sward DG, Bennett BL. Wilderness medicine. World J Emerg Med. 2014;5(1):5–15. https://doi.org/10.5847/wjem.j.issn.1920-8642.2014.01.001.
40. Sieker JW, Vilke GM, Schongalla MS, Mei-Dan O. Injury patterns and wilderness medical preparedness in BASE jumping. Muscles, Ligaments Tendons J. 2020;10(2):156–64. https://doi.org/10.32098/mltj.02.2020.01.
41. Mountain medical kits: epidemiology-based recommendations and analysis of medical supplies carried by mountain climbers in Colorado. J Travel Med. Oxford Academic. https://academic.oup.com/jtm/article/24/2/taw088/2930765. Accessed 6 Aug 2022.
42. Wernicki P, Szpilman D. Immobilization and extraction of spinal injuries. In: Bierens JJLM, editor. Drowning: Prevention, Rescue, Treatment. Springer; 2014. p. 621–8. https://doi.org/10.1007/978-3-642-04253-9_96.

GPSR Compliance

The European Union's (EU) General Product Safety Regulation (GPSR) is a set of rules that requires consumer products to be safe and our obligations to ensure this.

If you have any concerns about our products, you can contact us on ProductSafety@springernature.com

In case Publisher is established outside the EU, the EU authorized representative is:

Springer Nature Customer Service Center GmbH
Europaplatz 3
69115 Heidelberg, Germany

Batch number: 08315996

Printed by Printforce, the Netherlands